NMS Medicine Casebook

The National Medical Series for Independent Study

NMS Medicine Casebook

Tilak Shah, M.D.
Resident in Internal Medicine
Duke University Medical Center
Durham, North Carolina

Wolters Kluwer | Lippincott Williams & Wilkins
Health
Philadelphia • Baltimore • New York • London
Buenos Aires • Hong Kong • Sydney • Tokyo

Acquisitions Editor: Charles W. Mitchell
Senior Managing Editor: Stacey Sebring
Editorial Assistant: Oakley Julian
Marketing Manager: Jennifer Kuklinski
Production Editor: Beth Martz
Design Coordinator: Holly Reid McLaughlin

351 West Camden Street
Baltimore, MD 21201

530 Walnut Street
Philadelphia, PA 19106

Printed in the United States of America

9 8 7 6 5 4 3 2 1

Library of Congress Cataloging-in-Publication Data
Shah, Tilak.
NMS medicine casebook / Tilak Shah.
p. ; cm.—(The national medical series for independent study)
Includes index.
ISBN 978-0-7817-8468-9 (alk. paper)
1. Internal medicine—Case studies. I. Title. II. Title: Medicine casebook. III. Series.
[DNLM: 1. Internal Medicine—Case Reports. 2. Diagnostic Techniques and Procedures—Case Reports.
WB 293 S525n 2009]

RC66.S42 2009
616—dc22 2008029294

DISCLAIMER

Care has been taken to confirm the accuracy of the information present and to describe generally accepted practices. However, the authors, editors, and publisher are not responsible for errors or omissions or for any consequences from application of the information in this book and make no warranty, expressed or implied, with respect to the currency, completeness, or accuracy of the contents of the publication. Application of this information in a particular situation remains the professional responsibility of the practitioner; the clinical treatments described and recommended may not be considered absolute and universal recommendations.

The authors, editors, and publisher have exerted every effort to ensure that drug selection and dosage set forth in this text are in accordance with the current recommendations and practice at the time of publication. However, in view of ongoing research, changes in government regulations, and the constant flow of information relating to drug therapy and drug reactions, the reader is urged to check the package insert for each drug for any change in indications and dosage and for added warnings and precautions. This is particularly important when the recommended agent is a new or infrequently used drug.

Some drugs and medical devices presented in this publication have Food and Drug Administration (FDA) clearance for limited use in restricted research settings. It is the responsibility of the healthcare provider to ascertain the FDA status of each drug or device planned for use in their clinical practice.

To purchase additional copies of this book, call our customer service department at **(800) 638-3030** or fax orders to **(301) 223-2320**. International customers should call **(301) 223-2300**.

Visit Lippincott Williams & Wilkins on the Internet: http://www.lww.com. Lippincott Williams & Wilkins customer service representatives are available from 8:30 am to 6:00 pm, EST.

To my parents Upendra and Prerana,
who have always supported my every endeavor.

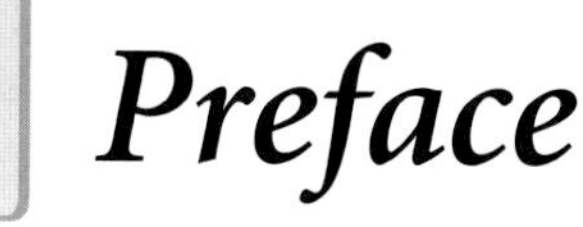

Preface

As a third-year medical student, I found a problem-based approach the most effective and efficient method to prepare for the wards and the National Board of Medical Examiners shelf examinations. Despite the plethora of review books available, there lacked an interactive yet comprehensive resource to prepare for the internal medicine clerkship. Available casebooks lacked the depth to serve as a primary source for learning. On the other hand, comprehensive texts and review books were written in a format that did not simulate real-life patient encounters or shelf and board exam questions.

The *NMS Medicine Casebook* covers all the information necessary to excel on the medicine clerkship in an interactive, case-based format. Although no text can cover all of internal medicine, this book is intended to serve as a comprehensive source for shelf exam review. The text emphasizes "next steps in management" and includes case variations to distinguish between similarly presenting conditions. The conversational approach along with numerous algorithms, tables, mnemonics, and images facilitate rapid accumulation of large amounts of information in the short span of the clerkship.

The depth and format of the book is also ideally suited to prepare for the United States Medical Licensing Examination (USMLE) Step 2 CK and USMLE Step 3 examinations. Nurse practitioners and physician assistants may find this text helpful early in their careers. Clinician educators can use the cases in this book as tools for instruction during pathophysiology courses and the medicine clerkship.

To those of you beginning your medicine clerkship, I wish you the best of luck. I hope this book can help you get the most out of your rotations and ace the shelf!

Tilak Shah, M.D.

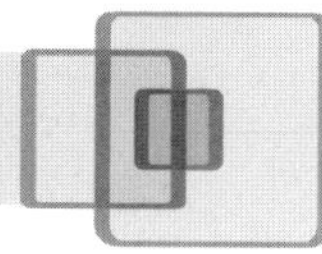

Acknowledgments

I would like to thank Donna Balado, Liz Stalnaker, Stacey Sebring, Jennifer Clements, and everyone else at Lippincott Williams & Wilkins who was involved in the production of this book. I appreciate the helpful feedback from the student and faculty reviewers. For the educational opportunities that provided the foundation for this book, I am grateful to the faculty and house staff at my medical school, the University of North Carolina. Finally, I thank my fiancée Nipa, not only for the countless hours spent editing the manuscript, but also for her constant encouragement throughout the writing process. As my very first "customer" to use the manuscript to study for her internal medicine clerkship, her support really sustained this project.

T.S.

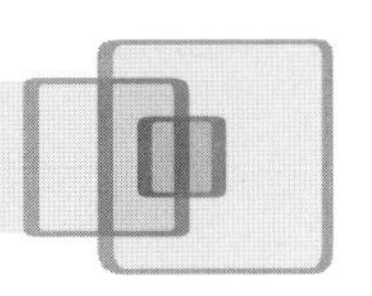

Contents

chapter **1**

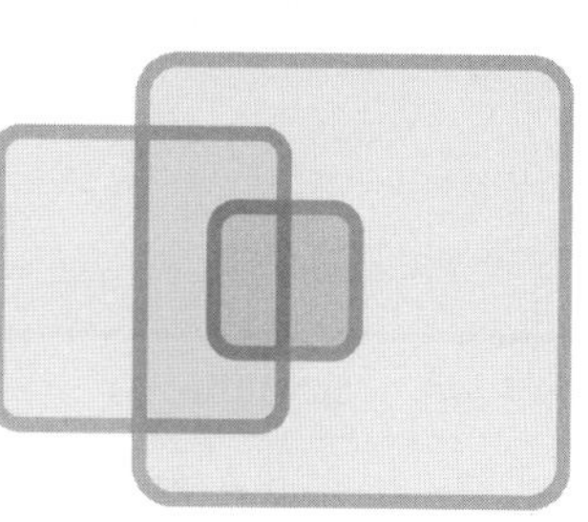

Health Maintenance and Statistics

CASE 1–1 IMMUNIZATIONS

An 18-year-old male is brought to the emergency department 3 hours after he was involved in a motor vehicle crash. There are a number of dirty wounds. Some of them are stellate and >1 cm. Sensation is intact. His immunization status is unknown.

What vaccine should you administer immediately?

Wounds with the following characteristics have increased risk of clostridium tetanus wound infection (mnemonic is "*SIC SOD*"): **S**tellate, **I**nfected, **C**ontaminated, decreased **S**ensation over wound, **O**lder than 6 hours, **D**eeper than 1 cm. Patients with any of these features and unknown immunization status should receive human tetanus immune globulin (HTIG) and an initial dose of Tetanus, diphtheria, and pertussis (Tdap) vaccine (Tables 1-1, 1-2, and 1-3).

> Motor vehicle accidents are the leading cause of death in young adults.

Would you administer tetanus vaccine if the records showed that he had received a Tdap booster 7 years ago?

Consider administering a tetanus booster if a patient with a tetanus-prone wound has not received a booster in the last 5 years.

The patient requires a splenectomy. What additional vaccines should you administer?

Asplenic patients should receive a single dose of pneumococcal vaccine (PPV23) and meningococcal vaccine 14 days after emergency splenectomy.

> **Elective splenectomy**: Administer vaccines 14 days prior to surgery.

TABLE 1–1 Live Attenuated Vaccines

Vaccine	General Indications	Schedule	Contraindications
MMR (measles, mumps, and rubella)	• All children • Unvaccinated adults born after 1957	2 doses at least 4 weeks apart	Standard[a] Pregnancy Immunocompromised[b]
Varicella	• All children • Unvaccinated adults with no history of chicken pox and no varicella antibodies	2 doses at least 4 weeks apart	Standard Pregnancy Immunocompromised
Oral typhoid vaccine	• Travel to endemic area	4 capsules taken every other day	Standard Pregnancy Immunocompromised
Intranasal influenza vaccine	• Age $\geq$ 50 • Consider in all patients	Single dose	Standard Pregnancy Immunocompromised History of anaphylactic reaction to eggs Chronic medical conditions

Adapted from Agebegi S, Derby E. *Step-up to medicine*. 2005. Lippincott Williams and Wilkins.

[a] Standard contraindications are history of anaphylactic reaction to vaccine and severe illness after vaccination (mild illness is not a contraindication).

[b] MMR is the only live vaccine not contraindicated in HIV-positive patients.

TABLE 1–2 Inactivated (killed virus) Vaccines

Vaccine	Indications	Schedule	Contraindications
Inactivated polio vaccine (IPV)	• All children • Unvaccinated adults who plan to travel to an endemic area	2 doses at least 4 weeks apart and a third dose 6–12 months after second dose	Standard
Intramuscular influenza vaccine	• Age $\geq$ 50 years • Chronic medical conditions (e.g., diabetes mellitus, chronic renal failure, etc.) • Healthcare workers • Second or third trimester pregnancy during "flu season" (October to May) • Consider in all patients	Annual	Standard History of anaphylactic reaction to eggs
Hepatitis A (HAVRIX)	• Chronic liver disease • Clotting factor disorder • Risk factors for hepatitis B or hepatitis C infection (Chapter 5) • Travel to endemic area	2 doses 6–12 months apart	Standard

Adapted from Agebegi S, Derby E. *Step-up to medicine*. 2005. Lippincott Williams and Wilkins.

Sickle cell anemia: Usually administered PPV23 and meningococcal vaccine because these patients are functionally asplenic.

Would you re-administer meningococcal vaccine if medical records indicated that the patient had elected to receive the meningococcal vaccine 1 year ago when he first moved into a college dormitory?

Patients who have already received the meningococcal vaccine do not require repeat vaccination, even after splenectomy.

TABLE 1–3 Toxoid and Component Vaccines

Vaccine	Recommended Recipients	Schedule	Contraindications
Diphtheria, tetanus, and pertussis (Tdap)	• All children • Unvaccinated adults with a major dirty wound • Unvaccinated adult who plans to travel to an epidemic area	2 doses at least 4 weeks apart and a third dose 6–12 months after second dose; then, booster every 10 years	Standard
Meningococcus	• Persons who plan to travel to an epidemic area • All asplenic patients • Consider in college students who live in a dormitory and military personnel	Single dose	Standard
Hepatitis B	• All infants • Unvaccinated healthcare workers • Unvaccinated adults with risk factors for hepatitis B infection	2 doses at least 4 weeks apart and a third dose 6–12 months after second dose	Standard
Pneumococcus (PPV23)	• Age ≥ 65 years • Chronic medical conditions (e.g., diabetes mellitus, chronic renal failure, etc.) • Asplenia	Single dose	Standard
Intramuscular typhoid vaccine	• Travel to endemic area	Single dose	Standard

Adapted from Agebegi S, Derby E. *Step-up to medicine*. 2005. Lippincott Williams and Wilkins.

College students living off-campus: Risk of meningococcal infection is similar to general population; vaccination is not cost-effective.

Would you re-administer PPV23 if the patient had received this vaccine in the past?

Yes, consider a single repeat PPV23 dose in these patients. Other indications for a single repeat dose of PPV23 are:

1. Patient is ≥65 years and received PPV23 ≥10 years ago before the age of 65.
2. Immunocompromised patient received PPV23 ≥5 years ago.

The patient tells you he has never had sexual intercourse and does not use illegal drugs. He is in college studying finance. He is up to date with all his childhood immunizations except hepatitis B. Should he receive any vaccines at this time?

This patient does not appear to have any indications for the hepatitis B vaccine. However, he should consider annual influenza vaccine if he wishes to avoid getting the “flu” during “flu season” (October to May). Killed intramuscular and live attenuated intranasal versions of the influenza vaccine are available, both of which are equally effective.

During a follow-up appointment 1 year later, the patient reveals he has been injecting heroin for the last 3 months. What additional vaccines should you consider?

Intravenous drug use is a risk factor for hepatitis B and hepatitis C infection, which can cause chronic cirrhosis. Test the patient for human immunodeficiency virus (HIV) and hepatitis B virus. If hepatitis B virus serology is negative, administer hepatitis B vaccine. Also, consider hepatitis A vaccine. There is no vaccine against hepatitis C.

Serology for HIV-1 (enzyme immunoassay) and hepatitis B (HbsAg) is negative. The patient receives all three doses of hepatitis B vaccine; he declines hepatitis A vaccine. Two years later, he tells you he is planning to go to India in a couple of months. What immunizations should you recommend?

Offer a polio booster, hepatitis A vaccine, and typhoid vaccine to patients who plan to travel to the Indian subcontinent. A live, attenuated, oral vaccine and an intramuscular polysaccharide vaccine are available to protect against salmonella typhi. Unless the patient does not wish to receive an injection, the intramuscular preparation is generally preferred.

> **Traveller's diarrhea:** Antibiotic prophylaxis is not recommended for immunocompetent patients; consider ciprofloxacin if the patient develops any of the following: ≥4 unformed stools per day, bloody stools, or mucus in stool.

> **Malaria prophylaxis:** Consider mefloquine or atovaquone-proguanil, with doxycylcine as an alternative; chloroquine is not recommended except in Central America and the Caribbean because of the high prevalence of resistant *Plasmodium falciparum.*

CASE 1–2 TUBERCULOSIS SCREENING

A 20-year-old patient visits the clinic for the first time. She is asymptomatic. She emigrated from Mexico 3 years ago and works with the state prison system.

Would you recommend tuberculosis (TB) screening for this patient?

Annual TB screening is indicated in any of the following asymptomatic patients (mnemonic is "***Mycobacterium*** = ***SIC Lungs***"):

1. **M**edical risk factor: Chronic renal failure, diabetes mellitus, and immune suppression (HIV, organ transplant, blood cancer, and chronic steroid use)
2. **S**ocioeconomic risk factor (e.g., homelessness, alcoholism, intravenous drug use)
3. **I**mmigration <5 years ago from area with increased TB prevalence (e.g., India, Mexico)
4. **C**areer with high potential for close contact with active TB patient (healthcare worker, prison guard)
5. **L**ong-term care facility resident (nursing home, mental care facility, prison)

This prison guard, who recently emigrated from a high-prevalence country, should undergo annual screening.

> Perform TB screening once if a person has a single potential exposure (e.g., infected family member) or an incidentally detected fibrotic lung lesion.

What test is used to screen asymptomatic patients for TB?

Use the Mantoux test to screen asymptomatic patients. Inject purified protein derivative into the patient's arm and measure the transverse length of induration (not erythema) 48 to 72 hours later.

There is 11 mm of induration 60 hours later. How would you interpret this finding?

On the basis of this patient's risk factors, the Mantoux test is considered positive because she has >10 mm of induration (Table 1-4).

How would your interpretation of the Mantoux test differ if the patient mentioned that she had received the Bacilli Calmette-Guerin (BCG) vaccine as a child, and her medical records mentioned that her baseline level of induration was 7 mm?

Many patients from countries with a high TB prevalence have been immunized with the BCG vaccine as children to prevent childhood TB, meningitis, and miliary TB. Interpret the Mantoux test as follows in BCG-vaccinated patients:

1. Age <35 years: Test is positive if there is an increase of 10 mm induration from baseline

TABLE 1-4 Interpretation of Mantoux Test (intradermal PPD injection)

Induration	Considered Positive in the Following Patients
>5 mm	1. Immunosuppression or HIV positive 2. Recent close contact with known active TB patient 3. Fibrotic changes on chest radiograph that suggest prior TB
>10 mm	1. Socioeconomic risk factor 2. Immigrant <5 years ago from an area with high TB prevalence 3. Career with increased potential for close contact with active TB patient 4. Long-term care facility resident
>15 mm	Considered positive in all persons

2. Age >35 years: Test is positive if there is an increase of 15 mm induration from baseline

If this 20-year-old patient's baseline induration was 7 mm, the Mantoux test is negative because she has an increase of only 4 mm induration from baseline.

> Most individuals in the United States do not receive BCG vaccine because overall prevalence is low, the vaccine's efficacy is variable, and it interferes with the purified protein derivative test.

How would your interpretation of the Mantoux test differ if the patient mentioned that she received the BCG vaccine as a child but did not know her baseline induration?

If the patient does not know her baseline level of induration, interpret and treat skin test reactivity just like you would an unvaccinated person. This patient would therefore have a positive Mantoux test.

What is the next step in management of an asymptomatic patient with a positive Mantoux test?

The next step is to obtain a chest radiograph (CXR) to exclude active infection. If CXR shows signs of active infection, treat with combination therapy (refer to Chapter 3).

What is the next step in management if CXR of a patient with a positive Mantoux test does not show any signs of active infection?

If CXR does not demonstrate active infection, treat with a 6- to 12-month course of isoniazid (INH) to prevent reactivation of latent infection.

> **3 months of INH + rifampin:** Alternative if compliance is a concern.
> **4 months of rifampin monotherapy:** Reserved for known exposure to INH-resistant TB.

What other infectious diseases should you screen for in adults?

1. HIV-1: The U.S. Centers for Disease Control (CDC) recommends screening all persons ≥13 years old. The U.S. Preventive Services Task Force (USPSTF) makes no recommendation for or against universal HIV screening.
2. Human papillomavirus: Refer to case 1-3.
3. Chlamydia: Routinely test all sexually active women <25 years old; use nucleic acid amplification assays of cervical swabs or urine samples. Screen women >25 years old if they have a history of sexually transmitted diseases or multiple sexual partners.

> Also screen high-risk women for gonorrhea and syphilis.

CASE 1–3 CANCER SCREENING

A 22-year-old woman presents for a routine evaluation. She saw a breast cancer documentary on television and wants to know if she should undergo any screening for breast cancer. She is particularly interested in learning breast self-examination (BSE). Her father was diagnosed with colon cancer at age 55. There is no other cancer history in her family. She reports that she has never had sexual intercourse.

What screening should you recommend for early detection of breast cancer at this time?

Perform clinical breast exam (CBE) every 3 years in women between the ages of 20 and 40 to screen for breast cancer (Table 1-5). After the age of 40, she should undergo annual CBE and mammography. BSE is an adjunctive option for patients who express interest, but this method is not a substitute for CBE.

Family history of early breast cancer: Discuss the risks and benefits of aggressive screening, and then tailor screening protocol based on patient preference; the main risk of mammography is over-diagnosis (requires unnecessary invasive testing).

TABLE 1–5 American Cancer Society Guidelines for Early Cancer Detection

Breast Cancer	Women aged 20–40 years: Perform clinical breast exam every 3 years. Women aged 40–70 years: Perform annual clinical breast exam and mammography. Women >70 years: Discontinue screening if the woman's life expectancy is <10 years.
Colorectal Cancer	Initiate screening at age 50 in all average-risk persons. Any one of the following five options are acceptable:[a] 1. Annual fecal occult blood test or fecal immunochemical test[b] 2. Flexible sigmoidoscopy every 5 years 3. Annual fecal occult blood test or fecal immunochemical test plus flexible sigmoidoscopy every 5 years 4. Double-contrast barium enema every 5 years 5. Colonoscopy every 10 years Refer to Chapter 4 and table 1-6 for screening recommendations in patients with greater than average risk.
Cervical Cancer	Begin annual Pap test in women 3 years after the first episode of sexual intercourse or at age 21 (whichever is earlier).[c] After age 30, women with at least three normal Pap smears in a row can decrease screening interval to every 2–3 years. After age 70, women with at least three normal Pap smears in a row and normal Pap tests for the last 10 years can discontinue screening.
Prostate Cancer	Discuss the risks and benefits of early prostate cancer detection in all males at age 50 as long as their estimated life expectancy is >10 years.[d] If the patient wishes to undergo screening or asks the physician to decide, test with annual digital rectal exam and prostate specific antigen.
Other	Starting at age 20, perform the following physical exam maneuvers during periodic health exams: 1. Thyroid palpation to screen for thyroid cancer 2. Bimanual pelvic exam to screen for ovarian cancer 3. Mouth and skin inspection to screen for oral and skin cancers 4. Lymph node palpation

[a] Follow up on a positive result in options 1 to 4 with colonoscopy.
[b] Examine two samples from each of three consecutive stools.
[c] Perform every two years rather than annually if using the newer, liquid-based Pap test.
[d] Initiate the discussion and possible screening at age 45 if the patient is African American or has a family history of prostate cancer before age 65 in one or more family members.

Is any other cancer screening test recommended at this time?

Perform annual Papanicolaou testing (Pap test, Pap smear) to screen for cervical cancer in all females by the age of 21 even if they report never having had sexual intercourse (Table 1-5).

Gardasil: Vaccine against cervical cancer that protects against human papillomavirus serotypes 6, 11, 16, and 18; guidelines for immunization are unclear.

When should she start colorectal cancer screening?

Colorectal cancer in at least one first-degree family member or at least two second-degree family members is associated with a greater than average risk of colon cancer. Colonoscopy is the screening test of choice in such patients. This patient should start screening colonoscopy at age 40 (Table 1-6).

At the age of 48, the patient asks whether she needs to continue with Pap testing. She had a subtotal hysterectomy for menstrual migraines 11 months ago. She has been in a monogamous relationship with her husband for the last 25 years. Her prior Pap tests were all negative.

Because the cervix is left in place after subtotal hysterectomy, the recommendations regarding Pap testing are not changed in her situation. She should continue to undergo regular Pap testing. If this patient had a total hysterectomy (cervix excised), then she would no longer require screening for cervical cancer.

The results of a Pap test at age 50 are "unsatisfactory for evaluation." What is your recommendation regarding follow-up testing?

A satisfactory specimen contains at least 8000 to 12,000 squamous cells, as well as both squamous metaplastic and endocervical cells (indicates adequate sampling of the transformation zone of the cervix, the area at greatest risk for neoplasia). Always repeat unsatisfactory Pap smears in 2 to 4 months.

The patient undergoes repeat testing two more times, and both times the specimen is labeled as unsatisfactory. What is the next step in management?

Women with repeated unsatisfactory Pap smears have increased risk of cervical intraepithelial lesions. The next step in management is colposcopy ± biopsy.

Colposcope: lighted, binocular microscope that provides enlarged view of the cervix, vagina, and vulva.

Colposcopy and biopsy are negative. Over the next 22 years, she regularly undergoes Pap testing. All subsequent Pap tests are negative. She has not had sexual intercourse since her husband passed away 5 years ago. Can she discontinue Pap testing?

Yes, she can discontinue cervical cancer screening at this time (Table 1-5).

TABLE 1-6 Colorectal Cancer Screening in Persons with a Positive Family History

Family Member	Earliest Age at Diagnosis	When to Start Screening Colonoscopy
One or more first-degree relatives	≥50 years	40 years
One or more first-degree relatives	<50 years	10 years before earliest age at diagnosis
Two or more second-degree relatives	Any	40 years
One second-degree relative	Any	50

Suppose the patient's subtotal hysterectomy at age 48 was performed to treat stage-2 cervical carcinoma in situ rather than menstrual migraines. Can she discontinue cervical cancer screening at age 70 if all her Pap tests are negative after age 48?

The following situations pose an increased risk for cervical cancer (DICE):

1. **D**ES (Diethylstilbestrol) exposure *in utero*
2. **I**mmune compromise
3. **C**ervical cancer, history of CIN II or CIN III (Cervical intraepithelial neoplasia)
4. **E**ndocervical cells repeatedly absent or obscured on Pap tests

Patients with any of these risk factors should undergo annual screening after age 30 and should continue screening after age 70 even if prior Pap tests are all negative.

The 70-year-old patient has regularly undergone CBE and mammography, which have always been normal. She has mild hypertension but is otherwise healthy and active. Should she discontinue breast cancer screening?

The patient has a strong chance of living ≥10 more years. She should not discontinue annual CBE and mammography unless life expectance is <10 years (Table 1-5).

The 70-year-old patient's 45-year-old daughter has a 25-pack-year history of cigarette smoking. She asks about lung cancer screening. What should she be told?

Lung cancer screening with low dose helical (spiral) CT ± sputum cytology does detect lung cancer at an earlier stage, but it is unclear whether early detection improves mortality (lead-time bias). On the other hand, screening detects a number of benign pulmonary nodules that require invasive testing to rule out cancer. The American Cancer Society and USPSTF do not make any recommendation for or against screening.

CASE 1–4 PREVENTION OF CORONARY HEART DISEASE

A 54-year-old male presents to the clinic for the first time. He has not visited a healthcare provider in many years. He is asymptomatic. His father died of a myocardial infarct at age 70. His mother died after a stroke at age 80. He has a 30-pack-year history of cigarette smoking. Physical activity is limited to walking 15 minutes daily to catch the train to work. He does not eat fruits and vegetables often. Blood pressure is 150/90 mm Hg.

On the basis of history and physical exam alone, how many major risk factors does this patient have for coronary heart disease (CHD)?

The patient has two major risk factors for CHD: smoking and hypertension (Table 1-7). On the basis of his history and physical exam, he also has three nonmajor risk factors for CHD (male sex, sedentary lifestyle, and diet).

> **CHD:** Stable angina, unstable angina, and myocardial infarct; synonymous with coronary artery disease (CAD).

When should you start screening patients for hypertension?

Measure blood pressure in all patients ≥18 years of age at every clinical encounter.

When should you start screening patients for dyslipidemia (hyperlipidemia)?

National Cholesterol Education Project (NCEP) recommends a fasting lipid profile at age 20. If values are normal, recheck fasting lipid profile every 5 years. If the patient has a borderline measurement, recheck within 1 to 2 years. If the patient has not fasted prior to testing, obtain nonfasting total and high-density lipoprotein cholesterol.

> Most other organizations recommend initial fasting lipid profile at age 35.

TABLE 1–7 Risk Factors for Coronary Heart Disease

Major risk factors	Hypertension Diabetes mellitus Dyslipidemia (↑ low-density lipoprotein and ↓ high-density lipoprotein) Smoking
Other risk factors	Age: male, >45 years; female, >55 years Male gender First-degree family history of coronary heart disease: male, <55 years; female, <65 years Lab markers: increased homocysteine, c-reactive protein, fibrinogen, and estrogen Sedentary lifestyle and abdominal obesity Diet: inadequate fruits and vegetables

Note: DM, chronic renal failure, and peripheral arterial disease are CHD equivalents.

When should you start screening patients for DM?

The American Diabetes Association recommends screening everyone ≥45 years for DM every 3 years. The USPSTF recommends this screening interval only for patients with hypertension or hyperlipidemia.

> Aggressive control of major risk factors decreases mortality from CHD.

The patient's fasting lipid profile is normal. Fasting blood sugar is 150 mg/dL on 2 repeat measurements, which indicates he has DM. He starts taking hydrochlorothiazide, lisinoprol, and metformin. He quits smoking. In addition to lifestyle measures and medications that help control risk factors, what drug could lower his risk of developing CHD?

Aspirin can lower the risk of developing CHD in patients without known CHD (primary prevention).

Should this asymptomatic patient take aspirin?

Although aspirin lowers the risk of developing overt CHD, it also carries a risk of gastrointestinal bleeding. The benefits of aspirin outweigh the risks when the 10-year risk of developing CHD exceeds 10%. The risk of CHD is >10% in patients with DM and at least one other risk factor. Therefore, because this patient has DM and more than one other risk factor, he should consider aspirin for primary prophylaxis.

> Risk factors used to calculate CHD probability are major risk factors + age.

Would you recommend aspirin if he were asymptomatic and had no CHD risk factors?

The 10-year risk of CHD is <1% in asymptomatic patients with no CHD risk factors, so aspirin is not recommended for primary prevention in these patients.

Suppose the patient has stable angina. Would you recommend aspirin?

Patients with stable angina already have CHD. Aspirin can prevent further cardiovascular events in these patients (secondary prevention). Because the 10-year risk of a future cardiovascular event is well over 10% in patients with known CHD, he should take aspirin for secondary prevention.

CASE 1–5 SCREENING AND PREVENTION OF OSTEOPOROSIS

A 34-year-old white female presents for a routine evaluation. She is concerned about her risk of osteoporosis because her 67-year-old mother recently had a compression fracture. The patient is asymptomatic. She has regular menstrual periods. She has never had a fracture. She does not get much time to exercise and smokes a pack of cigarettes every day.

TABLE 1–8 Risk Factors for Osteoporosis (National Osteoporosis Foundation)

KEY RISK FACTORS THAT DETERMINE RISK OF HIP FRACTURES

- Personal history of fracture as an adult
- Family history of fracture in first-degree relative
- Cigarette smoking
- Low body weight (<58 kg)

OTHER RISK FACTORS (MNEMONIC: *"OLD WHITE FEMALE FALLS DOWN AND FRACTURES SECOND VERTEBRA"*):

- **O**ld age
- **W**hite race
- **F**emale sex
- **F**alls (recurrent)
- **D**ementia
- **A**lcoholism
- **F**rail (poor overall health)
- **S**edentary
- ↓ **E**strogen
- ↓ **C**alcium intake
- **V**ision poor despite adequate correction

What measures should you recommend at this time to prevent osteoporosis?

Discuss risk factors for osteoporosis (Table 1-8), and advise all women to adopt lifestyle measures to prevent this condition. Lifestyle measures include:

1. Adequate calcium and vitamin D intake: Premenopausal women should consume ≥100 mg of calcium and 400 IU of vitamin D. Consider supplements if dietary intake is insufficient.
2. Weight-bearing physical activity: Perform activities that require the body to work against gravity (e.g., walking, tennis, resistance training, etc.).
3. Stop smoking and avoid excessive alcohol intake.

Non–weight-bearing exercise: Activities such as swimming and riding a bicycle do not reduce risk of osteoporosis.

The patient asks if she should undergo screening for osteoporosis. What should you recommend to her?

Screen men and premenopausal women only if they have a history of fragility fracture. Screening is not indicated in this premenopausal woman because she has no fracture history.

Fragility fracture: Fracture that occurs after a fall from standing height or less; most common sites are neck of femur, wrist, and vertebrae.

Over the next 20 years, the patient performs weight-bearing exercise regularly but continues to smoke. She is postmenopausal. Is any osteoporosis screening indicated?

Postmenopausal women <65 years old with at least one osteoporosis risk factor should consider dual-energy x-ray absorptiometry (DXA) to screen for osteoporosis. If the DXA T-score is >–1 (normal), consider follow-up DXA after 3 to 5 years (not universally recommended). If the T-score is between −1 and −2.5 (osteopenia), consider follow-up DXA every 1 to 2 years. The optimum DXA measurement site is debatable, although the hip and spine are frequently used.

Use DXA to screen all women ≥65 years of age regardless of risk factors.

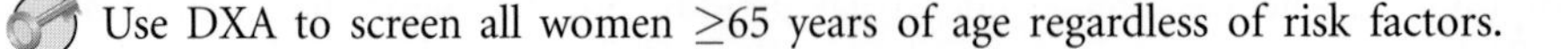

T-score is −1.5. Should this patient take any medications to prevent osteoporosis?

Discuss the risks and benefits of pharmacologic therapy with patients who have osteopenia and multiple osteoporosis risk factors (see Chapter 8: Endocrinology). First-line agents for primary prevention in patients who desire medications are raloxifene and bisphosphonates. Estrogen is a second-line agent if first-line agents are contraindicated or cause intolerable side effects.

> All postmenopausal women should continue lifestyle measures; recommended calcium and vitamin D intake in postmenopausal women is 1200 mg and 800 IU, respectively.

CASE 1–6 SMOKING CESSATION

A 60-year-old male with hypertension visits the clinic to follow up on his antihypertensive regimen.

What is the first step with regard to smoking cessation?

Ask all patients whether they smoke. A modified CAGE questionnaire or Fagerstrom test can help assess nicotine dependence in smokers:

1. Have you ever tried to, or felt the need to, **C**ut down on your smoking?
2. Do you ever get **A**nnoyed when people tell you to quit smoking?
3. Do you ever feel **G**uilty about smoking?
4. Do you ever smoke within one-half hour of waking up (**E**ye-opener)?

For the modified CAGE questionnaire, two "yes" responses constitute a positive screening test. To assist with patients who are attempting to quite smoking, use the Five As of Office-Based Smoking Cessation Counseling:

- **Ask** all patients whether or not they smoke.
- **Advise** them about the risks of smoking and the benefits of quitting.
- **Assess** their willingness to quit smoking.
- **Assist** the patient (set quit date, provide pharmacologic therapy, etc.).
- **Arrange** follow-up to reassess smoking status.

> Doctors are three times more likely to intervene if they know a patient smokes.

The patient has a 30-pack-year history of smoking. He does not feel that smoking is a problem and does not wish to quit at this time. What is the next step in management?

There are five stages of smoking cessation. In the precontemplation stage, the patient does not believe that smoking is a problem or refuses to consider smoking cessation. In the contemplation stage, the patient recognizes that smoking is a problem and wishes to quit. In the preparation stage, the patient makes specific plans to quit smoking (e.g., setting a quit date). In the action stage, the patient stops smoking. In the maintenance stage, the patient continues to abstain from smoking. Patients often cycle through these stages several times before reaching stable abstinence.

This patient is in the precontemplation stage. "Motivational interviewing" to encourage contemplation is the best strategy at this time:

1. Express concern about his habit.
2. Discuss the risks of smoking and the benefits of quitting (Table 1-9).
3. Recommend smoking cessation.
4. Arrange for a follow-up appointment.

TABLE 1–9 Hazards of Smoking

Cardiovascular	Smoking is responsible for >10% of cardiovascular deaths; smoking cessation reduces the risk of acute coronary events.
Cancer	1. Pulmonary (nasopharynx, pharynx, larynx, bronchogenic cancer, mesothelioma) 2. Gastrointestinal (esophagus, stomach, liver, pancreas) 3. Renal and reproductive (kidney, bladder, renal pelvis, cervix) 4. Heme (leukemia)
Pulmonary	Smokers with chronic obstructive pulmonary disorder have an accelerated decline in FEV1 (forced expiratory volume in 1 second). Smoking cessation slows this rate of decline and may lead to remission of certain interstitial lung diseases such as Langerhans histiocytosis. Finally, smoking increases the risk of pneumonia and tuberculosis infections.
Peptic ulcer disease	Smoking cessation decreases the risk of developing peptic ulcer disease and accelerates the rate of healing in established disease.
Reproductive disorders	Smoking increases the risk of infertility, spontaneous abortion, ectopic pregnancy, and premature menopause.
Osteoporosis	Smoking accelerates bone resorption and is a risk factor for hip fracture in women; 10 years of smoking cessation reduces this risk.
Mortality	Smoking is the leading cause of preventable death among all patients in the United States. Smoking cessation decreases mortality from all causes.

Six months later, the patient returns for a follow-up appointment. When questioned about smoking, he reports that he wishes to quit because his uncle was recently diagnosed with lung cancer. What are the next steps in management?

The patient is now in the contemplation stage. The next steps are:

1. Set a quit date, typically within 2 to 3 weeks.
2. Prepare the environment: Ask patient to remove cigarettes and smoking-related paraphernalia from home, office, and vehicle; have patient tell others not to smoke in his presence.
3. Avoid triggers and recommend healthy substitute activities.
4. Prescribe pharmacologic therapy if the patient desires.
5. Arrange follow-up 3 to 7 days after the quit date.

The patient decides to quit smoking in 2 weeks. His wife and children support his decision. He prepares the environment and decides to restart his prior hobby of woodworking. He presents 4 days after the quit date with irritability, difficulty concentrating, and insomnia. What is the most likely cause of these symptoms?

Smoking cessation can lead to nicotine withdrawal. Symptoms include depression, anxiety, irritability, restlessness, insomnia, difficulty concentrating, increased appetite, and weight gain. These symptoms typically resolve within a few weeks of cessation. Pharmacologic therapy can reduce but not completely eliminate symptoms.

What pharmacologic options exist to decrease symptoms of nicotine withdrawal?

1. Nicotine replacement: Available in five forms (see Table 1-10). All five forms are equally effective, so patient preference decides which method to use. Nicotine pharmacotherapy reduces rate of relapse by 50%.
2. Bupropion (Zyban): Bupropion inhibits dopamine and norepinephrine reuptake in the central nervous system. Bupropion is as effective as nicotine at reducing relapse. Nicotine + bupropion may be superior to either agent alone.
3. Varenicline (Chantix): This recently approved drug is designed to partially activate nicotinic acetylcholine receptors while displacing nicotine at its sites of action in the brain.

TABLE 1–10 Pharmacotherapy for Nicotine Withdrawal

Drug	Duration	Drawbacks
Nicotine gum/lozenge	3–6 months	Requires patient education because it is difficult to use correctly. Many smokers become chronic gum/lozenge users.
Nicotine patch	2–3 months	Can cause vivid, disturbing dreams. The combination of cigarettes and the nicotine patch causes discomfort due to high nicotine levels (associated with almost 100% relapse rate).
Nicotine inhaler/spray	2–3 months	Highest potential for nicotine dependence.
Bupropion	2–3 months	Can cause seizures in 0.1% of patients.
Varenicline	3–6 months	Can cause nausea, headache, insomnia, and vivid dreams.

Behavioral programs: Associated with decreased relapse rates; pharmacotherapy plus behavioral therapy is associated with lower relapse rates than either method alone.

CASE 1–7 ALCOHOL ABUSE AND DEPENDENCE

A 38-year-old woman tells you she drinks two to three 5-ounce glasses of wine every night. She works as a lawyer and was recently promoted to partner. She does not feel like her alcohol use is a problem and does not feel guilty about her drinking. Her husband sometimes tells her she needs to cut down on the wine, which she finds annoying.

What is the next step in management?

Women who consume >7 drinks a week or ≥3 drinks per occasion are considered to be at risk for future adverse consequences. The next step for at-risk patients is brief intervention, which can vary from a single discussion to multiple sessions of counseling and follow-up sessions.

1 drink: 0.5 oz alcohol (12 oz beer, 5 oz wine, or 1.5 oz 80-proof spirit).

At-risk men: >14 drinks per week or ≥4 drinks per occasion.

After a brief discussion, the patient tells you she is not interested in cutting down on her alcohol intake and does not want any further discussions on the topic. One year later, she is arrested for driving under the influence of alcohol. Her husband has threatened to leave her if she doesn't stop drinking. She continues her usual intake of alcohol. How would you classify her pattern of alcohol use?

Substance use is classified as abuse if the patient meets any of the following criteria:

1. Failure to fulfill obligations (at work, school, home, etc.)
2. Continued use despite social or interpersonal problems caused by substance use
3. Use in dangerous situations (e.g., driving a car)
4. Recurrent substance-related legal problems

Alcohol abuse screening: suspect if two or more criteria on CAGE questionnaire are present.

Two years later, the patient tells you she now consumes 25 glasses of wine per week to achieve the same effect. She doesn't get out of the house much because she prefers to drink alone in her free time. She realizes she has a drinking problem and is very depressed because she is unable to stop drinking. How would you classify her pattern of alcohol use?

Three out of seven criteria are required to diagnose dependence on alcohol or any other substance:

1. Tolerance (patient requires an increased amount of substance to achieve the desired effect)
2. Withdrawal (see Chapter 7: Fluids, Electrolytes and Acid Base Disorders)
3. Significant time spent getting, using, or recovering from the substance
4. Using substance more than originally intended
5. Persistent desire to cut down on use
6. Decreased social, occupational, or recreational activities as a result of substance use
7. Continued use despite physical or psychological problems

> Legally, blood alcohol level >80 mg/dL is classified as intoxication; chronic users may not experience signs of intoxication until much higher levels.

What treatment should you recommend?

Set a quit date. Monitor the patient for withdrawal and treat if necessary (see Chapter 7: Fluids and Electrolytes). Recommend an Alcoholics Anonymous (AA) program, which is a cost-effective alternative to professional outpatient alcohol treatment.

> AA emphasizes recovery through belief in a higher power; other non-faith programs are available but have not been studied rigorously.

The patient agrees on a quit date. She experiences minor tremors and nausea within a few hours of her last drink, which is successfully treated with outpatient diazepam. She remains abstinent for 12 days and enrolls in an AA program. She constantly experiences cravings for "just one" alcoholic beverage. What additional therapy can you offer?

Consider a 4-month course of naltrexone for patients who have stopped drinking but need additional support to remain abstinent. This opioid antagonist reduces alcohol cravings. Before prescribing this drug, check serum creatinine and liver function tests because naltrexone is contraindicated in patients with chronic liver or kidney disease.

> **Alcohol withdrawal:** inpatient therapy is recommended if the patient has seizures, hallucinations, or delirium tremens (see Chapter 7: Fluids, Electrolytes, and Acid-Base Disorders).

CASE 1–8 CLINICAL STATISTICS

The CDC estimated that in 2002 there were about 700,000 people in the United States living with HIV/AIDS. They also estimated that there were 40,000 new infections that year. The population of the United States at that time was approximately 280 million people.

On the basis of the CDC report, what was the prevalence of HIV/AIDS in 2002?

Prevalence is the total number of cases of a disease in the population at a given time, so the prevalence of HIV/AIDS in 2002 was 700,000. Prevalence can also be expressed as (total number of cases) / (total population) = 700,000 / 280 million = 0.025%.

On the basis of the CDC report, what was the incidence of HIV/AIDS in 2002?

Incidence is the number of new cases of disease in the population at a given time, so the incidence of HIV/AIDS in 2002 was 40,000. Incidence can also be expressed as (total new cases) / (total population at risk) = 40,000 / (280 million − 700,000) = 0.00014%.

Which measure is more useful when describing a disorder such as infectious mononucleosis?

Incidence is far more useful than prevalence to describe acute, short-lived disorders such as infectious mononucleosis.

Western blot is the gold standard test to detect HIV-1 infection. Enzyme immunoassay (EIA) is the most frequently used screening test. Table 1-11 describes the findings of a study that compared EIA to the gold standard test in 10,000 persons. On the basis of this study, what is the sensitivity of EIA?

Sensitivity tells us how good a test is at correctly identifying people with disease. Therefore, a very sensitive test helps rule out disease.

Sensitivity = TP / (TP + FN) = 9990 / (9990 + 10) = 0.999 = 99.9%.

SNOUT = SeNsitivity rules OUT

On the basis of this study, what is the specificity of EIA?

Specificity tells us how good a test is at correctly identifying people without disease. Therefore, a very specific test helps rule in disease.

Specificity = TN / (TN + FP) = 9990 / (9990 + 10) = 0.999 = 99.9%.

SPIN = SPecificity rules IN

On the basis of this study, what is the positive predictive value (PPV) of EIA?

PPV tells us what proportion of positive results is correct.

PPV = TP / (TP + FP) = 9990 / (9990 + 10) = 99.9%.

On the basis of this study, what is the negative predictive value (NPV) of EIA?

NPV tells us what proportion of negative results is correct.

NPV = TN / (TN + FN) = 9990 / (9990 + 10) = 99.9%.

The prevalence of HIV/AIDS in Malawi is about 20%. How would this increased prevalence affect sensitivity, specificity, PPV, and NPV?

Sensitivity and specificity are unaffected by prevalence; however, increased prevalence leads to increased PPV and decreased NPV (and *vice versa*).

What is the probability that a randomly chosen person in Malawi will be HIV-positive?

The probability that a person will have a disorder before the results of a test are known is called pretest probability. The pretest probability that a randomly chosen person in Malawi will be HIV-positive is 20%.

Increased pretest probability does not affect sensitivity or specificity of a test; however, increased pretest probability leads to increased PPV and decreased NPV (and *vice versa*).

TABLE 1–11 EIA *versus* Western Blot

	Western Blot (+)	Western Blot (–)
EIA (+)	9990 = True positive (TP)	10 = False positive (FP)
EIA (–)	10 = False negative (FN)	9990 = True negative (TN)

What are the odds that a randomly chosen person in Malawi will be HIV-positive?

Pretest odds = Pretest probability / (100 − pretest probability) = 20 / (100 − 20) = 20:80 = 0.25.

> Odds of a:b correspond to a probability of a / (a + b).

Diagnostic testing for HIV is not available in the Mulanje district of Malawi. A 32-year-old patient presents with fever, cough, lymphadenopathy, and an abnormal lung exam. You read in a journal that these findings carry a positive likelihood ratio of 8 for HIV seropositivity in this district. How can you use this positive likelihood ratio to calculate the probability of AIDS?

In this case, the "test" is compatible clinical features:

$$\text{Posttest odds} = \text{likelihood ratio} \times \text{pretest odds}$$
$$\text{Posttest odds} = 8 \times 0.25 = 2 = 2 / 1$$
$$\text{Posttest probability} = 2 / (2 + 1) = 2 / 3 = 66\%.$$

Therefore, on the basis of clinical findings alone, this patient has a 66% chance of AIDS.

You also read that absence of these findings carries a negative likelihood ratio of 0.2. What is the probability that a person with none of these findings will be HIV-positive?

$$\text{Posttest odds} = 0.2 \times 0.25 = 0.05 = 0.05{:}1$$
$$\text{Posttest probability} = 0.05 / (0.05 + 1) = 0.05 / 1.05 = 0.047 = 4.7\%.$$

You see another patient in Malawi who presents with purple nodules on his face and trunk. The nodules bleed easily. You read in a journal that the sensitivity and specificity of these findings for HIV seropositivity are 80% and 85%, respectively. How can you calculate the probability that the patient is HIV-positive?

$$\text{Positive likelihood ratio} = \text{sensitivity} / (1 - \text{specificity}) = 0.8 / (1 - 0.85) = 5.3$$
$$\text{Posttest odds} = \text{pretest odds} \times \text{positive likelihood ratio} = 0.25 \times 5.3 = 1.325$$
$$\text{Posttest probability} = 1.325 / 2.325 = 0.57 = 57\%.$$

> Negative likelihood ratio = (1 − sensitivity) / specificity = (1 − 0.8) / 0.85 = 0.24

An HIV-positive patient presents with mild fatigue. The pretest probability of pneumonia in a patient with fatigue and no other clinical findings is 5%. The test threshold to order a CXR is 10%, and the test-treat threshold is 15%. What is the next step in management?

If the pretest probability is less than the test threshold, do not order the test or initiate treatment.

What would have been the next step in management if the pretest probability were 8%?

If the pretest probability is greater than the test threshold but less than the test-treat threshold, the next step is to order the diagnostic test (CXR).

What would have been the next step in management if the pretest probability were 20%?

If the pretest probability is greater than the test-treat threshold, the next step is to initiate treatment without ordering any diagnostic tests.

chapter **2**

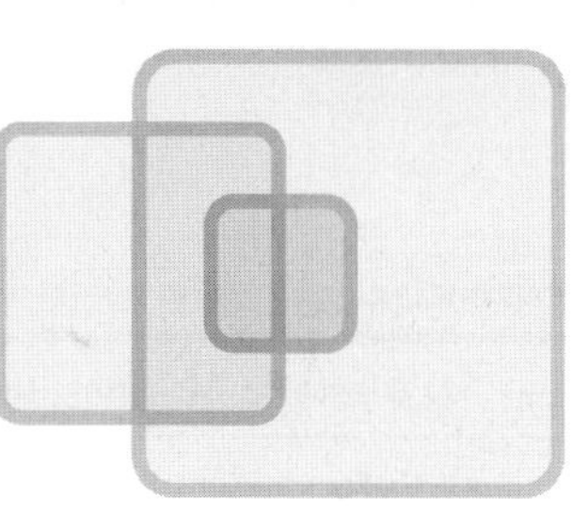

Cardiology

CASE 2-1 HYPERTENSION

A 50-year-old man presents to the clinic for an annual physical. He does not have any prior medical history, hospitalizations, or surgeries. He smokes half a pack of cigarettes a day and drinks a glass of wine every night. Physical examination is unremarkable. Temperature, pulse, and respirations are within normal limits. Blood pressure is 135/80. The patient asks if his blood pressure is normal.

What should you tell this patient?

This patient with no other medical conditions has prehypertension (HTN), defined as systolic blood pressure of 120 to 139 mm Hg or diastolic pressure of 80 to 89 mm Hg (Table 2-1). His risk of cardiac disease is elevated compared to patients with optimal blood pressure. However, antihypertensive therapies do not reduce cardiovascular (CV) risk in otherwise healthy patients

TABLE 2-1 Classification of Hypertension

Systolic BP (mm Hg)	Diastolic BP (mm Hg)	Classification
<120	<80	Normal
<120–139	80–89	Prehypertension
140–159	90–99	Stage 1
≥160	≥100	Stage 2

Abbreviation: BP, blood pressure.

with pre-HTN. He should adopt nonpharmacological measures to reduce his blood pressure. Also, arrange a follow-up appointment to recheck his blood pressure in a year.

Nonpharmacological measures to control HTN are **SAAD**:

1. **S**moking cessation
2. **A**ctivity: aerobic activity at least 30 minutes a day, most days of the week
3. **A**lcohol moderation: <2 drinks a day for men and <1 drink a day for women and light-weight patients)
4. **D**iet: Consume a diet high in fruits and vegetables and low in saturated and total fat. Limit sodium intake to <2.4 g/day

The threshold to initiate anti-HTN medications is >130/80 mm Hg if the patient has congestive heart failure (CHF), coronary artery disease (CAD), or CAD equivalents (e.g., peripheral artery disease (PAD), diabetes, or chronic renal failure).

The patient quits smoking and begins to walk for 30 minutes every day. He reduces his intake of saturated fat. During his follow-up appointment 1 year later, his blood pressure is 145/90. What is the next step in management?

Do not diagnose HTN on the basis of a single blood pressure measurement. In the absence of end-organ damage, confirm the diagnosis by obtaining at least three elevated measurements on separate occasions within the next 2 months. Ask patients to avoid caffeine or nicotine for at least 30 minutes prior to blood pressure measurement.

Confirm the diagnosis within 1–4 weeks in patients with initial measurements corresponding to stage 2 HTN.

The patient's blood pressure is 150/92 during a follow-up visit 1 month later. He is surprised because he has been measuring his blood pressure at the local Wal-Mart frequently and has never had a reading >130/80. What is the next step in management?

This patient may have "white coat HTN." An option in this case is ambulatory blood pressure monitoring (ABPM) using a device that measures the patient's blood pressure every 15 to 20 minutes over a 24- to 48-h period. The patient has HTN if either:

1. Average blood pressure over 24 hours is >135/85 mm Hg.
2. Average blood pressure during the day is >140/90 mm Hg.
3. Average blood pressure during the night is >125/75 mm Hg.

ABPM confirms the diagnosis of HTN. What additional work-up should you perform?

The goal of the initial evaluation of a patient with confirmed HTN is to search for clues suggesting secondary causes (Table 2-2), assess CV risk, and detect end-organ damage (Table 2-3). The following work-up is indicated:

TABLE 2–2 Secondary Causes of Hypertension in Adults

Renal	Renal artery stenosis (most prevalent cause of secondary HTN) Renal parenchymal disease
Endocrine	Pheochromocytoma Primary hyperaldosteronism (Conn's syndrome) Cushing's syndrome Hypo- or hyperthyroidism, hyperparathyroidism
Other	Sleep apnea Medications (e.g., oral contraceptive pills)

Abbreviation: HTN, hypertension.

TABLE 2–3 End-Organ Damage Caused by Hypertension

Organ System	Complications
Central nervous system	Intracerebral hemorrhage (hypertension is the major cause) Encephalopathy when blood pressure is severely elevated Stroke caused by accelerated atherosclerosis
Eyes	Early changes: Arteriovenous (AV) nicking (thick retinal arteries compress retinal vein) Cotton wool spots (yellow-white discoloration of the retina due to ischemic injury and swelling of retinal nerve layers) Late changes: Hemorrhage Exudates Papilledema when blood pressure is severely elevated
Heart	LV hypertrophy and congestive heart failure (due to increased afterload) Coronary artery disease and MI (due to accelerated atherosclerosis) Aortic dissection and aortic aneurysm
Kidneys	Chronic renal failure (due to hypertensive nephrosclerosis caused by sclerosis of glomerulus, afferent, and efferent arterioles) Worsening of other causes of chronic kidney disease
Extremities	Peripheral vascular disease (due to accelerated atherosclerosis)

Abbreviation: AV, arteriovenous; LV, left ventricular; MI, myocardial infarction.

1. Physical examination to screen for end-organ damage and to search for clues to suggest a secondary cause of HTN (e.g., abdominal bruits suggest renal artery stenosis (RAS); an abdominal mass suggests pheochromocytoma; arteriovenous (AV) nicking and cotton wool spots indicate end-organ damage to the eyes).
2. Evaluate renal function with blood urea nitrogen (BUN), creatinine, and urinalysis.
3. Screen for left ventricular (LV) hypertrophy with resting electrocardiogram (EKG).
4. Measure blood glucose to screen for diabetes mellitus (DM).
5. Obtain fasting lipid profile to screen for hyperlipidemia.

Laboratory test results are normal. The patient does not have any physical signs to suggest a secondary cause or end-organ damage caused by HTN. What therapy is most appropriate?

All antihypertensive drugs are equally effective at lowering blood pressure. This patient does not have any compelling indications for a specific drug (Table 2-4). Initiate therapy with a low-dose thiazide diuretic such as hydrochlorothiazide (HCTZ) because of its low cost (see Fig. 2-1).

TABLE 2-4 JNC-7 Guidelines for Antihypertensive Therapy

COMPELLING INDICATIONS FOR SPECIFIC DRUG CLASSES	
Stable systolic heart failure or asymptomatic LV dysfunction	ACE inhibitor, a β-blocker ± an aldosterone antagonist[a]
Heart failure with fluid overload	Add a loop diuretic to the regimen
Postmyocardial infarct	ACE inhibitor and a β-blocker
Angina or atrial fibrillation	β-Blocker or a nondihydropyridine CCB
Diabetes or chronic renal failure	ACE inhibitor
RELATIVE INDICATIONS FOR SPECIFIC DRUG CLASSES	
Benign prostatic hypertrophy	α-Blocker
Hyperthyroidism, essential tremor, glaucoma, or perioperative hypertension	β-Blocker
Migraine headaches	β-Blocker or CCB
Raynaud's syndrome, esophageal spasm	CCB
Osteoporosis	Thiazide diuretic
ABSOLUTE CONTRAINDICATIONS TO SPECIFIC DRUG CLASSES	
β-Blockers	Cardiogenic shock or hypotension Bradycardia with heart rate <50 beats per minute Second- or third-degree AV block Decompensated heart failure Active asthma or reactive airways disease
CCBs	Cardiogenic shock or hypotension Bradycardia with heart rate <50 beats per minute Second- or third-degree heart block Decompensated heart failure Avoid short-acting CCBs after MI
ACE inhibitors/ARBs	History of angioedema Bilateral renal artery stenosis Pregnancy

Abbreviation: ACE, angiotensin-converting enzyme; ARB, angiotensin receptor blocker; CCB, calcium channel blocker.
[a] If the patient has a compelling indication for an ACE inhibitor but cannot tolerate the associated cough, switch to an ARB.

The patient begins taking a low dose of HCTZ. One month later, his blood pressure is 145/91. What is the next step in management?

If the initial dose fails to adequately reduce the patient's blood pressure to <140/90, optimize the diuretic dose. If the blood pressure is still not within normal limits, options are to maximize the dose of the single drug, switch to another drug, or add a second drug. Combinations should almost always include a thiazide diuretic because they minimize volume expansion and thereby improve the antihypertensive response to other drugs.

> Diuretics can cause hypokalemia, hyperuricemia, and hyperglycemia; angiotensin-converting enzyme (ACE) inhibitors and angiotensin II receptor blocker (ARBs) minimize these electrolyte abnormalities.

> β-Blockers may mask hypoglycemic symptoms in insulin-dependent diabetics; however, do not withhold β-blockers if the patient has a compelling indication.

> Avoid using β-blockers and rate-limiting calcium channel blockers (CCBs) together (verapimil and diltiazem) because the combination can cause bradycardia and heart block.

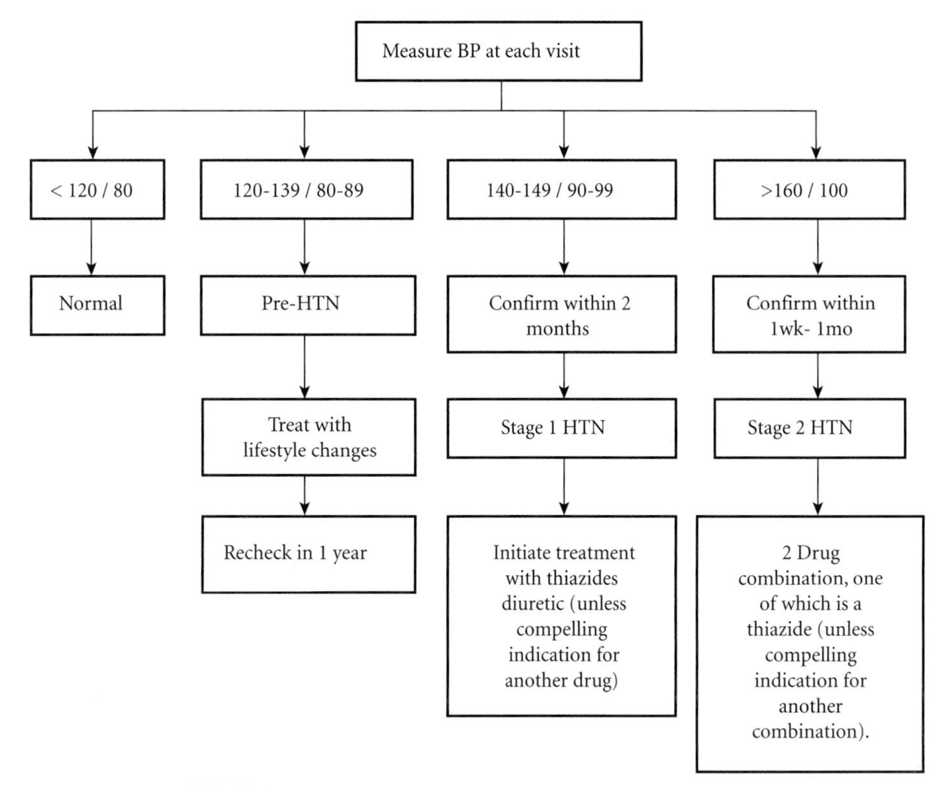

FIGURE 2–1 Algorithm for work-up and diagnosis of hypertension.

The patient's blood pressure is well-controlled with a thiazide diuretic over the next 7 years. Blood pressure during his last visit 6 months ago was 120/78. During this visit, however, blood pressure is 165/100. An ACE inhibitor is added to his regimen; 2 weeks later, the patient presents to the emergency department with new onset of dyspnea at rest. Physical examination is significant for bilateral rales and a bruit over the left abdomen. Extremities are warm. There is no JVD, peripheral edema, extra heart sounds, or murmurs. Temperature is 37°C, pulse is 90 beats per minute (bpm), and blood pressure is 175/110. Serum creatinine is 2.5, and chest radiograph reveals bilateral infiltrates. What is the most likely cause of his symptoms?

Suspect RAS in this patient with sudden, marked elevation in previously stable blood pressure, lateral abdominal bruit, noncardiogenic pulmonary edema, and acute renal failure after starting an ACE inhibitor. RAS reduces blood flow to the glomeruli, which activates the renin-angiotensin-aldosterone system and causes HTN.

> Suspect a secondary cause of HTN if the patient has any of the following: age <30 or >55 years, severe or refractory HTN, or sudden rise in blood pressure over a previously stable value.

> 90% of renovascular HTN is caused by atherosclerosis in older patients; the other 10% occurs in young women with fibromuscular dysplasia.

> Noncardiogenic pulmonary edema: rales and chest infiltrates without signs of fluid overload (described in Chapter 7: Fluids and Electrolytes).

What is the next step in management?

This patient has a very high probability for RAS. He should undergo digital subtraction angiography. Treatment is surgery or angioplasty with or without stent placement.

> **Low pretest probability**: First screen using captopril renal scan, magnetic resonance (MR) angiography, computed tomography (CT) angiography, or duplex Doppler ultrasound; perform digital subtraction angiography only if the screening tests are positive.

> **Renal arteriography**: Gold standard to diagnose RAS, but this test is invasive and the contrast dyes used are nephrotoxic.

How would management differ if RAS were clinically suspected on the basis of lateral abdominal bruit in an asymptomatic patient with well-controlled HTN?

Although diagnosis of RAS is possible on the basis of a physical exam, screening and specific treatment for RAS is only indicated if HTN is difficult to control or renal function is affected.

CASE 2–2 HYPERTENSIVE URGENCY AND EMERGENCY

A 55-year-old man presents to the emergency department with an 8-hour history of slowly progressing headache, nausea, and vomiting. He has a 5-year history of stage 2 HTN that is poorly controlled as a result of nonadherence with medications. He appears restless and confused. He is oriented to person but not to place and time. Examination of the eyes is significant for retinal hemorrhages and papilledema. Blood pressure is 240/140. Remaining vital signs are within normal limits.

What is the most likely cause of his symptoms?

A sudden rise in blood pressure to >180/120 mm Hg that is associated with end-organ damage is termed a hypertensive emergency. This patient has malignant HTN associated with hypertensive encephalopathy, most likely caused by noncompliance with medication.

How does malignant HTN differ from accelerated HTN and hypertensive encephalopathy?

Accelerated HTN, malignant HTN, and hypertensive encephalopathy are all possible presentations of hypertensive emergency:

1. Accelerated HTN is a sudden, marked elevation in blood pressure associated with end-organ damage but no papilledema (although retinal hemorrhage and exudates are often present).
2. Malignant hypertension is a sudden, marked elevation in blood pressure accompanied by end-organ damage including papilledema.
3. Hypertensive encephalopathy is a malignant HTN accompanied by cerebral edema, which presents with headache, nausea, vomiting, restlessness, and confusion.

> **Hypertensive encephalopathy versus stroke**: Onset is usually sudden in ischemic or hemorrhagic stroke but insidious in hypertensive encephalopathy.

How is hypertensive emergency managed?

The initial steps are:

1. Intravenous (IV) antihypertensives: First-line choices in this patient are nitroprusside, nicardipine, fenoldopam, or labelalol (Table 2-5).
2. Head CT: Obtain in patients with hypertensive encephalopathy to rule out hemorrhage.
3. Admit the patient to the intensive care unit (ICU).

The initial goal of treatment is to lower diastolic blood pressure to 100 to 105 mm Hg over 2- to 6 hours. After the patient reaches this goal he can switch to oral therapy. Consider screening for secondary causes of HTN after discharge from the ICU.

> Malignant HTN causes defective blood pressure autoregulation, so very rapid blood pressure reduction can lead to myocardial ischemia and ischemic stroke.

TABLE 2–5 Blood Pressure Management in Hypertensive Emergencies

Etiology	Recommended Antihypertensive Therapy	Antihypertensive Drugs to Avoid
Acute pulmonary edema	Nitroprusside and nitroglycerin	β-Blockers (decrease contractility), hydralazine (increases cardiac work)
Angina or acute MI	Labetalol, nitroprusside, and nitroglycerin	Hydralazine (increases cardiac work)
Aortic dissection	Nitroprusside plus propanalol or labetalol	
Increased sympathomimetic activity (e.g., cocaine, amphetamines, Guillian Barre, pheochromocytoma)	Phentolamine, labetalol, or nitroprusside	Do not use a β-blocker alone to avoid unopposed α-adrenergic vasoconstriction.
Antihypertensive drug discontinuation	Re-administer withdrawn drug; if necessary, administer nitroprusside, labetalol, phentolamine, nicardipine, or fenoldopam.	
Pregnancy	Hydralazine is first choice; nicardipine and labetalol are alternatives if hydralazine is unsuccessful.	Do not use nitroprusside and ACE inhibitors because they can harm the fetus.
Ischemic or hemorrhagic stroke	Refer to Chapter 12: Neurology.	Do not treat hypertension unless it is very elevated because hypertension helps maintain cerebral perfusion.

Alternative 2.2.1

The patient has a blood pressure of 200/120 but is asymptomatic. He has not adhered to his outpatient antihypertensive regimen of HCTZ and lisinopril. He does not have any other medical conditions. Physical examination is unremarkable.

How would you label this patient's HTN?

Blood pressure <180/120 that is not associated with end-organ damage is called hypertensive urgency.

How is hypertensive urgency managed?

The first step is to repeat the blood pressure measurement after a short period of rest. Because the patient has not been compliant, reinstitute his outpatient regimen. If blood pressure is still markedly elevated after repeat measurement, reduce blood pressure to <160/100 over several hours to days. Closely follow the patient over the next 1 to 2 days. If close follow-up is not possible, admit the patient for overnight observation. Over the next few weeks to months, tailor therapy to reach target blood pressure of >140/90.

> Do not aggressively reduce blood pressure with IV drugs in hypertensive urgency because the risk of organ hypoperfusion outweighs the benefits of blood pressure reduction.

CASE 2–3 HOARSENESS AND MURMUR

A 25-year-old man presents to the clinic with a 2-month history of hoarseness. He is tall and thin. His arms and legs are disproportionately long compared to the rest of his body. There are numerous stretch marks on his skin. He recalls that his father had a similar physical appearance. Auscultation of the heart is significant for a blowing diastolic murmur heard best at the upper sternal border. Vital signs are normal. Chest radiograph (CXR) is obtained which demonstrates a thoracic aneurysm of the ascending aorta.

What are the clinical manifestations of thoracic aortic aneurysms?

These aneurysms are frequently asymptomatic and are often detected incidentally. However, an ascending aneurysm can cause aortic root dilatation, which leads to aortic regurgitation and heart failure. The aneurysm can erode into the mediastinum to cause hoarseness (recurrent laryngeal nerve compression), hemidiaphragm paralysis (phrenic nerve compression), dysphagia (esophageal compression), cough, wheezing, dyspnea, or hemoptysis.

> Classification of thoracic aortic aneurysms:
>
> 1. Ascending aortic aneurysms (arise from aortic root to innominate artery)
> 2. Aortic arch aneurysms (affect brachiocephalic vessels)
> 3. Descending aortic aneurysms (arise distal to subclavian vein)

What is the next step in management?

Obtain a transesophageal echocardiogram (TEE) and either CT scan with IV contrast or MR angiography. Contrast angiography provides the best resolution, but this technique is invasive and potentially nephrotoxic.

> A high index of suspicion is needed to detect thoracic aortic aneurysm. Consider thoracic aorta imaging in any patient admitted with chest pain and no obvious cause.

TEE and MR angiography detect an ascending aortic root aneurysm that is 3 cm long. What condition likely predisposed this young patient to aortic aneurysm?

Thoracic aortic aneurysm is most common in older men with HTN. However, patients with Marfan's syndrome, Ehlors Danlos syndrome, and bicuspid aortic valve have an increased risk of thoracic aortic aneurysm at a young age. This patient's tall, thin body habitus with large extremities, stretch marks, and a positive family history are consistent with Marfan's syndrome.

What management should you recommend for this aneurysm?

Surgically resect symptomatic thoracic aneurysms regardless of size because they have a high risk of rupture.

Alternative 2.3.1

A 3-cm ascending aortic aneurysm is detected incidentally in a 65-year-old patient. The patient is asymptomatic and has no signs of aortic regurgitation or mediastinal extension. He has a 10-year history of HTN. Vital signs are temperature 37.1°C, pulse 75 bpm, respirations 18, blood pressure 160/100. How should you manage this aneurysm?

The risk of rupture is low in an asymptomatic patient with a thoracic aneurysm <6 cm. Treat asymptomatic aneurysms with β-blockers and monitor frequently for symptoms or growth. Indications for surgery are:

1. Aneurysm ≥ 5.5 cm on follow-up.
2. Aneurysm grows >1 cm per year.
3. Patient becomes symptomatic.

> **Marfan's syndrome**: Surgery is indicated when aneurysm grows to 5 cm.

The patient does not return to monitor his aneurysm and is lost to follow-up. He returns 1 year later with tearing chest pain. He has a blowing diastolic murmur along the right sternal border. Blood pressure is 180/110 in his right arm and 80/60 in the left arm. Pulse is 120 bpm, temperature is 36°C, and respirations are 25/minute. CXR is obtained (see Fig. 2-2). What is the most likely complication?

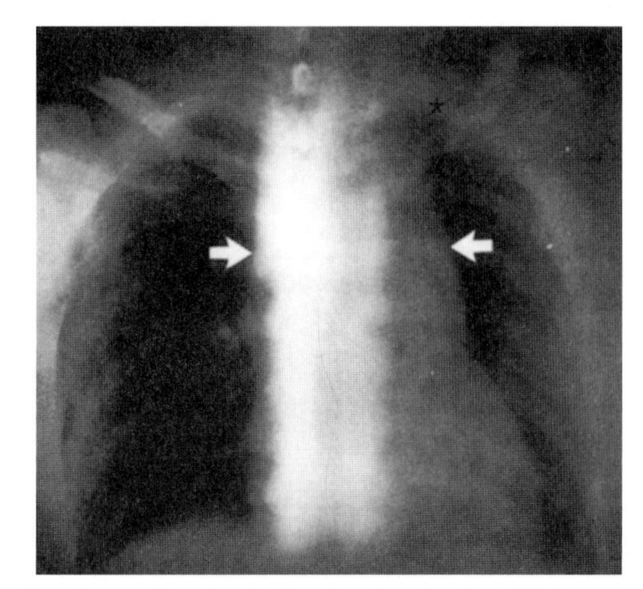

FIGURE 2–2 Chest radiograph suggestive of aortic dissection. From Jarrell B. *NMS Surgery Casebook,* 1st ed. Lippincott Williams & Wilkins, 2003.

Tearing chest pain and pulse deficits should always raise suspicion for aortic dissection, particularly if the patient has a history of longstanding HTN or aortic aneurysm. The CXR demonstrates the characteristic features of a dissected thoracic aorta (widened mediastinum and tracheal deviation).

> CXR is not a sensitive test to detect aortic aneurysm or dissection, so further testing is necessary if CXR is nondiagnostic and these diagnoses are suspected.

> 70% of patients with aortic dissection have a history of HTN.

What are the next steps in management?

1. Stabilize: Admit the patient to the ICU and administer IV propanalol or labetalol (target systolic blood pressure of 100 to 120 mm Hg). If β-blockers do not control the blood pressure, administer IV nitroprusside.
2. Pain control: Administer morphine while stabilization measures are being carried out.
3. Confirmatory testing: When the patient is stable, confirm the diagnosis with TEE.
4. Other: Obtain an EKG and measure cardiac enzymes to rule out myocardial infarction (MI).

TEE shows an ascending aortic dissection. What is the next step in management?

Patients with ascending aortic dissections (Type A) require emergent surgery.

> Type **A** = **A**scending thoracic aortic dissection: presents with sharp, tearing chest pain; management is surgical (mnemonic: ***Type A*** personalities are attracted to ***surgery***).
> Type **B** = Descending thoracic aortic dissection: presents with interscapular **B**ack pain; management is **β**-blockers.

CASE 2–4 DYSLIPIDEMIA

A 50-year-old woman with no prior medical history presents for her annual physical. She had breakfast 2 hours ago. She does not have any family history of CV disease. She does not smoke or drink alcohol, and she exercises 5 days a week for 30 minutes. She does not take any medications. Blood pressure is 120/80 mm Hg; blood glucose is 120 mg/dL.

What tests should you request to screen for hyperlipidemia?

Obtain a fasting lipid profile in patients who have fasted for at least 8 hours. This patient has not fasted, so obtain nonfasting total cholesterol (TC) and high-density lipoprotein (HDL) counts. If these are normal, further testing is not necessary.

TC is 240 mg/dL and HDL is 42 mg/dL. What is the next step in management?

If TC is >200 mg/dL or HDL is <40 mg/dL, obtain a fasting lipid profile, which includes triglycerides (TG) and a calculated low-density lipoprotein (LDL).

TG is 120 mg/dL, and LDL is 170 mg/dL. Does this patient require pharmacotherapy?

LDL cholesterol is the primary target of lipid management because it is the most atherogenic lipoprotein. The target LDL in a patient with no CV risk factors is 160 mg/dL, so no pharmacotherapy is necessary (Table 2-6).

> TC = LDL + HDL + (TG/5)

What measures are recommended to manage her cholesterol at this stage?

1. Diet and exercise: Initiate a step 1 diet. If cholesterol remains above goal (<160 mg/dL) 6 to 12 weeks later, consider a step 2 diet (more restrictive). Also consider increasing dietary intake of omega-3-fatty acids (found in fish oil).
2. Laboratory tests: Measure thyroid-stimulating hormone, liver function tests, glucose, BUN, creatinine, and urinalysis to establish a baseline; evaluate for secondary causes of dyslipidemia (Table 2-7).

> - **Step 1 diet**: <10% of calories from saturated fat, <300 mg/day of cholesterol.
> - **Step 2 diet**: <7% of calories from saturated fat, and <200 mg/day of cholesterol.
> - Limit fat intake to <30% of total calories in both step 1 and step 2 diets.

The patient initiates lifestyle measures and is able to lower her LDL to 150 mg/dL within 1 month. Two months later, DM is diagnosed and the patient initiates metformin. LDL is 150 mg/dL, HDL is 42 mg/dL, and TG is 170 mg/dL. What is the next step?

Diabetes is a coronary heart disease (CHD) equivalent, so her target LDL cholesterol is now 100 mg/dL. Statins are the initial drug of choice for patients with elevated LDL levels (Tables 2-8 and 2-9). Statins improve mortality when used for both primary and secondary prevention of CV disease. The patient should continue regular exercise and follow a step 2 diet even after initiating drug therapy. She should discontinue fish oil because it may worsen glycemic control.

TABLE 2–6 National Cholesterol Education Program Guidelines for Management of Hyperlipidemia

CV Risk Factors[a]	Target LDL (mg/dL)	LDL Level to Start Lifestyle Measures (mg/dL)	LDL Level to Start Drug Therapy (mg/dL)
0–1	≤160	≥160	≥190
≥2	≤130	≥130	≥130–160
DM or CHD	≤100	≥100	≥130

Abbreviation: CV, cardiovascular; DM, diabetes mellitus; LDL, low-density lipoprotein; HDL, high-density lipoprotein.

[a] CV risk factors are smoking, HTN, family history, age, male sex, and HDL < 40 mg/dL. If you count male sex as a risk factor, do not count age. Remove one risk factor if HDL cholesterol is ≥60 mg/dL. Diabetes, peripheral artery disease, and chronic renal failure are coronary artery disease equivalents.

TABLE 2–7 Secondary Causes of Dyslipidemia

Categories	Disorders	LDL	HDL	TG
Endocrine	Hypothyroidism	↑		↑
	DM		↓	↑
	Cushing's disease	↑		
Liver	Acute hepatitis			↑
	Primary biliary cirrhosis	↑		
Kidney	Nephrotic syndrome	↑		
	Uremia			↑
Other	Alcohol			↑
	Oral contraceptive pills			↑
	Cigarettes		↓	
	Obesity, sedentary lifestyle		↓	↑

Adapted from Sabatine M. *Pocket Medicine*, 2nd ed. Lippincott William & Wilkens, 2001.

TABLE 2–8 Side Effects and Contraindications of Dyslipidemia Drugs

Class	Examples	Side Effects	Contraindications
Statins	Atorvastatin Pravastatin	Myopathy ↑ LFTs	Liver disease (active or chronic)
Cholesterol absorption inhibitors	Ezetimibe	↑ LFTs	None
Bile acid binding resins	Cholestyramine Colestipol Cholesevalam	GI distress, ↓ Drug absorption	TG > 400 mg/dL
Niacin	Nicotinic acid	Flushing Hyperuricemia Hyperglycemia ↑ LFTs GI distress	Chronic liver disease Severe gout
Fibrates	Gemfibrozil Fenofibrate	Dyspepsia Gallstones Myopathy	Severe liver disease Severe kidney disease

Abbreviation: LFT, liver function tests; TG, triglyceride. Adapted from O'Rourke et al. *Hurst's The Heart: Manual of Cardiology*. 11th ed.

TABLE 2–9 Effect of Dyslipidemia Drugs on Lipoprotein Levels

Drug Class	LDL	HDL	TG
Statins	↓↓↓	↑	↓
Ezetimibe	↓↓	↑	↔
Bile acid binding resins	↓↓	↑	↑
Niacin	↓	↑↑	↓↓
Fibrates	↓	↑↑	↓↓

The patient initiates lovastatin, which brings her LDL to 90 mg/dL. Over the next 3 years, her LDL remains well controlled, but her triglycerides increase to 250 mg/dL; HDL is 30 mg/dL. Glycosylated hemoglobin is 6.0%. What is the next step in management?

Add a fibrate or niacin if the LDL cholesterol is well controlled by a statin but serum triglycerides are >200 mg/dL or HDL cholesterol is >40 mg/dL (Table 2-10). Do not use niacin if DM is not well controlled (glycosylated hemoglobin >6.5%).

DM and niacin: If niacin is chosen in a well-controlled diabetic, use the crystalline form because it has a smaller adverse impact on glycemic control.
Fibrates and statin: Use fenofibrate because it has fewer pharmacological interactions with statins than gemfibrozil.
Bile acid binding resins: Use of these resins is relatively contraindicated if TG >200 mg/dL.

Alternative 2.4.1

The patient is a 30-year-old man who presents with painless yellow nodules on his finger extensors and painless yellow plaques on his eyelids. His father had similar masses before he died of MI at the age of 42. He recalls that his paternal grandmother had an MI at the age of 40. Yellow deposits are seen in the peripheral cornea bilaterally. Serum LDL is 450 mg/dL, TG is 130 mg/dL, and HDL is 60 mg/dL. What is the diagnosis?

This patient has familial hypercholesterolemia (FH), an autosomal condition that leads to defective LDL receptors. Both homozygotes and heterozygotes are affected, although the clinical manifestations are more severe in homozygotes. Patients with FH have very high LDL levels at a young age; TG levels are usually normal. Excess LDL can deposit on eyelids and form yellow plaques (xanthelasma). LDL can also form yellow nodules on finger extensor tendons, the Achilles tendon, and plantar tendons (xanthoma). Most importantly, LDL can accumulate on arteries and form atheromas that predispose the patient to MI at a young age.

Corneal arcus: Bilateral yellow deposits in the peripheral cornea are common in older patients, but they should prompt an evaluation of serum lipids in patients <40 years old.

50% of homozygotes with FH develop aortic stenosis as a result of atheroma formation.

Familial defective apolipoprotein B-100: This relatively rare condition presents with findings identical to FH; genetic testing is the only way to distinguish the two conditions.

TABLE 2–10 TG Management

Level (mg/dL)	Classification	Treatment
<150	Normal	None
150–199	Borderline	Main goal is to control LDL cholesterol with statin; if LDL is normal, then only lifestyle measures are recommended.
200–499	High	Main goal is to control LDL cholesterol with statin; if patient has coronary heart disease equivalent and statin does not also lower TG, add niacin or fibrate.
≥500	Very high	First initiate treatment with fibrate or niacin to prevent pancreatitis; when TG level is controlled, address LDL target.

What treatment should this patient receive?

Options for initial therapy are high-dose statin or statin with a bile acid binding resin. If these regimens do not adequately lower LDL, add niacin to the regimen.

The patient asks if the yellow lesions will go away with treatment. What should you tell him?

Xanthomas and xanthelasmas usually resolve with treatment. If they are refractory, consider probucol. This antioxidant does not affect LDL but helps resolve xanthomas.

Alternative 2.4.2

The patient is a 32-year-old woman who presents with nausea, vomiting, and acute epigastric pain radiating to the back. Amylase and lipase levels are elevated, and acute pancreatitis is diagnosed in the patient. She recently initiated oral contraceptive pills (OCP). She does not drink alcohol, and right upper quadrant ultrasound does not show any gallstones. Physical examination reveals pimple-like plaques behind both knees and xanthomas on palmar creases. The patient's triglyceride level is 4000 mg/dL; BUN, creatinine, serum glucose, thyroid-stimulating hormone, and transaminase levels are within normal limits. Body mass index is 22.

What is the most likely cause of her symptoms?

Serum TG levels >1000 mg/dL can precipitate acute pancreatitis for unclear reasons. Eruptive xanthomas (pimple-like plaques on extensor surfaces) are a common physical finding when TG >1000 mg/dL. The most likely reason for acutely elevated TG in this patient is a familial condition superimposed with a secondary cause (oral contraceptives).

What familial condition is most likely in this patient?

Palmar crease xanthomas are pathognomic for familial dysbetalipoproteinemia.

> Familial conditions associated with elevated triglycerides:
>
> 1. Mixed hypertriglyceridemia
> 2. Familial hypertriglyceridemia
> 3. Familial combined hyperlipidemia
> 4. Familial dysbetalipoproteinemia

How should you treat this patient?

In addition to treating acute pancreatitis (refer to Chapter 5: Hepatology), administer fibrates or niacin and discontinue oral contraceptive pills.

> When DM is the precipitating secondary cause of hypertriglyceridemia, insulin is part of the acute treatment plan.

CASE 2–5 SCREENING FOR CAD

A 50-year-old woman visits her primary care physician for an annual physical. Her husband recently had a myocardial infarct and she is worried about her risk of a heart attack. She asks if she should have a stress test to make sure she does not have heart disease. She does not have any chest pain, shortness of breath, diaphoresis, nausea, or vomiting. She does not have any medical problems. Her father died of a myocardial infarct at the age of 80. She does not smoke or drink alcohol. Physical examination and vital signs are normal.

Should she undergo exercise stress testing?

This asymptomatic patient does not have any significant risk factors for CHD. Her pretest probability of CHD is very low, so a positive stress test in her case is more likely to be a false positive result. In general, do not screen asymptomatic, low-risk patients for CHD.

The patient returns to the clinic for a scheduled appointment 6 years later. She has had HTN for the last 2 years and received a diagnosis of DM 5 months ago. She does not have any chest pain, dyspnea, diaphoresis, nausea, or vomiting. She takes HCTZ and metformin. She plans to train for a marathon with her new boyfriend. She has been fairly sedentary for the last 30 years. Physical exam and vital signs are normal. Is any screening for heart disease warranted before she starts training for the marathon?

This patient now has three major risk factors for CHD (see Table 1-7). Of these, her history of DM is most concerning because asymptomatic diabetics with no history of MI have the same risk for coronary mortality as nondiabetic patients who have had an MI. She should undergo an exercise stress test on a treadmill or bicycle to screen for CHD before starting an exercise program. Obtain a baseline resting EKG before the exercise stress test to evaluate for changes that might obscure the results of a stress test.

> Screening asymptomatic, intermediate- to high-risk patients for CHD is controversial. Consider an exercise stress test to screen for CHD in the following asymptomatic patients:
>
> 1. High-risk occupations (pilots, firefighters, law enforcement officers)
> 2. Older patients (women, >50 years; men, >40 years) who plan to engage in vigorous exercise
> 3. More than two CV risk factors or CHD equivalents such as DM or chronic renal failure

Baseline EKG is normal, and she is ready to undergo an exercise treadmill test (ETT). How is this test performed and interpreted?

At least two EKG leads are monitored continuously while the patient exercises on a treadmill. The treadmill speed and inclination is increased according to a set protocol. Blood pressure is measured before the test and at the end of each increase in exercise intensity. If the patient reaches 80% to 90% of her target rate without positive findings, the test is negative. Positive findings for ischemia are any of the following:

1. A drop in systolic blood pressure ≥10 mm Hg
2. Angina or angina equivalents
3. A new murmur, S3, or S4
4. EKG findings: ST segment depression ≥1 mm or ST elevation ≥1 mm, T wave inversion, frequent or multifocal premature ventricular contractions

Can she take all of her medications the morning of the test?

Withhold the following medications 24 hours before an ETT:

1. Insulin and oral hypoglycemics: Exercise combined with these medications can precipitate hypoglycemia.
2. β-Blockers and CCBs: It can be difficult to reach a target heart rate while on these drugs.

The patient develops T wave flattening and has 2 to 3 premature ventricular contractions near the end of the study. The remainder of the study is normal. She reached 10 metabolic equivalents (METS) without any signs of angina. What is the next step in management?

Patients who develop severe ST depression (>2 mm) at low workloads (<6 minutes) are likely to have a true-positive study. Such patients should undergo coronary angiography. In contrast, this asymptomatic patient has a good exercise capacity as shown by a high number of METS and equivocal findings on EKG. The next step in a patient with equivocal ETT is exercise myocardial perfusion scintigraphy or exercise echocardiography.

> 10% to 30% of patients with ≤1 mm of ST depression on ETT have a false-positive result.

1 to 4 METS: Performs activities of daily living.
4 to 10 METS: Climbs a flight of stairs, performs heavy housework, and mild exercise.
>**10 METS**: Plays sports.

How is exercise myocardial perfusion scintigraphy performed?

Inject radionuclides such as thallium or technetium during exercise. Record images soon after exercise and after a 3- to 4-hour rest period. Because radionuclide uptake is proportional to blood flow, areas of hypoperfusion represent either ischemia or scar tissue. If the defect reverses with rest, the cause is ischemia. Defects that are present 3 to 4 hours after injection indicate scar tissue from an old MI or severe ischemia.

Echocardiogram or echocardiograph: Noninvasive image of the heart created with high-frequency (ultrasound) sound waves.

Alternative 2.5.1

The patient is 56 years old and has diabetes. She wishes to begin training for a marathon. Physical exam and vital signs are within normal limits, but resting EKG demonstrates LV strain and 0.8 mm of ST segment depression.

How should you screen this patient for CHD?

Exercise EKG testing is the preferred initial test in most patients to screen for heart disease. There are two exceptions to this preference:

1. Baseline EKG changes: Wolf-Parkinson syndrome, ST-segment changes, and LV hypertrophy can obscure interpretation of ETT. Evaluate these patients with exercise myocardial perfusion scintigraphy or exercise echocardiography.
2. Impaired exercise capacity: Patients with leg claudication, arthritis, deconditioning, or severe pulmonary disease should undergo either pharmacological stress scintigraphy or pharmacological stress echocardiography. Pharmacological stress scintigraphy is performed with the vasodilators adenosine or dipyridamole. Dobutamine is used to pharmacologically stress the heart during echocardiography.

This patient, who has LV hypertrophy, mild ST-segment changes, and no difficulty exercising, should undergo exercise myocardial perfusion scintigraphy or exercise echocardiography.

What test would you recommend if she had a left bundle branch block on EKG?

Transient septal defects can cause false-positive results on exercise myocardial perfusion scintigraphy in patients with left bundle branch block. Perform pharmacological stress test in this group of patients.

CASE 2–6 EXERTIONAL CHEST DISCOMFORT THAT RESOLVES WITH REST

A 58-year-old woman presents with an 8-week history of substernal chest tightness and pressure that radiates to the left arm. The discomfort occurs predictably after 5 minutes of exercise and causes her to stop all activity. Her symptoms gradually increase in intensity and resolve with 3 to 4 minutes of rest. Breathing and position do not change her symptoms. She does not have any dyspnea, diaphoresis, nausea, or vomiting. She does not currently have any symptoms. She has a history of HTN that is controlled with HCTZ. Her father has diabetes and both parents have HTN. She has one younger sibling who has no known medical conditions. She has smoked a pack of cigarettes a day since she was 25 years old. Physical examination, vital signs, and resting EKG are normal.

What is the most likely cause of her symptoms?

This patient's symptoms are characteristic of angina caused by myocardial ischemia (Tables 2-11 and 2-12). Angina that occurs predictably and reproducibly at a certain level of exertion and is relieved with rest or nitroglycerin is called stable angina.

TABLE 2–11 Characteristics of Chest Pain Due to Myocardial Ischemia

O	**O**nset	Gradual
P	**P**rovokes, Palliates	Provoked by exercise or exertion, Palliated by rest or nitroglycerin.
Q	**Q**uality	"Crushing" or "squeezing" discomfort rather than pain. Symptoms are difficult to localize because angina is referred pain from dermatomes that supply the same sections of the spinal cord as the heart. The classic description of the location is a clenched fist placed over the center of the chest (Levine sign).
R	**R**adiation	Because angina is referred pain, symptoms can radiate to the upper abdomen, shoulders, arms, wrist and fingers, neck and throat, lower jaw and teeth (but not upper jaw), and rarely to the back (specifically the interscapular region).
S	**S**everity	Angina associated with nausea, vomiting, or sweating should raise suspicion for acute coronary syndrome.
T	**T**iming	Stable angina usually lasts 2 to 5 minutes. Suspect acute coronary syndrome if pain lasts >20 minutes and is not relieved with rest or nitroglycerin.

TABLE 2–12 Differential Diagnosis of Chest Pain

Organ System	Disorders
Cardiac	Myocardial ischemia (angina, MI), pericarditis, myocarditis, aortic dissection
Pulmonary	Pulmonary embolism, pneumothorax, pneumonia, pulmonary hypertension
Gastrointestinal	Gastroesophageal reflux, esophageal spasm, Mallory-Weiss tear, peptic ulcer disease, biliary diseases, pancreatitis
Musculoskeletal	Costochondritis, osteoarthritis/cervical spine disease
Other	Herpes zoster, anxiety

Visceral pain: Dull aching, tightness, or burning that is poorly localized is more common with myocardial ischemia and gastrointestinal causes.
Pleuritic pain: Sharp pain increased with movement, position, inspiration, and cough is more common with pulmonary causes, pericarditis, and musculoskeletal causes.

> The characteristic EKG change with angina is horizontal or down-sloping ST segment depression that reverses after the symptoms disappear. T wave flattening or inversion can also occur.

How is stable angina managed?

Patients with stable angina should adopt certain general measures, take anti-ischemic medications, and undergo exercise stress test.

What general measures should patients with stable angina adopt?

1. Take 81 to 325 mg aspirin daily. Patients with aspirin allergy can take clopidogrel instead. Patients who have a gastrointestinal (GI) bleed while taking aspirin can often resume 81 mg aspirin daily after the bleeding has resolved only if they are also taking a proton pump inhibitor (see Chapter 4: Gastroenterology).
2. Exercise and aggressively control CV risk factors (stop smoking; monitor and treat DM, HTN, and hyperlidipidemia).

What anti-ischemic drugs are generally instituted in patients with stable angina?

Anti-ischemic drugs for patients with stable angina are known as "**NBC**":

1. **N**itrates: Sublingual nitroglycerin is the treatment of choice to relieve acute episodes of angina and as prophylaxis prior to activities known to elicit angina. Nitrates cause

systemic vasodilatation, which reduces LV wall stress. Chronic oral or transdermal nitrate therapy is a second-line measure if the initial regimen does not successfully control symptoms. With chronic therapy, a 12- to 14-hour nitrate-free interval is required to avoid tolerance.

2. β-Blockers: These drugs reduce angina and improve exercise tolerance. Nonselective β-blockers inhibit peripheral vasodilatation and bronchodilation, so use long-acting β-1–selective agents such as Atendol or Metoprolol. Titrate the dose to achieve a heart rate between 50 and 60 beats per minute.
3. CCBs: Long-acting CCBs also reduce angina and improve exercise tolerance. Prescribe CCBs if β-blockers are contraindicated, or combine them with β-blockers if β-blocker monotherapy is not successful. Do not use short-acting CCBs because they increase the risk of MI in hypertensive patients and the risk of death after an MI.

Common CCBs:

1. Verapimil (long-acting)
2. Diltiazem (long-acting)
3. Dihydropyridines: amlodipine and felodipine (long-acting); nifedipine (short-acting)

None of the anti-ischemic drugs reduce mortality in stable angina patients with no history of MI.

Why is an exercise stress test recommended in patients with stable angina?

A stress test is generally recommended in intermediate- to high-risk patients such as the person in this case because the test can identify the subset of patients with stable angina who have a high risk of MI. The test can also assess the efficacy of anti-angina therapy.

The exercise stress test is positive for 2 mm of ST segment depression after 5 minutes of exercise. What is the next step in management?

Although it is the gold standard for diagnosing CAD, coronary angiography is not indicated in most low- to intermediate-risk patients with stable angina because it is expensive and invasive. There are two exceptions to this general rule:

1. Angina that significantly interferes with the patient's lifestyle despite maximum tolerable medical therapy, and
2. High-risk criteria on noninvasive testing, regardless of angina severity.

This patient should undergo coronary angiography because significant ST depression appeared <6 minutes into the study (high-risk criteria). Angiography can identify whether she would benefit from a revascularization procedure.

Coronary angiography: Thread a catheter through the femoral artery into the heart. Inject contrast into the coronary vessels and take x-ray images (fluoroscopy) to detect occlusion.

During coronary angiography, 65% stenosis is seen in the left main coronary artery. What is the next step in management?

Perform revascularization if a patient with stable angina has any of the following:

1. Angina that significantly interferes with a patient's lifestyle despite maximum tolerable medical therapy.
2. Left main coronary artery stenosis >50% (this patient).
3. ≥70% stenosis in three coronary vessels.
4. ≥70% stenosis in two coronary vessels and one of them is the proximal left anterior descending artery.

How is revascularization of the coronary arteries achieved?

There are two methods for revascularization:

1. **Percutaneous coronary intervention (PCI)**: Percutaneous transluminal coronary angioplasty (PTCA) is performed in a cardiac catheterization laboratory under local anesthesia at the same time as diagnostic coronary angiography. A balloon is inflated under high pressure to dilate the area of stenosis. A bare-metal or drug-eluting intracoronary stent is usually placed after the procedure to prevent restenosis.
2. **Coronary artery bypass graft (CABG)**: Grafts from the internal mammary artery or saphenous vein are used to bypass the area of stenosis.

Should this patient undergo PCI or CABG?

In most patients, infarction and mortality rates are similar with PCI and CABG. However, CABG is superior to PCI in three groups of patients:

1. Diabetics
2. Reduced left ventricle function
3. Left main CAD

This patient with left main CAD should undergo CABG.

> A major limitation of studies that compare PTCA and CABG is that they did not evaluate newer developments (drug-eluting stents after PTCA and internal mammary grafts during CABG).

> PCI in patients with stable angina is superior to medical therapy for symptom relief but not for preventing infarction or death.

Alternative 2.6.1

The patient is a 35-year-old woman who reports substernal chest discomfort radiating to the lower jaw. Her symptoms usually occur in the morning and often wake her up from sleep. She is a smoker, but she does not have any other risk factors for CHD. An EKG obtained when the patient is symptomatic is significant for ST segment elevation that disappears when the symptoms resolve. Physical exam and vitals signs are within normal limits.

What is the most likely diagnosis?

This patient has variant (Prinzmental) angina. It is caused by spasm in the coronary arteries (most commonly the right coronary artery) and is more common in women under the age of 50 who smoke. Symptoms usually occur early in the morning. The characteristic EKG finding is ST segment elevation that disappears when the symptoms resolve.

Is any other diagnostic test indicated for this patient?

Perform coronary angiography in patients with any chest pain syndrome associated with ST segment elevation to determine if stenotic lesions are present. If stenotic lesions are not seen and the examiner wishes to confirm the diagnosis of variant angina, administer ergonovine during angiography to precipitate and document vasospasm.

No stenosis is seen during angiography. Intravenous ergonovine administration confirms vasospasm. How is variant angina treated?

CCBs are the first-line treatment for variant angina. Add nitrates if the CCB does not completely relieve symptoms. Avoid nonselective β-blockers because they promote vasospasm.

> Cocaine can induce coronary artery vasospasm and is an important cause of MI in young patients.

> Women >35 years old should not smoke and take oral contraceptives at the same time because the combination additively increases the risk of MI.

CASE 2–7 PERSISTENT CHEST DISCOMFORT AT REST

A 65-year-old man presents to the emergency department with a 2-hour history of crushing, substernal, chest discomfort radiating to his left arm. He has a history of stable angina on exertion that is usually relieved with sublingual nitroglycerin. His current symptoms occurred at rest and have not responded to nitroglycerin at home. He has history of HTN and smoking. He is sweating and appears anxious. Vital signs are temperature 37.6°C, blood pressure 140/85, pulse 110 bpm, respirations 22/minute. Oxygen saturation is 98% on room air.

What is the most likely cause of his symptoms?

Suspect acute coronary syndrome (ACS) in a patient with angina that occurs at rest and persists for >20 minutes despite taking nitroglycerin. ACS is usually caused by disruption of an atherosclerotic plaque, which activates platelet aggregation and causes the formation of an intracoronary thrombus. Conditions categorized as ACS range from unstable angina (UA) and non-ST elevation MI (non-Q wave MI) caused by a partially occlusive thrombus to the more severe ST elevation MI (Q-wave MI) caused by a completely occlusive thrombus.

> Patients with angina should call emergency services if their symptoms have not improved or are worsening 5 minutes after taking a dose of sublingual nitroglycerin.

> Maintain a high level of suspicion for ACS in women, diabetics, and the elderly. These patients often present with atypical symptoms such as isolated dyspnea, jaw pain, nausea/vomiting, palpitations, and syncope.

What are the initial steps in the management of this patient with suspected ACS?

Within the first 10 minutes of presentation, carry out the following initial steps (mnemonic: *ABC, EKG, MONA, LABS*):

1. **ABC**: The first step is to assess and correct any **A**irway, **B**reathing or **C**irculation instability (see Case 16). Also, place the patient on a cardiac monitor and make sure resuscitation equipment is nearby.
2. **EKG**: A 12-lead EKG is the basis for initial diagnosis and management. If initial EKG is nondiagnostic, repeat EKG every 5 to 10 minutes if the patient is still symptomatic.
3. **M**orphine: Administration of 2- to 4 mg IV morphine reduces cardiac workload by decreasing sympathetic stimulation as a result of pain and anxiety.
4. **O**xygen (O_2): Maintain oxygen saturation (SaO_2) >90% with supplemental O_2.
5. **N**itrates: Administer three doses of 0.4 mg sublingual nitroglycerin every 5 minutes. Nitrates are contraindicated if the patient has taken a 5-PDE inhibitor such as Viagra or Cialis in the last 24 to 36 hours because the combination can cause severe hypotension.
6. **A**spirin: Give all patients 160 to 325 mg aspirin (antiplatelet therapy) unless it is contraindicated. Aspirin is the only MONA therapy that improves mortality.
7. **LABS**: Establish IV access and obtain cardiac enzymes (biomarkers that measure cardiac injury), serum electrolytes, lipids, and coagulation studies (prothrombin time, partial thromboplastin time (PTT), and International Normalized Ratio (INR)).

> Exercise stress testing is contraindicated if ACS is the suspected diagnosis.

> In the acute setting, pain relief with nitroglycerin or a "GI cocktail" (viscous lidocaine and antacids) does not reliably distinguish cardiac from noncardiac chest pain.

12-lead EKG is obtained (see Fig. 2-3). What is the diagnosis?

ST segment elevation ≥1 mm in two or more leads is diagnostic of an acute ST elevation MI (STEMI). This patient with lead II, III, and aVF ST elevation has an inferior STEMI (Tables 2-13, 2-14, and 2-15).

> Obtain EKG of right precordial leads (V4R, V5R, V6R) if the patient has an inferior MI to assess whether the right ventricle is affected.

Right precordial leads are normal. What are the next steps in management?

The patient should undergo prompt revascularization with PCI or thrombolytics. Before revascularization, administer the following medications:

1. **Clopidogrel**: This anti-platelet agent inhibits ADP receptors (see Chapter 10: Hematology and Oncology). Combined therapy with aspirin and clopidogrel improves outcomes compared to aspirin alone. Clopidogrel is also an alternative when aspirin is contraindicated.
2. **GPIIb/IIIa inhibitors**: Add a GPIIb/IIIa inhibitor (abciximab or eptifibatide) to the antiplatelet regimen prior to PCI but not prior to thrombolytics.

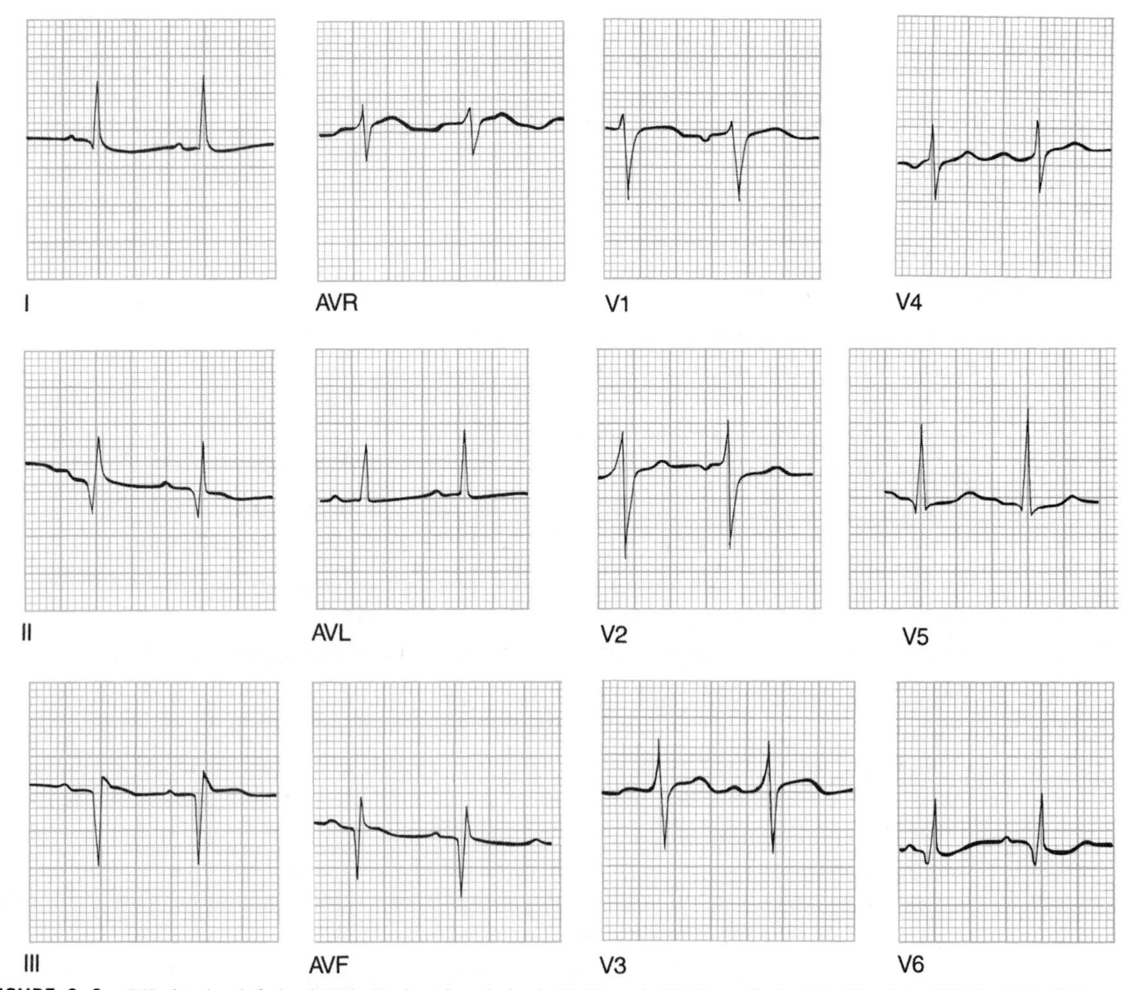

FIGURE 2–3 EKG showing inferior STEMI: ST elevations in leads II, III and aVF. From Thaler MS. *The Only EKG Book You'll Ever Need*, 5th ed. Lippincott Williams & Wilkins, 2007.

TABLE 2–13 Basic EKG Interpretation

Basics		Each little box is 0.04 seconds Each big box is 0.2 seconds (5 little boxes) P wave: represents atrial depolarization; normally upright except in aVR (inverted) and lead V1 (biphasic with upright initial deflection and inverted terminal deflection) QRS: represents ventricular depolarization Q wave: if first deflection of QRS is down, it is called a Q wave R wave: first upward deflection in the QRS complex S wave: any downward deflection that follows the R wave R′: second upward deflection after an S wave QRS nomenclature: small deflections are denoted in lowercase, large deflections in uppercase T wave: represents ventricular repolarization
Rate		Rate: 300/(number of large boxes between each R wave) Normal rate: 60 to 100 beats per minute Tachycardia: >100 beats per minute; bradycardia <60 beats per minute
Rhythm		Sinus rhythm: Similarly shaped p wave precedes every QRS; R-R interval is the same. Irregular rhythm: QRS not preceded by p wave or irregular R-R interval.
Axis		Normal axis: upright QRS complexes in leads I and aVF Left axis deviation: upright QRS in lead I, inverted QRS in aVF Right axis deviation: inverted QRS in lead I, upright QRS in lead Extreme right axis deviation: inverted QRS in leads I and aVF
Intervals	PR	Definition: time from beginning of P to beginning of QRS Normal PR interval: ≤1 big box PR interval >1 big box: suspect AV block PR interval <3 little boxes: suspect Wolf-Parkinson-White syndrome or Lown-Ganong-Levine syndrome
	QRS	Definition: time from beginning of QRS to end of QRS Normal QRS interval: <3 little boxes Abnormal (wide) QRS: suspect bundle branch block (p before QRS) or impulse originating in ventricle (no p before QRS)
	QT	Definition: time from start of QRS to the end of the T wave Normal QT interval: less than half the distance between 2 R's
Hypertrophy evaluation	LA	Lead V1: terminal downward deflection width or depth >1 mm
	RA	Lead II: initial half of p wave >2.5 little boxes (and larger than terminal part)
	LV	Left axis deviation V1 or V2: S wave: ≥6 big boxes in V1 or V2 V5 or V6: R wave: >5 big boxes in V5 or V6 or S wave (in V1) + R wave (in V5 or V6) >7 big boxes
	RV	Right axis deviation V1: R wave ≥7 little boxes V1 to V6: R wave size progressively decreases
Evaluation for bundle branch block (BBB)	Right BBB	Wide QRS preceded by p wave V1: rSR′; R′ > S (see Fig. 2-24) V6: large wide S wave in lead V6
	Left BBB	Wide QRS preceded by p wave V1: normal small R wave is absent V5 and V6: RR′ (see Fig. 2-25)
Infarct evaluation		Larger than normal Q waves: > one fourth the size of R wave or >1 little box. ST elevation > 1 mm above baseline[a] (see Tab. 2-15) T wave inversion: T wave deflection in opposite direction as R wave
Ischemia evaluation		ST depression >1 mm T wave inversion
Other important patterns		Pulmonary embolism: S1Q3T3 (see Chapter 3: Pulmonary) Hypokalemia: U wave (small upward deflection after T wave) Hyperkalemia: peaked T waves, wide QRS, flattened p wave Pericarditis: diffuse ST elevation and down-sloping PR interval

[a] ST segment elevation is an unreliable finding in patients with left bundle branch block.

TABLE 2-14 EKG Changes During an STEMI

Within Minutes	ST Elevation
Hours	ST elevation + Q wave
Day 1–2	ST elevation + Q wave + T wave inversion
Days later	ST normalizes, T wave inversion and Q wave persist
Weeks later	ST segment and T wave normal but Q wave persists

Abbreviation: STEMI, ST elevation MI.

TABLE 2-15 Location of Infarct Based on Abnormal EKG Leads

Abnormal EKG leads	Location	Coronary Artery
ST depression and large R wave in V1 and V2	Posterior	Right coronary
Inferior leads (II, III, aVF)	Inferior	Right or left coronary
Leads I and aVL and leads V4–V6	Lateral	Circumflex
V1–V3	Anteroseptal	Left anterior descending
One or more precordial leads (V1–V6)	Anterior	Distal left anterior descending
V4R, V5R, V6R	Right ventricle	Right coronary

A patient is presumed to have a STEMI if he/she has a new left bundle branch block in the presence of symptoms.

3. **β-Blockers**: Administer a β-1–selective agent to all hemodynamically stable STEMI patients (reduce myocardial O_2 consumption and have antiarrhythmic effects).
4. **IV nitroglycerin**: Administer if the patient continues to have pain despite sublingual nitroglycerin. Unlike β-blockers, nitrates do not improve mortality, so stop nitrates if the resulting drop in blood pressure prevents β-blocker administration.
5. **Potassium (K^+) and magnesium (Mg^{+2})**: Maintain serum K^+ >4 mEq/L because hypokalemic patients have an increased risk of ventricular fibrillation. Maintain Mg^{+2} >2 mEq/L because serum potassium will not rise with concurrent hypomagnesemia.
6. **Heparin**: Although there is limited data to support its efficacy, heparin is generally administered prior to revascularization to prevent thrombus progression.

The patient is at a small hospital, with no experienced interventional cardiologist on-site to perform PCI. The hospital is 4 hours away from a center where PCI is available. What revascularization method should this patient undergo?

PCI is preferred to thrombolytics if the patient presents within 12 hours of symptom onset and the hospital can ensure a "door to balloon time" <90 minutes (time lapse between entering the hospital and inflation of the PTCA balloon). Although this patient presents <12 hours after symptom onset, transporting him to a center where PCI is available would entail a "door to balloon time" >90 minutes. He should receive thrombolytics instead.

Thrombolytics in STEMI: Effective up to 12 hours after symptom onset (most effective in first 4 hours). Goal is "door to needle time" <30 minutes.

CABG in STEMI: This is an infrequent revascularization strategy in STEMI. Indications are failure of PCI or thrombolytics, STEMI associated with cardiogenic shock, and life-threatening ventricular arrhythmias in patients with left main or three-vessel disease detected on angiography.

Which thrombolytic should this patient receive?

Tenecteplase, lanotleplase, and alteplase have equivalent efficacy. Tenecteplase is usually preferred because it the easiest to use (single bolus) and has a lower rate of bleeding complications.

> **Heparin and thrombolytics**: Heparin is usually continued for 24 to 48 hours. Monitor using PTT (maintain between 1.5 and 2 times upper limit of normal).

> **Heparin and PCI**: Large doses are given during the procedure, and monitored using activated clotting time (maintain between 250 and 350 seconds). Heparin is usually not continued after an uncomplicated procedure.

While tenecteplase is being administered, the initial troponin and creatine kinase (muscle/brain type) (CK-MB) values return as normal. How should you interpret these values?

Virtually all patients with MI have at least one elevated cardiac biomarker (troponin I and T, CK-MB, myoglobin, and lactate dehydrogenase). Serum troponins are the preferred marker because they are more specific for cardiac muscle damage than the other enzymes. However, their sensitivity in the first 4 to 6 hours is low. In fact, troponin elevation may take up to 12 hours. Because initial measurements are often negative, obtain a second set of cardiac biomarkers 4 to 6 hours later, and a third set of cardiac biomarkers 4 to 6 hours after the second. Do not delay revascularization because of delayed or normal initial cardiac biomarkers in this patient with symptoms of ACS and an STEMI documented on EKG.

Subsequent troponin and CK-MB levels are elevated. The patient is admitted to the coronary care unit. His symptoms resolve. He does not have any further complications over the next 5 days and is ready for discharge. What tests are recommended prior to discharge for risk stratification?

1. **Echocardiography**: Cardiac ischemia can lead to systolic or diastolic heart failure, which is associated with a worse prognosis. Perform echocardiography to evaluate contractility and stiffness of the heart.
2. **Stress test**: Exercise stress testing detects residual ischemia and helps assess exercise capacity for subsequent cardiac rehabilitation. Most patients undergo submaximal exercise stress right before discharge from the hospital and a maximal exercise stress test after 3 to 6 weeks.

What medications should this patient take after STEMI?

There are several discharge medications suitable after STEMI (mnemonic: "***ABC N' ACE, STAT!***"):

1. **ABC**: **A**spirin, **β**-1 Blockers, and **C**lopidogrel reduce mortality after STEMI.
2. **N**itrates are used for symptom relief but do not reduce mortality.
3. **ACE** inhibitors reduce mortality after STEMI. The mechanism is decreased LV remodeling, which lowers risk of subsequent CHF and recurrent MI. Initiate ACE inhibitors within 24 hours as long as they are not contraindicated. If the patient cannot tolerate an ACE inhibitor, substitute with an ARB (specifically valsartan or candesartan).
4. **STAT**ins.

> Aggressive control of CV risk factors reduces mortality after MI (smoking cessation, blood pressure <130/80, LDL <70, and tight glycemic control).

What additional therapy would you recommend if the patient had evidence of systolic heart failure with an ejection fraction of 30% on echocardiography?

1. **K^+-Sparing diuretics** improve survival after an MI in patients with DM or heart failure. The first-line K^+-sparing diuretic is spironolactone (because it is less expensive). If the patient

suffers endocrine side effects, switch to eplerenone. Regularly monitor serum K^+ in patients taking spironolactone or eplerenone.

2. **Implantable cardioverter-defibrillator** (**ICD**) improves survival after in MI in all patients with LV ejection fraction <30% and in patients with LV ejection fraction <35% with New York Heart Association (NYHA) class II or II heart failure.

Alternative 2.7.1

The patient is a 65-year-old man with 2 hours of crushing, substernal discomfort radiating to the left arm that was not relieved with nitroglycerin at home. He has a history of stable angina. Blood work is obtained after IV access is established. He is placed on a monitor and a 12-lead EKG is obtained. The EKG shows 1 mm of ST segment depression and T wave inversion in leads V1, V2, and V3. He receives aspirin, sublingual nitroglycerin, and morphine.

What is the most likely cause of his symptoms?

Both UA and non-ST elevation MI (NSTEMI) cause symptoms of ACS without the characteristic ST elevation and Q waves seen in STEMI. ST depression and T wave inversion may or may not be observed in either (if present, they tend to be transient in UA and persistent in NSTEMI). The primary difference between UA and NSTEMI is that myocardial injury is sufficient to cause a detectable elevation in cardiac enzymes in NSTEMI but not in UA. Because an elevated troponin or CK-MB level may not be detected for up to 12 hours after presentation, the initial management of UA and NSTEMI is the same.

> Technically, any worsening of stable angina symptoms is referred to as UA.

What is the next step in management?

1. Administer the same medications given prior to revascularization in STEMI. Low molecular weight heparin is preferred to unfractionated heparin.
2. Risk-stratify this patient on the basis of TIMI risk score as low, intermediate, or high risk. This patient has an intermediate TIMI risk score (Table 2-16).

How would you manage the patient based on his TIMI score?

Intermediate- to high-risk patients should undergo coronary angiography within 48 hours. Perform PCI or CABG on the basis of coronary angiography findings (indications for CABG over PCI are the same as those in patients with stable angina). Before the patient is discharged, perform echocardiogram, submaximal stress test, and medications (ABC N' ACE, STAT).

> With low-risk TIMI, angiography not necessary; obtain stress test before discharge.

TABLE 2–16 TIMI Risk Score for NSTEMI and UA

Risk Factor	Points
Age ≥ 65 years	1
≥3 risk factors for CHD	1
Prior coronary stenosis ≥50%	1
ST segment depression	1
At least 2 angina episodes in last 24 hours	1
Elevated serum cardiac biomarkers	1
Use of aspirin in last 7 days	1

Abbreviation: NSTEMI, non-ST elevation MI; UA, unstable angina.
Note: Low risk score = 0–2, Intermediate risk = 3–4, High risk = 5–7.

Do not administer thrombolytics for UA or NSTEMI. This is because the thrombi are nonocclusive and platelet-rich. Such thrombi do not respond to thrombolytics like the fibrin-rich thrombi in STEMI.

Alternative 2.7.2

The patient is a 65-year-old man with 2 hours of crushing, substernal discomfort radiating to the left arm that was not relieved with nitroglycerin at home. He has 12 cm of JVD and a holosystolic murmur at the left sternal border that increases with inspiration. Lungs are clear to bilateral auscultation. Blood pressure is 98/60, heart rate is 50 beats per minute. Blood work is obtained after IV access is established. He is placed on a monitor and a 12-lead EKG is obtained, which shows 2 mm of ST elevation in leads II, III, and aVF. ST elevation (2 mm) is also seen in the right precordial leads (V4R, V5R, and V6R).

Where is the infarct located?

This patient has a right-ventricle infarct that is most commonly caused by occlusion of the right coronary artery. A right ventricle infarct usually occurs in association with an inferior infarct. A hemodynamically significant right-ventricle infarct can present with signs of right heart failure (JVD, hypotension, and tricuspid regurgitation). The infarct can affect the AV node and cause bradycardia.

How does management of a right-ventricle MI differ from that of a left-ventricle MI?

Cardiac output is highly dependent on preload in right-ventricle STEMI. In general, avoid nitrates, β-blockers, and CCBs because they decrease preload, which could decrease cardiac output and cause severe hypotension. If symptoms of angina are intolerable, an option is to administer normal saline to expand intravascular volume and then use nitrates judiciously.

Alternative 2.7.4

The patient is a 25-year-old man who presents with signs and symptoms of ACS. His medical history is significant for an upper respiratory infection 2 weeks ago. The patient denies cocaine use, and urine drug screen is negative. EKG shows ST elevation in leads V1-V5. However, coronary angiography is normal.

What diagnosis should you suspect?

Suspect viral myocarditis in patients who present with unexplained signs and symptoms of MI, heart failure, or cardiac arrhythmias. The classic patient is a young man with a recent viral infection. Many viruses can cause myocarditis, but the most common one is coxsackie B. Viral myocarditis can sometimes cause elevated troponins and EKG findings of STEMI, but coronary angiography is normal. Diagnosis is primarily clinical.

How is myocarditis managed?

Obtain a CXR and echocardiogram to evaluate for heart failure, and treat heart failure if present. Otherwise, treatment is supportive. The patient should avoid exercise. If his symptoms persist, consider endomyocardial biopsy to confirm the diagnosis, although even biopsy is not very accurate.

CASE 2–8 COMPLICATIONS AFTER STEMI

A patient is given a diagnosis of right-ventricle STEMI. He undergoes PCI and is admitted to the coronary care unit. His symptoms resolve. Ten hours later he has an episode of ventricular tachycardia (VT) that lasts for 10 seconds.

What is the next step in management?

Arrhythmias are a common complication during and after the acute phase of STEMI. Treat arrhythmias according to Advanced Cardiac Life Support protocols. This patient had an episode of nonsustained VT. Treat VT only if it is sustained (i.e., lasts >30 seconds). Limit arrhythmia prophylaxis to β-blockers and correction of electrolyte imbalances.

Seventeen hours after diagnosis, the patient has a recurrence of angina symptoms. Troponin levels are elevated. What is the next step in management?

Repeat the 12-lead EKG to look for changes suggestive of re-infarction in this patient with recurrent ischemia. Increase the nitrate and β-blocker dose to reduce myocardial oxygen demand. Initiate heparin and perform coronary angiography followed by CABG or PCI ("rescue PCI") depending on the lesion, even if transfer to another center where PCI is available takes longer than 2 hours.

Elevated troponins within the first 18 hours after STEMI are not diagnostic of reinfarction.

The patient undergoes rescue PCI and is admitted to the coronary care unit. Three days later, his blood pressure drops to 80/60. On examination, there is 13 cm of JVD. A harsh, loud holosystolic murmur is heard at the right and left sternal borders. A palpable thrill is present and the precordium is hyperdynamic. Extremities are cool and clammy. What is the most likely cause of these symptoms?

Suspect a life-threatening mechanical complication when a patient develops hemodynamic compromise and a new, loud murmur in the first 2 to 12 days after STEMI. The major mechanical complications are ventricular free-wall rupture, interventricular septum rupture, and rupture of the papillary muscles (Table 2-17). This patient's murmur is consistent with interventricular septal rupture. The right coronary artery supplies the inferior one third and the left anterior descending artery supplies the superior two thirds of the septum, so STEMIs that occlude these arteries pose a higher risk for this complication.

Alternative 2.8.1

A patient with chest discomfort at rest has ST elevation in V1-V5, and an anterior STEMI is diagnosed. He undergoes PCI and is admitted to the coronary care unit. Twenty-four hours later he complains of sharp chest pain that increases on inspiration, improves on leaning forward, and radiates to the left shoulder. Physical examination is significant for a three-component friction rub heard over the left sternal border. Vital signs are within normal limits.

TABLE 2–17 Mechanical Complications After MI

Complication	Distinguishing Symptoms	Management
Rupture of left ventricle free wall	Hemopericardium and cardiac tamponade	Diagnose with echocardiogram-directed pericardiocentesis; if blood is detected on pericardiocentesis, then emergent surgery is necessary.
Rupture of interventricular septum	Harsh, loud, holosystolic murmur, hyperdynamic precordium and palpable thrill	Diagnose with Doppler echocardiogram or pulmonary artery catheter to document left to right shunt; unstable patients require prompt surgical repair, whereas stable patients can undergo elective surgical repair at a later time.
Papillary muscle rupture	Apical or parasternal systolic murmur and pulmonary edema; hyperdynamic precordium but no thrill	Diagnose with Doppler echocardiogram followed by cardiac catheterization; after diagnosis, reduce afterload with nitrates, diuretics, and intra-aortic balloon counterpulsation. If the patient is still unstable, perform emergent surgery; if the patient stabilizes, surgery can be delayed.

Note: All mechanical complications can present with hypotension and cardiogenic shock. Initial steps always include stabilizing the patient (airway, breathing, and circulation).

What is the cause of these signs and symptoms?

Infarction pericarditis presents with pleuritic chest pain that radiates to the trapezius ridges and improves on leaning forward. Three-component friction rub is a very specific sign. This complication is more common with anterior STEMI and usually develops in the first 1 to 2 days. STEMI changes usually overshadow EKG findings of pericarditis.

How is infarction pericarditis managed?

Aspirin or indomethacin is sufficient to treat this complication. Perform echocardiography in all patients who develop pericarditis after STEMI to evaluate for a pericardial effusion. Discontinue anticoagulation if echocardiography detects an effusion >1 cm to minimize the risk of cardiac tamponade.

No effusion is detected on echocardiography. The symptoms and friction rub resolve. Two months after discharge from the hospital, he returns to the clinic with fever, malaise, and symptoms of pericarditis. A three-component friction rub is again heard on physical examination. Temperature is 39°C. What is cause of these findings?

This patient has developed postinfarct injury syndrome (Dressler's syndrome). Unlike infarction pericarditis, the symptoms of fever, malaise, and pericarditis do not appear for weeks to months after STEMI (Table 2-18). Cardiac muscle injury releases antigens that stimulate the formation of immune complexes. These immune complexes deposit on the pericardium and induce inflammation, which leads to Dressler's syndrome. Diagnosis is clinical, although elevated erythrocyte sedimentation rate (ESR) is a common finding. Treat with nonsteroidal anti-inflammatory drugs (NSAIDs). Use corticosteroids if symptoms are refractory.

> **Complications of MI**: The "**MAD PALS**" of an infarct are **M**echanical complications, **A**rrhythmia, **D**ressler's syndrome, **P**ericarditis, **A**neurysm of LV (predisposes to embolus from a mural thrombus), **L**V failure and pulmonary edema, and **S**hock (cardiogenic).

Alternative 2.8.2

A 65-year-old man undergoes PCI for an anterior MI. A drug-eluting stent is placed in the left anterior descending artery. One week after discharge, he stops taking aspirin and clopidogrel. Two weeks after discharge, he has another anterior STEMI. Angiography demonstrates no flow through the stented lesion.

What is the most likely cause of the second STEMI?

Stent thrombosis is a feared complication of PCI that presents with sudden occurrence of MI as a result of complete stent occlusion. Stent thrombosis can be acute (within 24 hours), subacute (within 30 days), or late (more than 30 days). This complication occurs as a result of the formation of a blood clot over the region where the stent damages the intimal wall. Antiplatelet therapy (lifelong aspirin and clopidogrel for at least a year) markedly reduces the incidence of stent thrombosis. Premature cessation of antiplatelet therapy greatly increases the risk of stent thrombosis. Treatment is emergent PCI.

TABLE 2-18 Characteristic EKG Findings in STEMI Versus Acute Pericarditis

	STEMI	Pericarditis
ST segment	Elevated and upwardly convex in regional leads	Elevated and upwardly concave ("saddle shaped") in all leads
PR segment	Not depressed	Depressed
Q waves	Q waves	No Q waves
T waves	Inverted	Not inverted

Types of drug-eluting stents: sirolimus-eluting stents (Cypher) and paclitaxel-eluting stents (Taxus)

What diagnosis is more likely if the patient received a bare metal stent (BMS) and presents with a 3-week history of increasing angina 6 months later?

Gradually worsening angina after BMS placement should raise concern for in-stent restenosis. Unlike stent thrombosis, this complication is caused by smooth muscle proliferation in the region of the stent, which leads to gradually worsening angina. Consider repeat PCI if the patient's symptoms are refractory to medical therapy.

In-stent restenosis risk: BMS > drug-eluting stents
Stent thrombosis risk: drug-eluting stent > BMS
Stent thrombosis risk with antiplatelet therapy: drug-eluting stent = BMS = low

CASE 2–9 PLEURITIC CHEST PAIN AND FRICTION RUB IN AN OTHERWISE HEALTHY PATIENT

A 24-year-old man presents with a 2-day history of fever, malaise, and pleuritic chest pain radiating to the left shoulder and left trapezius muscles. The chest pain improves on leaning forward. He denies any weight loss, anorexia, cough, or hemoptysis. He does not have any prior medical history and does not take any medications. He has never had sexual intercourse. Auscultation of the heart demonstrates a three-component friction rub. Temperature is 38°C. Other vital signs are normal. Figure 2-4 is the patient's EKG.

What is the most likely diagnosis?

The patient has acute pericarditis. Typical symptoms are fever, malaise, and pleuritic chest pain that may radiate to the shoulder and trapezius and improves on leaning forward. The classic physical finding is a three-component friction rub. This patient's EKG demonstrates the characteristic down-sloping PR segment and diffuse ST segment elevation (as opposed to

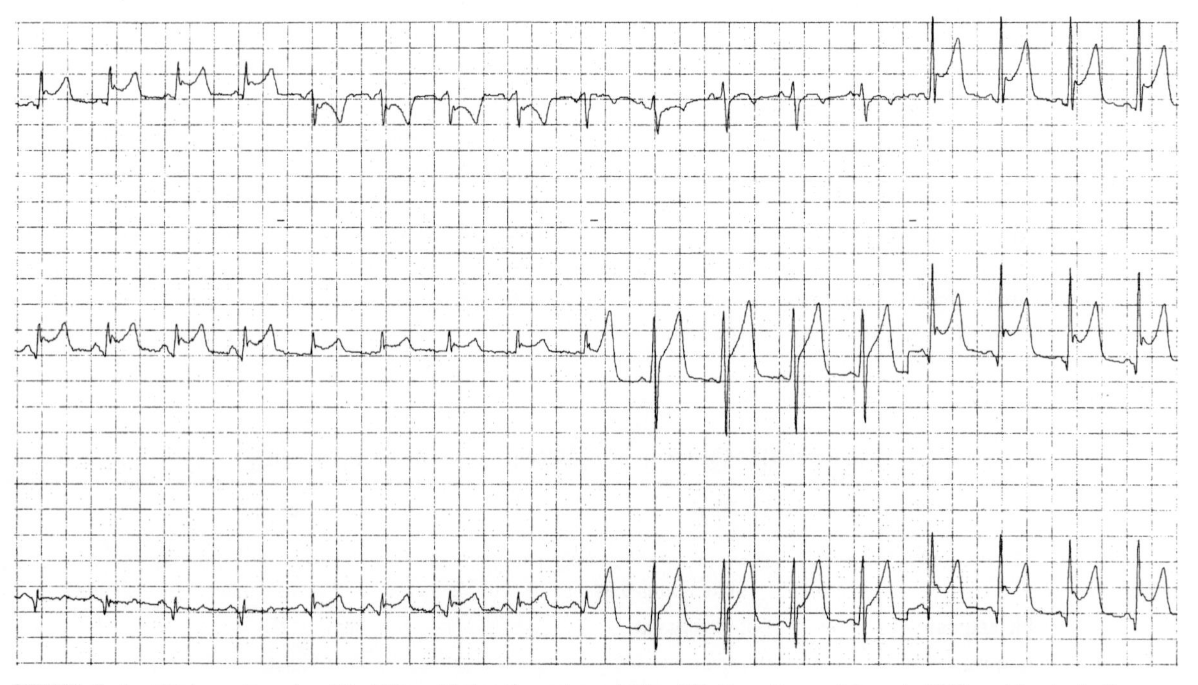

FIGURE 2–4 EKG in acute pericarditis (diffuse ST elevations, down-sloping PR). From Harwood-Nuss A, Wolfson AB, et al. *The Clinical Practice of Emergency Medicine*, 3rd ed. Lippincott Williams & Wilkins, 2001.

MI, where ST elevations occur in specific leads). The patient has the classic signs, symptoms, and EKG findings of acute pericarditis.

What causes acute pericarditis?

1. Infections: In otherwise healthy patients, viral infection is the most common cause of pericarditis; tuberculosis, HIV, bacteria, and fungi are other, less common infectious causes.
2. Uremia (see Chapter 6: Nephrology)
3. Autoimmune disorders (e.g., rheumatoid arthritis)
4. Malignancy
5. MI
6. Other medical causes (iatrogenesis): drugs, cardiac surgery or procedures, and radiation

> Acute pericarditis can cause mild elevation in CK-MB and troponin-I. This transient elevation does not indicate a worse prognosis.

> **Acute pericarditis caused by uremia**: Diffuse ST elevation is often absent.
> **Acute pericarditis caused by rheumatoid arthritis**: Chest pain is often absent.

What is the next step in management?

Perform echocardiography in all patients with acute pericarditis to evaluate for a pericardial effusion ("wet" pericarditis). If the patient has a small pericardial effusion, repeat echocardiography 1 to 2 weeks later to assess whether more fluid has accumulated. If the pericardial effusion is large, perform diagnostic pericardiocentesis even if the patient is hemodynamically stable.

Echocardiography does not show any pericardial effusion. What treatment is indicated?

An exhaustive search for the cause of acute pericarditis is unnecessary in patients with dry pericarditis and no obvious clues to suggest a nonviral cause. Outpatient treatment with an NSAID to relieve symptoms and colchicine to prevent recurrence is sufficient. Symptoms should resolve within 1 week of onset.

> Symptoms recur in 15% to 30% of acute pericarditis patients who do not receive colchicine.

The patient returns 2 weeks later with continued symptoms. What is the next step in management?

If symptoms do not resolve after 1 week, admit the patient to the hospital and conduct a more thorough investigation for underlying causes of pericarditis. If no underlying cause is found, consider a short course of high-dose systemic corticosteroids.

No underlying cause is found. His symptoms resolve over the next few days after a short course of steroids. He presents 1 year later with a 3-month history of fatigue and dyspnea on exertion. There is 2+ peripheral edema and ascites. The liver edge is felt 6 cm below the costal margin. Neck veins are distended even during inspiration (Kussmaul sign). Auscultation of the heart reveals a loud S3 (pericardial knock). What is the most likely cause of his symptoms?

The initial insult in acute pericarditis may trigger fibrous scarring of the pericardium. The scar tissue leads to a rigid pericardium with impaired filling during late diastole. This condition is called constrictive pericarditis. Patients present with signs of right heart failure as a result of impaired filling. Jugular venous distension (JVD) is the most common initial finding. Advanced disease leads to peripheral edema and ascites. Other common findings are Kussmaul sign and pericardial knock (basically a loud S3).

Restrictive cardiomyopathy: Findings similar to constrictive pericarditis, except patients have S3 gallop instead of loud S3 (softer; occurs later in diastole).
Cirrhosis: Presents with ascites and peripheral edema but no JVD.

EKG in constrictive pericarditis: Nonspecific; ~25% have decreased voltage and atrial fibrillation.

What is the next step in management?

Perform Doppler echocardiography to distinguish constrictive pericarditis from restrictive cardiomyopathy and cirrhosis. If this test is inconclusive, consider cardiac CT or MR imaging.

Cardiac catheterization: Occasionally required to establish the diagnosis. Findings are elevated and equal diastolic pressures in all chambers, and the "square root sign" (rapid y descent on ventricular pressure tracing).

Echocardiography and gated cardiac MR imaging confirm the diagnosis of constrictive pericarditis. What treatment is recommended?

This patient with severe symptoms of advanced disease should undergo surgical pericardiectomy (removal of the pericardial sac). Close observation is sufficient for patients with mild symptoms like isolated ascites.

Alternative 2.9.1

The patient with signs, symptoms, and EKG findings indicating acute pericarditis is found to have a 1-cm pericardial effusion. Repeat echocardiogram is scheduled 7 days from this time, but 3 days later he presents to the emergency department with sudden onset of dyspnea at rest and pleuritic chest pain radiating to the left shoulder that improves somewhat on leaning forward. Physical examination is significant for 12 cm of JVD, distended forehead and scalp veins, weakened carotid pulse during inspiration, muffled heart sounds, and a friction rub. Vitals signs are temperature 37°C, pulse 120 bpm, respirations 27/minute. Blood pressure is 100/80 on expiration but decreases to 80/60 on inspiration (pulsus paradoxus). EKG now shows low voltage and sinus tachycardia.

What is the cause of his clinical deterioration?

Excessive accumulation of pericardial fluid can impair ventricular filling and lead to hypotension (caused by decreased cardiac output). This condition is termed cardiac tamponade and is the most likely diagnosis in this patient. The classic triad (Beck's triad) of tamponade is JVD, muffled heart sounds, and hypotension. Other findings may include:

1. Symptoms: dyspnea and pleuritic chest pain
2. Vital signs: tachycardia and tachypnea
3. Physical signs: distended scalp veins and weakened carotid pulse during inspiration, friction rub, and pulsus paradoxus
4. EKG: low voltage and sinus tachycardia with or without electrical alternans

Electrical alternans: Beat-to-beat variation in the amplitude or axis of the QRS complex caused by swinging of the heart within the pericardial space. It is an insensitive but relatively specific sign for cardiac tamponade.
Pulsus paradoxus: Greater than normal decrease in systolic blood pressure during inspiration (>12 mm Hg decrease). The paradox is that S1 is audible with all beats during inspiration, but the pulse is weak or cannot be felt. A number of cardiac and pulmonary conditions can cause this phenomenon.
Ewart sign: Dullness and bronchial breath sounds near the angle of the scapula is neither sensitive nor specific for tamponade.

> **Cardiac tamponade versus constrictive pericarditis:** Both conditions cause JVD. Pulsus paradoxus is rare in constrictive pericarditis. Kussmaul sign is rare in cardiac tamponade.

What causes cardiac tamponade?

Any cause of pericardial effusion can theoretically progress to tamponade. The most common causes of cardiac tamponade are malignancy and trauma (including iatrogenic tamponade caused by pericardiocentesis, central line placement, etc.). Free-wall rupture is an important cause in the post-MI setting.

What work-up and management is indicated?

Diagnosis is clinical, although echocardiography is usually performed to confirm the diagnosis. Treat this hemodynamically unstable patient with emergent catheter pericardiocentesis to drain fluid from the pericardial sac.

CASE 2–10 CHRONIC, PROGRESSIVE DYSPNEA

A 58-year-old man with a 10-year history of HTN presents with dyspnea and dry cough that has been progressively worsening over the last 6 months. Initially he experienced dyspnea only after a brisk 1-mile walk. He now has dyspnea climbing up the flight of stairs to his bedroom. Lying down worsens symptoms, and he often needs three to four pillows to fall asleep (orthopnea). Auscultation of the heart reveals an S3, S4, and a 1/6 blowing holosystolic murmur heard best at the apex that radiates to the axilla. Point of maximal impulse is displaced to the left. There are scattered rales and wheezes on lung exam. There is 9 cm of JVD. The liver edge is tender and 4 cm below the costal margin (tender hepatomegaly). He has marked peripheral edema. Blood pressure is 170/100, and pulse is 80 bpm and regular.

What are the most common causes of chronic dyspnea?

Two thirds of chronic dyspnea (duration >1 month) is caused by pulmonary or cardiac causes. Remember the five most common causes using the mnemonic "***Chronic Cigarette Addicts Can't Inhale***" (**C**hronic obstructive pulmonary disease (COPD), **C**HF, **A**sthma, **C**HD, and **I**nterstitial lung disease). Other important pulmonary causes are lung cancer, pleural effusion, and bronchiectasis. Other important cardiac causes are arrhythmias and deconditioning. Anemia is a common noncardiopulmonary cause.

What is the most likely cause of progressive dyspnea in this patient?

The most likely diagnosis is CHF. Although no single physical finding establishes the diagnosis, suggestive findings include:

1. Symptoms: dyspnea and orthopnea
2. Fluid overload: elevated JVD, peripheral edema, and ascites
3. Heart exam: S3, S4, displaced point of maximal impulse, or murmur suggesting valve disease (Table 2-19).
4. Lung exam: normal or rales and wheezes

> Distension of the internal jugular vein is a marker for central venous pressure (CVP) (normally <6 cm). The four causes of JVD >6 cm are cardiac tamponade, constrictive pericarditis, CHF (biventricular or isolated right heart failure), and superior vena cava syndrome.

What causes CHF?

CHF is the final and most severe manifestation of almost every type of heart disease. In descending order, the most common causes of CHF are CAD, HTN, and valvular heart disease (Table 2-20).

TABLE 2–19 Murmurs Caused by Valvular Heart Disease and Other Select Conditions

EARLY DIASTOLIC MURMURS	
Aortic regurgitation	Decrescendo murmur heard best at left lower sternal border
Pulmonic regurgitation	Decrescendo murmur heard best at upper sternal border that increases with inspiration
MID-LATE DIASTOLIC MURMURS	
Mitral stenosis	Opening snap followed by rumble heard best at apex when patient is in left lateral decubitus position; loud S1
Tricuspid stenosis	Opening snap followed by rumble heard best at left sternal border that increases with inspiration; canon "a wave" may be present if severe.
Atrial myxoma (benign tumor)	Murmur similar to mitral stenosis but changes with body position
HOLOSYSTOLIC MURMURS (SOUND THE SAME THROUGHOUT SYSTOLE)	
Mitral regurgitation	Blowing murmur heard best at apex and radiates to the axilla
Tricuspid regurgitation	Blowing murmur heard best at left lower sternal border that increases with inspiration and decreases with expiration or valsalva
OTHER SYSTOLIC MURMURS	
Mitral valve prolapse	Mid systolic click followed by rumble that increases with standing, sustained handgrip, and valsalva. The click and murmur decrease with squatting
Aortic stenosis	Harsh crescendo-decrescendo murmur at right upper sternal border that radiates to carotids; carotid upstroke is diminished and delayed (parvus et tardus)
Pulmonic stenosis	Harsh crescendo-decrescendo murmur
MURMURS CAUSED BY SELECT PEDIATRIC CONDITIONS	
Atrial septal defect	Mid-systolic murmur with fixed and widely split S2
Ventricular septal defect	Loud holosystolic murmur heard best at left lower sternal border and often accompanied by a thrill
Hypertrophic cardiomyopathy	Harsh crescendo-decrescendo systolic murmur that increases with standing and valsalva, and decreases with squatting and sustained handgrip
Patent ductus arteriosus	Machine-like murmur heard in systole and diastole
Rumbling sound = low-pitched	
Blowing sound = high-pitched	

Note: Other classic signs of aortic regurgitation are widened pulse pressure (markedly increased systolic BP and decreased diastolic BP), water-hammer pulse (rapidly increasing pulse that collapses suddenly in late diastole and systole), Austin-Flint murmur (late diastolic rumble due to relative mitral stenosis), Duroziez sign (pistol-shot sound over femoral arteries), and DeMusset sign (rhythmic head jerking).

Systolic heart failure: Decreased ejection fraction as a result of increased afterload (e.g., HTN) or decreased contractility (e.g., myocardial damage caused by MI, myocarditis, etc.).

Diastolic heart failure: Decreased ventricular filling (i.e., decreased preload) as a result of impaired relaxation.

Clinical distinction between systolic and diastolic CHF: It is very difficult to distinguish between systolic and diastolic CHF on the basis of signs and symptoms alone.

Systolic or diastolic CHF can affect the left heart, right heart (cor pulmonale), or both. Left heart failure is the most prevalent cause of right heart failure. Chronic obstructive pulmonary disease (COPD) is the most prevalent cause of cor pulmonale.

TABLE 2–20 Causes of Heart Failure

DCM: left ventricular dilatation and systolic heart failure.

Secondary DCM ("HIV"):
HTN: Prognosis is better than other patients with DCM, as long as hypertension is controlled.
Ischemia: Coronary artery disease is the most common cause of heart failure. DCM is also a common complication after MI. Prognosis is worse with ischemic DCM than nonischemic causes of DCM.
Valvular heart disease
Note: The above conditions can cause isolated diastolic heart failure or both systolic and diastolic heart failure.

Primary DCM (I4P): Accounts for 90% of primary cardiomyopathies.
Idiopathic
Infections: viral myocarditis, HIV, *Trypanosoma cruzi* (Chagas disease), Lyme disease (transient dilated cardiomyopathy).
Ingestions: Alcohol, cocaine, HIV drugs, chemotherapy drugs (**ADD** = **a**nthracyclin, **d**oxorubicin, **d**aunorubicin).
Inherited: muscular dystrophies, thalassemias
Postpartum cardiomyopathy: Occurs in the last trimester or first 6 months after pregnancy; most patients recover but, because of the risk of recurrence, advise against future pregnancies.

Hypertrophic cardiomyopathy (diastolic heart failure, sometimes also systolic heart failure)

Restrictive cardiomyopathies (diastolic heart failure). Many cases are idiopathic or familial. Other causes are **CRASSH** = **C**ancer (carcinoid, multiple myeloma), **R**adiation, **A**myloidosis, **S**arcoidosis and **S**cleroderma, **H**emochromatosis.

What tests should you order initially in a patient with suspected CHF?

The goal of initial testing is to distinguish heart failure from pulmonary etiologies and to detect the underlying cause of heart failure. Order the following tests initially:

1. **CXR**: Findings in CHF include cardiomegaly, cephalization of the pulmonary vessels, Kerley B-lines, and pleural effusions (see Fig. 2-5).
2. **EKG**: The EKG can detect underlying causes of CHF, such as arrhythmias that are causing or exacerbating CHF. A normal EKG is unusual in patients with symptomatic heart failure.
3. **Echocardiogram**: Echocardiography is the most helpful test in the evaluation of heart failure suggested by history, physical, and chest radiography. Ejection fraction <40% indicates systolic heart failure. Ejection fraction >40% in a symptomatic patient suggests diastolic heart failure (as a result of impaired relaxation). Many clinicians confirm the diagnosis of diastolic heart failure by documenting decreased end-diastolic volume on Doppler echocardiography.

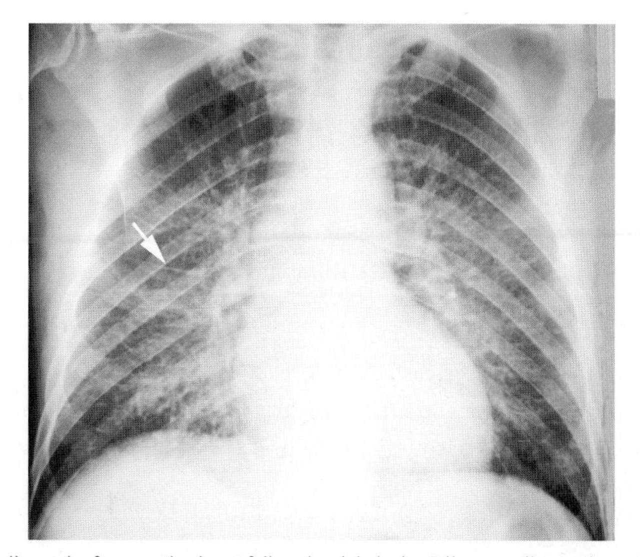

FIGURE 2–5 Chest radiograph of congestive heart failure (explain kerley B lines, cardiomegaly, and cephalization of the pulmonary vessels. From Webb WR, Higgins CB. *Thoracic Imaging*. Lippincott Williams & Wilkins, 2005.

4. **Plasma BNP (bone natriuretic peptide) or n-terminal BNP**: Plasma BNP is usually >100 pg/ml in CHF. BNP <100 pg/ml suggests a pulmonary etiology is more likely. Note that BNP does not help distinguish systolic from diastolic heart failure.
5. **Complete blood count, serum electrolytes, and liver function tests**: These tests are not diagnostic of heart failure, but they are used to detect exacerbating conditions such as anemia and to establish a baseline.
6. **Stress tests**: These tests are used to evaluate all patients with heart failure for CAD.

> CHF is a clinical diagnosis, made on the basis of clinical, radiographic, and laboratory findings. There is no single test to diagnose heart failure.

CXR shows cardiomegaly, cephalization, and Kerley B lines. EKG shows biventricular hypertrophy. Echocardiography reveals biventricular hypertrophy, left ventricle dilatation, and an ejection fraction of 30%. What is the pathophysiology behind the signs and symptoms of systolic heart failure?

1. Cardiac output is proportional to stroke volume and heart rate. Stroke volume is inversely proportional to afterload and directly proportional to preload and contractility. Therefore, increased afterload (e.g., HTN) or decreased contractility (e.g., myocardial damage caused by MI, myocarditis, etc.) reduces stroke volume.
2. Compensatory mechanisms to maintain stroke volume are myocardial hypertrophy (to increase contractility) and dilatation (to increase preload). Physical signs of hypertrophy are S4 and displaced point of maximal impulse (caused by the resulting cardiomegaly). The physical sign of dilatation is S3. Progressive dilatation can also lead to mitral regurgitation.
3. As long as stroke volume is adequate, symptoms of CHF are absent. However, as CHF progresses, compensatory mechanisms become inadequate to maintain stroke volume. Systolic emptying ceases at a higher end-systolic volume than normal, which increases end-systolic pressure in the LV. During diastole (when the mitral valve is open), this increased pressure is transmitted to the left atrium and pulmonary vasculature. Pulmonary HTN causes transudation of fluid into the pulmonary interstitium (pulmonary edema), which leads to the loud pulmonic component of S2, dyspnea, orthopnea, paroxysmal nocturnal dyspnea, and a nonproductive cough.
4. Eventually, increased pulmonary pressure is transmitted to the right ventricle, which leads to worsening right heart failure. Signs of right heart failure are right ventricular heave, tricuspid regurgitation, and fluid retention (JVD, tender hepatomegaly, ascites, nocturia, and pitting edema).
5. Decreased cardiac output leads to progressive fatigue and weakness. Also, decreased perfusion of the kidneys (as a result of decreased cardiac output) stimulates the renin-angiotensin-aldosterone system, which leads to sodium and fluid retention.

How would you classify this patient's disease severity?

Disease severity is generally classified using the NYHA system (Table 2-21). This patient's symptoms correspond to NYHA class II CHF.

TABLE 2–21 New York Heart Association Classification of Heart Failure

Class	Severity
I	Symptoms occur only with vigorous activities, like playing sports.
II	Symptoms occur with moderate exertion, like climbing a flight of stairs or carrying heavy packages.
III	Symptoms occur with usual activities of daily living, such as getting dressed or walking across the room.
IV	Symptoms occur at rest.

Stress testing is equivocal. The patient then undergoes coronary angiography, which does not reveal any significant CAD. He denies any recent infections or ingestions. What is the most likely cause of this patient's systolic heart failure?

Echocardiography findings of a dilated, hypertrophic LV with decreased ejection fraction indicate that he has dilated cardiomyopathy (DCM). Ischemic heart disease is the most common cause of heart failure, but he has a negative work-up for CAD. The most likely cause of CHF in this patient is HTN. The prognosis of dilated cardiomyopathy secondary to HTN is better than with other primary and secondary causes of dilated cardiomyopathy.

> Coronary angiography is often performed in the initial evaluation of CHF to rule out ischemic cardiomyopathy (the most prevalent cause of CHF).

How is stable systolic heart failure treated?

1. Initiate loop diuretics (e.g., furosemide) first to control symptoms caused by fluid overload. Loop diuretics improve symptoms more rapidly than other therapies (hours to weeks), although they do not improve long-term survival.
2. During diuretic therapy, initiate an ACE inhibitor, which decreases preload and afterload. Use an ARB if the patient cannot tolerate the ACE inhibitor. ACE inhibitors/ARBs improve symptoms and survival in all groups of patients with systolic heart failure. Patients taking ACE inhibitors should monitor serum K+, BUN, and creatinine regularly.
3. Initiate a β-blocker when the patient is stable on an ACE inhibitor and signs and symptoms of fluid overload have resolved. "Start low and go slow" to minimize the risk of cardiac decompensation that may occur initially with β-blockers. β-blockers also improve symptoms and survival in all groups of patients with systolic heart failure.
4. Consider the use of digoxin if the patient continues to have symptoms despite maximal doses of loop diuretics, ACE inhibitor, and β-blockers. Digoxin improves symptoms and reduces hospitalizations but does not increase survival. Patients taking digoxin should regularly monitor serum levels digoxin to ensure that blood content is in the therapeutic but not the toxic range.
5. If digoxin does not control symptoms, add spironolactone or the combination of hydralazine and a nitrate. Hydralazine and nitrates may improve survival in African Americans with NYHA class III or IV systolic heart failure. Spironolactone may improve survival in select patients with NYHA class III or class IV systolic heart failure.
6. All patients with systolic heart failure should alter their lifestyle: consume <2 g of sodium per day and increase physical activity.

> Medications for stable systolic heart failure are made in **Dr HyNi'S LAB** (**D**igoxin, **Hy**dralazine, **Ni**trates, **S**pironolactone, **L**oop diuretics, **A**CE inhibitors/ARBs, and **β**-blockers).

When is implantation of an ICD recommended in patients with nonischemic CHF?

ICD implantation improves survival in patients with NYHA class II to class IV heart failure and ejection fraction <35%. On the basis of these criteria, this patient qualifies for an ICD.

> **Combined resynchronization therapy (CRT)**: Consider an ICD plus a biventricular pacemaker in patients with NYHA class IV CHF and ejection fraction <35% who also have a wide QRS complex on EKG (>120 ms).

Why are ACE inhibitors started before β-blockers in CHF?

ACE inhibitors provide rapid hemodynamic benefit and do not exacerbate CHF. The hemodynamic benefit of β-blockers is delayed, and cardiac function may initially worsen. For this reason, start β-blockers after the patient is stable on ACE inhibitor therapy.

Dyspnea, peripheral edema, and JVD improve with furosemide. Enalapril (2.5 mg twice a day) is then initiated. The enalapril is titrated over the next few weeks to 20 mg twice a day without any hypotension or laboratory abnormalities. Carvedilol (3.125 mg/day) is started. One week after starting carvedilol, the patient gains 5 lbs. He has 9 cm of JVD and bilateral pedal edema. What is the next step in management?

Symptoms can transiently worsen when the patient initiates or increases the dose of a β-blocker. Rather than discontinuing the β-blocker, increase the dose of the loop diuretic to minimize fluid overload during this short period.

> Unexplained weight gain is an early sign of worsening CHF.

Two weeks later, the patient's blood pressure is 98/70. What is the next step in management?

Excessive diuresis can cause volume contraction, which increases the risk of hypotension and renal failure from ACE inhibitors. Decrease the diuretic dose and/or the ACE inhibitor dose at this time.

Over the next two years, digoxin and then spironolactone are added to the heart failure regimen. He now presents to the emergency department with nausea, vomiting, anorexia, and blurry vision. He recently started taking paroxetine for depression. EKG is significant for ventricular ectopic beats. He is oriented to person but not place and time. There is no JVD or peripheral edema. Lungs are clear. Temperature, blood pressure, and respirations are within normal limits. What is the most likely cause of his symptoms?

GI symptoms, visual disturbances, and disorientation coupled with a rhythm disturbance should raise suspicion for digoxin toxicity. The most likely cause is the recent initiation of a selective serotonin reuptake inhibitor, which decreases renal digoxin excretion. Check a digoxin level at this time. Also obtain serum electrolytes because hyperkalemia is an ominous finding in the setting of digoxin toxicity.

> "**DIVERT**": Drugs that commonly predispose to digoxin toxicity are **DI**litiazem, **V**erapimil, **E**rythromycin, **R**ifampin, and **T**etracycline.

> Digitalis toxicity can cause almost any kind of arrhythmia, although Mobitz type II AV block, atrial fibrillation, and atrial flutter are less likely.

Serum digoxin level is 6 ng/ml (normal <2 ng/ml), and serum potassium is 5.5 mEq/L. What is the next step in management?

Digibind (digoxin-specific Fab fragments) is indicated for the following patients with digoxin toxicity:

1. Patients with digoxin level >10 ng/L
2. Patients with plasma potassium >5 mEq/L
3. Patients who are hemodynamically unstable
4. Patients with digoxin-induced arrhythmia

This patient with ventricular ectopy and plasma K^+ >5 mEq/L should receive Digibind.

The patient improves with Digibind. One year later, he presents to the emergency department with dry cough and dyspnea at rest. He ran out of his medications 4 weeks ago, and he was unable to obtain more after losing insurance coverage. Lung examination reveals bilateral crackles. Auscultation of the heart is significant for an S3 gallop, S4, loud P2, and mitral regurgitation. There is 13 cm of JVD and peripheral edema bilaterally. The liver is tender and can be palpated 4 cm below the costal margin. He is using accessory muscles to breathe. Vital signs are temperature 37.1°C, pulse 120 bpm, respirations 24/minute, blood pressure 150/95, and SaO_2, 89%. CXR shows bilateral infiltrates in a butterfly pattern. What is the cause of his symptoms?

The most likely explanation for his symptoms is acute decompensated CHF (cardiogenic pulmonary edema). Acute decompensated heart failure is characterized by signs of acutely worsening volume overload and decreased cardiac output.

> **Noncardiogenic pulmonary edema**: Common causes are volume overload in renal failure or increased afterload in hypertensive emergency. Unlike cardiogenic pulmonary edema, patients typically have a warm periphery and a bounding pulse.
> **Flash pulmonary edema**: Sudden and dramatic onset of cardiogenic pulmonary edema.

What is the most likely cause of decompensation in this patient?

The most common cause of acute decompensation is nonadherence with lifestyle measures, followed by nonadherence with drug therapy. Nonadherence to prescribed medication appears to be the most likely cause in this patient. Other causes of acute decompensated heart failure include the six I's and high-output heart failure:

1. **I**schemia/infarction
2. **I**nflammation of heart (myocarditis, etc.)
3. **I**nfection (endocarditis, etc.)
4. **I**nability to take medications or adhere to lifestyle measures (noncompliance)
5. **I**ngestions (alcohol or drugs such as β-blockers, CCBs, and chemotherapy drugs)
6. **I**nappropriate rhythm (arrhythmias)

High-output conditions are those that increase cardiac output requirements to maintain peripheral oxygenation: anemia, pregnancy, AV fistulas, hyperthyroidism, wet beriberi (B1 deficiency), Paget's disease, and mitral and aortic regurgitation.

How is cardiogenic pulmonary edema?

Key measures in acute cardiogenic pulmonary edema are "***LMNOP***":

1. **L**oop diuretics: IV loop diuretics reduce volume overload and have an initial morphine-like effect. Measure daily weight and 24-hour fluid balance to assess the efficacy of diuresis.
2. **M**orphine: Reduces anxiety → decreased work of breathing → decreased sympathetic outflow → arteriolar and venous dilation → decreased cardiac filling pressure.
3. **N**itrates: Transdermal nitroglycerin (vasodilator) reduces cardiac filling pressure. Consider IV nitroglycerin if transdermal nitroglycerin is not sufficient. Nitroprusside is another alternative, but it is used less frequently because of the risk of cyanide toxicity.
4. **O**xygen: Maintain oxygen saturation >90% with supplemental oxygen. If the patient progresses to respiratory failure, attempt noninvasive positive pressure ventilation. If this is not successful, intubate and mechanically ventilate the patient.
5. **P**osition: Have patients sit up with their legs dangling over the side of the bed.

> Do not initiate ACE inhibitors for the first time during the initial 12 to 24 hours of acute cardiogenic pulmonary edema (risk of hypotension and renal failure). If the patient is already on an ACE inhibitor, he can continue the drug.

The patient with systolic heart failure continues to have dyspnea at rest despite maximal outpatient therapy. He has repeated admissions for exacerbations and is currently hospitalized with cardiogenic pulmonary edema that is refractory to maximal therapy with loop diuretics, morphine, nitrates, oxygen, and position. What additional options exist for patients with refractory, NYHA class IV, systolic heart failure?

1. **IV dobutamine (β-1 agonist) or milrinone (phosphodiesterase inhibitor)**: Helpful for inpatient management of refractory cardiogenic pulmonary edema.
2. **Nesiritide**: This vasodilator may help heart failure patients with refractory pulmonary edema who are not hypotensive or in cardiogenic shock.

3. **Hemodialysis**: Helps reduce volume overload and may improve responsiveness to loop diuretics.
4. **Mechanical circulatory support**: Intraaortic balloon pump, LV assist devices, and a recently approved total artificial heart can serve as a bridge to transplantation. A long-term LV assist device is available for patients who are not candidates for cardiac transplantation.
5. **Cardiac transplantation**: Most of the above therapies are intended as a bridge to transplantation. One-year survival is close to 80% and 5-year survival is 65% to 70% after heart transplant.

Alternative 2.10.1

A 40-year-old woman presents with progressive dyspnea on exertion over the last 3 months. She denies recent infection, cigarette, or alcohol use. Her father died of heart failure at the age of 45, and her brother died of sudden cardiac arrest while practicing for a triathlon as a teenager. There is 12 cm of JVD and a positive "a" wave. There is 2+ pedal edema. Auscultation of the heart reveals a harsh crescendo-decrescendo systolic murmur that increases with standing and valsalva, and decreases with squatting and sustained handgrip. Carotid pulse is bifid with a brisk upstroke.

What is the most likely cause of this patient's symptoms?

This patient presents with signs and symptoms of heart failure caused by hypertrophic cardiomyopathy (idiopathic subaortic stenosis). Approximately 30% of patients have obstruction of the LV outflow tract as a result of hypertrophy of the ventricular septum, which causes the characteristic murmur (see Table 2-19). This is an autosomal dominant condition with variable penetrance, and often presents with sudden cardiac arrest in young athletes.

Aortic stenosis: Crescendo-decrescendo murmur that radiates to carotids and does not change with maneuvers. Carotid upstroke is diminished and delayed (parvus et tardus).
Hypertrophic cardiomyopathy: Crescendo-decrescendo murmur that does not radiate to carotids. Intensity changes with maneuvers. Carotid upstroke is brisk and bifid.

What findings would you expect to find on echocardiography?

Typical findings are asymmetric left-ventricle hypertrophy without dilatation, preserved systolic function but decreased end-diastolic volume (diastolic heart failure). Because this patient has the characteristic murmur of LV outflow tract obstruction, you should expect the anterior septum of the mitral valve to contact the ventricular septum during systole.

Screen all first-degree family members with echocardiography every year during adolescence and then every 5 years until the sixth or seventh decade.

Echocardiography confirms the diagnosis of hypertrophic cardiomyopathy with diastolic dysfunction and LV outflow tract obstruction. In general, how should you approach the treatment of diastolic heart failure?

Management of diastolic heart failure can be extremely challenging. The left ventricle is small and stiff, so medications that decrease preload such as diuretics and venodilators can drastically reduce left ventricle filling, resulting in decreased cardiac output and hypotension. Control HTN, atrial fibrillation, volume overload, and CAD when they present. Monitor the patient closely for hypotension and syncope if you are using diuretics or venodilators such as nitrates, dihydropyridine CCBs, and ACE inhibitors.

What are the specific recommendations regarding management of hypertrophic cardiomyopathy?

1. For asymptomatic patients, all patients with outflow tract obstruction should take prophylactic antibiotics before dental, genitourinary, or other invasive procedures to decrease risk of mitral valve infective endocarditis. No other treatment is necessary for asymptomatic patients.

2. For symptomatic patients, the preferred initial therapy for dyspnea on exertion is a β-blocker. If symptoms persist, add verapamil or disopyramide (an anti-arrhythmic). Consider surgery (septal myomectomy) for patients with outflow tract obstruction and symptoms refractory to medical therapy. Alternatives to septal myomectomy are alcohol septal ablation and dual-chamber pacing.

> Use of an ICD may prevent sudden cardiac death in high-risk patients with hypertrophic cardiomyopathy.

CASE 2–11 FEVER, SYSTEMIC SYMPTOMS, AND A MURMUR

A 15-year-old African woman presents to a mission clinic in Malawi with a 3-week history of joint pain. The pain initially began in her legs. That pain resolved itself, and then she experienced pain in her knees followed by her wrists. She recalls having a sore throat 2 weeks before her symptoms began. Physical examination is significant for three firm, symmetric, and painless subcutaneous nodules over the olecranon processes. There are erythematous, nonpruritic plaques with a pale center on the trunk. Auscultation of the heart reveals a 2/6 blowing holosystolic murmur that is heard best at the apex and radiates to the axilla. Vital signs are temperature 38.9°C, pulse 90 bpm, respirations 12/minute, blood pressure 110/70, and oxygen saturation, 95%.

What is the most likely diagnosis?

The most likely diagnosis is rheumatic fever. Diagnosis of rheumatic fever is clinical based on the Jones criteria. To make the diagnosis, a patient must have either two major and one minor or one major and two minor criteria. Remember the major criteria for acute rheumatic fever with the mnemonic "***J♥NES***":

1. **J**oints: Migratory polyarthritis that predominantly affects the large joints is usually the first manifestation of acute rheumatic fever.
2. Carditis (♥): Acute rheumatic fever can cause pancarditis (pericarditis, epicarditis, and myocarditis). Mitral regurgitation is a common finding. The cardiac manifestations are often subtle.
3. **N**odules: Firm, painless, subcutaneous nodules over a bony surface or tendons that can be moved under the skin.
4. **E**rythema marginatum: A pink, nonpruritic rash with a central clearing located on the trunk and limbs but not the face.
5. **S**ydenham chorea: Neurological disturbances include inappropriate behavior, weakness, and abrupt, purposeless, nonrhythmic involuntary movements. This is usually a late manifestation, occurring months after the initial infection.

Minor criteria for rheumatic fever include:

1. Clinical findings of fever, arthralgias, or history of acute rheumatic fever in the past.
2. Laboratory findings of prolonged PR interval, elevated ESR, and elevated C-reactive protein (CRP).

> ESR and CRP are general markers for inflammation. They are not specific for any one condition.

What causes rheumatic fever?

Rheumatic fever is an immune-mediated condition that occurs 2 to 4 weeks after untreated streptococcal pharyngitis in 3% of patients. This complication most frequently affects children between the ages of 6 and 15 years.

How can you establish that the sore throat was secondary to group A streptococcal infection?

Either increased antistreptolysin O (or other streptococcal antibodies), positive throat culture, positive rapid streptococcal antigen test, or recent scarlet fever can establish the diagnosis.

Throat culture is usually negative by the time the patient develops acute rheumatic fever. At this stage, the best test, if available, would be antistreptolysin O, which peaks 5 weeks after the initial infection.

> **Scarlet fever** presents with fever; chills; cervical lymphadenopathy; sore throat; and an erythematous, maculopapular, sandpaper-like rash on trunk and abdomen for 2 to 5 days.

How is acute rheumatic fever treated?

Acute rheumatic fever is a self-limiting condition, and NSAIDs such as aspirin are sufficient for symptomatic treatment. It is important to treat the streptococcal infection with oral penicillin-V to prevent rheumatic heart disease. Use intramuscular benzathine penicillin-G if compliance is an issue. Erythromycin is an alternative for patients allergic to penicillin. Continue antibiotic prophylaxis until the patient is 18 to 20 years of age to prevent recurrence of acute rheumatic fever.

> Patients with a history of rheumatic fever should take erythromycin or amoxicillin before dental, genitourinary, and other invasive procedures to prevent infective endocarditis.

> Antibiotic treatment of streptococcal pharyngitis has dramatically reduced the incidence of rheumatic fever and rheumatic heart disease in the United States.

There is no penicillin-G in the clinic, and the patient loses the penicillin-V on her way home. She does not return to the clinic. She moves to the United States the next year. Fifteen years later, she presents to the clinic with gradually progressive dyspnea and orthopnea over the last 3 months. She finds it difficult to climb stairs and walk to her mailbox. Auscultation of the heart reveals a mid-diastolic opening snap followed by a 3/6 rumble heard best at the apex. The murmur is followed by a loud S1. Bilateral rales are heard on lung examination. There is 2+ pedal edema. What is the most likely diagnosis?

This patient has rheumatic heart disease, which presents 10 to 20 years after the original infection in untreated patients. Immune-mediated damage to the mitral valves causes fusion of the valve commissures, leading to mitral stenosis ("fish mouth orifice"). Mitral stenosis causes elevated left atrial pressure, which leads to pulmonary HTN and right heart failure. The condition is typically asymptomatic until the mitral valve area decreases to <1.5 cm^2 (normal: 4cm^2 to 5 cm^2). Atrial fibrillation and atrial thrombus formation are important complications of mitral stenosis.

> Rheumatic heart disease can also lead to aortic stenosis. Tricuspid and pulmonary valve stenoses are possible but uncommon.

Echocardiography shows a mitral valve area of 1 cm^2. There is no left atrial thrombus, valve calcification, or mitral regurgitation. Ejection fraction is 28%. How is mitral valve stenosis treated?

1. Asymptomatic patients: No specific treatment is required for asymptomatic patients except periodic monitoring with echocardiography.
2. Mild fluid overload: Diuretics are sufficient for patients with mild fluid overload.
3. NYHA class II to class IV heart failure: Perform surgical valve replacement or catheter balloon commissurotomy.

What treatment should this patient receive?

This patient has NYHA class II CHF. Surgery is recommended in this patient because of the mitral regurgitation. Other indications for surgery are calcified valves or left atrial thrombus. Catheter balloon commissurotomy is indicated in patients with none of these indications for surgery.

Alternative 2.11.1

The patient is a 30-year-old man who presents to the clinic with a 3-week history of low-grade fever, malaise, and arthralgias. He has a history of IV cocaine and heroin use. He has no other prior medical history. Physical examination is significant for a 1/6 blowing murmur heard best at the left lower sternal border that increases with inspiration and decreases with expiration. There are numerous recent injection marks on his right and left arms. Vital signs are temperature 39°C, pulse 90 bpm, respirations 15/minute, blood pressure 110/75.

What cause should you suspect on the basis of his symptoms?

Suspect infective endocarditis in any patient with unexplained fever and a new murmur. Infective endocarditis often affects heart valves, which is why patients develop a murmur. IV drug abuse is an important risk factor, particularly for right-sided (tricuspid valve) endocarditis. With fever, murmur, and flu-like symptoms for >2 weeks, this patient is more likely to have subacute than acute bacterial endocarditis (Table 2-22).

> Murmur and physical signs are often absent, so infective endocarditis is an important diagnostic consideration in fever of unknown origin.

What are other physical signs of infective endocarditis?

Important physical findings of infective endocarditis (often not present) are:

1. Petechiae: Although not specific, petechiae on the skin, mucous membrane, and conjunctiva are the most common skin findings.
2. Splinter hemorrhages: Nonblanching, red-brown lines under the nail bed.
3. Janeway lesions: Erythematous, painless, blanching macules on palms and soles.
4. Osler nodes: Painful violaceous nodules on the pulp of fingers and toes.
5. Roth spots: Retinal hemorrhage and exudates.

> Janeway lesions, Osler nodes, and Roth spots are specific but not sensitive.

In addition to careful physical examination, what tests should you order for this patient with suspected subacute infective endocarditis?

1. **Blood cultures**: These are the most important diagnostic tests for infective endocarditis. Draw three sets of cultures at least 1 hour apart to maximize diagnostic yield.
2. **Echocardiography**: Transthoracic echocardiography (TTE) is sufficient for most patients. If transthoracic echocardiography is negative or equivocal and clinical suspicion is high, perform TEE, which is more accurate albeit more invasive. If the patient has a prosthetic valve or staphylococcus aureus bacteremia, skip transthoracic echocardiography and go straight to TEE. The test is positive if echocardiogram detects vegetation.

TABLE 2–22 Acute Versus Subacute Bacterial Endocarditis

	Acute Bacterial Endocarditis	Subacute Bacterial Endocarditis
Heart valve	Healthy native valve	Damaged or prosthetic valve
Presentation	High fever and systemic symptoms over the course of a few days	Low-grade fever and nonspecific symptoms such as fatigue, weakness, malaise, anorexia, and arthralgias lasting weeks to months.
White cell count	Leukocytosis with a left shift	White count may or may not be elevated
Microbiology	*Staphylococcus aureus* (most common), *Staphylococcus epidermis,* and Gram-negative bacilli	*Streptococcus viridans* (most common). *Streptococcus bovis, enterococcus,* and HACEK organisms
Prognosis	Fatal in <6 weeks if left untreated	Takes >6 weeks to cause death if untreated

3. **EKG**: EKG is not diagnostic for endocarditis, but it helps determine whether the vegetation has spread into the conducting system and caused heart block or conduction delays.
4. **CXR**: CXR is not diagnostic, but small, patchy infiltrates suggest septic pulmonary emboli.
5. **Laboratory tests**: Although of limited diagnostic utility, patients with infective endocarditis usually have elevated ESR and CRP, anemia of chronic disease, increased rheumatoid factor, and microscopic hematuria. In acute bacterial endocarditis, white blood cell count is elevated with a leftward shift.

What causative organism is most likely in this patient?

The most common organism responsible for endocarditis in IV drug users is *Staphylococcus aureus* followed by streptococcus and enterococcus. Gram-negative rods (especially pseudomonas) and fungi (like candida) are less common causes.

> Staphylococcus aureus usually causes acute bacterial endocarditis except in IV drug users with native healthy valves, in whom the infection tends to be more indolent.

Two of three blood cultures are positive for Staphylococcus aureus. TEE indicates tricuspid valve vegetation and tricuspid regurgitation. EKG is normal. ESR, CRP, and rheumatoid factor is elevated. Serum electrolytes are normal. What are the diagnostic criteria for infective endocarditis?

Infective endocarditis is a clinical diagnosis based on the Duke criteria (Table 2-23). This patient has all three major criteria and three minor criteria for infective endocarditis.

What treatment should this patient receive?

Bacterial endocarditis is usually fatal if left untreated. This patient with uncomplicated, native valve, right-sided staphylococcus infection should receive a 2-week course of IV nafcillin (or oxacillin) and gentamycin (Table 2-24).

> Monitor acute phase reactants during therapy. Normalization of ESR and CRP indicates successful antibiotic treatment.

How would treatment differ if cultures grew methicillin-resistant Staphylococcus aureus?

If the culture results show methicillin-resistant *Staphylococcus aureus*, treat with a 6-week course of vancomycin instead.

TABLE 2–23 Duke Criteria for Diagnosis of Infective Endocarditis

Major criteria
1. At least 2 blood cultures positive for *Staphylococcus aureus*, *Streptococcus viridans* or *bovis*, *enterococcus*, or HACEK strains[a]
2. Echocardiogram shows a vegetation, abscess, valve perforation, or partial dehiscence of the prosthetic valve
3. Echocardiogram documents a new valvular regurgitation.

Minor criteria
1. Predisposing condition (abnormal heart valve or intravenous drug use)
2. Fever >38°C
3. Vascular phenomena (septic emboli, mycotic aneurysms, intracranial hemorrhage, Janeway lesions)
4. Immune phenomena (glomerulonephritis, Osler nodes, Roth spots, elevated rheumatoid factor)
5. Positive blood cultures not meeting major criteria
6. Positive echocardiogram not meeting major criteria

To make the diagnosis, the patient must fulfill one of the three options:
1. At least 2 major criteria and 1 minor
2. At least 1 major criterion and 2 minor criteria
3. At least 5 minor criteria

[a] HACEK strains are Hemophilus species, *Actinobacilli actinomycete*, *Cardiobacterium hominis*, Eikenella, and Kingella species. Single positive blood culture or IgG titer >1:800 is sufficient for *Coxiella burnetii*.

TABLE 2-24 Empiric Treatment for Infective Endocarditis

	Organisms	Intravenous Antibiotics
Native valve endocarditis	*S. viridans, S. aureus,* enterococci	Nafcillin + ampicillin + gentamycin
Right-sided endocarditis in IV drug users	*S. aureus*	Nafcillin + gentamycin
Early prosthetic valve endocarditis (<60 days)	Staphylococci	Vancomycin + gentamycin
Late prosthetic valve endocarditis (>60 days)	Same as native valve endocarditis	Same as native valve endocarditis

Adapted from O'Rourke et al. *Hurst's The Heart: Manual of Cardiology*. 11th ed. McGraw Hill, 2005.

Treatment duration of left-sided bacterial endocarditis is 6 weeks.

The patient continues to remain febrile despite 2 weeks of antibiotics, and EKG shows a prolonged PT. What complication should you suspect?

Suspect paravalvular abscess in patients who continue to remain febrile or develop new conduction abnormalities despite appropriate antibiotics. This complication is more common in infective endocarditis as a result of IV drug use. Obtain a repeat TEE to evaluate for this complication. If TEE is positive, treatment is prompt surgery and IV antibiotics.

What are some other common complications of untreated infective endocarditis?

Remember common complications with the mnemonic "***Endocarditis Complications May Never Go Away***":

1. **E**mbolization: Left-sided vegetations can cause systemic emboli. Right-sided lesions can throw septic pulmonary emboli.
2. **C**HF is the most common cause of death as a result of infective endocarditis.
3. **M**ycotic aneurysm: Infection can weaken and dilate blood vessel walls. The classic presentation is a painful, pulsatile mass in a febrile patient. Rupture of a cerebral mycotic aneurysm can lead to intracerebral hemorrhage. Treatment is prompt surgery and 4 to 6 weeks of IV antibiotics.
4. **N**eurological complications occur in 25% to 30% of patients.
5. **G**lomerulonephritis is mediated by the immune complex.
6. **A**bscess (paravalvular).

Alternative 2.11.2

A 70-year-old man presents with a 2-day history of high fever and rigors. He has a history of aortic stenosis (caused by calcification) that required placement of a porcine valve 30 days ago. The murmur has increased in intensity compared to when he was discharged after surgery. Temperature is 39.3°C, pulse is 120 bpm, respirations are 18/minute, and blood pressure is 100/75.

What diagnosis should you suspect?

Suspect acute bacterial endocarditis in a patient with acute onset of high fever, rigors, and a new or worsening murmur. The most common organisms responsible for endocarditis within 60 days of prosthetic valve placement are *Staphylococcus epidermis* and *Staphylococcus aureus* (see Table 2-24).

Mechanical valve (ball, disk, St. Jude) is usually selected for younger patients or those who need anticoagulation.

Biologic valve (human or porcine) is usually selected in older patients with a short life expectancy or those who cannot tolerate anticoagulation.

What is the next step in management?

Do not delay treatment in an attempt to isolate a specific organism because acute bacterial endocarditis is a fulminant condition. Draw the first set of blood cultures and then initiate empiric IV vancomycin and gentamycin without waiting for the culture results.

What are important noninfectious causes of heart valve vegetations?

1. **Marantic (thrombotic) endocarditis** occurs in patients with advanced malignancies. Vegetations consist of platelets and fibrin. Suspect this condition when a cancer patient develops unexplained acute stroke. Diagnose with TEE and treat with unfractionated or subcutaneous heparin.
2. **Libman-Sachs (verrucous) endocarditis** occurs in patients with systemic lupus erythematosus. Vegetations consist of platelets, fibrin, and immune complexes. Although asymptomatic, these vegetations can throw systemic emboli. Also, the damage they cause to heart valves predisposes to infectious endocarditis. Consider anticoagulation for this condition.

CASE 2–12 BRADYCARDIA

A 20-year-old man presents to the university health clinic with chest pain localized to his right ribs that worsens with deep inspiration. The pain is consistently reproducible with deep palpation. He does not have any other symptoms. He plays varsity basketball. An EKG is obtained (see Fig. 2-6).

What is the next step in management?

Chest wall tenderness that increases with inspiration and is reproducible with palpation is consistent with a musculoskeletal cause. In young patients with no risk factors, further work-up is not necessary. In his case, the EKG that was obtained showed sinus bradycardia. Sinus bradycardia is a common finding in many well-trained athletes (results from increased vagal tone). No further work-up or treatment is indicated in asymptomatic patients with sinus bradycardia.

What are other causes of sinus bradycardia?

1. **2 As:** Athletic training and **A**dvanced age
2. **Hypos:** **H**ypokalemia and **H**ypothyroidism
3. **Medications** that depress sinus node function include β-blockers, CCBs, digitalis, clonidine, lithium, and anti-arrhythmic drugs (amiodarone, quinidine, lidocaine, and procainamide).

Alternative 2.12.1

A 70-year-old man presents with resting angina that does not respond rapidly to sublingual nitroglycerin. EKG shows ST elevation in leads II, III, and aVF, as well as sinus bradycardia. Blood pressure is 80/60.

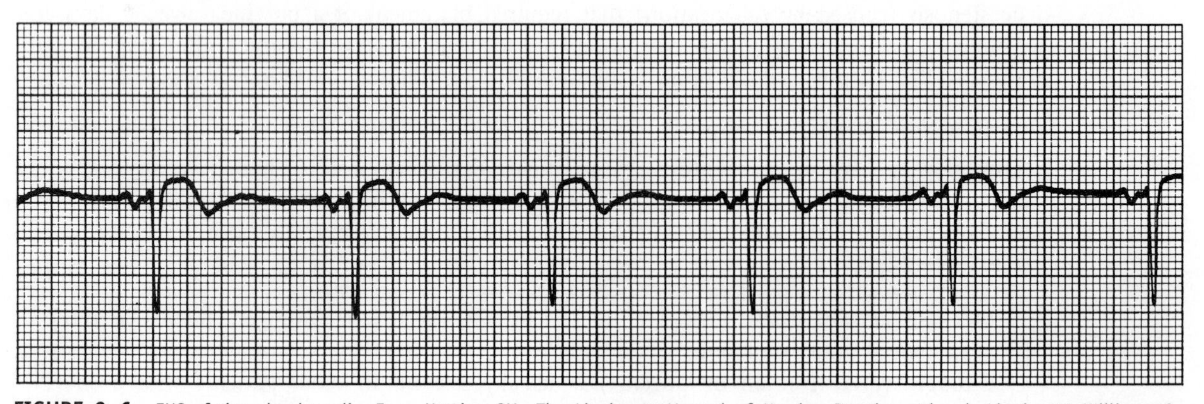

FIGURE 2–6 EKG of sinus bradycardia. From Nettina SM. *The Lippincott Manual of Nursing Practice*, 7th ed. Lippincott Williams & Wilkins, 2001.

What treatment is indicated for the sinus bradycardia?

This patient has an inferior-wall MI, which often involves the right coronary artery. Because the right coronary artery supplies the SA node, sinus bradycardia is a common, transient finding that resolves within 24 hours. This patient, who is hemodynamically unstable, requires prompt treatment. Prepare for transcutaneous pacing. While awaiting the pacemaker, administer IV atropine (see Fig. 2-7).

> **FASTropine**: Atropine makes the heart beat faster.
> **AdenoSLOW**: Adenosine makes the heart beat slower.

Alternative 2.12.2

The patient is a 78-year-old man with a history of HTN and systolic heart failure. He began experiencing fatigue and light-headedness shortly after initiating metoprolol. He does not have any other medical conditions. EKG shows left-ventricle hypertrophy and sinus bradycardia with a heart rate of 45 beats per minute. Vital signs are normal.

What is the next step in management?

Some patients with sinus bradycardia experience symptoms of fatigue, light-headedness, syncope, and worsening angina and heart failure. The first step in stable symptomatic patients is to identify and discontinue medications that can depress sinus node function (e.g., metoprolol). Consider using an antihypertensive that does not depress sinus node function such as an ACE inhibitor.

The patient continues to have episodes of lightheadedness and syncope despite discontinuation of metoprolol. Serum electrolyte and thyroid-stimulating hormone levels are normal. What is the next step in management?

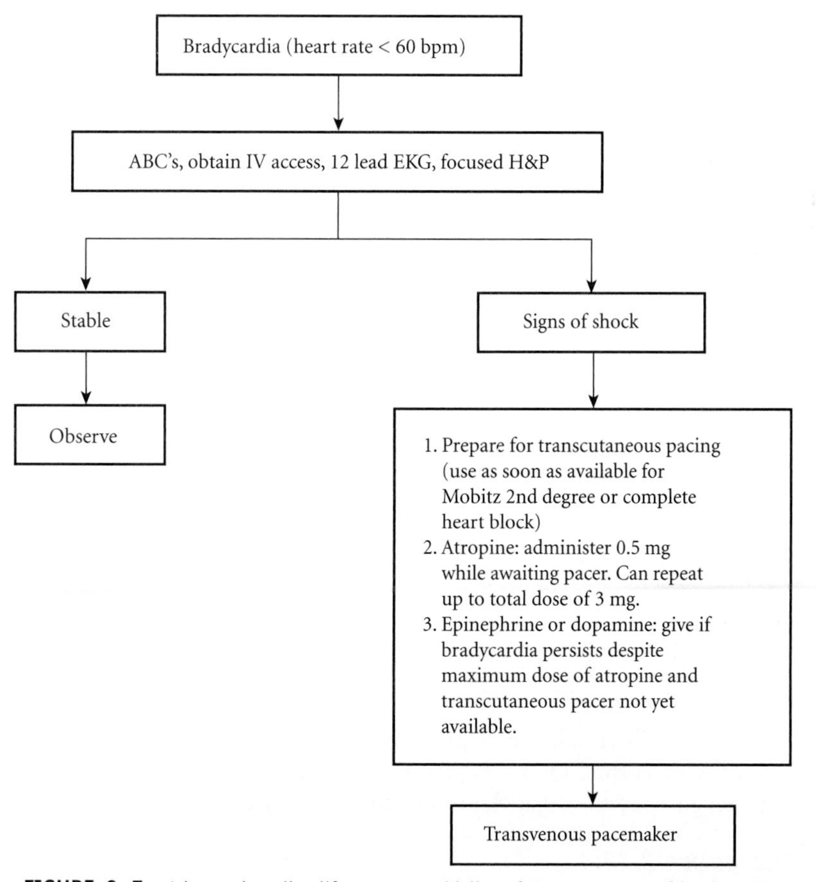

FIGURE 2–7 Advanced cardiac life support guidelines for management of bradycardia.

First, perform carotid sinus massage (vagal maneuver) for 5 to 10 seconds. A pause in heartbeat >3 seconds indicates carotid sinus hypersensitivity as the cause of bradycardia. If carotid sinus massage is negative, consider ambulatory EKG monitoring (Holter monitor or cardiac event monitor) to correlate symptoms with EKG changes.

> Make sure there are no carotid bruits prior to auscultation and do not massage both sinuses at the same time (risk of precipitating cerebral ischemia).

> **Holter monitor**: Portable device that continuously monitors EKG for ≥24 hours.
> **Cardiac event monitor**: Portable device that continuously monitors EKG for ≥1 month.

Carotid sinus testing is negative. The patient is placed on ambulatory EKG monitoring. During symptomatic periods, EKG shows supraventricular tachycardia alternating with sinus bradycardia. What diagnosis should you suspect?

Suspect sick sinus syndrome in elderly patients with heart disease and marked sinus bradycardia without any obvious cause. Sick sinus syndrome is caused by SA node dysfunction together with dysfunctional atrial and junctional foci that are unable to use their normal escape beats, which means that patients can present with recurrent sinus block or sinus arrest. More than 50% of patients experience alternating atrial tachycardia and bradycardia (tachy-brady syndrome), as is the case with this patient.

What treatment should this patient receive?

Patients with persistent, symptomatic sinus bradycardia or sick sinus syndrome should receive a pacemaker to artificially stimulate the heart. This patient should also receive a β-blocker or CCB after the pacemaker is implanted to control the tachyarrhythmia.

> A pacemaker is also indicated if a symptomatic patient has a compelling indication not to discontinue a drug that depresses sinus node function.

What are the different methods of cardiac pacing?

1. Transcutaneous pacing: Place pads on the external chest wall (one on the sternum and the other on the left axilla). Electrical impulses travel between the two pads and stimulate the heart muscle between them. Used only for temporary stabilization in unstable patients.
2. Transvenous pacing: A wire is inserted into the right heart using a central venous catheter. The other end of the wire is attached to the pacemaker generator outside the body. Transvenous pacemakers serve as a bridge to permanent pacemaker placement.
3. Permanent pacemaker: Wires are placed in the chambers of the heart as desired. The other ends of the wires usually connect to a titanium generator placed beneath the subcutaneous fat of the chest wall.

> Pacemaker stimuli appear on an EKG as narrow vertical spikes.

Alternative 2.12.3

A 55-year-old man is given a diagnosis of HTN. As part of the evaluation, an EKG is performed (see Fig. 2-8). The patient is asymptomatic.

What is the diagnosis?

The EKG abnormality is a prolonged PR interval, which indicates that he has an AV block. Because a normal QRS complex follows every p wave, he has a first-degree AV block. This is a benign condition that does not require any treatment.

Alternative 2.12.4

A 55-year-old man is given a diagnosis of HTN. As part of the evaluation, an EKG is performed (see Fig. 2-9). The patient is asymptomatic.

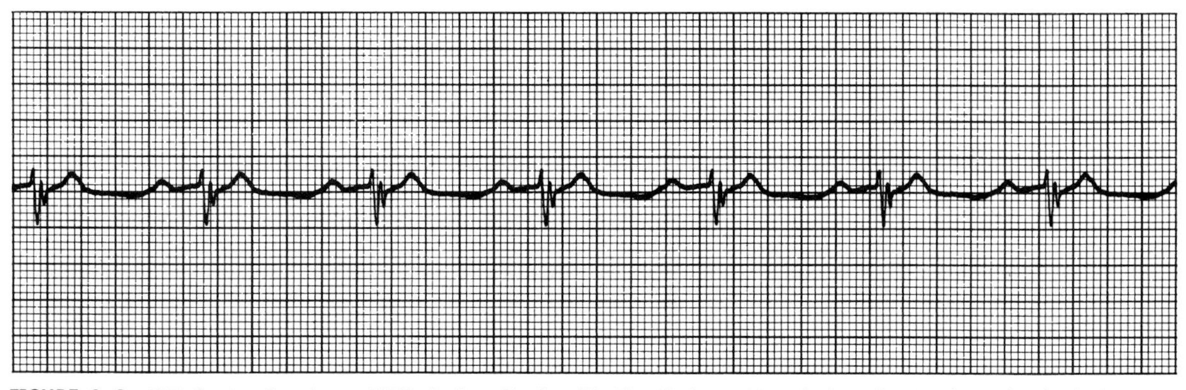

FIGURE 2–8 EKG showing first-degree AV block. From Nettina SM. *The Lippincott Manual of Nursing Practice,* 7th ed. Lippincott Williams & Wilkins, 2001.

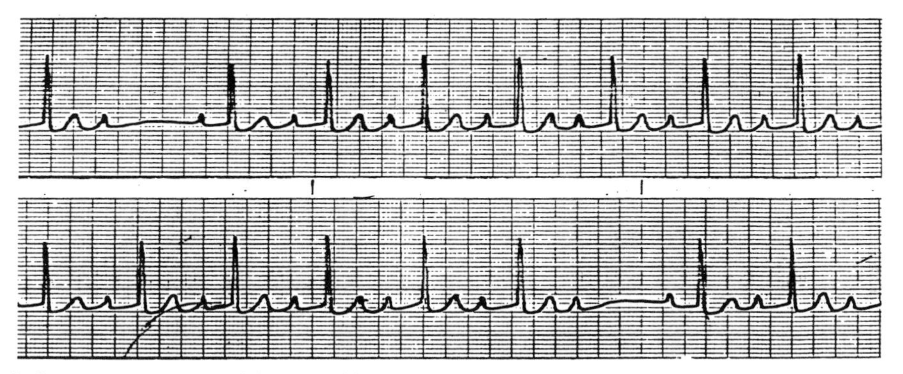

FIGURE 2–9 EKG showing second-degree AV block (type I mobitz). From Harwood-Nuss A, Wolfson AB, et al. *The Clinical Practice of Emergency Medicine,* 3rd ed. Lippincott Williams & Wilkins, 2001.

What is the diagnosis?

In this EKG, the PR interval progressively lengthens until finally an impulse is blocked and a QRS complex does not follow the p wave. The patient has Type 1 (Wenkebach) second-degree AV block. No treatment is necessary.

Alternative 2.12.5

The patient is a 70-year-old man with a history of systolic heart failure. An EKG is performed (see Fig. 2-10).

What arrhythmia does this patient have?

He has Type II (Mobitz) second-degree AV block. There is no PR interval lengthening, and a number of normal impulses are conducted. Suddenly, the P wave fails to conduct and there is no QRS complex. This condition results from a His bundle block or a block in the Purkinje fibers and usually occurs in patients with underlying heart disease. He should receive a permanent pacemaker to prevent progression to complete heart block.

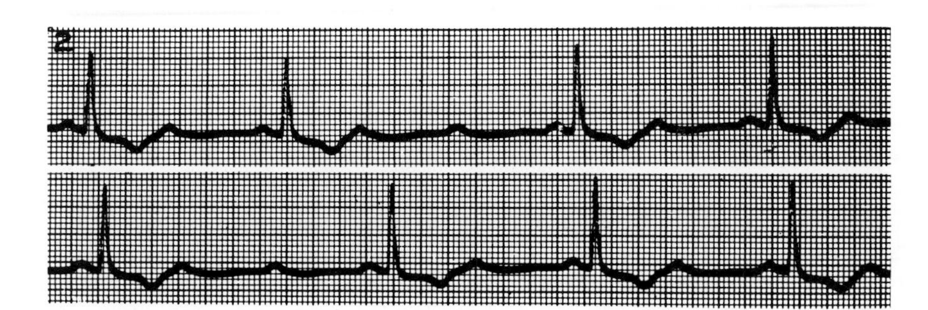

FIGURE 2–10 EKG showing second-degree AV block (type 2 mobitz). From Harwood-Nuss A, Wolfson AB, et al. *The Clinical Practice of Emergency Medicine,* 3rd ed. Lippincott Williams & Wilkins, 2001.

Alternative 2.12.6

The patient is a 60-year-old man who was admitted to the hospital 24 hours ago with an anterior STEMI. In the cardiac care unit, the monitor detects an abnormal rhythm (see Fig. 2-11).

What arrhythmia does this patient have?

This patient has third-degree or complete heart block. No p waves are conducted to the ventricles, so ventricular automaticity foci take control of ventricular pacemaking at a rate of 20 to 50 beats per minute. As a result, p waves and QRS complexes are completely asynchronous. Treat this patient with atropine and transcutaneous pacing followed by transvenous pacing (see Fig. 2-7). Complete heart block in the setting of an anterior MI is often permanent, so place a permanent pacemaker after the patient is stable.

> Complete heart block in the setting of an inferior MI is often transient, so a permanent pacemaker is usually not necessary.

CASE 2–13 IRREGULAR NARROW COMPLEX TACHYCARDIA

A 76-year-old man presents with a 1-week history of intermittent palpitations. He is currently asymptomatic. He has a history of HTN that is treated with HCTZ and lisinopril. He is alert and oriented. Heart rate is 120 beats per minute, and pulse is irregular. He is afebrile. Blood pressure is 130/80. An EKG is obtained (see Fig. 2-12).

What is the abnormal rhythm?

The patient has the characteristic "irregularly irregular" rhythm of atrial fibrillation (AF). Multiple irritable foci fire rapidly, but the impulses do not travel very far, so EKG records a wavy baseline but no identifiable p waves. Occasional depolarizations near the AV node conduct to the ventricles, which accounts for the random narrow QRS complexes.

> Symptoms of AF and other tachyarrhythmias are palpitations, shortness of breath, weakness, dizziness, and worsening angina or heart failure; however, 90% of atrial fibrillation episodes are asymptomatic.

FIGURE 2–11 EKG showing third-degree AV block. From Harwood-Nuss A, Wolfson AB, et al. *The Clinical Practice of Emergency Medicine*, 3rd ed. Lippincott Williams & Wilkins, 2001.

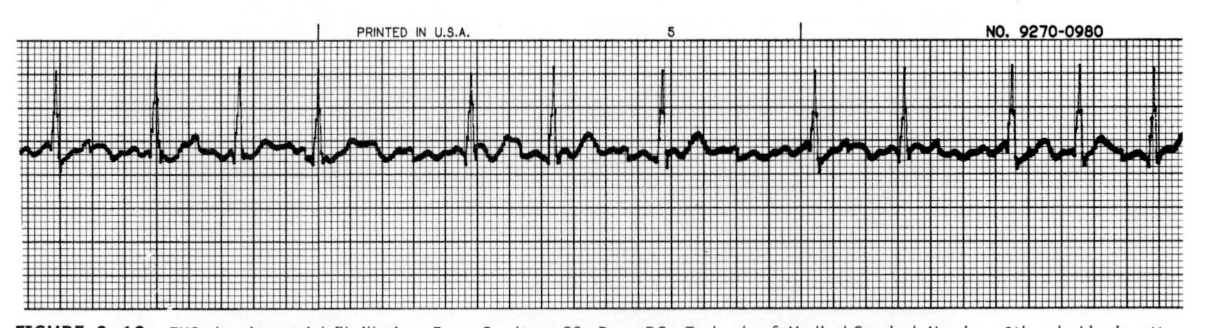

FIGURE 2–12 EKG showing atrial fibrillation. From Smeltzer SC, Bare BG. *Texbook of Medical-Surgical Nursing*, 9th ed. Lippincott Williams & Wilkins, 2000.

What are the underlying causes of atrial fibrillation?

Atrial fibrillation is the most common arrhythmia in adults. It is more common in older patients, especially if they have underlying cardiac conditions such as HTN (the most common underlying disorder), CHF, CAD, MI, sick sinus syndrome, Wolf-Parkinson-White syndrome, or cardiac surgery. Noncardiac risk factors for atrial fibrillation are:

1. Lungs: pulmonary embolism, COPD, pneumonia, and obstructive sleep apnea.
2. Endocrine: hyperthyroidism and pheochromocytoma (caused by increased β-adrenergic tone).
3. Alcohol and caffeine intake: atrial fibrillation that occurs after binging on alcohol during the weekend or holidays is termed "holiday heart syndrome."

> **Lone atrial fibrillation**: AF in patients without underlying cardiac or pulmonary disease. These patients have a lower risk of thromboembolism and mortality.
> **Persistent atrial fibrillation**: AF that fails to self-terminate for >7 days.
> **Paroxysmal atrial fibrillation**: Episodes last <7 days, but may recur.
> **Permanent atrial fibrillation**: AF that lasts for at least 1 year.

What is the next step in management?

The next step in this stable patient is to control the heart rate with β-blockers or CCBs (verapimil or diltiazem). Digoxin is a second-line agent for rate control except in patients with heart failure (see Fig. 2-13). Also, obtain CXR, echocardiogram, and thyroid function tests to identify possible precipitants.

> Approximately 75% of patients spontaneously revert to normal sinus rhythm.

Why is cardioversion not recommended initially in stable patients with atrial fibrillation?

The erratic motion of the atria leads to blood stasis, which predisposes to atrial thrombus formation. Pharmacological or electrical cardioversion can dislodge a clot from this thrombus and lead to systemic embolization, the most dangerous complication of AF.

How would initial management have differed if the patient presented with palpitations and tachycardia, and his blood pressure was 80/60 mm Hg?

Initial management of an unstable patient in atrial fibrillation is urgent synchronized cardioversion (see Fig. 2-14). In these patients, the risk of death from the irregular rhythm is greater than the risk of possibly dislodging a clot.

What is synchronized cardioversion? How does it differ from defibrillation?

Both synchronized electrical cardioversion and defibrillation transiently deliver electric current to depolarized cardiac cells, which allows the sinus node to resume normal pacemaker activity. External paddles or implanted devices deliver the current.

1. Cardioversion is used to terminate atrial fibrillation, atrial flutter, supraventricular tachycardias, and stable VT with a pulse. Current is delivered during the R or S wave of the QRS complex (i.e., synchronized with the R or S wave). This helps avoid delivering current during the period after ventricular depolarization (risk of precipitating VT). When used electively, patients are sedated beforehand to minimize discomfort.
2. Defibrillation is used to emergently terminate ventricular fibrillation or pulseless VT. Electric current is unsynchronized (delivered at any time in the cardiac cycle). Electricity levels are higher than with cardioversion.

> The ICD is surgically implanted under the skin. It detects abnormal rhythms and delivers the appropriate current. Originally designed to deal with ventricular fibrillation, it is now used to treat atrial and ventricular arrhythmias as well as for biventricular pacing.

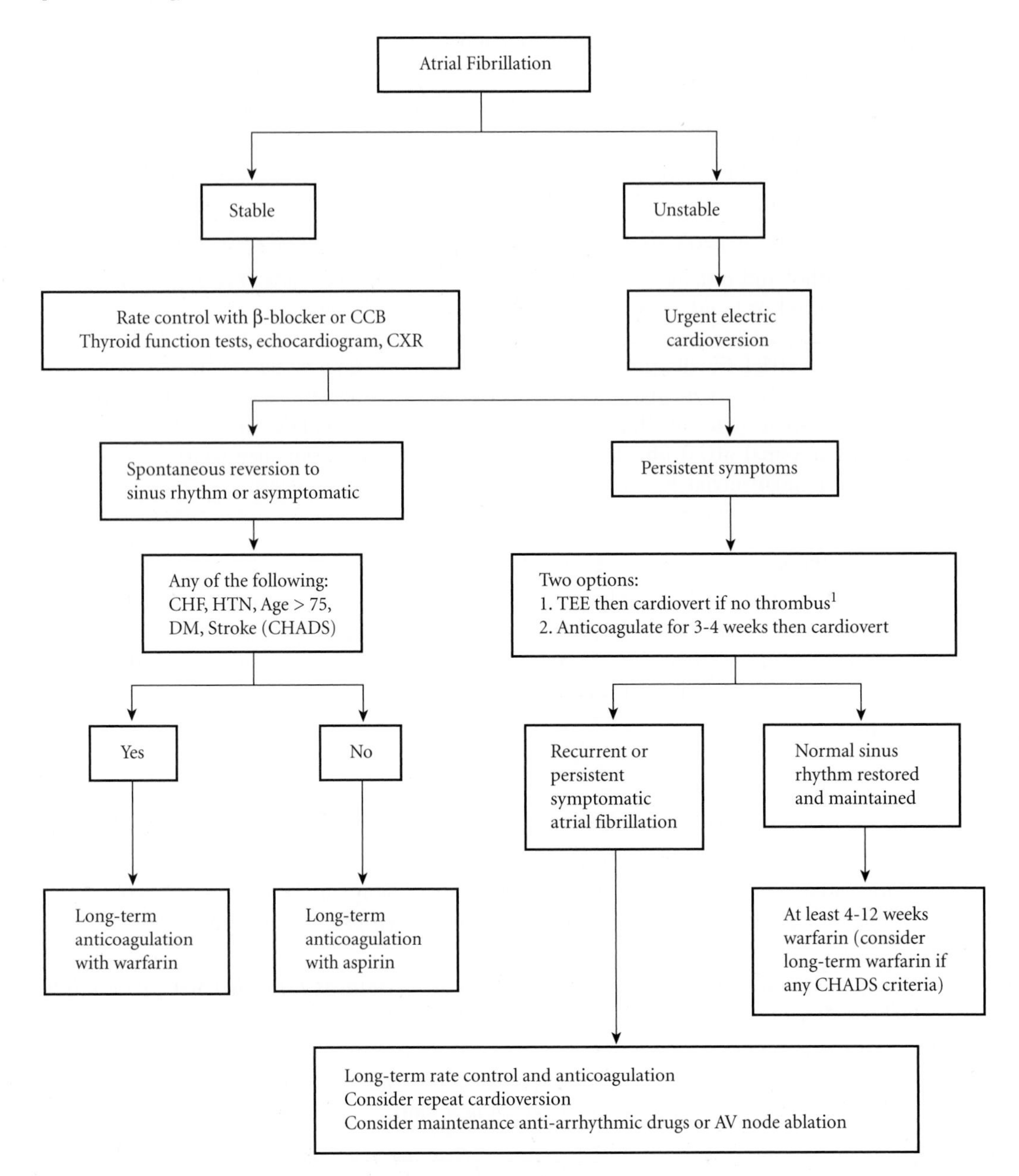

[1]If TEE detects thrombus, anticoagulate for 3-4 weeks then cardiovert.
If known duration < 48 hours, can cardiovert immediately without TEE.

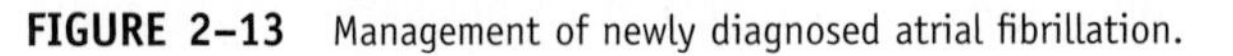

FIGURE 2–13 Management of newly diagnosed atrial fibrillation.

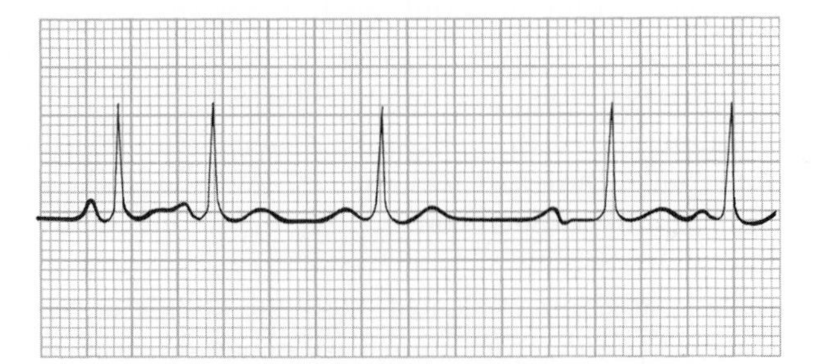

FIGURE 2–14 EKG showing MAT. From Thaler MS. *The Only EKG Book You'll Ever Need,* 5th ed. Lippincott Williams & Wilkins, 2007.

The stable patient's heart rate decreases to 86 beats per minute with metoprolol. The rhythm does not spontaneously convert. No underlying cause is detected. He remains asymptomatic with the β-blocker. Vital signs remain normal. What is the next step in management?

If heart rate is well controlled and the patient remains asymptomatic, cardioversion is not necessary. Consider chronic anticoagulation with warfarin (target INR 2 to 3) in patients with a history of any of the following (mnemonic: "***CHADS***"): **C**HF, **H**TN, **A**ge >75 years, **D**M, or **S**troke (or transient ischemic attack or systemic embolus). The goal of anticoagulation is to prevent stroke.

> **Low-risk patient (no CHADS):** Anticoagulation with aspirin is usually sufficient.

> The AFFIRM and RACE trials concluded that the combination of rate control and anticoagulation is preferred to rhythm control in patients with stable atrial fibrillation.

How would management differ if the stable patient continued to experience distressing episodes of palpitations and diaphoresis or was unable to achieve adequate rate control?

There are two options if a stable patient continues to experience distressing symptoms or is unable to achieve adequate rate control (see Fig. 2-13):

1. Anticoagulation followed by cardioversion: Initially administer heparin and warfarin. When the INR is 2 to 3, discontinue heparin and continue warfarin for 3 to 4 weeks. Then perform electric or pharmacologic cardioversion.
2. TEE followed by cardioversion: Obtain TEE to rule out atrial thrombus. If no thrombus is present, proceed with electric or pharmacologic cardioversion.

> **Atrial fibrillation duration <48 hours:** Cardiovert without anticoagulation or TEE.

Is anticoagulation necessary after successful cardioversion?

Atrial fibrillation often recurs and can once again place the patient at risk for left atrial thrombus and subsequent embolic stroke. Long-term warfarin is still recommended in patients with any of the CHADS criteria.

How can you manage patients who continue to experience symptoms because of recurrent atrial fibrillation after successful or unsuccessful cardioversion?

Consider maintenance anti-arrhythmic drugs in this subset of patients. Amiodarone is usually first-line except in patients with bradycardia. Other anti-arrhythmic options are flecainide, dofetilide, propafenone, and sotalol. Catheter AV node ablation is a final option for patients with refractory atrial fibrillation.

Alternative 2.13.1

The patient is a 75-year-old man with known COPD and HTN. He presents to the emergency department with dyspnea, palpitations, and light-headedness. Medications include inhaled albuterol and ipratropium, oxygen at night, inhaled steroids, and HCTZ. Vital signs are temperature 37°C, blood pressure 130/80, pulse 120 bpm, respirations 20/minute, and oxygen saturation 90%. An EKG is obtained (see Fig. 2-14).

What is the abnormal rhythm?

The patient has multifocal atrial tachycardia (MAT). At least three to four different atrial automaticity foci pace the heart at their inherent rates, but no single focus achieves pacemaking dominance. As a result, the patient develops a rapid, irregular heart rate with p waves of various shapes.

What conditions predispose to MAT?

COPD is the most common underlying disorder. Other predisposing conditions include pulmonary and cardiac diseases, DM, hypokalemia, and hypomagnesemia.

How should you manage this patient?

β-blockers or CCBs can help slow the heart rate. The primary treatment, however, is to correct the underlying cause.

> Cardioversion does not help convert MAT to normal sinus rhythm.

> **Wandering pacemaker**: Pacemaker activity wanders from SA node to nearby automaticity foci. Like MAT, p waves are of different shapes. Unlike MAT, heart rate is 60 to 100 beats per minute. No specific therapy is required.
> **Multifocal atrial bradycardia**: P waves are of different shapes but heart rate is <60 beats per minute. Patients may need a pacemaker if the rhythm is persistent and symptomatic.

CASE 2–14 REGULAR NARROW COMPLEX TACHYCARDIA

A 30-year-old man presents with palpitations and lightheadedness. An EKG is performed (see Fig. 2-15).

What is the abnormal rhythm?

The patient has a supraventricular tachycardia, which occurs when an irritable focus in the atria or the AV node takes over pacemaking activity, leading to a fast rate but regular rhythm. The narrow QRS complex indicates that the impulse originates above the His bundle. The lack of any discernible p waves indicates that the irritable focus is in the AV node or that the p waves are buried within the QRS complex (see Fig. 2-16).

What are the mechanisms of SVT?

1. **Atrioventricular nodal re-entrant tachycardia** (**AVNRT**): An atrial re-entry circuit that involves the AV node causes the arrhythmia. This is the most common mechanism of SVT, and is the likely cause of SVT in this patient.
2. **AV re-entrant tachycardia** (**AVRT**): Re-entry circuit uses a bypass tract that circumvents the AV node. The cause of this rhythm is Wolf-Parkinson-White syndrome, a condition in which ventricular pre-excitation produces a delta wave right before the QRS complex. The PR interval appears shorter because of this delta wave (see Fig. 2-17).

> Wolf-Parkinson-White syndrome can also cause atrial fibrillation and flutter. Avoid digoxin in Wolf-Parkinson-White syndrome because it can accelerate conduction through the AV node.

How should you manage this arrhythmia?

If the patient is unstable, perform synchronized cardioversion. Otherwise, the first step is carotid sinus massage, alone or in conjunction with the valsalva maneuver. If these vagal

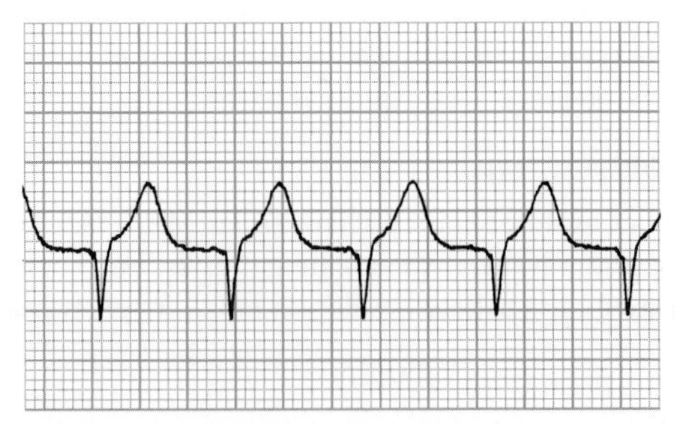

FIGURE 2–15 EKG showing supraventricular tachycardia. From Spellberg B, Ayala C. *Boards and Wards*, 3rd ed. Lippincott Williams & Wilkins, 2007.

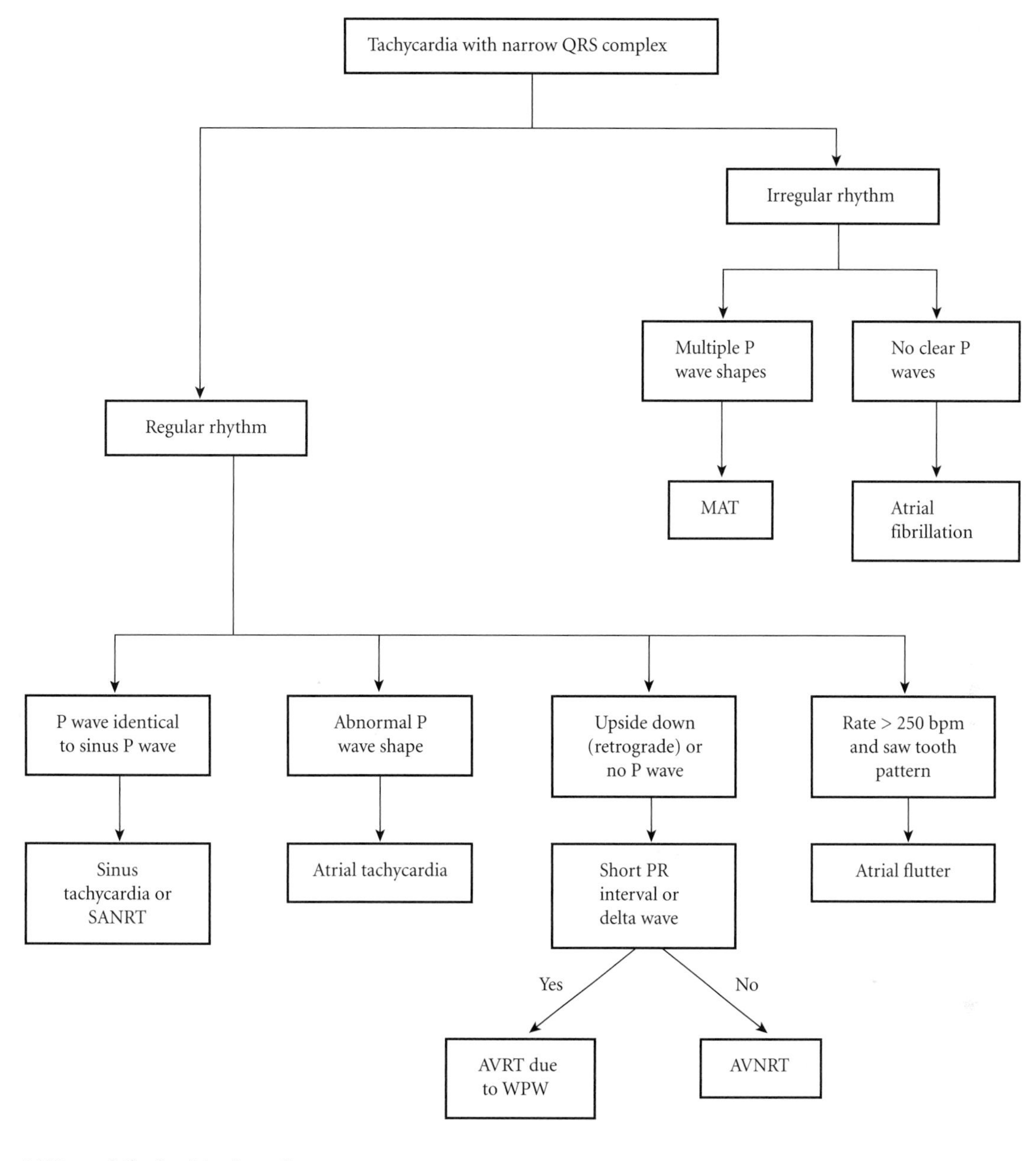

MAT = multifocal atrial tachycardia
AVNRT = AV nodal re-entrant tachycardia
AVRT = AV re-entrant tachycardia
WPW = Wolf-Parkinson-White syndrome
SANRT = SA node re-entrant tachycardia

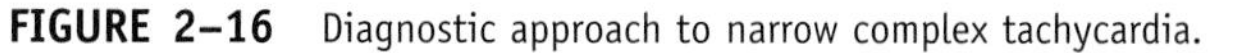

FIGURE 2–16 Diagnostic approach to narrow complex tachycardia.

maneuvers are not successful, administer adenosine. Intravenous verapimil, diltiazem, and β-blockers are second-line agents if the rhythm persists despite two doses of adenosine.

No chronic therapy is required for short-lived, well-tolerated attacks that respond to vagal maneuvers. Others require either long-term anti-arrhythmia drugs or radiofrequency ablation of the accessory tract.

SVT with wide QRS complexes: These can occur as a result of delayed conduction in the left or right bundle branch block. Unless you are sure this is the case, treat a wide QRS complex tachycardia as a VT. Verapimil can cause hemodynamic compromise when administered to a patient with VT.

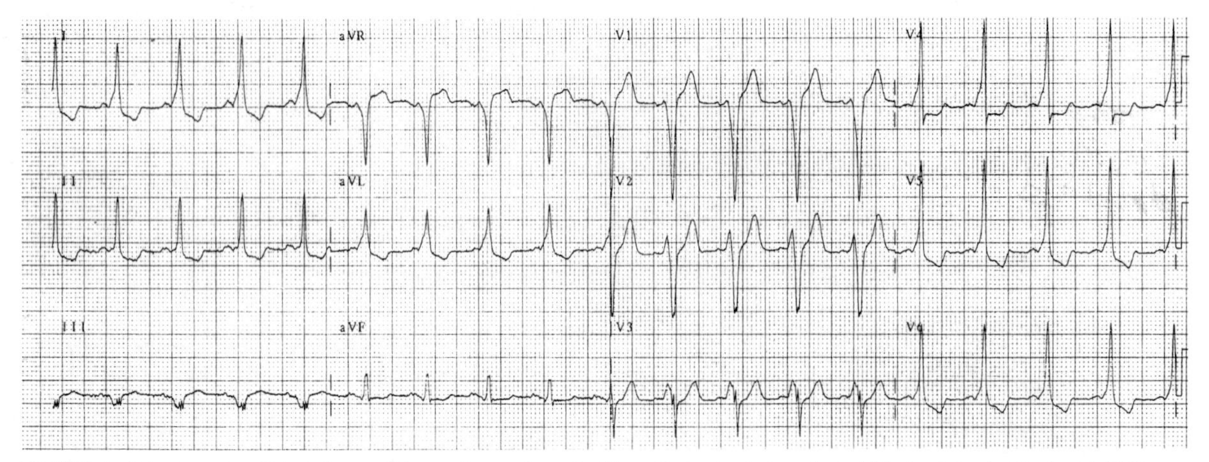

FIGURE 2–17 EKG of Wolf-Parksinson-White syndrome. From Spellberg B, Ayala C. *Boards and Wards*, 3rd ed. Lippincott Williams & Wilkins, 2007.

Alternative 2.14.1

A 75-year-old man with known CHF presents to the emergency department with a 2-hour history of palpitations and light-headedness. An EKG is obtained (see Fig. 2-18).

What is the abnormal rhythm?

The patient's EKG shows atrial flutter. One irritable atrial focus fires at a rate of 250 to 350 beats per minute, giving rise to the identical p waves in a "saw-tooth" pattern. The AV node only allows one out of every two to three atrial depolarizations to conduct to the ventricles (2:1 block or 3:1 block), leading to a regular, narrow QRS complex.

What conditions predispose to atrial flutter?

Predisposing factors for atrial flutter are similar to atrial fibrillation. Heart failure and COPD are the most common underlying causes. Atrial flutter in the absence of any predisposing cause (lone atrial flutter) is uncommon.

How is atrial flutter treated?

Management is similar to atrial fibrillation.

CASE 2–15 SUDDEN CARDIAC ARREST

A 69-year-old woman collapses in the local mall. She does not respond when a nurse who happens to be nearby asks if she can hear her.

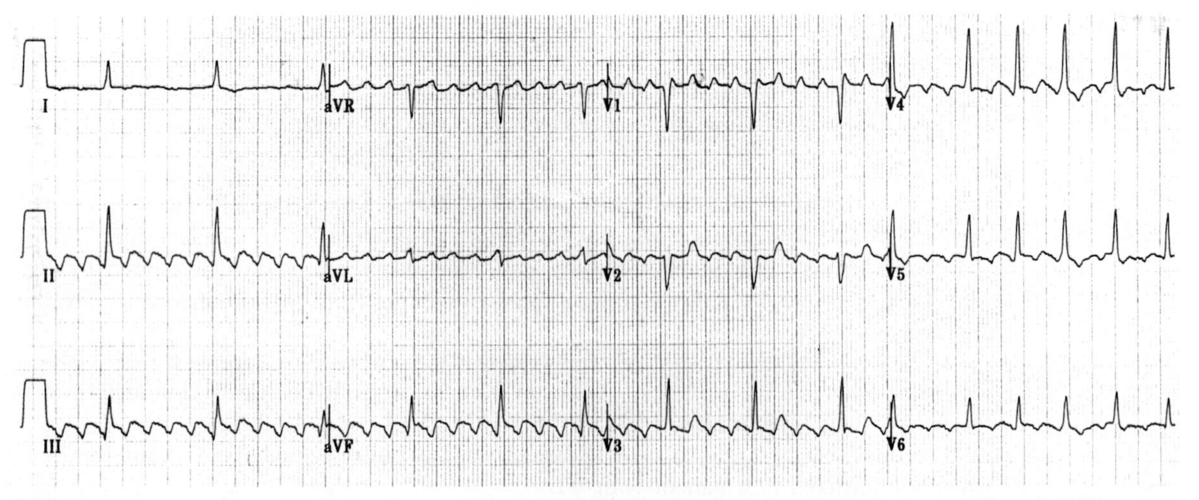

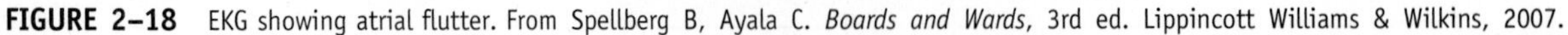

FIGURE 2–18 EKG showing atrial flutter. From Spellberg B, Ayala C. *Boards and Wards*, 3rd ed. Lippincott Williams & Wilkins, 2007.

What are the initial steps in management?

The initial step in an unresponsive patient is to assess whether the patient is breathing and has a pulse. Absent respirations or palpable pulses indicate cardiac arrest (abrupt cessation of normal circulation as a result of failure of the heart to contract effectively). The general sequence for cardiopulmonary resuscitation (CPR) is as follows:

1. Call for help: Ask someone to call 9-1-1 and to fetch an automated external defibrillator if available.
2. Airway and breathing: Open the patient's airway using the head tilt/chin lift maneuver. Then look, listen, and feel for breathing. If the patient is not breathing, deliver two breaths that make the patient's chest rise.
3. Circulation: Check for a carotid pulse. If no pulse is felt within 10 seconds, initiate chest compressions at a rate of 100 per minute. Chest compressions should compress the sternum at least 1.5 to 2 inches and allow for complete recoil.
4. Reassess: After 30 compressions, reassess breathing. If the patient is not breathing, deliver two breaths, and then reassess pulse. If there is no pulse, deliver 30 compressions. Continue this cycle of compression and ventilation until an automated external defibrillator or paramedics arrive.

> Lay persons performing CPR are advised not to check for a carotid pulse (unreliable) and instead proceed directly to chest compressions if the patient is unresponsive. Healthcare workers, however, should check for a pulse.

The patient does not have any signs of breathing or a pulse. There is no automated external defibrillator in the mall. The patient receives 30 cycles of compressions and ventilations before the paramedics arrive. The cardiac monitor shows an abnormal rhythm (see Fig. 2-19). What arrhythmia does the patient have?

The rhythm on the monitor is VT. VT is characterized by a succession of wide QRS complexes at a rate >100 beats per minute. VT that lasts >30 seconds is called sustained VT. Sustained VT is a life-threatening arrhythmia that can progress to ventricular fibrillation and sudden cardiac death if left untreated.

> **Ventricular fibrillation**: Multiple ventricular foci fire rapidly, which leads to chaotic quivering of the ventricles but no cardiac output. Most common rhythm in witnessed cardiac arrest.

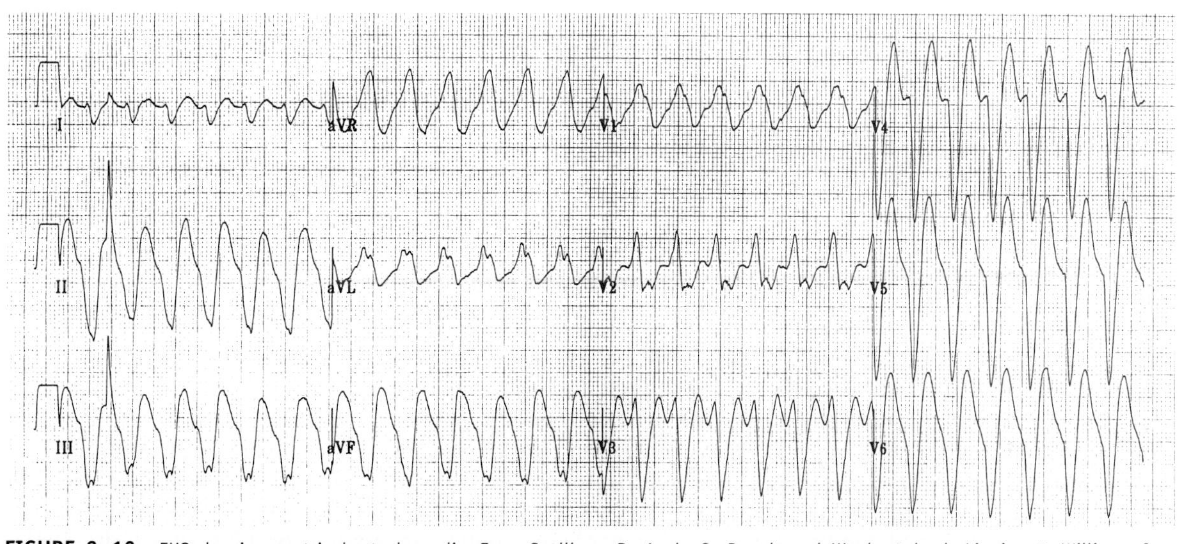

FIGURE 2–19 EKG showing ventricular tachycardia. From Spellberg B, Ayala C. *Boards and Wards*, 3rd ed. Lippincott Williams & Wilkins, 2007.

Monomorphic VT: All QRS complexes are identical.
Polymorphic VT: QRS complexes are different.

Fusion beat: Occasionally during VT, a p wave from the atria depolarizes a ventricle and produces a narrow QRS complex. This "fusion" beat confirms that the rhythm is VT and not wide-complex SVT.

What is the next step in management?

The most important step for an unresponsive patient in ventricular fibrillation or pulseless VT is defibrillation. Defibrillation is preferred to synchronized cardioversion because syncing the stimulus to the QRS complex would waste valuable time. Resume CPR soon after defibrillation for 2 minutes and then reassess breathing, pulse and rhythm (see Fig. 2-20).

Many steps are performed at the same time during a cardiac arrest. IV placement and basic labs are usually obtained while CPR is being performed.

What defibrillation current is recommended for ventricular fibrillation or pulseless VT?

Use 360 J if the defibrillator is monophasic or 200 J if the defibrillator is biphasic (mnemonic: "***Give TWO hundred joules with a BIphasic defibrillator.***").

Make sure nobody is in contact with the patient during defibrillation.

Two minutes later, the patient still does not have a pulse. An abnormal rhythm is seen on the cardiac monitor (see Fig. 2-21). What is the next step in management?

The rhythm on the monitor is ventricular fibrillation. Treatment for ventricular fibrillation is identical to treatment for pulseless VT. The next step is to deliver another defibrillation shock using the same current. Also consider IV epinephrine or vasopressin. After the shock, resume CPR immediately for 2 minutes and then reassess (see Fig. 2-20).

Epinephrine: Dose is 1 mg; can re-administer every 3 to 5 minutes.
Vasopressin: Dose is 40 units; can only administer once.

The patient receives another shock, and then CPR is resumed. She receives a dose of vasopressin once IV access is established. Two minutes later, the rhythm on the monitor still indicates ventricular fibrillation. What is the next step in management?

Defibrillate again and then resume CPR immediately. Also, consider an anti-arrhythmic drug such as amiodarone or lidocaine (amiodarone preferred before lidocaine).

If the patient recovers a pulse, consider an IV infusion of the anti-arrhythmic that helped break the *ventricular tachycardia/fibrillation* arrest during the recover period.

Two minutes later, the rhythm on the monitor indicates sinus tachycardia. The patient still does not have a pulse. What is the next step in management?

Any rhythm that is not VT or *ventricular fibrillation* in an unresponsive patient without a pulse is termed pulseless electrical activity (PEA). In PEA, the heart may produce adequate depolarizations, but the cardiac muscle is unable to respond to the electrical stimuli. Electric current plays no role in the management of PEA. The next step in the patient with tachycardia and PEA is epinephrine or vasopressin and continued CPR (see Fig. 2-20). Also, begin to search for the underlying reversible causes of PEA.

PEA and bradycardia: Atropine is another option in asystole or PEA with heart rate <60 beats per minute.

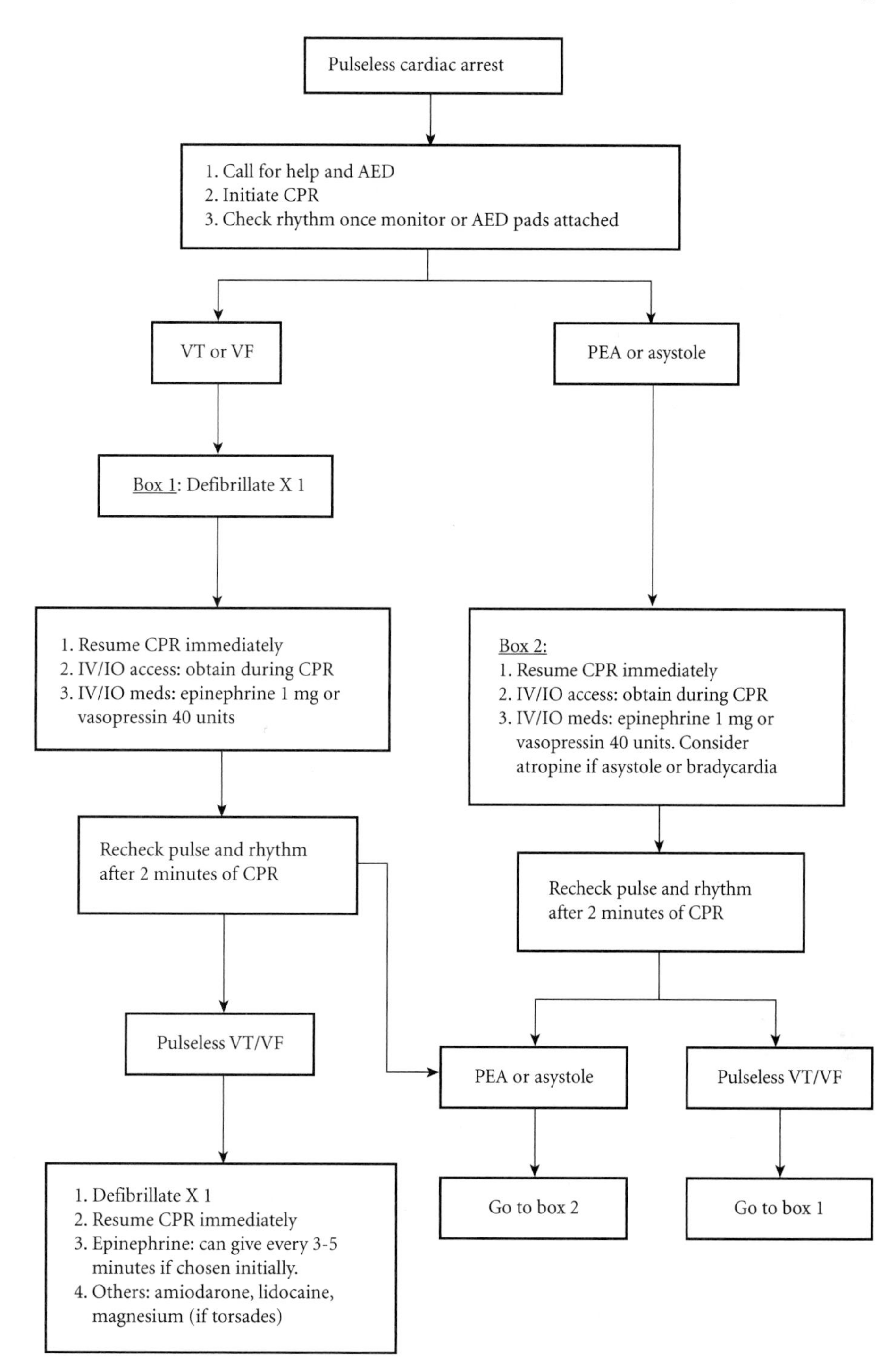

IV access is 1st line; intraosseous access (IO) is 2nd line.

FIGURE 2–20 Advanced Cardiac Life Support guidelines for management of pulseless cardiac arrest.

What are the underlying reversible causes of PEA?

Remember the six H's and the four T's:

1. **H**ypovolemia: Treat with volume infusion.
2. **H**ypoxia: Treat with oxygenation.
3. **H**ydrogen ions (acidosis): Treat with bicarbonate.
4. **H**yperkalemia: Treat with calcium gluconate, bicarbonate, and insulin.

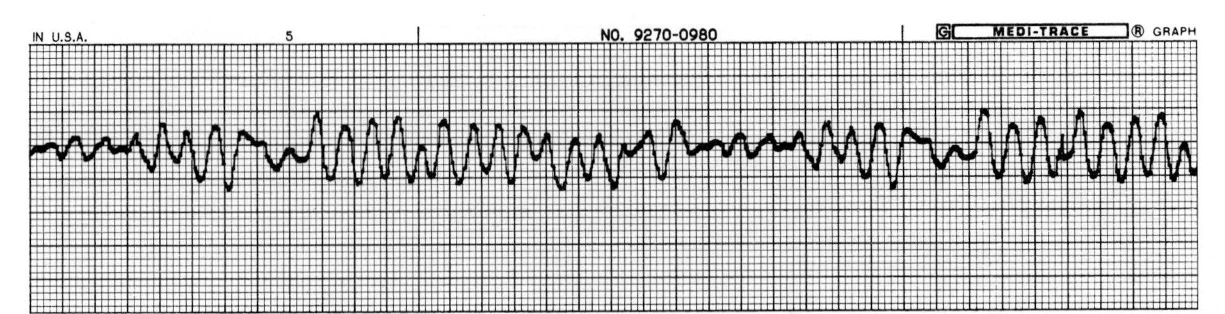

FIGURE 2–21 EKG showing ventricular fibrillation. From Smeltzer SC, Bare BG. *Texbook of Medical-Surgical Nursing*, 9th ed. Lippincott Williams & Wilkins, 2000.

5. **H**ypokalemia: Treat with potassium.
6. **H**ypothermia: Treat by keeping the patient warm.
7. **T**amponade: Treat with pericardiocentesis.
8. **T**ension pneumothorax: Treat with needle decompression and tube thoracostomy.
9. **T**hrombosis (cardiac thrombosis or MI, and pulmonary thrombosis caused by PEA)
10. **T**ablets (medications or drugs)

After 10 minutes of resuscitation, the monitor shows a flat line. What is the next step?

A flat line on the monitor is called asystole. Treatment of asystole is identical to PEA. Stop resuscitation efforts if asystole persists despite therapy. Only 1% to 2% of patients in asystole survive despite adequate resuscitation.

"Do not shock **SPAM**": Tachyarrhythmias with no role for cardioversion or defibrillation are **S**inus tachycardia, **P**EA, **A**systole, and **M**AT.

Alternative 2.15.2

A 68-year-old woman is admitted to the cardiac care unit after revascularization of an anterior STEMI. On day three, she is found unresponsive. Breath sounds are weak and pulses are absent. An abnormal rhythm is seen on the cardiac monitor (see Fig. 2-22).

What is abnormal rhythm?

The rhythm on the monitor is Torsades des pointes. Torsades is a specific type of polymorphic VT in which the QRS complexes change constantly such that the electrical activity looks like it has been twisted into a helix. QT interval is prolonged. This abnormal rhythm is more common in women and patients with underlying heart, liver, or kidney disease. Congenital long QT syndrome is also a risk factor.

What is the next step in management?

This patient is in cardiac arrest, so promptly defibrillate. The first-line medication for Torsades des pointes is IV magnesium sulfate. If IV magnesium is not successful, initiate

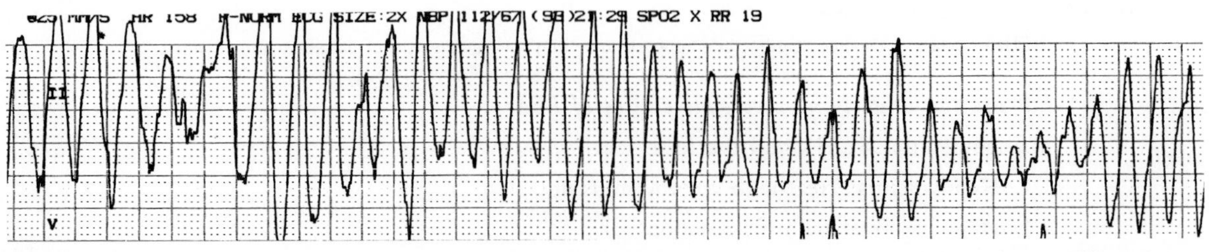

FIGURE 2–22 EKG showing torsades de pointes. From Spellberg B, Ayala C. *Boards and Wards*, 3rd ed. Lippincott Williams & Wilkins, 2007.

temporary overdrive pacing. When the rhythm is corrected, identify and remove precipitating causes.

> It is essential to distinguish Torsades from polymorphic VT because magnesium can worsen polymorphic VT.

What are common precipitating causes of Torsades des pointes?

1. **Medications**: five **Anti's** (tricyclic **Anti**depressants, **Anti**cholinergics, macrolide **Anti**biotics like erythromycin, **Anti**-arrhythmics, and nonsedating **Anti**histamines).
2. **Electrolyte abnormalities**: particularly hypokalemia and hypomagnesemia.

CASE 2–16 VT IN A STABLE PATIENT

A 47-year-old man is admitted to the hospital for acute pancreatitis. He also complains of palpitations. He does not have any history of CAD or CAD risk factors. EKG is normal, and the patient is placed on a cardiac monitor. The next day, the telemetry nurse mentions that he had five nonconsecutive beats of VT over the course of 30 seconds. Vital signs are normal.

How should you manage the abnormal rhythm?

Nonsustained VT (NSVT) is defined as three to five consecutive ventricular impulses or ≤ 6 ventricular impulses over the course of 30 seconds. Emergent treatment is not necessary for nonsustained VT. Obtain an echocardiogram and stress test on an elective basis to evaluate for CAD. Consider a β-blocker in all patients with nonsustained VT to prevent sudden cardiac death. Also consider ICD placement in patients with evidence of CAD.

> **Torsades in a stable patient**: Defibrillation is not required; treat with IV magnesium.

How would management differ if the stable patient had sustained VT?

Treat stable sustained VT with pharmacological or synchronized electrical cardioversion. Because the situation is not emergent, avoid defibrillation, which poses a risk of shocking the heart during the vulnerable period after the QRS. Consider an anti-arrhythmic drug such as amiodarone if the patient continues to experience symptomatic or recurrent VT despite cardioversion.

CASE 2–17 HYPOTENSION, TACHYCARDIA, AND ALTERED MENTAL STATUS (SHOCK)

A 25-year-old man is stung by a swarm of bees. His girlfriend brings him to the emergency department 25 minutes later. He complains of dyspnea and pruritis. He is oriented to person but not to place and time. His lips are swollen, and his skin is warm and flushed. Auscultation of the lungs reveals bilateral wheezes. Vital signs are temperature 37°C, blood pressure 90/60, respirations 25/minute, and pulse 130 bpm. Oxygen saturation is 90%. The attending mentions that the patient is in "shock."

What is shock?

Shock is a state of decreased tissue perfusion, which leads to decreased tissue oxygenation. Tissue hypoxia disrupts normal biochemical processes and causes end-organ failure and death unless treated promptly.

What are the three general mechanisms of shock?

1. **Hypovolemic shock**: Decreased blood volume → decreased preload → decreased cardiac output → decreased tissue perfusion.
2. **Distributive shock**: Decreased systemic vascular resistance (SVR) → decreased tissue perfusion.
3. **Cardiogenic shock**: Decreased heart muscle contractility → decreased cardiac output → decreased tissue perfusion.

What are the different sub-types of distributive shock?

1. Septic shock: Infection → massive inflammatory response → increased capillary permeability and vasodilation → decreased SVR.
2. Anaphylactic shock: Exposure to allergen → massive inflammatory response → increased capillary permeability and vasodilation → decreased SVR.
3. Neurogenic shock: central nervous system or spinal cord injury → decreased sympathetic output → vasodilation → decreased SVR.
4. Addison crisis and myxedema coma (see Chapter 8: Endocrinology).

What are the clinical features of shock?

The earliest stage is termed "warm" shock. During this period, compensatory mechanisms are able to compensate for decreased perfusion. Tachycardia is usually the earliest sign of shock. As the compensatory mechanisms are overwhelmed, patients develop four major features as a result of end-organ failure: marked hypotension (<90/40 mm Hg), lactic acidosis, oliguria (urine output <0.5 mg/kg per hour), and altered mental status.

> **Cardiogenic and hypovolemic shock**: Skin is cool and clammy because of decreased cardiac output.
> **Distributive shock**: Skin is warm and flushed because of vasodilation; however, in late-stage sepsis, the skin is cool and clammy.

Is this patient in shock? If so, what type of shock is he suffering from?

Marked hypotension, tachycardia, and altered mental status all indicate that this patient is in shock. Warm and flushed skin, angioedema, and dyspnea after a bee sting most likely indicates anaphylactic shock. Dyspnea commonly occurs in anaphylactic shock as a result of bronchoconstriction and laryngeal edema. Patients usually develop symptoms within minutes to hours of exposure.

> **Most common causes of anaphylactic shock (in descending order)**: insect bites, food allergy (especially to fish and nuts), drug reactions (especially to penicillins and NSAIDs), radiocontrast dyes, blood products, and latex.

What are the next steps in the management of this patient?

1. **ABCs** (Airway, Breathing, and Circulation): Administer 100% oxygen by facemask. Consider elective intubation in this patient with dyspnea and wheezing because laryngeal edema can make it difficult to secure the airway later. Establish IV access with two large-bore needles in each arm.
2. **Epinephrine**: Administer intramuscular epinephrine while securing ABCs. There are no contraindications to epinephrine in the setting of anaphylactic shock.
3. **Normal saline**: Attempt to correct hypotension with a 1- to 2-L rapid bolus if the patient does not respond to the first dose of intramuscular epinephrine.
4. **IV epinephrine**: Administer if the patient does not respond to intramuscular epinephrine and normal saline.
5. **Vasopressors**: Consider norepinephrine, dopamine, or phenylephrine if hypotension is refractory to fluids and epinephrine.
6. **IV antihistamines and inhaled albuterol**: Administered to all patients in anaphylactic shock; these drugs are not as vital as epinephrine.

> **Corticosteroids** are commonly administered to prevent delayed reactions; clinical trials have not demonstrated improved outcomes with this practice.

The patient responds to 100% oxygen, intramuscular epinephrine, normal saline, IV antihistamines, and inhaled albuterol. He is now breathing without any difficulties, and his blood pressure is 120/80. What discharge instructions should you give him?

Monitor the patient for at least 8 hours for a recurrence before discharge. Provide the patient with an epinephrine auto-injector pen and instruct him to use it if similar symptoms recur. Consider referring the patient to an allergy specialist.

Alternative 2.17.1

A 55-year-old man presents with fever and malaise. Skin is warm and flushed. Vital signs are temperature 39°C, blood pressure 69/40, pulse 125 bpm, respirations 25/minute.

What is the likely cause of shock in this patient?

Suspect an infectious cause of shock in this patient with fever (sepsis). Ninety percent of septic patients have fever. The other 10% of patients present with hypothermia (poor prognostic sign).

How is sepsis classified?

There is a clinical continuum that ranges from systemic inflammatory response syndrome to multiple-organ dysfunction syndrome:

1. Systemic inflammatory response syndrome: More than two of the following: fever or hypothermia, tachypnea, tachycardia, or leukocytosis.
2. Sepsis: systemic inflammatory response syndrome plus positive blood culture
3. Severe sepsis: sepsis plus hypotension
4. Septic shock: severe sepsis unresponsive to fluid resuscitation
5. Multiple-organ dysfunction syndrome: multi-organ failure

What are the initial steps in management of this patient with severe sepsis?

1. ABCs: Administer 100% oxygen and intubate if necessary. Establish IV access, preferably via a large central vein (internal jugular, subclavian, or femoral), and rapidly infuse a 1- to 2-L bolus of normal saline.
2. Cultures and antibiotics: Send specimens of blood and urine for Gram stain and culture. Then administer empiric IV antibiotics.
3. Arterial line: Allows healthcare staff to constantly monitor blood pressure and also provides easy access for frequent blood sampling.

> **Goals of initial resuscitation**: CVP 8 to 12 mm Hg, mean arterial pressure (MAP) ≥65 mm Hg, mixed venous oxygen ≥70%, and urine output ≥0.5 ml/kg per hour.

> **MAP** is the average arterial pressure during a single cardiac cycle; this is a better approximation of perfusion pressure than blood pressure. MAP > 60 is usually sufficient to sustain all organs of the body.

What antibiotics should you use?

Typical empiric coverage for severe sepsis/septic shock includes vancomycin for Gram-positive coverage and either a β-lactam/β-lactamase inhibitor such as piperacillin-tazobactam, a third- or fourth-generation cephalosporin such as ceftriaxone, or a carbapenem such as imipenem for Gram-negative coverage. If a causative microbe is identified later by Gram stain and culture, tailor antibiotics to the specific organism.

One hour later, blood pressure is 85/60 despite 2 L of normal saline. CVP is 3 mm Hg. What is the next step in management of the hypotension?

Continue to administer normal saline boluses until CVP is 8 to 12 mm Hg. Patients with severe sepsis often need 4 to 12 L of normal saline.

Peripheral edema: This is an expected complication of massive fluid resuscitation. Its presence does not guide fluid resuscitation or imply fluid overload.
Pulmonary edema: New lung crackles on auscultation or radiographic findings of pulmonary edema indicate the patient is fluid overloaded.

The patient receives 8 L of normal saline. CVP is 10 mm Hg, but 8 hours later MAP is still 54 mm Hg. What is the next step in management?

If hypotension persists despite adequate fluid resuscitation or the patient develops pulmonary edema, initiate vasopressors. Start with norepinephrine or dopamine, then use vasopressin and finally phenylephrine. Consider recombinant protein C (Xigris) if hypotension persists despite fluids and vasopressors. Recombinant protein C may improve mortality in septic shock, but it is extremely expensive.

Twenty-four hours later, MAP rises to 70 mm Hg with norepinephrine and vasopressin. Mixed venous oxygen saturation is 60%. Arterial lactate has risen from 2 to 4 mg/dL. What is the next step in management?

Arterial lactate is currently the most useful global measure of tissue perfusion. A rising lactate level and low mixed venous saturation indicates inadequate tissue perfusion despite normal CVP and MAP. Consider red blood cell transfusion at this stage.

What is the prognosis of septic shock?

Septic shock is the most common cause of death in the ICU. The mortality from septic shock is >40 %.

What are colloids and crystalloids?

Crystalloids (normal saline or lactated ringers) and colloids (albumin or hetastarch) are equally effective as resuscitation fluids. Because a greater proportion of colloids remain in the intravascular space, smaller quantities are required compared to crystalloids. Crystalloids are used far more frequently because they are less expensive, and there is some concern that colloids can harm critically ill patients.

Alternative 2.17.2

The patient is a 38-year-old woman with ovarian cancer who completed a course of taxol and carboplatin 7 days ago. She presents with a 7-day history of fatigue, poor appetite, and intractable vomiting. She did not take the ondansetron she was prescribed to control nausea after discharge from the hospital after chemotherapy because she lost the prescription. She has also had watery diarrhea for the last 3 days. On physical examination, she is oriented to person but not to place and time. Skin is cool and clammy. Vital signs are temperature 37°C, blood pressure 70/50, pulse 130 bpm, and respirations 25/minute. Oxygen saturation is 98% on room air.

What is the likely cause of shock in this patient?

The most likely cause in this patient with intractable vomiting and diarrhea is hypovolemic shock. Cisplatin and carboplatin tend to cause nausea in >90% of patients who do not receive anti-emetics.

What are the causes of hypovolemic shock?

Hypovolemic shock can result from hemorrhage (e.g., trauma, GI bleeding, hemorrhagic pancreatitis, etc.) or fluid loss (diarrhea, vomiting, burns, third spacing).

Third spacing: fluid accumulation outside the intravascular space (ascites, peritonitis, etc.).

How is hypovolemic shock treated?

Administer a 1- to 2-L bolus of normal saline. Continue to infuse boluses of normal saline to correct the fluid deficit. If the patient does not respond promptly, consider placing an arterial line to continuously monitor blood pressure. In patients with hypovolemic shock as a result of blood loss, fluid replacement should include blood products.

> Vasopressors are not helpful in hypovolemic shock because the mechanism does not involve vasodilation.

Alternative 2.17.3

The patient is a 65-year-old man who is admitted to the hospital after PCI for an anterior STEMI. Fifteen hours later, blood pressure is 90/60, pulse is 120 bpm, respirations are 25/minute, and oxygen saturation is 94%. Skin is cool and clammy, and 14 cm of JVD is present. New crackles are appreciated in both lung bases. Urine output is 0.2 mg/kg per hour.

What is the likely cause of shock?

The setting and clinical manifestations indicate that this patient is in cardiogenic shock. LV failure after MI is the most common cause of cardiogenic shock. The presence of elevated JVD distinguishes cardiogenic shock clinically from other types of shock. Two thirds of patients also have pulmonary edema.

What are the next steps in management?

1. ABCs: Place the patient on 100% oxygen. Intubation is not necessary at this time because oxygen saturation is 98% on room air.
2. Echocardiography helps determine the cause of cardiogenic shock (pump failure as a result of LV failure versus reinfarction versus mechanical complications).
3. Treat the underlying cause promptly once identified.

Echocardiography detects findings consistent with LV failure. There is no evidence of tamponade or other mechanical complications. What are the next steps in management?

1. Initiate vasopressors: Dopamine is the first-line agent; if hypotension persists, add norepinephrine and phenylephrine.
2. Consider a Swan-Ganz catheter and an intra-arterial catheter when the patient is stabilized for hemodynamic assessment to guide therapy.

> Dobutamine in combination with a vasodilator like nitroprusside or nitroglycerin is an option for patients in cardiogenic shock who are not hypotensive.

What is a Swan-Ganz catheter? What are the Swan-Ganz findings in different types of shock?

Swan-Ganz or pulmonary artery catheters are inserted into the right atrium and pulmonary artery. They record pulmonary capillary wedge pressure (PCWP), which is the pressure recorded when a balloon is inflated in a branch of the pulmonary artery. PCWP is a surrogate measure of left atrial pressure. The catheter also calculates hemodynamic parameters such as cardiac output and systemic vascular resistance using a thermistor that measures temperature change when warm venous blood mixes with cold injected fluid. Finally, Swan-Ganz catheters allow sampling of mixed venous blood. Swan-Ganz measurements help guide management in cardiogenic shock, and also help determine the cause of shock when unclear (Table 2-25).

> Despite the potential advantages, studies have not shown improved patient outcomes with Swan-Ganz catheterization.

PCWP is 21 mm Hg (normal 6 to 12). Hypotension, elevated PCWP, and other signs of shock persist despite vasopressors. Is there any other treatment for patients with refractory cardiogenic shock?

TABLE 2–25 Hemodynamic Parameters During Swan-Ganz Catheterization

Category of Shock	CO[a]	SVR	PCWP[b]	SVO_2
Hypovolemic	↓	↑	↓	↓
Cardiogenic	↓	↑	↑	↓
Distributive	↑	↓	↓	↓

Abbreviations: CO, cardiac output; PCWP, pulmonary capillary wedge pressure; SVO_2, systemic venous oxygen saturation; SVR, systemic vascular resistance.
[a] Normal CO = 4 to 8 mm Hg.
[b] Normal PCWP = 6 to 12 mm Hg.

Consider using an intra-aortic balloon pump. This mechanical device sits on the aorta and deflates just before systole (to reduce afterload) and inflates at the onset of diastole (to increase diastolic pressure). This counterpulsation helps increase cardiac output.

Hypovolemic shock: Treatment is ABCs and normal saline; give blood products if hypovolemia is caused by hemorrhage.
Septic shock: Treatment is ABCs, normal saline, and antibiotics; second-line treatment is vasopressors and recombinant protein C.
Anaphylactic shock: Treatment is ABCs, epinephrine, and normal saline; second-line treatment is vasopressors. All patients also get antihistamines and albuterol.
Cardiogenic shock: Treatment is ABCs, correct underlying cause, vasopressors, careful with fluids if LV pressure is increased.

CASE 2–18 ACUTE UNILATERAL LEG SWELLING AND TENDERNESS

A 40-year-old woman presents with a 10-hour history of gradually increasing pain and swelling in her left calf. There is no history of trauma to the leg. Past medical history is unremarkable. She started taking oral contraceptive pills (OCP) 1 week ago. Her left calf is erythematous, warm and tender to palpation, and is 4 cm thicker than the right calf. Vital signs are normal. Pulses are 2+, and there is 2+ lower extremity pitting edema.

What is the most concerning possibility at this time?

Acute onset of swelling >3 cm, erythema, warmth, and tenderness of a lower extremity should always raise suspicion for deep venous thrombosis (DVT), particularly in this patient with a history of OCP use. Other risk factors for DVT (mnemonic: "***SHEA stadium***") include:

Stasis: Prolonged bed rest, immobility, CHF

Hypercoagulability: Inherited thrombophilia, OCPs, pregnancy, malignancy

Endothelial injury: Trauma, recent surgery

Age: >60 years

The most common cause of acute unilateral leg swelling and tenderness is calf muscle injury. Patients usually recall an episode of lower extremity trauma.

Half the patients with DVT have no clinical findings. Half the patients with classic signs of DVT do not actually have DVT.

What is the next step in diagnosis?

Signs and symptoms of DVT are nonspecific, so confirm the diagnosis noninvasively using compression ultrasound of the lower extremity. Lack of compressibility is sensitive and specific for DVT.

Impedance plethysmography is an alternative, noninvasive test for DVT. Although cumbersome and not widely available, it is preferred over compression ultrasound in patients with recurrent DVT. The test uses electrodes to measure opposition to flow of electric current when a thigh cuff is inflated, which helps estimate blood flow.

Ultrasound detects DVT in the femoral and popliteal vein. What is the next step?

Lower extremity DVT is divided into calf vein thrombosis and proximal (thigh vein) thrombosis. Calf vein thrombosis is not clinically significant. On the other hand, proximal thrombi carry a high risk of breaking off emboli that can migrate to the pulmonary artery (pulmonary embolism). The next step is to discontinue OCPs and initiate anticoagulation with unfractionated or low molecular weight heparin and warfarin. Discontinue heparin on day five if the INR is between 2.0 and 3.0 (therapeutic range for warfarin). Continue warfarin for at least 3 months (Table 2-26).

If compression ultrasound is negative but there is a high clinical suspicion for DVT, repeat the test 5 to 7 days later.

Alternative 2.18.1

A 70-year-old man presents with a 12-hour history of unilateral leg swelling. He denies any dyspnea, chest pain, cough, or hemoptysis. He has a 50-year history of smoking one to two packs of cigarettes a day. He does not have any other identifiable risk factors for DVT. Compression ultrasound detects DVT in the right lower extremity.

What additional diagnostic tests are appropriate for this patient?

Occult neoplasm is often the cause of DVT in patients with no known risk factors (idiopathic DVT). However, it is not cost-effective to perform an extensive search for cancer in all patients with idiopathic DVT. Limit cancer screening to a careful history and physical examination that includes digital rectal exam, fecal occult blood testing, and pelvic examination in women. Routine laboratory testing in such patients should include a complete blood count, serum electrolytes, liver function tests, urinalysis, CXR, and, in men $\geq$50, prostate-specific antigen.

Alternative 2.18.2

A 25-year-old man presents with right lower extremity swelling. He has a history of left lower extremity DVT 10 years ago that was treated with a 6-month course of warfarin. His father died of a pulmonary embolism (PE) at the age of 45. Compression ultrasound demonstrates a thrombus in the right popliteal and femoral veins. He has no known risk factors for DVT.

What is the most likely underlying cause for this patient's recurring DVT?

Suspect an inherited thrombophilia in a young patient with recurrent DVT or PE and a positive family history of thromboembolism. Inherited thrombophilia is a genetic tendency to

TABLE 2–26 Duration of Anticoagulation for DVT

Patient Characteristics	Anticoagulation Period
Isolated symptomatic calf vein DVT	6–12 weeks
First episode in a patient with a reversible risk factor	3 months
First idiopathic episode	6–12 months
DVT due to malignancy	12 months to lifelong
Recurrent episodes	Lifelong
Inherited thrombophilia	Lifelong

Abbreviation: DVT, deep venous thrombosis.

develop DVT. Factor V Leiden is the most common cause of the syndrome accounting for 40% to 50% of cases. Other inherited thrombophilias are prothrombin gene mutation, deficiencies in protein S, protein C, antithrombin III (AT III), and the dysfibrinogenemias.

Inherited thrombophilia can cause recurrent unexplained fetal loss.

AT III deficiency: Heparin's mechanism involves activation of AT III, so patients with AT III deficiency do not respond appropriately to heparin anticoagulation.

Alternative 2.18.3

The patient is a 65-year-old man. He presents with tenderness, pain, and erythema along a vein on his right calf extending up to his thigh. There is a palpable, nodular cord with warmth and erythema. Compression ultrasound of the lower extremity is negative for the presence of DVT.

What is the most likely diagnosis?

This patient has signs and symptoms of superficial phlebitis (SP). A patient with SP can also have DVT because hypercoagulable states are predisposing factors for both. Rule out DVT in patients with SP extending above the knee. SP localized below the knee does not require further evaluation. Treatment of SP is supportive (heat, elevation, NSAIDs, and compression stockings).

Two weeks later, the patient develops high fever and purulent drainage at the site of the SP. What is the next step in management?

The patient has developed septic thrombophlebitis. The next step in management is antibiotics and surgical exploration.

Alternative 2.18.4

A 58-year-old man presents with pain in his right knee and calf. The pain began as tightness behind his right knee. He denies dyspnea or chest pain. He has a long history of osteoarthritis. There is a small hematoma over the medial malleolus. Effusions are seen in both knees. Vitals signs are normal.

What diagnosis is most likely?

This patient has a ruptured popliteal cyst (Baker's cyst). Popliteal cysts result from posterior herniation of a tense knee effusion in patients with underlying joint disease. The cyst causes a feeling of pressure or fullness behind the knee. Rupture of this cyst into the posterior calf muscles leads to pain and edema below the knee. The presence of a hematoma over the medial malleolus (crescent sign) distinguishes it from DVT and SP. Treatment is supportive (heat, elevation, NSAIDs, and compression stockings).

Alternative 2.18.5

A 60-year man with a history of chronic atrial fibrillation presents to the emergency department with severe pain in the left calf and foot that began suddenly 2 hours ago. There is no history of any prior pathology involving the legs. On physical examination, the extremity is pale and cold to touch. There is no palpable dorsalis pedis or popliteal pulse in the left lower extremity. Light touch, vibration and proprioception sensations are decreased to absent in the left foot. Left leg muscle strength is 1/5. On Doppler, venous signal is audible but arterial signal is not.

What is the most likely diagnosis?

This patient presents with the 6 P's of acute arterial occlusion:

1. **P**ain: Sudden onset of ischemic pain at rest.
2. **P**allor: Skin is pale below the site of occlusion.

3. **P**oikilothermia: The skin is cold below the site of the occlusion.
4. **P**ulseless: Sudden loss of previously palpable pulse distal to the occlusion; confirm lack of pulse using a Doppler device.
5. **P**aresthesia: Begins with a feeling of "pins and needles" and progresses to sensory loss; the degree of paresthesia is a clinical indicator of limb viability.
6. **P**aralysis: The degree of weakness also reflects the extent of ischemic damage.

What is the likely source of arterial occlusion in this patient?

Acute arterial occlusion can result from distant emboli, acute thrombosis of a previously patent artery, or direct trauma to an artery during CV procedures. On the basis of this patient's history of atrial fibrillation, an embolus from a left atrial thrombus is the most likely source of occlusion.

What is the next step in management?

This patient with rest pain, weakness, and widespread sensory loss is in acute danger of limb loss. The presence of an audible arterial signal on Doppler indicates that it is possible to salvage the limb with prompt treatment ("threatened extremity"). Initiate immediate revascularization with heparin followed by surgery. In the operating room, surgeons typically perform an embolectomy with the use of a Fogarty balloon catheter. They then perform arteriography to confirm vessel patency. If there are emboli in distal vessels, they may also administer thrombolytics.

How does management of a threatened extremity differ from management of a viable or a nonviable extremity?

1. **Viable extremity**: There is no muscle weakness or sensory loss. Arterial and venous pulses are clearly audible on Doppler. Administer heparin and then perform arteriography to plan treatment (intra-arterial thrombolytics versus surgery).
2. **Nonviable extremity:** There is no muscle strength or sensory function (i.e., paralysis and anesthesia). Neither arterial nor venous pulses are audible on Doppler. Prompt amputation is necessary to prevent infection, myoglobinuria and acute renal failure.

What diagnosis is more likely if the patient had pain, pallor, and poikilothermia in his toe but his feet and legs were warm with strong pedal pulses?

Blue toe syndrome results from atheroemboli that occlude small vessels. The clinical presentation is pain, pallor, and poikilothermia in the toe despite strong pedal pulses and warm feet. The first step is angiography to identify the source of emboli. Treatment is surgery (endarterectomy or bypass of atheroembolic area). If arteriography does not identify any source, assume cholesterol embolization as the underlying cause.

Acute cholesterol embolization: Atherosclerosis, anticoagulants, thrombolytics, or interventional vascular techniques damage intima and expose the bloodstream to subintimal cholesterol. Showers of cholesterol crystals cause symptoms that range from isolated blue toe syndrome to a diffuse multi-organ illness. The most common sign is livedo reticularis (blue-red skin mottling in a net-like pattern that blanches). Treatment is to control CV risk factors.

The surgeon performs Fogarty catheter embolectomy and documents reperfusion during intraoperative arteriography. Two hours after surgery, the nurse notices that the patient's leg is swollen and tense. What is the next step in management?

Suspect acute compartment syndrome if the patient develops a swollen tense extremity immediately after reperfusion. Reperfusion leads to muscle edema, which increases the volume and pressure within the fascial compartment. Treatment is immediate fasciotomy. Delaying fasciotomy can lead to decreased pulses, paralysis, and limb loss.

Acute compartment syndrome of the leg can also result from fractures, crush injury, a tight cast or dressing, and alcohol or drug use. The classic finding is pain on passive toe flexion that is out of proportion to the injury.

"**BAL**" and "**DISCC**": Differential diagnosis of acute unilateral leg pain or swelling is **B**aker cyst, **A**cute arterial occlusion, **L**ymphangitis, **D**VT, **I**njury to calf muscle, **S**P, **C**ellulitis, and acute **C**ompartment syndrome.

CASE 2–19 CHRONIC LEG PAIN

A 75-year-old man presents with a 3-month history of cramping pain in the upper two thirds of his calf. The pain begins after 10 minutes of brisk walking, causes the patient to stop walking, and resolves with rest. Popliteal and pedal pulses are diminished. The patient has smoked two packs of cigarettes a day since he was 20 years old.

What is the most likely diagnosis?

The most likely disease is PAD, which results from peripheral artery atherosclerosis. Risk factors for PAD are the same as those for CAD. The classic initial presentation is intermittent claudication.

Screening: Ask all patients >70 years old or patients >50 years old with CV factors about symptoms of claudication.

On the basis of this patient's symptoms, which artery is affected?

Cramping in the upper two thirds of the calf plus absent popliteal and pedal pulses indicates that the lesion is probably in the superficial femoral artery (Table 2-27). This is the most common location of peripheral atherosclerosis.

What is the next step in management?

Calculate the ankle brachial index (ABI) in both legs with a Doppler device. ABI is the ratio of the systolic pressure at the ankle to the systolic pressure in the brachial artery. A Doppler device also provides arterial waveform tracings, which helps isolate the site of occlusion. Normal waveform is triphasic. As occlusion increases, the waveform becomes diphasic, then monophasic, and finally disappears.

Diabetes: ABI can produce a false-negative because diabetics often have calcified vessels with decreased compressibility. Consider toe-brachial index instead.

ABI is 1.1. What is the next step in management?

ABI is borderline normal, but the patient's symptoms are very suspicious for PAD. The next step is to measure ABI before and after the patient has exercised on a treadmill (see Fig. 2-23).

TABLE 2–27 Clinical Findings Based on Location of Peripheral Atherosclerotic Lesion

Affected Artery	Location of Ischemic Pain (cramps)	Arteries With Decreased Pulses
Aortoiliac (Leriche's syndrome)	Hip and buttocks	Femoral, popliteal, and pedal (bilateral)
Aortoiliac and common femoral	Thigh	Femoral, popliteal, and pedal (unilateral)
Superficial femoral	Upper two thirds of the calf	Popliteal and pedal
Popliteal	Lower one third of the calf	Pedal
Tibial or peroneal	Foot	Pulses not diminished

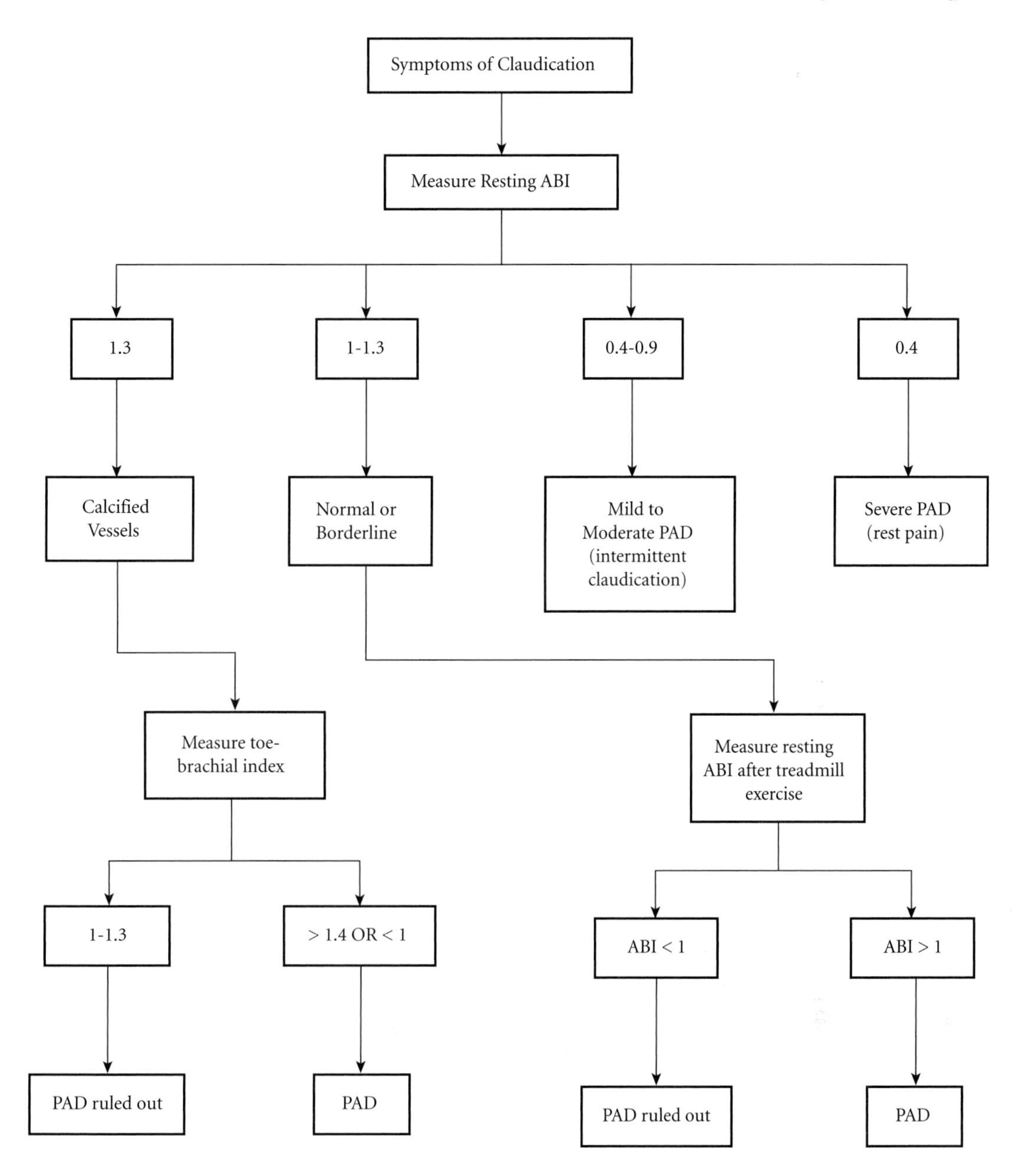

PAD = peripheral artery disease
ABI = ankle brachial index

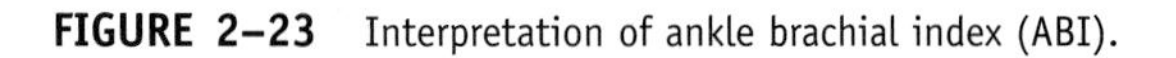

FIGURE 2–23 Interpretation of ankle brachial index (ABI).

ABI after exercise on a treadmill is 0.7. Doppler waveform is monophasic at the level of the superficial femoral artery. How should the patient manage his condition?

Initial management of a patient with PAD with intermittent claudication is conservative:

1. CV risk factor control: Evaluate for and control all CV risk factors.
2. Antiplatelet therapy: First-line is aspirin; use clopidogrel if aspirin is contraindicated.
3. Exercise: Supervised exercise rehabilitation (30 to 45 minutes at least three times a day).

PAD is a CAD equivalent.

The patient returns 9 months later. He now has cramping right calf pain at rest. The pain improves somewhat when he hangs his leg over the side of the bed. He has not quit smoking.

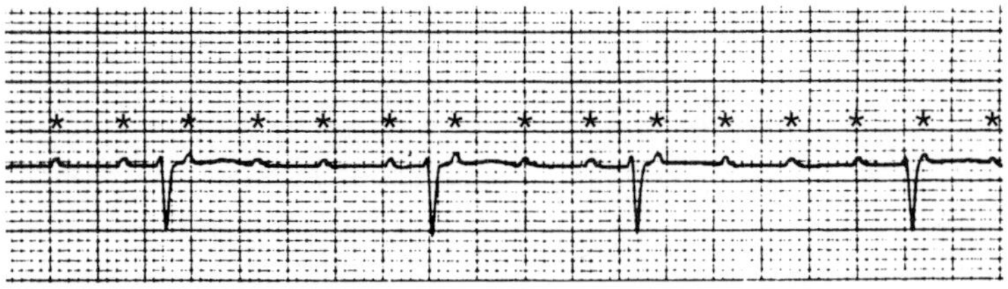

FIGURE 2–24 Right bundle branch block. From Spellberg B, Ayala C. *Boards and Wards*, 3rd ed. Lippincott Williams & Wilkins, 2007.

The right calf is smooth and shiny with very little hair on inspection. The right leg is cool to touch. There is an ulcer on the right toe and the toenail is thickened. What is the next step in management?

Rest pain and ulcers are signs of severe ischemia. Other signs of advanced disease are toenail thickening and cool, smooth, shiny skin with hair loss. Patients with rest pain, ulcers, or lifestyle-limiting symptoms refractory to conservative management should undergo a revascularization procedure (surgical bypass or angioplasty). Perform angiography before revascularization to define the anatomy and plan the procedure.

CT angiography or MR angiography: noninvasive alternative to conventional angiography; consider these methods in diabetics and patients with renal insufficiency to minimize the risk of contrast nephropathy.

Cilostazol: Phosphodiesterase inhibitor that causes vasodilation and inhibits platelet aggregation. It is an option for patients with lifestyle-limiting claudication who are not surgical candidates or who decline surgery.

Takayasu arteritis: Vasculitis that affects aorta and its branches. Suspect when a young Asian patient presents with systemic symptoms (fever, fatigue, weight loss, etc.) and large artery stenosis (RAS, PAD, etc.). ESR and CRP are elevated. Biopsy is not usually necessary, although histology is identical to temporal arteritis (see Chapter 9: Rheumatology). Treatment is corticosteroids.

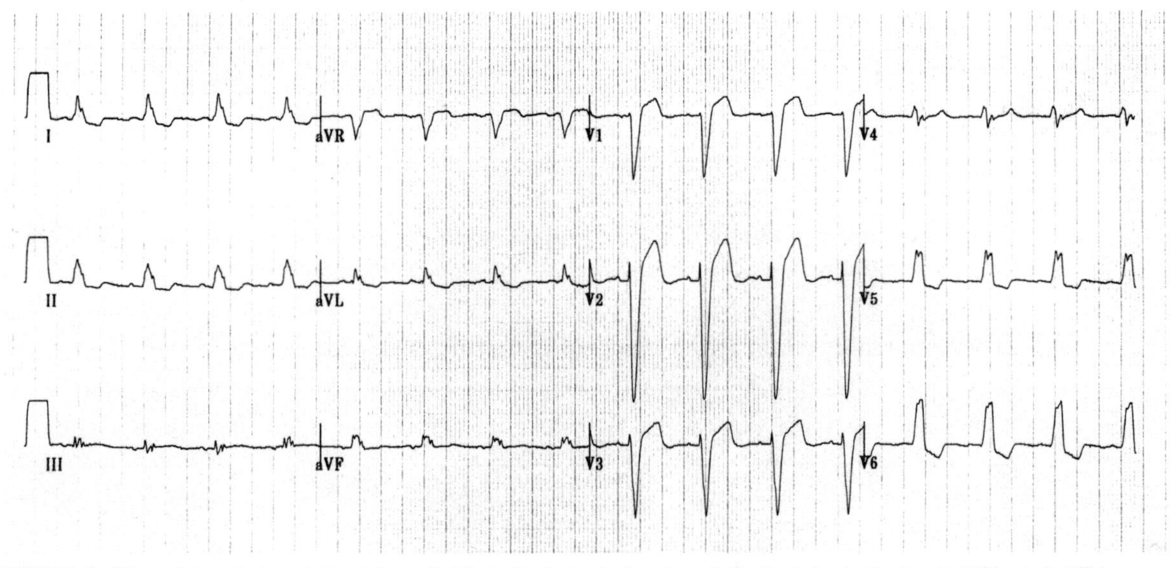

FIGURE 2–25 Left bundle branch block. From Spellberg B, Ayala C. *Boards and Wards*, 3rd ed. Lippincott Williams & Wilkins, 2007.

Alternative 2.19.1

A 75-year-old man presents with hip, buttock, and thigh cramps on exertion that resolve with rest. He also complains of impotence. Femoral, popliteal, and pedal pulses are absent. ABI is 0.6.

Where is the lesion most likely to be located?

The patient has the classic triad of Leriche's syndrome (absent femoral pulses, impotence, and claudication in hips, buttocks, and thighs) as a result of aortoiliac atherosclerosis.

How should you treat this patient?

Aortoiliac lesions tend to be more progressive than distal lesions. They also have a greater risk of distal embolization and blue toe syndrome. Most surgeons recommend a revascularization procedure before rest pain and ulceration develop.

What other conditions are often mistaken for Leriche's syndrome?

1. **Pseudoclaudication**: Lumbar spinal stenosis causes hip and buttock pain that occurs with standing and is relieved by sitting straight or lying down.
2. **Endofibrosis**: Professional cyclists can develop kinking of the iliac artery, which leads to symptoms of Leriche's syndrome.
3. **Osteoarthritis**: Symptoms vary from day to day and with the seasons.

Alternative 2.19.2

An 80-year-old woman presents with 4 months of right leg aching and swelling. The swelling is worse at the end of the day and improves when she lies down. There is pitting edema and numerous tortuous blue vessels in the right leg. The medial malleolus is hyperpigmented. Pedal pulses are palpable.

What is the diagnosis?

The patient has chronic venous insufficiency. This disorder is most prevalent among older women. Obstructed or incompetent venous valves cause venous HTN and leg tissue hypoxia and can lead to a spectrum of five clinical findings:

1. Pain: Ranges from asymptomatic to fullness and aching to bursting leg pain on standing.
2. Edema: Most patients present with unilateral calf edema that improves on lying down. The edema does not respond well to diuretics.
3. Varicose veins: Ranges from small, nonpalpable, bluish discoloration to large, tortuous, and palpable veins.
4. Hyperpigmentation: Venous HTN causes extravasation of red blood cells into the dermis, leading to dark red-brown discoloration. Hyperpigmentation usually begins at the medial malleolus but can spread to other areas of the foot.
5. Ulcers: These are typically painful, shallow, and red with irregular margins. The usual location is over the medial malleolus.

What tests should you order to confirm the diagnosis?

Findings of unilateral leg edema, varicose veins, and hyperpigmentation are sufficient to make the diagnosis, and no further testing is necessary in this case. If the presentation is less obvious, perform duplex ultrasound to confirm the diagnosis. If the patient has diminished pedal pulses, rule out coexisting PAD with ABI.

What treatment should she receive at this time?

First-line therapy is daily leg elevation and compression stockings. Consider intermittent pneumatic compression pumps or a short course of diuretics for severe edema.

> Compression stockings can cause severe skin necrosis in patients with co-existing PAD. Use horse chestnut seed extract instead.

Three months later, the patient complains of severe pruritis at the right medial malleolus. There is an area of dry, crusted skin over the hyperpigmented area, but no ulceration. How should you treat this complication?

The patient has venous stasis dermatitis, characterized by pruritic and dry crusted skin. This complication occurs as a result of progression of chronic venous insufficiency hyperpigmentation. Treat uncomplicated venous stasis dermatitis with zinc oxide paste and topical steroids.

> Patients who use bacitracin, neomycin, or sulfadiazine to treat stasis dermatitis often develop contact dermatitis to these substances. Treatment of contact dermatitis is avoidance and topical steroids.

Six months later, she presents with an ulcer on the medial malleolus. How are ulcers caused by chronic venous insufficiency treated?

Cover venous ulcers with a dressing and initiate aspirin to speed ulcer healing. The three main types of dressings used are nonadherent wet to dry saline dressings, occlusive dressings, and the unna boot (bandages with zinc oxide paste). All three are equally effective, but patients tend to find occlusive dressings the most convenient to use. Use systemic antibiotics only if the ulcer appears infected. Consider surgical referral for non-healing or recurrent ulcers.

How do venous ulcers differ in presentation from diabetic and PAD ulcers?

1. **Diabetic ulcers**: DM causes painless ulcers at areas of high pressure; foot sensation is often decreased (neuropathy).
2. **PAD**: causes painful ulcers on areas prone to trauma; pulses are often decreased.
3. **Venous ulcers**: causes painful ulcers associated with hyperpigmentation and edema; the most common location is the medial malleolus.

chapter 3

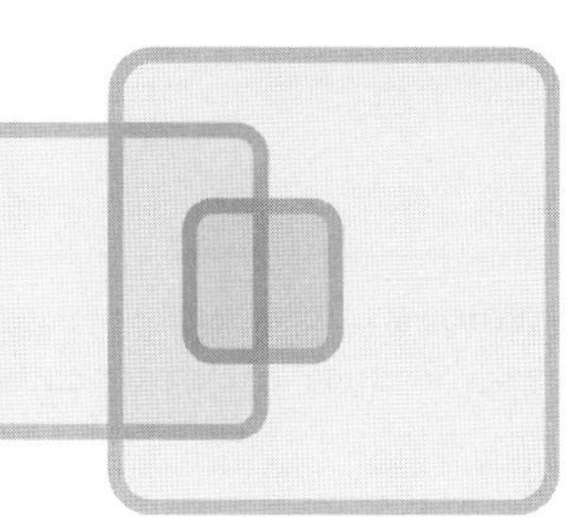

Pulmonary

CASE 3–1 UPPER RESPIRATORY SYMPTOMS

A 37-year-old man presents with a 3-day history of nasal congestion, runny nose (rhinorrhea), and cough in June. On the first day, his most troublesome symptom was a sore throat. Physical exam and vital signs are normal.

What is the most likely diagnosis?

The most likely diagnosis is an upper respiratory infection (URI). Also known as the "common cold" or "acute rhinosinusitis," this disorder is caused by viral infection. Rhinoviruses, coronaviruses, and respiratory synctial viruses are the most common pathogens. Patients typically report sore throat on the first day, followed by nasal congestion, rhinorrhea, and cough. Physical exam and vital signs are usually normal.

What is the next step in management?

URI is self-limiting, and no further diagnostic work-up is necessary. Treatment is symptomatic. Remember therapies that have demonstrated symptomatic benefit with the mnemonic "***A PINCH***" (**A**ntihistamines, **P**seudoephedrine, intranasal **I**pratropium, **N**onsteroidal anti-inflammatory drugs (NSAIDs), intranasal **C**romolyn, and **H**eated, humidified air).

> Ineffective URI therapies include vitamin C, vitamin E, echinacea, antitussives, and zinc.

> **Rhinitis medicamentosa**: Avoid using nasal vasoconstrictors such as pseudoephedrine or oxymetazoline for >1 week because they can cause rebound rhinitis.

The patient continues to have rhinorrhea, nasal congestion, and cough productive of clear sputum after 5 days. There is wheezing on forced expiration. Vital signs are normal. What is the next step in management?

Acute bronchitis is a possibility if patients have persistent cough after 5 days and/or signs of airway obstruction (wheezing). Initial symptoms are identical to URI. Diagnosis is clinical. Treatment is similar to viral rhinosinusitis ("***A PINCH***") because viral infections account for 95% of acute bronchitis. Antibiotics are not beneficial.

> Obtain a chest radiograph (CXR) to rule out pneumonia if the patient has a "***Vital Old Lung***": **V**ital signs are abnormal, **O**lder than 75 years, or **L**ung exam findings (Table 3-1).

> Consider spirometry to rule out asthma if a patient has repeated episodes of acute bronchitis. To avoid false positives, do not perform spirometry until symptoms resolve.

> Sputum characteristics do not help distinguish acute bronchitis from pneumonia because both can cause clear or purulent (yellow-green) secretions.

How would management differ if the patient presented with a 2-day history of rhinorrhea, nasal congestion, cough, fatigue, and a temperature of 38.9°C in January?

Unlike other viral causes of acute bronchitis and the common cold, influenza virus can also cause fever and constitutional symptoms such as fatigue and myalgias. The pretest probability of influenza virus infection in a patient with acute onset of fever, constitutional symptoms, and upper respiratory symptoms during "flu season" (winter) is high enough to warrant empiric therapy with a neuraminidase inhibitor (decreases symptom duration by 1 day). CXR is unnecessary unless the patient has abnormal findings on lung examination.

How would management differ if the patient with "flu-like" symptoms in January presented 3 days after symptom onset?

Neuraminidase inhibitors are not effective if used >48 hours after symptom onset. Only symptomatic therapy is warranted in these patients. Influenza virus–induced acute bronchitis is usually self-limited in the general population.

TABLE 3–1 Adventitious Lung Sounds

Sound	Pitch	Description	Continuity	Interpretation
Wheeze[a]	High	Whistling	Continuous	Upper or lower airway obstruction
Stridor	High	Harsh vibrating wheeze	Continuous	Inspiratory stridor suggests upper airway obstruction; expiratory stridor suggests lower airway obstruction
Rhonchi	Low	Snoring	Continuous	Secretions in large airways
Fine crackle[a]	High	Like rubbing a strand of hair	Intermittent	Infection/inflammation of the distal bronchi, bronchioles, or alveoli
Coarse crackle[a]	Low	Velcro-like	Intermittent	Infection/inflammation of the distal bronchi, bronchioles, or alveoli
Mediastinal crunch[b]	High	Coarse crackle synchronized with heart beat and increase during expiration	Intermittent	Air in the mediastinum (pneumomediastinum)

[a] Crackles are also referred to as rales or crepitus.
[b] Also called Hamman's crunch.

How would management differ if the patient presented with a 10-day history of nasal congestion and rhinorrhea and had experienced episodes of rapid coughing followed by a loud inspiratory sound?

The type of cough described is called a paroxysmal cough ("whooping cough"). Obtain cultures of nasopharyngeal swabs or aspirates to rule out *Bordetella pertussis* infection in any patient with paroxysmal cough (even if they have been vaccinated in the past). First-line therapy is a macrolide such as erythromycin.

The prevalence of acute bronchitis due to *Bordetella pertussis* fell dramatically with the advent of dTP vaccine. In recent years however, incidence has been rising.

Alternative 3.1.1

A 57-year-old woman presents with a 2-day history of nasal congestion and rhinorrhea. Viral rhinosinusitis is diagnosed in this patient. Two weeks later, she continues to have nasal congestion and rhinorrhea. In addition, she reports maxillary facial pain increased upon bending forward, discomfort in the upper teeth, and yellowish nasal discharge. Temperature is 38.3°C. Lung exam is normal.

What is the next step in management?

Most patients with viral URI have nose as well as sinus involvement. However, suspect secondary bacterial infection of the sinuses if symptoms persist for more than 7 to 10 days and the patient reports one or more of the following: maxillary facial pain increased on bending forward, maxillary tooth discomfort, or purulent (yellow or green) nasal discharge. Consider antibiotics for this patient with possible bacterial sinusitis. First-line choices are amoxicillin, doxycycline, or trimethoprim-sulfamethoxazole (TMP-SMX).

Imaging and diagnostic tests are not indicated for the diagnosis of acute sinusitis.

How would you manage the patient if symptoms of sinusitis persist for 3 months?

Sinusitis that lasts for $\geq$12 weeks is termed chronic sinusitis. First-line therapy is a 3-week course of amoxicillin-clavulonate or cefuroxime. Nasal irrigation with normal saline may provide symptomatic relief and hasten recovery. Order a computed tomography (CT) scan if the patient has fewer than three episodes of chronic sinusitis each year. If CT scan confirms the presence of sinus obstruction, consider endoscopic sinus surgery.

How would management differ if the patient with symptoms of acute sinusitis is a diabetic and nasal examination demonstrates a black eschar?

Maintain a high index of suspicion for mucormycosis (zygomycosis) in a diabetic or immunosuppressed patient with sinusitis. Infection of the nose and sinuses by these fungi can cause symptoms of sinusitis as well as:

1. Metabolic acidosis and altered mental status (due to diabetic ketoacidosis)
2. Facial or orbital swelling (if infection spreads rapidly throughout sinuses)
3. Blurry or decreased vision (if infection spreads to involve CN III, IV, or VI)
4. Nasal necrosis (visible as a black eschar)

The initial step in any diabetic or immunocompromised patient with sinusitis and one or more signs of mucormycosis is to initiate prompt, empiric, antifungal therapy (amphotericin B). Next, urgently refer the patient to a head and neck surgeon to obtain sinus tissue samples. Then, obtain a CT scan or a magnetic resonance imaging scan of the head to gauge the extent of head and neck involvement.

Mucormycosis histology: tissue necrosis and branched, septate hyphae.

Alternative 3.1.2

A 22-year-old man presents with chronic rhinorrhea, sneezing, and nasal congestion. The symptoms occur year-round, but they are worse in the spring. On physical exam there is a transverse nasal crease and excoriation around the nares. The nasal mucosa is pale. The turbinates are edematous. Vital signs are normal.

What is the most likely diagnosis?

Suspect allergic rhinosinusitis rather than viral rhinosinusitis if the patient has upper respiratory symptoms throughout the year or many times during a particular season. Patients frequently push the tip of their nose up with the back of their hand, which leads to the formation of a transverse nasal crease ("allergic salute"). Pallor of the nasal mucosa and turbinate edema are common findings.

> Allergic rhinosinusitis patients have increased incidence of other atopic disorders such as asthma.

How is allergic rhinosinusitis treated?

The first-line measure is to minimize exposure to allergens (pollen, pets, dust mites, etc.); these measures should decrease symptoms over the next few weeks. If symptoms persist, intranasal steroids are the next line of therapy. Less effective alternatives include antihistamine decongestants (e.g., loratidine with pseudoephedrine), intranasal antihistamines, and intranasal cromolyn.

> **Dust mites** are small organisms that feed on shed human skin; their waste products can induce an allergic response. Some measures to minimize exposure are: do not sleep on upholstery (e.g., sofas), wash clothes and bedding in hot water (cold water does not kill mites), and use dust-proof covers on pillows and mattresses.

How would management differ if the patient also reported watery eyes and had dark rings under his eyes?

Watery eyes and dark rings under the eyes ("allergic shiners") indicate that the patient also has concurrent allergic conjunctivitis. Allergen avoidance is still the first and most important measure. If symptoms persist despite weeks of allergen avoidance, first-line therapy is intranasal steroids plus antihistamine eye drops.

The patient takes steps to minimize allergen exposure, but symptoms persist. Over the next 12 months, he continues to report symptoms almost every day despite intranasal steroids and antihistamine decongestants. The symptoms affect his ability to sleep and work effectively. How should you manage this patient?

Perform allergy testing (skin prick test) to document the presence of atopy and to identify the offending allergen. If skin testing identifies a specific allergen, consider allergen immunotherapy (indicated for patients with symptoms more than five times per week that significantly affects daily activities and is refractory to allergen avoidance and medications).

What diagnosis should you suspect if the patient with perennial chronic rhinosinusitis reported that the symptoms were exacerbated by strong odors, alcohol, and rapid changes in temperature?

The reported history should raise suspicion for vasomotor rhinosinusitis, which occurs as a result of nasal autonomic nervous system dysfunction. First-line therapy is intranasal steroids and topical azelastine (an antihistamine).

CASE 3-2 PERSISTENT COUGH

A 41-year-old man presents with a 4-week history of persistent nonproductive cough. He also reports runny nose, frequent throat clearing, and a feeling of liquid dripping in the back of his throat. He does not have any recent history of other upper respiratory symptoms. He does not take any medications. On physical exam, his nasopharynx has a cobblestone appearance. Lung examination is normal. Vital signs are normal.

What are the most common causes of persistent cough in a nonsmoker?

In descending order, the most common causes of persistent cough (duration >3 weeks) in a nonsmoker are postnasal drip, asthma, and gastroesophageal reflux disease.

What is the most likely diagnosis?

This patient has the classic findings of postnasal drip. The most common underlying etiology of postnasal drip is rhinosinusitis (viral, allergic, drug-induced, or vasomotor).

> A more accurate term for postnasal drip is upper airway cough syndrome (UACS).

What treatment should this patient receive?

An antihistamine decongestant is the first-line medication for UACS. Ipratropium nasal spray or nasal corticosteroids are other acceptable treatments. If the patient identifies an environmental precipitant, eliminate or minimize exposure to the allergen.

> When no specific cause for cough is apparent, treat empirically for UACS. Symptoms should resolve within a week of treatment.

When is a CXR indicated in the evaluation of isolated persistent cough?

Obtain a CXR in all patients whose cough lasts for >8 weeks.

The patient returns 6 months later. His symptoms have not improved despite treatment for postnasal drip. His physical exam is unchanged. CXR is unremarkable. What is the next step in the workup of this patient?

Asthma is the second leading cause of persistent cough in adults. Although patients typically also have a history of episodic dyspnea and wheezing, cough can be the sole manifestation of asthma (cough-variant asthma). A pattern of airflow obstruction (forced expiratory volume in 1 second/forced vital capacity (FEV1/FVC < 75%)) that is partially reversible after inhaling a short-acting bronchodilator is consistent with asthma.

This patient undergoes spirometry, which is normal. What is the next diagnostic step?

Spirometry is often normal in patients with cough-variant asthma. Consider bronchoprovocation with methacholine or an exercise challenge in patients with suspected asthma and normal spirometry. Documentation of bronchial hyperresponsiveness is consistent with asthma, whereas a negative methacholine test excludes asthma from the differential diagnosis.

The patient undergoes methacholine testing. No bronchial hyperresponsiveness is demonstrated. What is the next step in the workup of this cough?

The next step is to test his sputum for eosinophils to evaluate for nonasthmatic eosinophilic bronchitis. If this is not possible, an empiric trial of high doses of inhaled or oral steroids is an acceptable alternative.

The induced sputum sample does not contain excess eosinophils. What is the next step in management?

Gastroesophageal reflux disease is the most common cause of persistent cough in nonsmokers after UACS and asthma. Even though this patient has no gastrointestinal symptoms, initiate a trial of proton pump inhibitors at this point.

Alternative 3.2.1

A 55-year-old patient presents with persistent cough. He has a history of hypertension and diabetes. His primary care physician started him on zestoretic (lisinopril and hydrochlorothiazide) 6 months ago.

What is the most likely cause of his cough?

Angiotensin-converting enzyme (ACE) inhibitors such as lisinopril can cause a nonproductive cough. If the patient cannot tolerate the cough, substitute the ACE inhibitor with an angiotensin receptor blocker. The cough should resolve within 1 day to 4 weeks of discontinuation of the ACE inhibitor.

Alternative 3.2.2

A 32-year-old man presents with cough that began after a viral URI 6 weeks ago. Physical examination of the lungs demonstrates mild wheezing on forced expiration.

What is the most likely diagnosis?

This patient's symptoms are probably due to postviral bronchial hyperresponsiveness. Like asthma, this transient condition can present with a persistent dry cough, dyspnea, and wheezing. Treatment is inhaled corticosteroids.

CASE 3–3 EPISODES OF COUGH AND DYSPNEA

A 30-year-old woman presents with episodes of dyspnea, chest tightness, and cough productive of clear sputum. She says that she has had similar episodes over the last 2 years. The episodes occur approximately twice per month, and they are sometimes triggered by vigorous exercise. She has more frequent episodes in the spring season. In addition, she reports frequent runny nose in the springtime. She has a history of eczema. This is the first time she has sought clinical attention for these episodes. She does not take any medications. She does not smoke cigarettes or drink alcohol. Physical examination is significant for bilateral wheezes on forced expiration. Vital signs are temperature 36.6°C, pulse 86 beats per minute (bpm), respirations 18/min, blood pressure 120/80.

What is the most likely diagnosis?

This patient has the classic asthma triad (episodes of dyspnea, cough, and wheezing). Symptoms are caused by bronchial hyperresponsiveness. Asthma is more common in patients with a history of other atopic diseases (atopic dermatitis, allergic rhinitis, etc.).

What is the next step in diagnosis?

The initial test in a patient with suspected asthma is spirometry (Fig. 3-1). If spirometry demonstrates an obstructive pattern, perform bronchoprovocation testing.

Office spirometry demonstrates an FEV1/FVC of 70% that increases to 90% after administration of inhaled albuterol. How would you manage her condition?

Outpatient asthma management involves administering medications and avoiding precipitants:

1. **Pharmacological therapy**: Guided by disease severity (Table 3-2). This patient with mild intermittent asthma should take a short-acting inhaled β-2 agonist (bronchodilator) such as albuterol to control her symptoms on an as-needed basis.
2. **Avoid precipitants**: Remember the six general categories of asthma triggers with the mnemonic "***Avoid PRECIpitants***" (Allergens, **P**hysical activity, **R**espiratory infections, **E**motional stress, **C**hemicals, and **I**rritants).

> As far as possible, avoid aspirin, NSAIDs, and β-blockers in patients with asthma because they can worsen bronchospasm.

> **Pollen avoidance**: Consider an air conditioner or filter during pollen season.

The patient does not wish to stop exercising because it is a very important part of her social life. What options exist for this patient?

She could take an extra dose of bronchodilator 10 minutes before exercising.

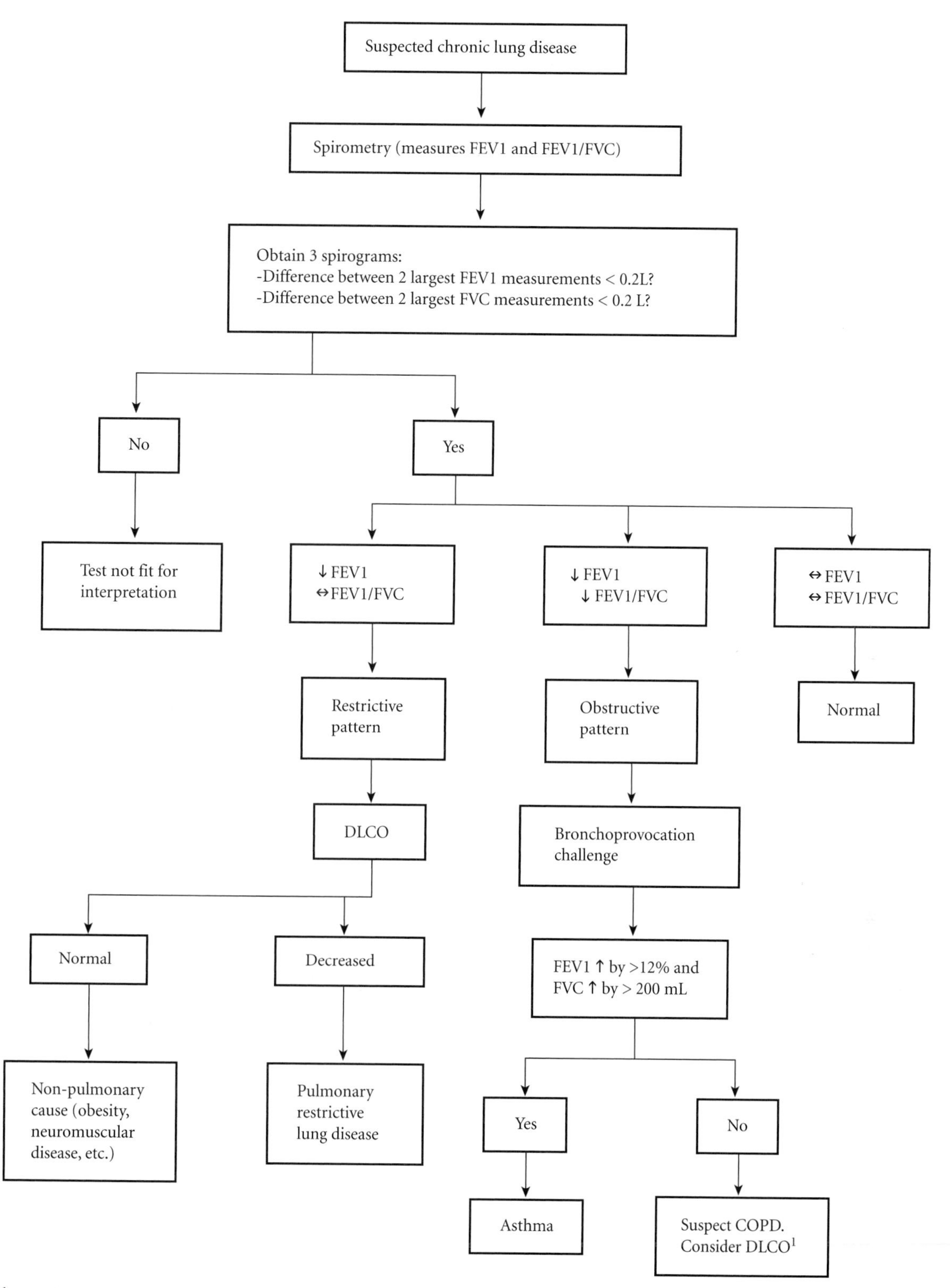

[1]Normal DLCO indicates asthma; Decreased DLCO suggests COPD

FIGURE 3–1 Approach to pulmonary function testing to diagnose chronic lung disease.

One month later, the patient is doing well. However, she is unable to tolerate the side effects of tremulousness and palpitations that accompany the additional pre-exercise β-agonist dose. Is there any alternative to her current regimen?

She can decrease her pre-exercise dose from two puffs to one and supplement her pre-exercise albuterol with a mast cell stabilizer such as cromolyn or nedocromil.

TABLE 3-2 Asthma Classification and Stepwise Therapy

Severity	Daytime Symptom Frequency	Nighttime Symptom Frequency	FEV1 or PEFR (% predicted)	Control Medications
Mild intermittent	≤2 times/week	≤ Twice a month	≥80% (normal between flares)	Inhaled short-acting bronchodilator as needed
Mild persistent	>2 times/week but <1 time/day	>2 times/month <1 time/week	≥80%	Add low-dose inhaled steroid
Moderate persistent	Daily	>1 time/week	60–80%	Add long-acting bronchodilator
Severe persistent	Continual plus flares	Frequent	≤60%	High-dose inhaled steroid + long-acting bronchodilator + systemic steroids (if needed)

Abbreviations: FEV1, forced expiratory volume in 1 second; PEFR, peak expiratory flow rate.
Note: Adapted from *National Asthma Education and Prevention Project Expert Panel Report,* 2002.

The patient returns 4 months later. She now has episodes approximately five times per week during the daytime, which she controls with her albuterol inhaler. She also has nighttime episodes of dyspnea and wheezing about once per week. What is the next step in management?

The patient now has mild persistent asthma. In addition to avoiding triggers and inhaled short-acting bronchodilators for symptom control, she should start taking a low-dose of inhaled steroids twice a day. Steroids reduce airway inflammation and remodeling.

The patient initially does well on her new regimen. Six months later however, she reports daily symptoms requiring the use of a bronchodilator despite her compliance with the prescribed regimen and avoidance of triggers. What is the next step?

Patients who remain symptomatic despite adequate treatment for mild persistent asthma have moderate persistent asthma. Increase her inhaled corticosteroid dose up to the lowest dose that controls her symptoms. Also add a long-acting bronchodilator such as salmeterol to the regimen. Patients with moderate to severe asthma should also measure their peak expiratory flow rate (PEFR) at home every day to monitor changes or trends in lung function.

Two months later, the patient presents to the emergency department complaining of increased dyspnea over the last hour that has not responded to β-agonist inhaler at home. On physical exam, she has bilateral expiratory wheezes. Vitals are: temperature 37.1°C, pulse 120 bpm, respirations 25/min, blood pressure 118/78. Peak flow is 60% of her baseline. Oxygen saturation is 88%. What should be done at this time?

Reduced peak flow and dyspnea that is unresponsive to home medications indicate that the patient is having an acute asthma exacerbation. The goal of treatment is to rapidly alleviate airflow obstruction (Fig. 3-2). Administer an inhaled, short-acting, β-2 agonist such as albuterol by nebulizer or metered-dose inhaler (MDI) every 20 minutes. If the response to albuterol is not immediate and marked, administer oral or intravenous (IV) steroids early. Also, administer supplemental oxygen to maintain SaO_2 >90% (Table 3-3). Monitor the response to therapy by measuring PEFR every 1 to 2 hours.

Ipratropium: There is some evidence that adding inhaled ipratropium to the bronchodilator improves outcomes; however, this is not confirmed, and ipratropium should not be a mainstay in the management of asthma exacerbation.

When is measurement of arterial blood gas (ABG) indicated in asthma exacerbation?

ABG analysis can be used to help assess tissue oxygenation and acid–base status (see Chapter 7: Fluids and Electrolytes). Obtain an ABG if PEFR is <25% despite initial therapy with inhaled bronchodilators, oxygen, and steroids. Obtain an ABG if the patient is too sick to perform PEFR.

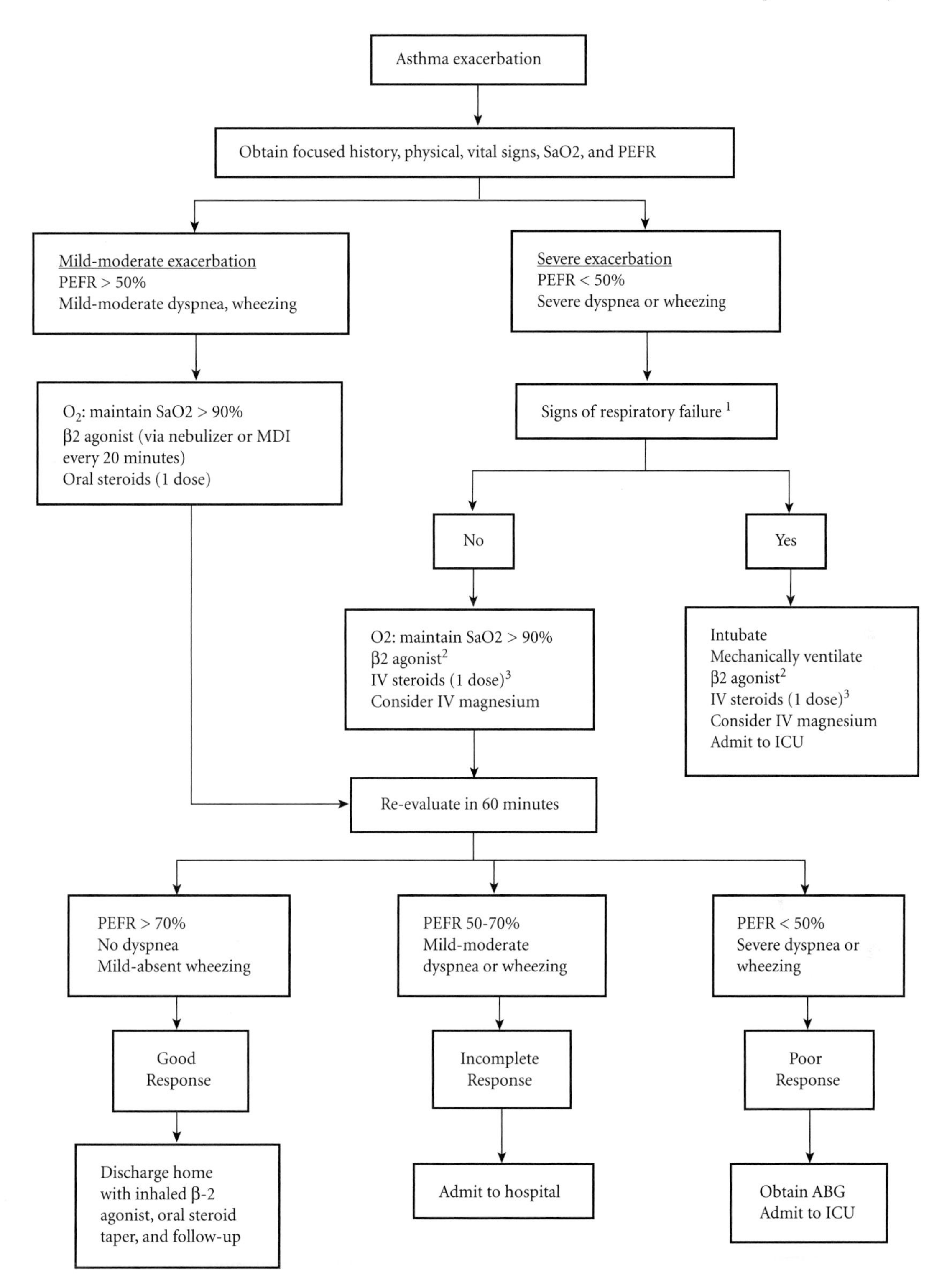

[1]Use of accessory muscles, hypoxia, altered mental status, pulsus paradoxus, etc.
[2]Inhaled every 20 minutes via nebulizer or continuously
[3]If IV access not available, administer oral or IM steroids

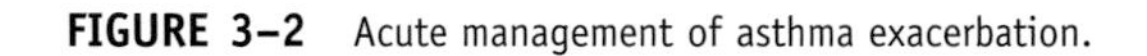

FIGURE 3–2 Acute management of asthma exacerbation.

TABLE 3–3 Common Supplemental Oxygen Delivery Methods

Delivery System	Maximum FiO_2	Maximum Flow Rate	Description
Nasal cannula	Up to 40%	6 L/min	Prongs placed in nostrils deliver oxygen at set flow rate. FiO_2 varies on the basis of rate of respirations.
Face mask	Up to 60%	10 L/min	Delivers oxygen at set flow rate. FiO_2 varies on the basis of rate of respirations.
Non-rebreather	Up to 80%	15 L/min	Facemask with a reservoir bag. Delivers oxygen at set flow rate. FiO_2 varies on the basis of rate of respirations.
Venturi mask	Up to 50%	10 L/min	High flow mask that can deliver oxygen at a set flow rate and FiO_2.

Abbreviation: FiO_2, fraction of inspired oxygen.

One hour later, she is still dyspneic to the point where she is unable to lie supine. She has bilateral inspiratory and expiratory wheezes in all lung fields. Heart sounds are distant. She is using accessory muscles of respiration. PEFR is 20% of baseline. Blood pressure is 118/70, which falls to 100/65 during inspiration. Respirations are 32/min and pulse is 160 bpm. ABG measurements on 70% oxygen by non-rebreather are pH 7.30, PaO_2 140, $PaCO_2$ 40. What is the next step in management?

This patient is in status asthmaticus (severe attacks of asthma that respond poorly to β-agonists and are associated with signs and symptoms of respiratory failure). Physical signs of severe asthma are decreased consciousness, inability to lie supine, diaphoresis, and use of accessory muscles to breathe. Vital signs may demonstrate tachypnea (>30/min), tachycardia (>120/min), and pulsus paradoxus (inspiratory fall in systolic blood pressure >15 mm Hg). This patient is in imminent danger of respiratory failure. The next step is intubation, mechanical ventilation, and admission to the intensive care unit.

"Normal" $PaCO_2$ in the setting of tachypnea and accessory muscle use indicates that airway narrowing is so severe that the ventilatory demands of the respiratory center cannot be met.

What are the recommended settings for the mechanical ventilator?

Patients in status asthmaticus have significant bronchoconstriction. Because bronchoconstriction limits exhalation, air can be trapped in the lungs and cause barotrauma. To prevent barotrauma, maintain a long expiratory phase, a low tidal volume, and a low rate even though these settings would allow increased $PaCO_2$. This is called permissive hypercapnia.

Air trapping is the cause of distant heart sounds in status asthmaticus.

The patient recovers after a brief hospitalization. What changes should you make to her home regimen at discharge?

After an oral prednisone taper, her inhaled corticosteroid dose may need to be increased. Also, discuss and write down an action plan for the patient that reviews what the patient should do if she has another exacerbation.

Base the action plan on PEFR rather than on symptoms, because patients with a history of intubation may have decreased ability to perceive dyspnea and airway narrowing.

Alternative 3.3.1

A 22-year-old woman presents with episodes of dyspnea, wheezing, and rhinorrhea approximately 1 hour after she consumes aspirin. Her medical history is significant for bacterial sinusitis that required a prolonged course of antibiotics. On physical examination, there are nasal polyps.

What is the most likely diagnosis?

Asthma, aspirin sensitivity, and nasal polyps are the classic triad of aspirin-induced asthma. Approximately 20% of steroid-dependent asthmatics have aspirin-induced asthma.

Is there any difference in the treatment strategy for such patients?

Leukotriene receptor antagonists such as montelukast are the cornerstone of therapy. This is because the pathophysiology of aspirin-induced asthma involves increased activity of leukotrienes via the 5-lipooxygenase pathway. Treat nasal polyps with nasal steroids if they are bothersome. These patients should avoid aspirin and other NSAIDs. They can usually tolerate acetaminophen and cyclooxygenase-2 inhibitors.

Alternative 3.3.2

A 45-year-old nurse has experienced diagnosed asthma for the last 6 years. Her symptoms began 1 year after she began using latex at her workplace. The symptoms improve during her days off. Last year, her symptoms resolved after a month-long vacation but resumed when she began working again.

What is the most likely diagnosis?

The patient's history is consistent with occupational asthma. Occupational asthma develops within 2 to 5 years of exposure to an irritant in the workplace. Symptoms are worse with exposure and improve when the patient is away from the irritant. The symptoms tend to worsen with continued exposure, and the most important step in management is removing the patient from exposure to the offending irritant.

Alternative 3.3.3

The patient works as a firefighter in New York. Immediately after exposure to the dust and fumes from the World Trade Center rubble on September 11, 2001, she felt a burning sensation in her throat and nose, chest pain, dyspnea, and wheezing. Since then she has had episodic dyspnea and wheezing. She has reversible airflow obstruction documented by spirometry.

What is the most likely diagnosis?

This patient likely has reactive airways dysfunction syndrome. In this condition, the respiratory symptoms described above develop within minutes to hours after a single accidental inhalation of high concentrations of irritant gas, aerosol, or particles. After the acute symptoms, patients have asthma-like symptoms and airway hyperresponsiveness for a prolonged period. Treatment is a 10- to 15-day course of oral steroids followed by high-dose, inhaled steroids.

> Unlike occupational asthma, the pathophysiology of reactive airways dysfunction syndrome does not involve immunological sensitization, so there is no latency period between exposure and the onset of symptoms.

CASE 3–4 CLINICAL SYNDROMES IN LONG-STANDING ASTHMA

A 36-year-old man has had asthma since he was 10 years old. He presents with a 2-day history of low-grade fever, malaise, and cough productive of brownish mucous cords. This is his fourth such episode in the last 2 years. CXR shows bronchiectasis. A complete blood count (CBC) is significant for eosinophilia.

What is the most likely cause of his symptoms?

Suspect allergic bronchopulmonary aspergillosis (ABPA) in a patient with asthma or cystic fibrosis who presents with these findings. Aspergillus colonizes the airways and incites a vigorous immunoglobulin E (IgE)-mediated response. The immune response leads to bronchial obstruction, bronchiectasis, and eosinophilia.

What is bronchiectasis?

Respiratory infections in patients with underlying lung disease can cause permanent dilation and destruction of bronchial walls and cilia. Bronchiectasis typically presents with chronic cough and foul-smelling, mucopurulent sputum. The major complications of bronchiectasis are recurrent pneumonia and hemoptysis. These complications can be prevented by adequate hydration, inhaled bronchodilators, and pulmonary toilet (chest percussion and postural drainage).

How can you confirm ABPA?

Perform a skin-prick test for reactivity to aspergillus. If the skin-prick test is positive, obtain serum IgE levels and serum precipitins to aspergillus. Serum IgE levels >1000 ng/ml and positive precipitins confirms the diagnosis. If the skin-prick test is negative, perform intradermal testing for aspergillus reactivity. If this test is negative as well, then the patient does not have ABPA.

The skin-prick test is positive, and serum IgE levels are 1200 ng/ml. ABPA is diagnosed in this patient. How is ABPA treated?

First-line therapy for ABPA is corticosteroids. Consider itraconazole as an adjunct to steroids in patients with recurrent symptoms or a slow response to therapy, or in an attempt to wean steroid-dependent patients from the steroids.

Alternative 3.4.1

A 52-year-old patient has had allergic rhinitis, atopic dermatitis, and asthma of increasing severity for the last 10 years. He also has hypertension and is being treated by a neurologist for a mononeuropathy multiplex of unknown cause. During his last hospital admission, a CBC was significant for 20% eosinophils, and a CXR was indicative of patchy opacities. On physical examination, subcutaneous nodules are seen on the extensor surface of his arms.

What diagnosis should you suspect?

Suspect Churg Strauss Syndrome (CSS) in this patient with asthma, eosinophilia, abnormal CXR, and skin lesions (particularly subcutaneous nodules or ulcers on the extensor surfaces of the arms and elbows).

What are the clinical manifestations of CSS?

There are three stages in the progression of this multisystem vasculitis:

1. Prodrome: Characterized by asthma, allergic rhinitis and atopy.
2. Eosinophilic phase: Peripheral blood eosinophilia and eosinophilic infiltrates in the lung and gastrointestinal tract.
3. Vasculitic phase: This life-threatening phase occurs 8 to 10 years after the prodromal phase and affects a number of organ systems including:
   - Cardiovascular: Leading cause of death in CSS; complications include pericarditis, heart failure, and myocardial infarction.
   - Central nervous system: Cerebral hemorrhage and infarct is the second leading cause of death after cardiovascular disease; 75% of patients have peripheral neuropathy.
   - Renal: Many patients develop hypertension (HTN) as a result of focal segmental glomerulosclerosis; 10% progress to chronic renal failure.
4. Gastrointestinal: Eosinophilic gastroenteritis can cause abdominal pain, diarrhea, and gastrointestinal bleeding.
5. Skin: Subcutaneous nodules or ulcers may form on the extensor surfaces of the arms and elbows.

How should you work this patient up for CSS?

Confirm the diagnosis of CSS with surgical lung biopsy. If there are no lung infiltrates, perform biopsy of other clinically affected tissues.

Antineutrophilic cytoplasmic antibodies (ANCA): limited utility in CSS because it is neither sensitive nor specific.

The lung biopsy shows eosinophilic infiltrates and necrotizing granulomas, which is characteristic of CSS. How is this condition treated?

First-line treatment is high-dose steroids. Patients who are steroid-resistant may benefit from cyclophosphamide, azothioprine, and IV immunoglobulin.

CASE 3–5 CHRONIC, PROGRESSIVE COUGH AND DYSPNEA

A 60-year-old man presents with a 6-month history of dyspnea on exertion. His dyspnea has progressively worsened to the point where he experiences shortness of breath after walking one block. He also reports increased cough productive of white-yellow sputum over the last 10 years. He has smoked two packs of cigarettes every day for the last 30 years. Physical examination demonstrates soft breath sounds, increased expiratory phase, hyperresonance on lung percussion, and inspiratory rales at the posterior lung bases. Vital signs are temperature 36.8°C, pulse 88 bpm, respirations 18/min, blood pressure 130/70. Body mass index (BMI) is 20.

What is the differential diagnosis of chronic progressive cough and dyspnea?

1. Cardiac: Congestive Heart Failure (CHF) or coronary artery disease
2. Pulmonary: asthma, chronic obstructive pulmonary disease (COPD), interstitial lung disease (ILD), or lung cancer.

What is the most likely cause in this patient?

Physical findings of hyperresonance, increased expiratory phase, and soft breath sounds are highly suggestive of COPD. Earlier definitions divided COPD into chronic bronchitis and emphysema (Table 3-4).

What is the next step in management?

History and physical exam alone is inaccurate in one third of patients. The test of choice to confirm COPD is spirometry. If spirometry demonstrates an obstructive pattern, perform bronchoprovocation challenge to distinguish between COPD and asthma (see Fig. 3-1). A patient is considered to have COPD if FEV1 is <80% predicted and FEV1/FVC is <70% predicted after bronchoprovocation.

What other tests should you order?

In addition to spirometry, obtain the following tests to rule out other common causes of chronic dyspnea:

1. CBC: Normal hematocrit rules out anemia.
2. CXR: Can detect larger lung cancers and interstitial lung disease (ILD).

TABLE 3–4 Chronic Bronchitis Versus Emphysema

	Chronic Bronchitis	Emphysema
Chief complaint	Productive cough	Dyspnea
Definition	Clinical diagnosis: productive cough for ≥3 months/year for ≥2 consecutive years; must have excluded other causes of cough	Pathological diagnosis: permanent enlargement of airspaces distal to the terminal bronchioles
Classic appearance	"Blue bloater": obesity and cyanosis without digital clubbing	"Pink puffer": thin patient who has dyspnea at rest but no cyanosis

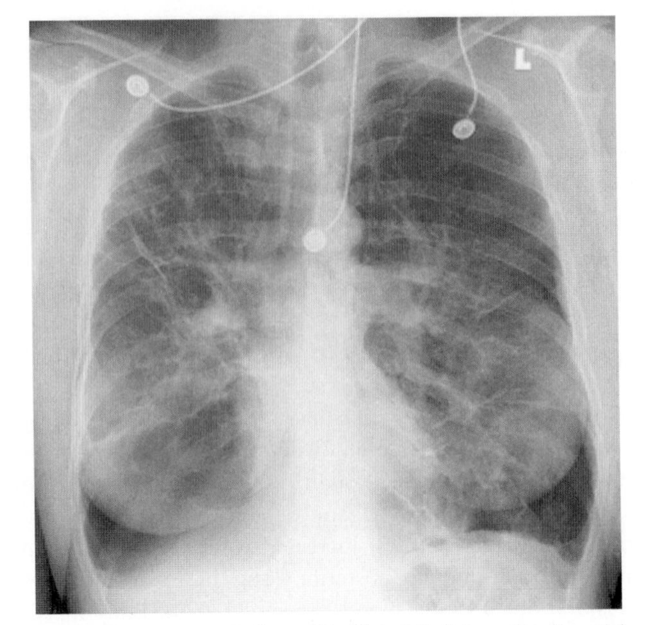

FIGURE 3–3 Chest x-ray of emphysema. From Daffner, RH. *Clinical Radiology: The Essentials*, 3rd ed. Lippincott Williams & Wilkins, 2007.

3. EKG: Normal EKG greatly decreases likelihood of cardiac causes.
4. 6-Minute walk test (6MWT): Monitor pulse oximetry with ambulation.

CXR is obtained (Fig. 3-3). Hematocrit is 42%. EKG is normal. Spirometry demonstrates FEV1 of 62% and FEV1/FVC that is 65% of predicted and not reversible with inhalation of bronchodilators. Pulse oximetry is 93% and falls to 90% with ambulation. How would you classify his disease severity?

Disease severity is staged using FEV1/FVC levels based on the GOLD criteria. On the basis of these criteria, this patient has moderate COPD (Table 3-5).

> **GOLD**: **G**lobal Initiative for Chronic **O**bstructive **L**ung **D**isease

How would you describe the patient's CXR?

CXR demonstrates hyperinflated lungs, flattened diaphragm, and a long, narrow heart shadow. These findings are characteristic of emphysema.

> **Lung volumes:** Total lung capacity (TLC) and functional residual capacity. Total lung volume in obstructive disease > normal > restrictive lung disease.

> CXR not sensitive for the diagnosis of mild and moderate COPD.

What measures are recommended initially in patients with COPD?

1. Smoking cessation: This is the most important step in management, because smoking cessation is the only measure that reduces the rate of lung function decline in COPD.
2. Medications: The initial therapy for COPD is a short-acting, inhaled β-agonist (e.g., albuterol) plus a short-acting inhaled anticholinergic (e.g., ipratropium) on an as-needed basis. Unlike asthma, combining the β-agonist and the anticholinergic has an additive symptomatic benefit in COPD. Unlike smoking cessation, medications do not reduce the rate of lung function decline.

TABLE 3–5 Classification of COPD Disease Severity (GOLD Criteria)

Stage	FEV1/FVC	FEV1
1 (mild)	<70%	≥80%
2A (moderate)	<70%	50–80%
2B (moderate)	<70%	30–50%
3 (severe)	<70%	<30% or respiratory failure or right heart failure

Abbreviation: COPD, chronic obstructive pulmonary disease; FVC, forced vital capacity; GOLD, Global Initiative for Chronic Obstructive Lung Disease.
Note: Adapted from Rabe KF, et al. Global Strategy for the Diagnosis, Management, and Prevention of COPD—2006 Update. *Am J Respir Crit Care Med*: 176: 532–555, 2007.

3. Vaccines: Administer a single pneumococcal vaccine and annual influenza vaccine (see Chapter 1: Health Maintenance and Statistics).
4. Pulmonary rehabilitation: Use this method to improve symptoms in patients with stage 2 or greater COPD but does not reduce rate of lung function decline.

Monitoring: Perform annual spirometry to monitor response to therapy in stable COPD. Use FEV1 rather than FEV1/FVC to monitor rate of lung function decline.

High-calorie supplements: Weight loss occurs in 20% of patients with moderate to severe emphysema. Some clinicians advocate high-calorie supplements, although studies have not documented any long-term benefit.

What therapy could you add if symptoms persist despite smoking cessation and as-needed, short-acting albuterol and ipratropium?

The next step is to add a scheduled dose of tiotropium (long-acting, inhaled anticholinergic). If symptoms persist despite tiotropium, consider adding a scheduled dose of a long-acting, β-2 agonist such as salmeterol. Like short-acting bronchodilators, long-acting bronchodilators improve dyspnea and reduce COPD exacerbations but do not reduce mortality or rate of lung function decline.

MDI versus nebulizer: Both methods of bronchodilator delivery are equally effective in both COPD and asthma.

What therapy can you consider if symptoms persist despite maximal doses of as-needed, inhaled albuterol and ipratropium as well as scheduled tiotropium and salmeterol?

Consider inhaled steroids if the patient has continued symptoms or severe airflow limitation despite maximal doses of short and long-acting bronchodilators. Do not initiate steroids unless spirometry documents airflow improvement with steroids.

When is oxygen therapy indicated in patients with stable COPD?

Oxygen is the only therapeutic intervention that decreases mortality in patients with COPD. Home oxygen therapy is indicated in the following patients with stable COPD:

1. Resting PaO_2 of 55 mm Hg ($SaO2 \leq 88\%$)
2. Exercise induced desaturation to ≤88%
3. Cor pulmonale or erythrocytosis

Stable COPD measures: drugs (inhaled bronchodilators, inhaled steroids), smoking cessation, pulmonary rehabilitation, oxygen, and high-calorie supplements.

The patient begins to take scheduled albuterol and ipratropium by MDI but does not stop smoking. Eight months later, he presents to the emergency department with increasing dyspnea over the last 6 hours. He is unable to lie supine because of breathlessness. He has been coughing more over the last 2 days with an increased amount of yellow sputum. Vital signs are temperature 38.7°C, pulse 125 bpm, respirations 20/min, blood pressure 120/80. Oxygen saturation is 87%. ABG is pH 7.36, PaO_2 54, $PaCO_2$ 44. What is the differential diagnosis of acute dyspnea?

Common causes of acute dyspnea are:

1. Psychiatric: panic attack
2. Cardiac: decompensated heart failure, acute corinary syndrome (ACS), cardiac tamponade
3. Pulmonary: **P**neumothorax, **P**ulmonary embolism (PE), **P**neumonia, **C**OPD exacerbation, **A**sthma exacerbation, **O**bstruction of the upper airway, **B**ronchitis (mnemonic: "***Poor Paul's Pneumonia Causes Acute Onset Breathlessness***")

What is the next step in management?

First, correct ABCs (airway, breathing, circulation). Then perform bedside spirometry to confirm the diagnosis. Also, obtain CXR, EKG, bone natriuretic peptide (BNP), CBC, and d-dimer to rule out other causes of acute dyspnea.

FEV1 and FEV1/FVC have declined from his baseline. EKG, cardiac BNP, and d-dimer are normal. CXR is unchanged from baseline. What acute cause of dyspnea is most likely in this patient?

The most likely cause of his symptoms is COPD exacerbation, defined as an acute worsening of symptoms accompanied by decreased lung function. COPD exacerbation usually occurs after a stressful precipitating event such as infection (bacterial or viral), bronchospasm, or excessive sedation from medications. Fever and increased purulent sputum suggest that an infection has triggered his deterioration.

How is COPD exacerbation treated?

Treat COPD exacerbation with "***BOCA***" (**B**ronchodilators, **O**xygen, **C**orticosteroids ± **A**ntibiotics):

1. Bronchodilators: Administer inhaled, short-acting β-2 agonists and inhaled anticholinergics every 1 to 2 hours via MDI or nebulizer.
2. Supplemental oxygen: Include this critical component of acute therapy, because hypoxemia is a defining feature of a COPD exacerbation; target arterial oxygen saturation is 60 to 65 mmHg ($SaO_2 \geq 90\%$).
3. Corticosteroids (IV or oral).
4. Empiric antibiotics: These are indicated if the patient has fever or increased volume and purulence of secretions; choose a 10-day course of amoxicillin, doxycyline, or TMP-SMX.

> A beneficial response to steroids during an acute COPD exacerbation does not predict benefit from the chronic use of steroids.

When is hospitalization indicated for patients with COPD exacerbation? Does this patient require hospitalization?

Indications for hospitalization are:

1. Marked increased in symptom intensity
2. Multiple comorbidities or severe background disease
3. Poor social support at home
4. No response to initial therapy

This patient with marked increase in symptom intensity requires hospitalization.

PaO_2 rises to 68 mm Hg on 3 L of oxygen by facemask, but $PaCO_2$ also rises to 59 mm Hg. The patient reports improved dyspnea and is alert and oriented to person, place, and time. What should be done about the elevation in $PaCO_2$?

Patients with COPD sometimes develop hypercapnia after receiving supplemental oxygen. Do not withdraw supplemental oxygen because this hypercapnia is generally well tolerated.

Two hours later, the patient's dyspnea worsens. The pH is 7.29, PaO_2 is 55, $PaCO_2$ is 61, and oxygen saturation is 88%. Is there any alternative to intubation and mechanical ventilation for this patient?

An alternative to intubation and mechanical ventilation in patients with COPD exacerbation is noninvasive positive pressure ventilation (NPPV). NPPV reduces the risk of nosocomial pneumonia and results in shorter hospital stays compared with intubation in select COPD patients. Indications for NPPV are:

1. Moderate to severe dyspnea
2. Arterial pH <7.35 with $PaCO_2$ >45 mm Hg
3. Respiratory rate ≥ 25/minute

> NPPV contraindications: decreased consciousness, hemodynamic instability, and arrhythmias.

The patient is ready for discharge after a 3-day hospitalization. What follow-up measures should you recommend to reduce the risk of another exacerbation?

Similar to asthma exacerbation, an oral steroid taper and a written action plan is recommended at the time of discharge after a COPD exacerbation.

The patient begins pulmonary rehabilitation. He is on continuous oxygen therapy at home, and he takes inhaled albuterol, ipratropium, and inhaled steroids. He does not quit smoking. Over the next 10 years, his dyspnea and cough continue to worsen. He now complains of chest tightness, fatigue, and lethargy. On physical examination, he appears thin, and his lips are pursed during expiration. His lower interspaces retract during inspiration. His neck veins are distended; he has 2+ pitting edema in his lower extremities. Abdominal examination is significant for ascites and his liver is felt 2 cm below the costal margin. Auscultation of the heart reveals a split S2 with a loud pulmonic component. The point of maximal impulse is in the epigastrium. Vital signs are temperature 37.2°C, pulse 120 bpm, respirations 25/min, blood pressure 150/90. FEV1 is 30% of predicted, and FEV1/FVC is 50% of predicted. Hematocrit is 60%. ABG measurements are pH 7.31, PaO_2 52, $PaCO_2$ 52. CXR shows enlarged pulmonary arteries, and EKG is significant for right axis deviation, a tall R wave in V1, S waves in V5 and V6, inverted T waves and ST depression in V1-V3, peaked P waves in lead II. What complication of COPD has he developed?

The clinical findings, CXR, EKG, and laboratory tests are characteristic of right heart failure (cor pulmonale). COPD is the most common cause of cor pulmonale, which occurs as a result of pulmonary hypertension (Fig. 3-4).

> Obtain Doppler echocardiography to confirm cor pulmonale noninvasively.

What are other causes of pulmonary HTN?

Pulmonary HTN is defined as pulmonary artery pressure >25 mm Hg at rest or >30 mm Hg after exercise (as measured by right heart catheterization). The World Health Organization classifies pulmonary HTN on the basis of mechanism into five groups (Table 3-6).

What is the treatment for cor pulmonale caused by COPD?

The key initial measure in pulmonary HTN is to treat the underlying cause. Thus, the most important measures in cor pulmonale due to COPD are bronchodilators and oxygen. Other therapeutic options are:

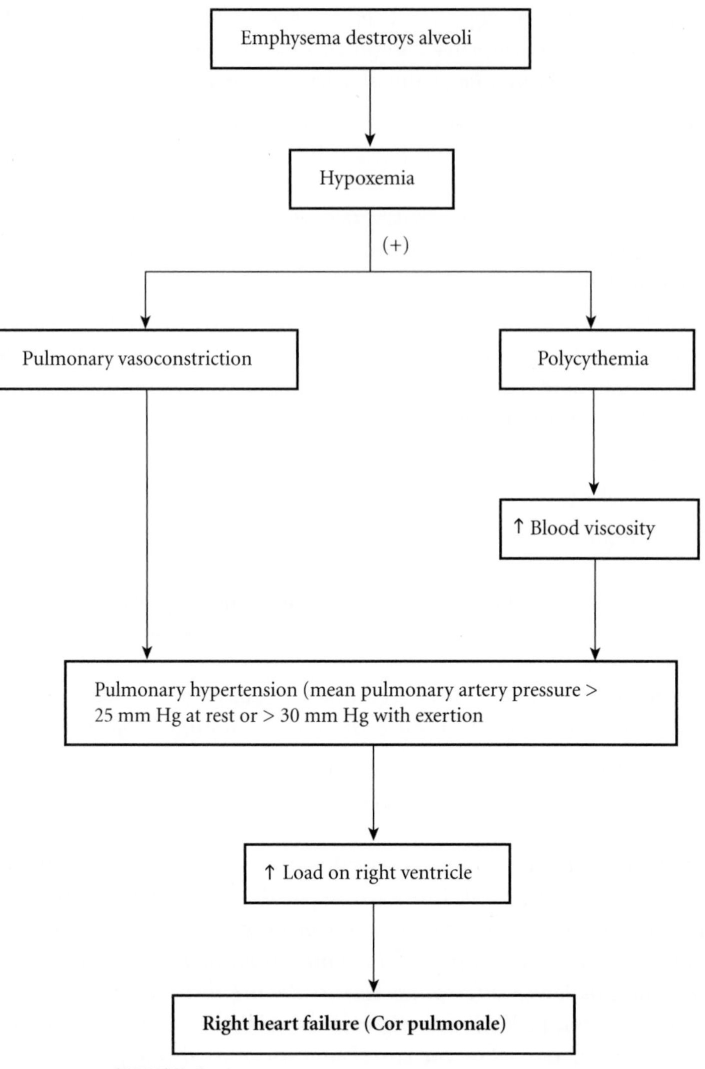

FIGURE 3–4 Mechanism of cor pulmonale in COPD.

1. Diuretics: Use carefully because excess volume depletion can decrease cardiac output in the preload-dependent right ventricle. Discontinue diuretics if the patient develops an unexplained increase in serum blood urea nitrogen or creatinine.
2. Phlebotomy: Adjunct therapy in the subset of patients with significant polycythemia (HCT > 55%) that is resistant to reduction of hypoxemia with long-term oxygen.
3. Vasodilators: Consider in pulmonary HTN and New York Heart Association class III or IV CHF refractory to oxygen and bronchodilators. Before initiating advanced therapies, perform right heart catheterization to obtain baseline pulmonary artery pressure. A calcium-channel blocker is usually the initial vasodilator therapy attempted. If pulmonary HTN persists, consider advanced vasodilator therapies (e.g., IV prostacyclin, oral bosentan, or oral sildenafil). Of these, the most widely studied advanced vasodilator therapy is IV prostacyclin (epoprostenol).

Digitalis and β-blockers are generally not effective in cor pulmonale.

Are there any surgical options for patients with severe COPD?

Lung volume reduction surgery may play a role in patients with upper-lobe predominant disease and decreased exercise capacity. Lung transplantation is an option for select patients under the age of 65, although it does not improve mortality.

TABLE 3–6 WHO Classification of Pulmonary Hypertension

Group	Category	Causes
1	Pulmonary artery HTN	Idiopathic pulmonary HTN Collagen vascular diseases HIV infection Atrial or ventricular septal defect
2	Pulmonary venous HTN	Left-sided CHF
3	Pulmonary HTN due to 1° lung disease	COPD ILD Obstructive sleep apnea
4	Pulmonary HTN due to pulmonary thrombosis or embolism	Chronic PE Schistosomiasis
5	Rare causes	Histiocytosis X is one example

Abbreviations: CHF, congestive heart failure; HTN, hypertension; ILD, interstitial lung disease; PE, pulmonary embolism; WHO, World Health Organization.

Alternative 3.5.1

The patient with progressive dyspnea and cough productive of sputum is 46 years old. He has never smoked cigarettes. His father died of lung disease in his 40s. His grandfather and paternal uncle died of liver failure in their 30s. Spirometry reveals an obstructive pattern not reversible with bronchodilators. CXR shows bullous changes in lung bases.

What is the cause of COPD?

The development of COPD at an early age in a nonsmoker with a family history of lung disease and liver failure should raise suspicion for α-1-antitrypsin deficiency. This autosomal, recessive, inherited condition predisposes to liver disease by the second decade and emphysema by the fourth decade of life. Treatment is IV or inhaled pooled human α-1 anti-protease. Lung transplant is an option for end-stage lung disease.

> Bullous changes in emphysema due to α-1 antitrypsin deficiency tend to be more prominent in the lung bases (panacinar) compared to the apices (centrilobular).

CASE 3–6 RESTRICTIVE LUNG DISEASE

A 55-year-old man complains of increasing dyspnea on exertion and a dry cough for the last 12 months. He does not take any medications. He has never smoked cigarettes, and occupational history does not reveal any workplace irritants. Physical examination reveals fine bibasilar crackles and digital clubbing. Pulmonary function tests show decreased FEV1, decreased FVC, ↔ FEV1/FVC, decreased TLC. CXR shows diffuse interstitial opacities with basal predominance and reduced lung volume.

What category of lung diseases is he suffering from?

ILDs are a heterogeneous group of disorders that are characterized by certain common features including progressively increasing dyspnea, a dry cough, and a restrictive pattern on spirometry. Fine crackles are the most common physical examination finding. The typical CXR will show reticular or reticulonodular infiltrates with diminished lung volumes.

> CXR can be normal in some patients with biopsy-proven ILD. Obtain high-resolution CT if there is a high index of suspicion for ILD but CXR is normal.

What are the causes of ILD?

There are almost 200 different ILDs. The major causes are:

1. Pneumoconioses: Years of exposure to inorganic dusts leads to chronic inflammation with resulting scarring and fibrosis. Asbestosis, silica, coal, and beryllium are among the more common etiologic agents.
2. Hypersensitivity pneumonitis (HP): Deposition of organic antigens leads to the formation of antigen-antibody complexes in the alveoli. The presentation can either be acute (4 to 6 hours after exposure, resolving within 12 hours), subacute, or chronic. Examples of hypersensitivity pneumonitis are farmer's lung (exposure to thermophilic actinomycetes in hay), pigeon fancier's lung (exposure to bird feathers and excreta), humidifier lung (exposure to thermophilic bacteria), and ABPA.
3. Sarcoidosis and collagen vascular disorders
4. Iatrogenic: cancer drugs, radiation, antibiotics, NSAIDS, β-blockers, anti-arrhythmics.
5. Idiopathic: Idiopathic pulmonary fibrosis (IPF), acute interstitial pneumonia, desquamative interstitial pneumonia (DIP), and respiratory bronchiolitis-associated ILD are pathologically different idiopathic causes of ILD.

Asbestosis symptoms tend to occur 15 to 20 years after the initial exposure.

Patients with silicosis have an increased risk of tuberculosis.

Which ILD is most likely responsible for this patient's symptoms?

This patient with basal infiltrates and no known exposures or connective tissue disorders most likely has IPF (Table 3-7). This condition tends to present in the fifth or sixth decades and is two times more common in females.

Digital clubbing is a common physical examination finding in IPF and asbestosis, but less common in other ILDs.

Analysis of the lung biopsy specimen shows areas of normal lung alternating with cystic fibrotic areas (honeycomb change), which confirms the diagnosis of IPF. What is this patient's prognosis?

Unfortunately, IPF usually follows a relentlessly progressive course, with most patients dying of respiratory failure within 5 to 10 years of diagnosis. Treatment options are limited, and these patients should be referred early for lung transplantation.

Alternative 3.6.1

A 60-year-old female presents with a 2-week history of worsening dyspnea and dry cough. Physical exam demonstrates bilateral crackles; CXR shows diffuse interstitial infiltrates. EKG, BNP, and CBC are normal. Spirometry demonstrates a restrictive pattern. No precipitant is identified.

TABLE 3–7 Typical Anatomic Location of ILD Infiltrates

Upper lung zones	Silicosis, beryliosis Hypersensitivity pneumonitis Sarcoidosis
Lower lung zones	Asbestosis Collagen vascular disease associated ILD Idiopathic pulmonary fibrosis (usual interstitial pneumonia)

Note: Adapted from Young VB, Kormos WA, Goroll AH. *Blueprints Medicine*, 2nd ed. Blackwell Publishing, 2001.

What diagnosis should you suspect?

The most likely diagnosis is acute interstitial pneumonia, which presents with explosive onset of respiratory symptoms and diffuse infiltrates and can rapidly progress to respiratory failure.

Alternative 3.6.2

A 50-year-old patient presents with chronic dyspnea, cough, interstitial infiltrates, and a restrictive pattern on spirometry. The patient has a 20-pack-year smoking history. Lung biopsy shows numerous mononuclear cells within most of the distal air spaces, and minimal fibrosis.

What are the most likely diagnoses?

This patient has either desquamative interstitial pneumonia or respiratory bronchiolitis-associated ILD. Both conditions tend to affect cigarette smokers in the fourth or fifth decade of life and have pathological features different from IPF. Treatment is smoking cessation and corticosteroids. Prognosis is good with adequate treatment.

Alternative 3.6.3

A 29-year-old African-American man presents with a 2-month history of dyspnea and dry cough. He does not have any environmental exposures. Spirometry reveals a restrictive pattern. CXR shows bilateral hilar adenopathy and upper lung field reticular opacities. Lung biopsy reveals noncaseating granulomas.

What is the diagnosis?

Bilateral hilar adenopathy and reticular opacities in the upper lung fields are highly suggestive of sarcoidosis. The presence of noncaseating granulomas on biopsy confirms the diagnosis. This multisystem disease of unknown cause is most common in African Americans between the ages of 20 and 40 (although worldwide, 75% of those affected are white). The lungs are the most commonly affected organ system (90%).

> 50% of sarcoid is detected incidentally on CXR in asymptomatic patients.

What stage of sarcoidosis does this patient have?

Sarcoidosis is staged based on CXR findings:

1. Stage 1: Bilateral hilar adenopathy
2. Stage 2: Bilateral hilar adenopathy + reticular opacities in upper lung fields
3. Stage 3: Reticular opacities in upper lung field ± mild bilateral hilar adenopathy
4. Stage 4: Reticular opacities in upper lung field ± bronchiectasis

This patient with bilateral hilar adenopathy and reticular opacities has stage 2 disease.

> **Nodular sarcoid**: Multiple bilateral nodules with minimal hilar adenopathy. Often mistaken for lung metastates; biopsy helps differentiate between the two.

What other organ systems can sarcoidosis affect?

Noncaseating granulomas can infiltrate almost any organ system. Commonly affected organs are:

1. **Lymph nodes**: painless hilar and peripheral lymphadenopathy occurs in ~90%.
2. **Eyes**: eye lesions occur in ~25% (presenting symptom in 5%). The most common eye lesion is uveitis followed by chorioretinitis.
3. **Skin**: Skin lesions occur in ~20%. The most common lesions are erythema nodosum (tender erythematous nodules on the shins as a result of inflammation of subcutaneous fat) and lupus pernio (violaceous lesions on the nose, cheeks, and ears).
4. **Kidneys**: Patients often develop hypercalcemia, which leads to calcium stones. Kidney granulomas cause glomerulonephritis in <1%.

5. Other: Liver (mild increase in liver function tests), bones (polyarthralgias), heart (arrhythmias and conduction defects), and parotid gland (dry mouth), etc.

Lofgren's syndrome: Variant of sarcoidosis that presents with fever, erythema nodosum, bilateral hilar adenopathy, and migratory polyarthralgias. Females > males. Good prognosis.

What laboratory abnormalities commonly occur in sarcoidosis?

Obtain the following laboratory studies in all patients. Although no single laboratory test is diagnostic, they help support the diagnosis, particularly if biopsy findings in lungs or other affected organs are inconclusive.

1. **Serum ACE level**: Elevated in 75% of patients.
2. **Immune tests**: Patients commonly have increased serum gamma globulins and decreased skin reactivity (due to decreased delayed hypersensitivity). Nonspecific markers of inflammation such as erythrocyte sedimentation rate (ESR) and rheumatoid factor (RF) are often elevated.
3. **Serum and urine calcium**: Sarcoidosis increases conversion of inactive to active vitamin D. Vitamin D increases intestinal calcium absorption, which can cause hypercalcemia and hypercalciuria.
4. **Other**: Reflects organ system involvement (restrictive pattern on spirometry with lung involvement, mild increase in alkaline phosphatase with liver involvement, etc).

Is treatment indicated for this patient with sarcoidosis? If so, how is sarcoidosis treated?

No treatment is necessary for asymptomatic patients with stage 1 or stage 2 disease on CXR. All patients with symptoms and/or stage 3 or stage 4 disease require treatment. This patient with symptomatic stage 2 disease requires treatment. First-line therapy is oral steroids. Also, correct increased urine or serum Ca^{+2} if present to prevent nephrolithiasis.

CASE 3–7 ACUTE ONSET OF DYSPNEA AND PLEURITIC CHEST PAIN

A 40-year-old woman presents with a 3-hour history of shortness of breath and chest tightness that is worse on inspiration. She was on a 15-hour bus ride 2 days ago. She does not have any known medical conditions. Her only medications are oral contraceptive pills. Her right calf is swollen and tender. Heart and lung findings are within normal limits. Stool is guaiac negative. Vital signs are temperature 38.2, pulse 121 bpm, respirations 30/min, blood pressure 142/90. SaO_2 is 93% on 2 L of oxygen via nasal cannula. CXR shows atelectasis; EKG shows sinus tachycardia with nonspecific ST and T wave changes. Cardiac BNP is 20. ABG shows pH 7.45, PCO_2 30, and PO_2 88.

What is the differential diagnosis of acute dyspnea and chest pain?

Common causes of dyspnea and chest pain arising over a matter of minutes to hours are:

1. Cardiac: e.g., myocardial infarction, CHF exacerbation, cardiac tamponade
2. Pulmonary: e.g., PE, pneumonia, pneumothorax, and asthma exacerbation
3. Psychogenic: panic disorder

What is the most likely diagnosis in this patient?

The most concerning diagnosis in this patient with a acute onset of dyspnea and pleuritic chest pain along with a history of immobility (long bus ride), oral contraceptive pill use, and unilateral leg swelling is PE. Cardiogenic causes are less likely in this patient with nonspecific EKG and CXR findings and a BNP of 20. Pneumothorax is less likely because typical CXR findings are absent. Asthma is less likely because there is no history of episodic symptoms.

Where do emboli to the pulmonary artery typically originate?

More than 90% of pulmonary emboli originate from a thrombus in the proximal deep venous system of the lower extremities (popliteal, femoral, or iliac veins). Calf-vein thrombosis is less likely to result in PE.

What are other possible sources of emboli to the lungs?

Sources of emboli to the lungs other than deep vein thrombosis (DVT) are:

1. Fat embolism after long bone fractures
2. Air embolism after central venous catheterization and trauma
3. Amniotic fluid embolism after delivery
4. Septic embolism resulting from infective endocarditis
5. Schistosomiasis

What are the signs, symptoms, CXR, EKG, and ABG findings of PE?

1. Symptoms: Up to 40% of patients with PE are asymptomatic. The most commonly reported symptoms are nonspecific and include dyspnea, pleuritic chest pain, cough, and hemoptysis.
2. Signs: Signs of PE are also nonspecific. The most common signs are tachypnea, tachycardia, low-grade fever, a fourth heart sound, and an accentuated pulmonic component of S2. DVT can cause pain and swelling in the affected lower extremity, but this finding is present in <30% of patients.
3. CXR: The most frequent findings are nonspecific atelectasis and pleural effusion. Classic but uncommon findings are Westermark sign (increased lung lucency in the area of the embolus) and Hampton's hump (wedge-shaped pleural infiltrate).
4. EKG: The classic but uncommon finding of PE is the S1Q3T3 pattern (S wave in lead I, Q wave in lead 3, and T-wave inversion in lead 3). More common findings are sinus tachycardia or nonspecific ST and T wave changes.
5. ABG: usually show respiratory alkalosis due to hyperventilation.

Is there any decision rule to help estimate the probability that this patient has PE on the basis of history and physical findings alone?

The Well's rule classifies patients solely on the basis of seven history and physical findings as low, intermediate, or high risk (Table 3-8). This patient has a score of 7.5, which places her in the high-risk category.

What is the next step in management of this patient?

Untreated PE carries a 30% risk of mortality. Most patients who die do so within the first few hours of the event. Therefore, it is important to initiate simultaneous anticoagulation with heparin (unfractionated or low molecular weight) and oral warfarin early in medically stable patients with a high likelihood of PE before losing precious time with confirmatory diagnostic testing.

TABLE 3-8 Well's Rule for Predicting Pretest Probability of PE

Variable	Point Score
Clinical signs or symptoms of DVT	3
HR > 100 beats per minute	1.5
Immobilization (bed rest ≥3 days) or surgery within last 4 weeks	1.5
Prior DVT or PE	1.5
Hemoptysis	1
Malignancy	1
PE as likely or more likely than alternative diagnosis	3

Abbreviations: DVT, deep vein thrombosis; HR, heart rate.
Note: Low risk = 0–2 points, intermediate risk = 2–6 points, high risk = >6 points.

Heparin and warfarin are initiated. How can you confirm the diagnosis of PE?

Evaluate this patient with a high probability for PE using helical CT angiography of the chest and compression ultrasound of the lower extremities (Fig. 3-5).

What is helical CT angiography?

Helical (spiral) CT is an advancement in standard CT technology. Unlike traditional CT, images are acquired more rapidly (single breath). This noninvasive test provides much better visualization of pulmonary vasculature (hence the term "angiography": "angio" = vessel and "graph" = description or recording).

> **V/Q scan:** Have subjects inhale a radionuclide like such as technetium or xenon, or inject subjects with technetium-99, and obtain an x-ray image. Suspect PE if x-ray shows V/Q mismatch, i.e., wedge-shaped area of decreased technetium-99 circulation in pulmonary vasculature (decreased perfusion due to blockage) but normal inhaled radionuclide uptake in the same area (adequate ventilation). This method is less frequently used for detection of PE since the advent of helical CT angiography.

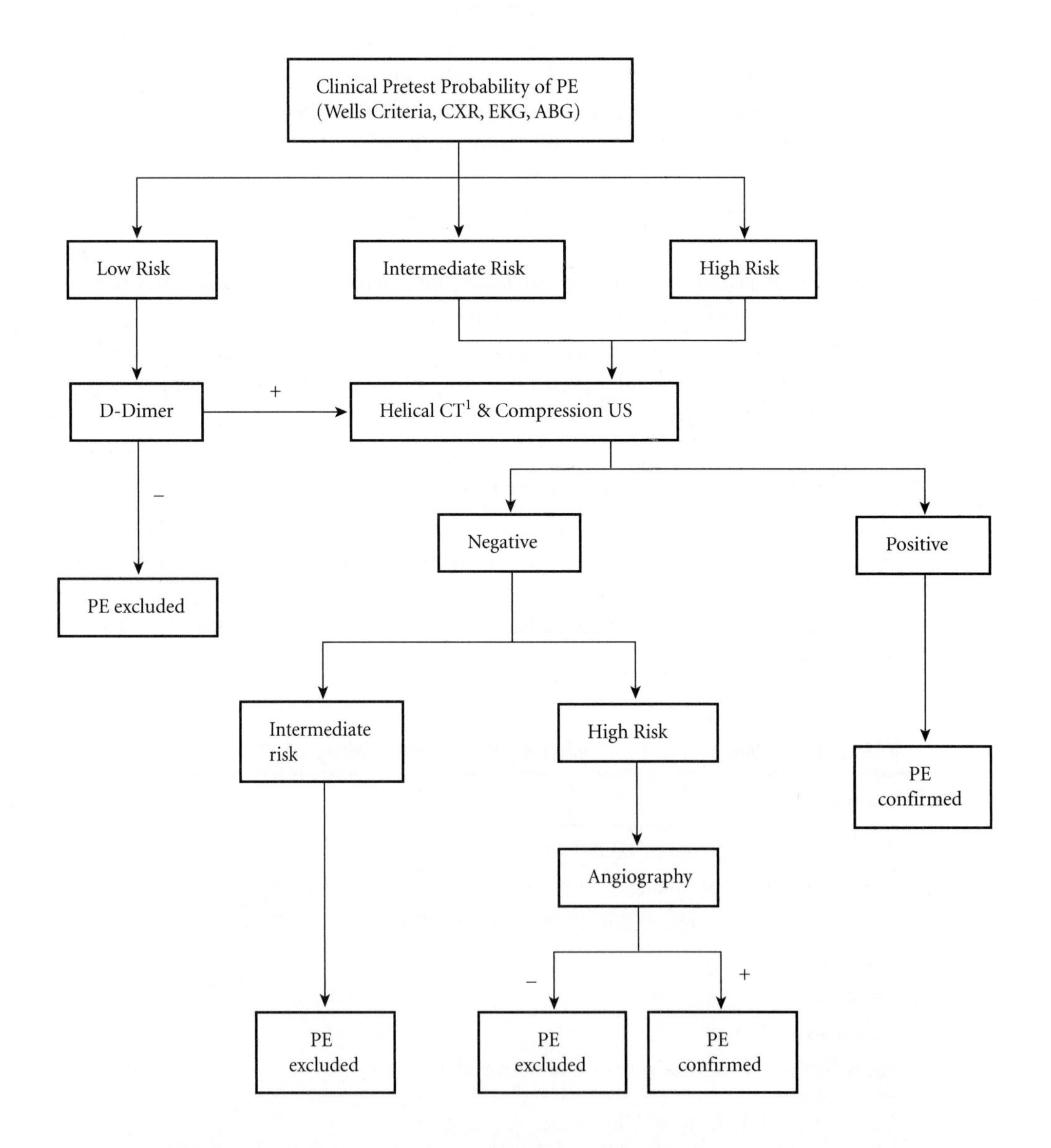

[1]If center does not have helical CT use V/Q scan instead.

FIGURE 3–5 Diagnostic algorithm for suspected pulmonary embolism.

Helical CT shows an intraluminal filling defect in the segmental pulmonary arteries, which confirms the diagnosis of PE. Lower extremity compression ultrasound identifies a thrombus in the right popliteal and femoral veins. The patient is admitted to the hospital. How are heparin and warfarin therapy typically titrated?

1. IV unfractionated heparin: Titrate on the basis of PTT level (see Chapter 10: Hematology and Oncology). Partial thromboplastin time (PTT) between 1.5 and 2.5 times the normal range is considered therapeutic (usually occurs within 24 hours after starting therapy).
2. Warfarin: Titrate on the basis of International Normalized Ratio (INR) level. INR between 2.0 and 3.0 is considered therapeutic (usually takes 48 to 72 hours). Discontinue heparin when warfarin levels have been therapeutic for 2 to 3 days.

INR: standardized reference value for prothrombin time.

Why does warfarin take 2 to 3 days to reach therapeutic levels?

Warfarin's mechanism of action involves inhibition of vitamin K–dependent clotting factors. Its anticoagulant action is delayed until normal clotting factors are cleared from the system. This is why it takes 2 to 3 days to reach therapeutic levels.

Is there any alternative to IV unfractionated heparin?

An alternative to IV unfractionated heparin in this medically stable patient is low molecular weight heparin (LMWH). Like unfractionated heparin, it is overlapped with warfarin and should be discontinued when INR levels are between 2.0 and 3.0 for 2 days.
Advantages of LMWH are:

1. Outpatient management: Because LMWH administration is subcutaneous, administration does not require hospitalization.
2. Monitoring: Unlike unfractionated heparin, there is no need to monitor PTT.
3. Complications: LMWH carries a lower risk of severe bleeding and heparin-induced thrombocytopenia (see Chapter 10: Hematology and Oncology).

Protamine: reverses bleeding caused by unfractionated heparin but not LMWH.

How long should this patient receive warfarin?

Patients with a single episode of DVT and/or PE due to identifiable and preventable risk factors should continue anticoagulation with warfarin for at least 3 months. Maintain INR between 2.0 and 3.0 during anticoagulation.

Two months later, the patient presents to her primary care physician for routine monitoring. She has not experienced any signs of bleeding while on warfarin. INR is 5.5. What is the next step in management?

The next step in this asymptomatic patient with supratherapeutic INR is to withhold the next 1 to 2 doses of warfarin and administer oral vitamin K (Table 3-9).

TABLE 3-9 Management of Supratherapeutic INR

INR	Bleeding	Recommended Management
3.0–5.0	No	Decreased warfarin dose or omit a dose
5.0–9.0	No	Omit 1–2 doses ± oral vitamin K
9.0–20.0	No	Omit 1–2 doses + oral vitamin K + resume at lower dose
>20.0	No	Hold warfarin + IV vitamin K ± FFP
Any	Yes	Hold warfarin + IV vitamin K ± FFP

Abbreviation: FFP, fresh frozen plasma; INR, International Normalized Ratio; IV, intravenous.
Note: Adapted from The Sixth ACCP Consensus Conference on Antithrombotic Therapy. *Chest* 119: 33S–34S, 2001.

Eight months later, the patient presents at the emergency department with dyspnea, chest tightness, tachypnea, and tachycardia. Helical CT shows a new, nonmassive, pulmonary embolus. She receives IV heparin and oral warfarin. PTT is 2.0 within the first 24 hours. On day 2, she again reports dyspnea, and a repeat helical CT shows a new PE. How should you manage this patient?

This patient developed a new PE despite adequate anticoagulation with heparin. In such patients, place an inferior vena cava (IVC) filter to prevent further migration of clots from the deep venous system to the lungs. Both long-term and short-term (retrievable) filters are available.

What are other indications for an IVC filter?

Indications for an IVC filter are failure, damage, and contraindications:

1. Failure: There is a new PE or DVT despite adequate conventional anticoagulation.
2. Damage: Pulmonary vessels are significantly damaged.
3. Contraindications: Recent surgery, hemorrhagic stroke, and active bleeding are absolute contraindications to conventional anticoagulation.

How long should this patient receive anticoagulation with warfarin?

Patients with recurrent thromboembolism require indefinite anticoagulation.

Alternative 3.7.1

A patient has a Well's score of 8 and is suspected to have a PE. Blood pressure is 86/60 and SaO_2 is 82%.

What are the first steps in the management?

Hypotension and severe hypoxemia in the setting of a PE should raise suspicion for a massive PE. The initial step in an unstable patient is to correct abnormalities in the ABCs (airway, breathing, circulation):

- Airway and breathing: Administer supplemental oxygen; intubate and mechanically ventilate the patient if necessary.
- Circulation: Administer normal saline judiciously because increased right ventricular afterload in this setting predisposes to right ventricular failure; if hypotension persists after 500 to 1000 mL of normal saline, consider norepinephrine (a vasoconstrictor and an inotrope).

> **Pathophysiology**: Massive PE obstructs pulmonary blood flow, leading to ↑ pulmonary artery pressure, leading to ↓ right ventricular outflow leading to ↓ cardiac output, leading to hypotension.

What test should you order to confirm the diagnosis?

Perform diagnostic testing and hemodynamic stabilization simultaneously. The initial diagnostic test for suspected massive PE is helical CT angiography or V/Q scan. If initial tests are nondiagnostic, perform pulmonary angiography (gold standard to detect PE).

> **Pulmonary angiography**: invasive procedure similar to coronary angiography. A catheter is threaded from the femoral artery to the heart, and dye is injected into the pulmonary arteries; x-ray images are obtained to detect occlusion.

V/Q scan shows multiple large, unmatched segments of ventilation and perfusion. What is the most appropriate treatment?

Treat a documented massive PE with thrombolytics. If thrombolytics are contraindicated or unsuccessful, options include catheter or surgical embolectomy.

> Absolute contraindications to thrombolytics are "***BSBS***": **B**leeding (active), **S**troke (hemorrhagic), **B**rain tumor, and **S**urgery within the last 2 months.

Alternative 3.7.2

A patient with acute onset of dyspnea has noticed gross blood in her stool for the last 3 weeks. Stool is guaiac-positive. Blood pressure and oxygen saturation are normal. Helical CT and compression ultrasound confirm a PE and a DVT in the lower right extremity.

What treatment should this patient receive for PE?

Active gastrointestinal bleeding is a contraindication to conventional anticoagulation. This patient should receive an IVC filter instead.

Alternative 3.7.3

A 22-year-old woman presents with chest tightness and dyspnea. Symptoms began after she learned that she had been laid off from her job. Her only physical findings are tachycardia and tachypnea. EKG and CXR are within normal limits. She has a history of panic disorder.

What is the next step in the evaluation of this patient?

Panic attack is more likely than PE in this situation. Her Well's score is 1.5. Consider serum d-dimer to rule out PE in this low-risk patient. This test is sensitive, so a negative d-dimer essentially rules out PE in low-risk patients. It is not specific, so an elevated d-dimer level in a low-risk patient warrants further evaluation with helical CT and compression ultrasound before initiating potentially dangerous anticoagulation.

Malignancy or history of surgery in last 3 months: d-Dimer is not useful in this population because majority will have a positive d-dimer even if DVT is absent.

Alternative 3.7.4

A tall, thin 25-year-old man with no risk factors for PE presents with sudden onset of dyspnea and right-sided chest pain. He describes the chest pain as sharp and worse with inspiration (pleuritic). Symptoms began 2 hours ago when he was out working in the yard and smoking a cigarette. He has decreased breath sounds on the right. SaO_2 is 81%. CXR is obtained (Fig. 3-6).

What is the diagnosis?

The patient has a right-sided primary spontaneous pneumothorax. This condition commonly occurs in tall, thin young smokers during strenuous activity as a result of rupture of a

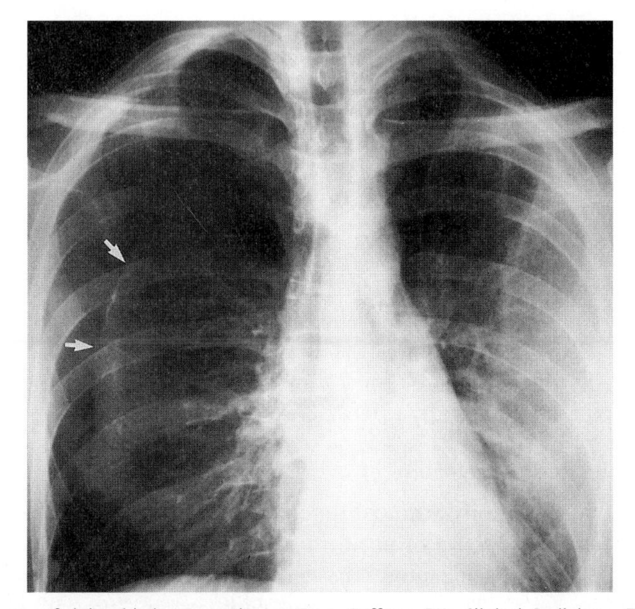

FIGURE 3–6 Chest x-ray of right-sided pneumothorax. From Daffner, RH. *Clinical Radiology: The Essentials,* 3rd ed. Lippincott Williams & Wilkins, 2007.

subpleural bleb into the pleural space, which causes air to leak into the pleural space. Pleural air can collapse the lung, which causes decreased breath sounds on the affected side. CXR is diagnostic, showing loss of normal lung markings in the periphery of the hemithorax and a well-defined, visceral pleural line between the chest wall and the hilum.

How is a pneumothorax treated?

1. Stable patient with small pneumothorax: Observation and supplemental oxygen is usually sufficient in a stable patient with a pneumothorax that occupies <15% of the hemithorax.
2. Stable patient with a large pneumothorax: Aspirate a larger pneumothorax with a catheter threaded through an 18-gauge needle.
3. Unstable patient or unsuccessful aspiration: If aspiration is ineffective or if the patient is unstable, insert a chest tube via an incision at the fourth or fifth intercostal space in the anterior axillary or mid-axillary line (tube thoracostomy). Tube thoracostomy is indicated in this unstable patient with a large pneumothorax.

> **Pneumomediastinum**: a complication of primary spontaneous pneumothorax. Suspect this condition if a patient has mediastinal crunch (see Table 3-1) or subcutaneous emphysema (bulging area of skin that crackles on palpation).

Alternative 3.7.5

The patient is a 55-year-old man with end-stage liver disease. He is undergoing central venous catheterization. During the procedure, the intern positions the patient upright. The catheter connection is detached during the procedure, so he decides to remove the catheter. He notices that the patient took a deep breath while he was removing the catheter. Within a few minutes, the patient becomes extremely short of breath. Blood pressure falls to 88/60. ABG indicates hypoxemia and hypercapnia.

What is the likely cause of these symptoms?

Suspect air embolism in patients who develop respiratory and hemodynamic compromise shortly after central venous catheterization. The risk of catheter-related venous air embolism is increased in this patient because he was placed upright during the procedure, the catheter connection was detached, and the patient took a deep breath during catheter removal (which increases negative pressure in the thorax). It is difficult to confirm this diagnosis. Echocardiography may document air in the right ventricle. Creatinine kinase is often elevated.

How is an air embolus treated?

Maintain the ABCs (airway, breathing, circulation) with mechanical ventilation, fluids, and vasopressors. Place the patient in the left lateral decubitus position (left side down), with the head positioned lower than the pelvis. If hemodynamic instability persists, consider hyperbaric oxygen.

CASE 3–8 ACUTE ONSET OF DYSPNEA, PLEURITIC CHEST PAIN, FEVER, AND COUGH

A 32-year-old man presents with a 2-day history of fever, shaking chills (rigor), cough productive of yellow sputum, dyspnea, and pleuritic chest pain. Past medical history is unremarkable. He has crackles, decreased breath sounds, dullness to percussion, increased tactile fremitus, and egophony at the left upper lobe. Vital signs are temperature 39°C, HR 110, respirations 25, blood pressure 110/80. SaO_2 is 92%.

What is the most likely cause of these symptoms?

"Typical" community-acquired pneumonia (CAP) classically presents with abrupt onset of fever, cough productive of purulent sputum, and pleuritic chest pain along with physical findings of lobar consolidation. The term "pneumonia" implies infection of the alveoli (lower respiratory tract). The most common pathogen in "typical" CAP is *Streptococcus pneumoniae*, followed by *Hemophilus influenza* and *Moraxella catarrhalis*.

Egophony: Ask the patient to say the letter "e" while you ascultate the lungs. Suspect an area of consolidation if "e" sounds like "a" over a particular area.
Tactile fremitus: Ask the patient to say "boy oh boy" while you palpate the lungs. Suspect consolidation if increased vibration is palpated over a particular area. Suspect pneumothorax or pleural effusion if there is an area of decreased vibration.

What are "atypical" signs of pneumonia?

Pneumonia can also present insidiously with atypical signs such as a dry cough, headache, myalgias, sore throat, and gastrointestinal symptoms (nausea, vomiting, diarrhea, and abdominal pain). *Mycoplasma pneumoniae* and *Chlamydia pneumoniae* are the most common causes of community-acquired "atypical" pneumonia.

What is the next step in management?

Obtain a CXR in all patients with clinical features suggestive of CAP to determine whether an infiltrate is present.

Clinical and CXR findings do not reliably differentiate typical from atypical pathogens.

CXR shows a left upper lobe consolidation (Fig. 3-7). How can you gauge the severity of this patient's pneumonia?

Use the pneumonia severity index (PSI) derived from the Prospective Investigation of Pulmonary Embolism Diagnosis (PIOPED) study to gauge pneumonia severity and appropriate triage (Table 3-10).

How should you manage this patient's pneumonia?

On the basis of clinical and demographic findings alone, this patient has a PSI of 32. Further testing is unlikely to raise his PSI score >70. Hence, further laboratory testing is unnecessary. Treat the patient empirically with a course of macrolide or doxycycline as an outpatient (Table 3-11). Symptoms should improve within 72 hours, although crackles may persist for 3 weeks.

Alternative 3.8.1

A 70-year-old nursing home resident presents with clinical findings identical to the previous patient. He has a history of end-stage liver disease secondary to hepatitis C, as well as chronic

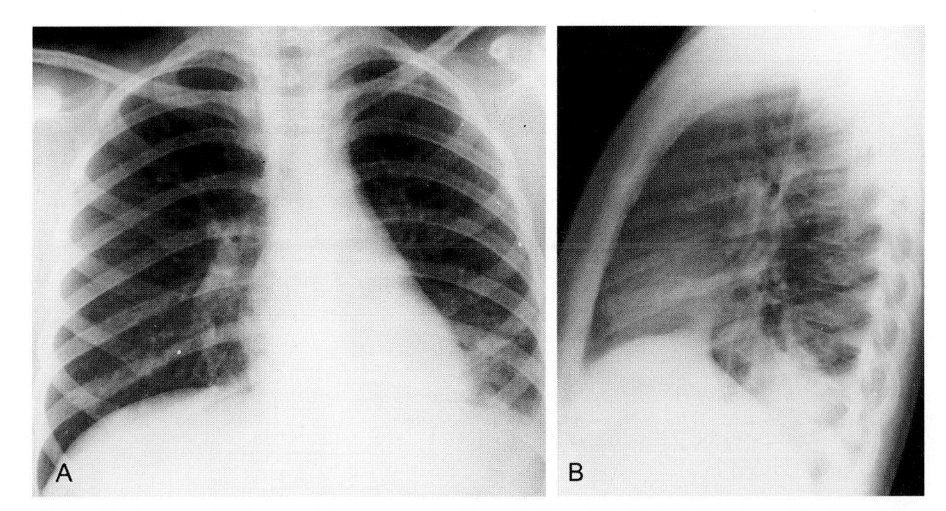

FIGURE 3–7 Chest x-ray of left upper lobe pneumonia. From Daffner, RH. *Clinical Radiology: The Essentials*, 3rd ed. Lippincott Williams & Wilkins, 2007.

TABLE 3-10 Pneumonia Severity Index Clinical Decision Rule

Class	Score	Mortality	Suggested Triage
I	Age <50, no comorbidities	<1%	Outpatient
II	≤70	<1%	Outpatient
III	71–90	2.8%	Brief inpatient
IV	91–130	8.2%	Inpatient
V	>130	29.2%	Intensive care unit

Variables	Points
Demographics	Men (age in years), women (age - 10), nursing home (+10)
Co-existing problems	Neoplasm (+30), liver disease (+20), CHF (+10), CVA (+10), renal disease (+10)
Physical exam	ΔMS (+20), RR interval > 30 (+20), SBP < 90 (+20), T < 35°C or T > 40°C (+15), HR > 125 (+10)
Laboratory	pH < 7.35 (+30), BUN > 30 (+20), Na < 130 (+20), glucose > 250 (+10), HCT < 30 (+10), PaO_2 < 60 or SaO_2 < 90 (+10), pleural effusion (+10)

Abbreviations: CVA, cerebrovascular accident; MS = mental status; SBP = systotic blood pressure; T, temperature; BUN, blood urea nitrogen; HCT, hematocrit.
Note: Adapted from Sabatine M. *Pocket Medicine*, 2nd ed. Lippincott Williams & Wilkins, 2000.

renal failure treated with intermittent hemodialysis. Physical exam, vital signs, and CXR are similar to the previous patient.

What is the next step in management?

This patient has a PSI score of 110 even without laboratory evaluation and therefore requires hospitalization. Obtain a CBC, serum chemistry, ABG, Gram stain, and blood and sputum culture specimens in any patient with pneumonia who requires hospitalization. After obtaining blood culture specimens, initiate empiric antibiotic therapy (target door-to-antibiotic time is 4 hours).

> Elderly patients frequently present with nonspecific signs and symptoms. Tachypnea is the most sensitive finding in elderly patients with pneumonia.

The only abnormal laboratory finding is leukocytosis with a leftward shift (many band forms). What is his revised PSI score?

Leukocytosis with a left shift is the most common laboratory abnormality in pneumonia. White blood cell findings are not a part of the PSI criteria, so his score remains 110.

> **Leukopenia** sometimes occurs with pneumonia (worse prognosis).

Would you classify this patient's pneumonia as community-acquired?

The following patients with pneumonia are considered to have healthcare-associated pneumonia (HCAP):

1. Healthcare workers
2. Residents of long-term care facilities

TABLE 3–11 Empiric Treatment Guidelines for Pneumonia

Triage	Suggested Antibiotics and Rationale	
CAP (outpatient)	No comorbidities	Macrolide[a] (preferred) or doxycycline *Rationale: cover most common typical and atypical pathogens in CAP*
	Comorbidities *or* antibiotic use in last 3 months *or* area with high prevalence of macrolide resistant *S. pneumoniae*	**Option 1:** (macrolide[a] or doxycycline) + β-lactam effective against *S. pneumoniae*[b]) **Option 2:** Fluoroquinolone[c] *Rationale: adds coverage against macrolide resistant S. pneumoniae*
CAP (hospitalized)	Not in intensive care unit	**Option 1:** azithromycin + third-generation cephalosporin[d] **Option 2:** fluoroquinolone[c] *Rationale: adds potent coverage against macrolide resistant S. pneumoniae*
	Intensive care unit	(Azithromycin or fluoroquinolone[c]) PLUS third-generation cephalosporin *Rationale: adds potent coverage against macrolide resistant S. pneumoniae and legionella*
Aspiration (outpatient)	Clindamycin *Rationale: covers oropharyngeal flora (anaerobes)*	
Nosocomial pneumonia or HCAP	β-Lactam effective against pseudomonas[e] + fluoroquinolone[f] + vancomycin *Rationale: Vancomycin adds coverage against MRSA. Other drugs add coverage against pseudomonas.*	

Abbreviations: CAP, community-acquired pneumonia; HCAP, healthcare-associated pneumonia; MRSA, methicillin-resistant *Staphylococcus aureus*.
[a] Macrolides: use azithromycin or clarithromycin; gastrointestinal side effects and need for multiple daily doses limit usefulness of erythromycin.
[b] β-Lactams with activity against *S. pneumoniae*: amoxicillin-clavulonate or second-generation cephalosporin such as cefuroxime.
[c] Fluoroquinolone: Choose between moxifloxacin, gatifloxacin, or levofloxacin.
[d] Third-generation cephalosporin: Use ceftriaxone or cefotaxime.
[e] β-Lactams effective against pseudomonas: Options are piperacillin-tazobactam, imipenem, meropenem, cefepime, or ceftazidime.
[f] Fluoroquinolones for nosocomial pneumonia: Use ciprofloxacin or levofloxacin.

3. Patients who were administered antimicrobials, dialysis, or chemotherapy within 30 days of infection.
4. Patients who were hospitalized for at least 2 days within 90 days of infection.

This nursing home resident on hemodialysis has HCAP and not CAP. Patients with HCAP have an increased risk of methicillin-resistant *S. aureus* (MRSA).

What antibiotics should you initiate?

Treat with a β-lactam effective against pseudomonas plus a fluoroquinolone (ciprofloxacin or levofloxacin) plus vancomycin (see Table 3-11). Tailor therapy once culture and susceptibility results return.

Nosocomial (hospital acquired) pneumonia: patients who develop pneumonia 48 hours after admission to the hospital. Empiric therapy is similar to HCAP.

Ventilator associated pneumonia: patients who develop pneumonia 48-72 hours after mechanical ventilation. Empiric therapy is similar to nosocomial pneumonia and HCAP.

Blood culture shows Gram-positive diplococci in chains. Sputum culture grows mixed flora with many epithelial cells. What organism should antibiotics target?

A good sputum sample has >25 polymorphonuclear leukocytes but <10 squamous epithelial cells. This patient's sputum sample is probably contaminated with oropharyngeal flora. Blood cultures are not sensitive, but a positive culture has a high positive predictive value. Tailor antibiotics against the organism identified on blood culture (*S. pneumoniae*).

Two thirds of positive blood cultures in pneumonia grow *S. pneumoniae.*

How would you interpret the blood culture if only one of two bottles shows Gram-positive cocci in clusters?

Typically two sets of blood cultures are obtained. Suspect contamination of the specimen with skin flora if only one of two bottles shows Gram-positive cocci in clusters.

Alternative 3.8.2

A 50-year-old homeless man with a history of alcoholism is brought to the emergency department after he was found unconscious on the street. After regaining consciousness, the patient admits that he passed out after drinking a large amount of alcohol. He has had multiple similar episodes in the past. He also reports that over the last 2 weeks he has had slowly worsening fevers, chills, dyspnea, and cough. He denies any rigors. Dentition is poor, and sputum is foul smelling. CXR detects a right middle lobe infiltrate. PSI score is 50.

What is the likely cause of his pneumonia?

The patient has clinical features highly suggestive of aspiration pneumonia, which results from aspiration of oral anaerobic flora into the lungs (Table 3-12). Unlike "typical" pneumonia, symptoms tend to evolve over days to weeks rather than hours. Patients do not usually experience rigors. Foul-smelling sputum is a common finding. Right middle lobe infiltrates are the classic finding on CXR.

What risk factors does this patient have for aspiration pneumonia?

1. Alcoholism: Impaired consciousness is one of the most important risk factors for aspiration pneumonia. Alcoholism predisposes to impaired consciousness.
2. Poor dentition: Patients with poor dentition tend to have increased anaerobic flora in their oropharynx.

Edentulous patients: Anaerobes normally reside in gingiva, so a patient with no teeth will not aspirate anaerobes.

TABLE 3–12 Classic Demographic and Sputum Findings in Pneumonia

Organism	Demographic	Sputum
Klebsiella pneumoniae	Alcoholics	Dark red, mucoid ("currant jelly" appearance)
Streptococcus pneumoniae	All ages	Purulent with blood ("rusty")
Hemophilus influenzae	Smokers, COPD	Purulent
Mycoplasma pneumonia	Younger patients	Scant, may be purulent
Aspiration	Alcoholics, altered mental status	Foul smelling
Staphylococcus aureus	Previous influenza infection	Bloody

Note: Adapted from Young VB, Kormos WA, Goroll AH. *Blueprints Medicine*, 2nd ed. Blackwell Publishing, 2001.

What antibiotic should you prescribe for this patient?

First-line empiric antibiotic for aspiration pneumonia is clindamycin (see Table 3-11). Alternatives include amoxicillin-clavulonate and amoxicillin plus metronidazole.

The patient's symptoms improve after a course of clindamycin. Two months later, he presents with a 3-hour history of dyspnea and cough. His friend states that he vomited after drinking a large amount of rum and may have swallowed some of his vomitus a couple of hours before his symptoms began. There are diffuse crackles over the right middle lobe. Temperature is 38.3°C. What is the most likely cause of his symptoms?

The most likely cause of his symptoms is chemical pneumonitis, which frequently results from aspiration of acidic gastric contents. Unlike aspiration pneumonia, patients tend to present with abrupt onset of dyspnea, cough, low-grade fever, and infiltrates a couple of hours after the aspiration event. Treatment of chemical pneumonitis is supportive, i.e., treat the ABCs (airway, breathing, and circulation). Many clinicians also prescribe antibiotics because bacterial pneumonia is still a part of the differential diagnosis.

CASE 3–9 SOLITARY PULMONARY NODULE

A 55-year-old nonsmoker presents with symptoms of acute bronchitis. His physician thinks he may have heard some fine crackles and orders a CXR (Fig. 3-8). Past medical history is unremarkable.

What is the finding on CXR?

This patient has a solitary pulmonary nodule (coin lesion). A coin lesion is defined as a single visible lesion <3 cm wide and surrounded by normal lung parenchyma on all sides.

What is the differential diagnosis of coin lesions?

1. Benign causes: e.g., infectious granulomas or hamartomas
2. Malignant causes: e.g., primary lung cancer, metastases, or pulmonary carcinoid

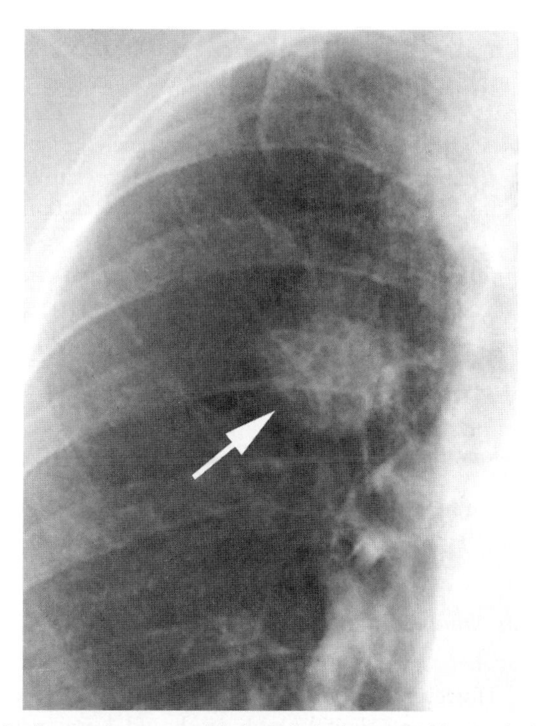

FIGURE 3–8 Chest x-ray of solitary pulmonary nodule (coin lesion). From Webb WR, Higgins CB. *Thoracic Imaging: Pulmonary and Cardiovascular Radiology*. Lippincott Williams & Wilkins, 2005.

What is the likelihood that this coin lesion is malignant?

Factors that increase the likelihood that a coin lesion is malignant are **C**hest imaging (irregular, spiculated border or irregular calcifications), **A**ge >50 years (risk that a coin lesion is 50% after age 50), **S**moking, and **E**nvironmental exposures (mnemonic: ***CASE***).

> **Benign lesions** typically have a smooth and discrete border. Suggestive calcification patterns are central, concentric, homogenous, or popcorn.

What is the next step in management?

Try to obtain an old chest film. If there is no old chest film or the lesion appears to have grown in the interval period, obtain a chest CT (Fig. 3-9).

Chest CT shows a 2-cm lesion with popcorn calcification but no lymph nodes. A history of environmental exposure is unrevealing. He denies any chronic cough, hemoptysis, fevers, chills, or weight loss. What is the next step in management?

The patient has an intermediate risk of malignancy because of his age. The next step in this patient with a 2-cm nodule is positron emission tomography (PET scan).

> **PET scan:** Inject fluorodeoxyglucose (FDG), which is a metabolically active substance (sugar) combined with a radioactive tracer. Cancers tend to demonstrate increased uptake of metabolically active substances.

The lesion does not show increased FDG uptake on PET scan. What is the next step?

Follow the lesion with serial CT scans for at least 2 years. The screening interval generally varies depending on the size of the lesion. Lesions <4 cm are generally followed with annual CT scans.

CASE 3–10 DYSPNEA AND HEMOPTYSIS IN A LONG-TIME SMOKER

A 55-year-old man with a history of chronic bronchitis presents with a 2-month history of increasing dyspnea and cough that has changed in character and is tinged with blood. His voice has become hoarse, and he has unintentionally lost 15 lbs in the last 2 months. He often wakes up drenched in sweat. He works as an occupational therapist. Annual PPD (i.e., purified protein derivative test, a tuberculosis (TB) skin test) was negative 1 week ago. He has a 25-pack/year history of smoking. On examination, there is digital clubbing. Vital signs are normal.

What is the differential diagnosis of hemoptysis (blood-tinged cough)?

The most common cause of hemoptysis is chronic bronchitis, followed by lung cancer and bronchiectasis. Less common causes include:

1. Infections of lung parenchyma: e.g., bacterial pneumonia, TB, mycetoma
2. Autoimmune disorders: e.g., Goodpasture's syndrome, Wegener's granulomatosis
3. Pulmonary vascular disorders: e.g., PE, left heart CHF, arteriovenous malformations
4. Airway trauma and iatrogenic injury: e.g., Swan-Ganz catherization
5. Cryptogenic (approximately 30% of cases)

What diagnosis should you suspect in this patient?

This patient has a history of chronic bronchitis, which is the most common cause of hemoptysis. However, the change in the character of cough along with weight loss, night sweats, hoarseness, and digital clubbing should raise suspicion for lung cancer. The next step is to obtain a CXR in addition to CBC, serum chemistry, and liver function tests.

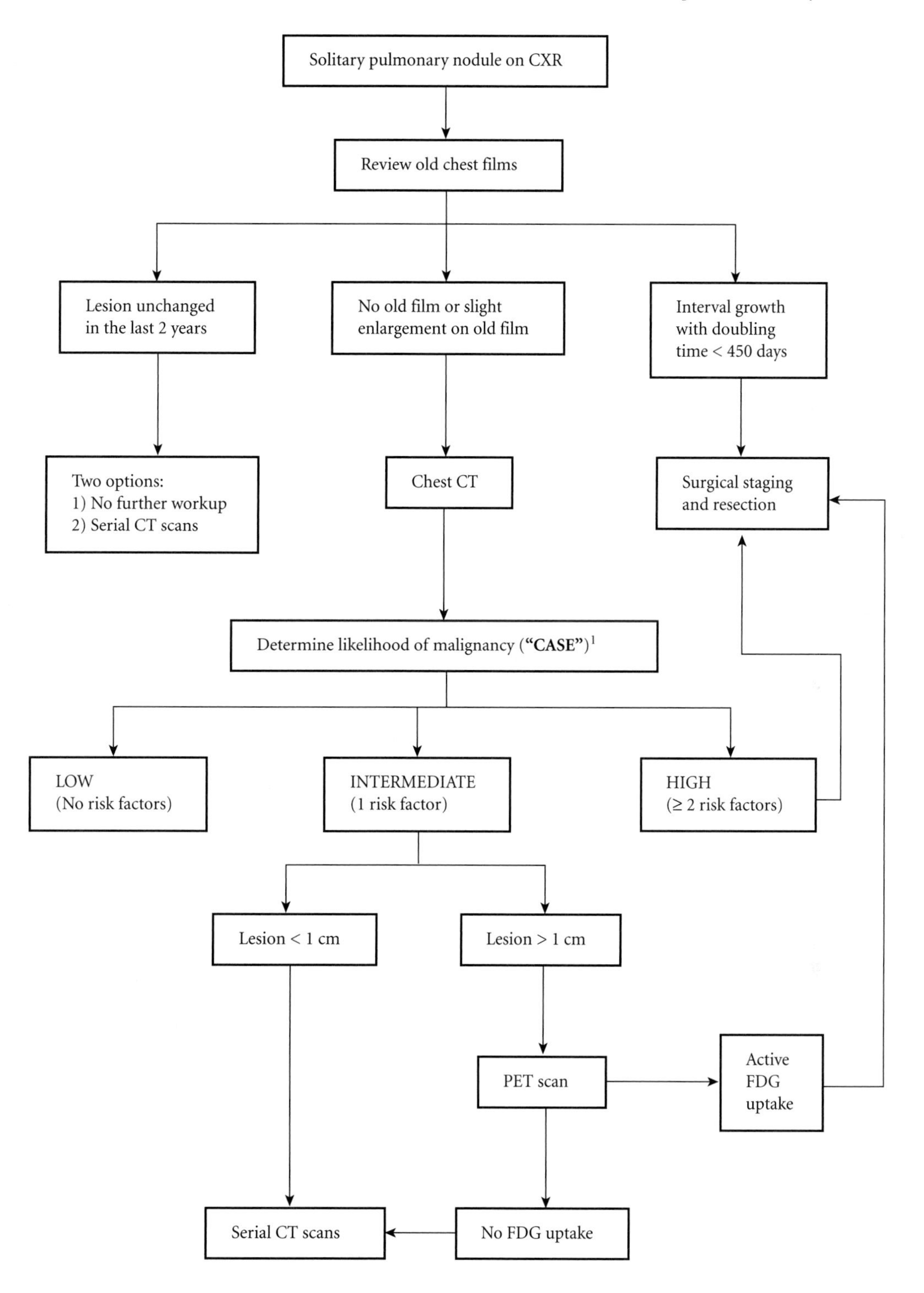

[1]**CASE:** Chest imaging findings, Age > 50, Smoking history, Environmental exposures

FIGURE 3–9 Diagnostic approach to solitary pulmonary nodule.

CXR shows mediastinal adenopathy and a 5-cm central pulmonary nodule with irregular borders. Abnormal laboratory findings are elevated calcium and anemia. What is the next step in the evaluation of this lesion?

Perform chest CT with contrast to define the extent of the mass and to detect intrathoracic lymph node metastases. Lung cancer most commonly metastasizes to the liver, adrenal glands, brain, and bones. Therefore, extend the chest CT to include the liver and adrenal glands. Also, obtain a head CT and a radionuclide-enhanced bone scan.

> Evaluation can be limited to chest CT in asymptomatic patients with no clinical, laboratory, or CXR findings to suggest advanced disease.

CT scan shows a spiculated central mass and two lymph nodes. No extrathoracic metastases are seen. What is the next step in management?

Tissue samples of the lesion and associated lymph nodes are necessary to define the type and stage of lesion. Cytology of an early morning sputum specimen occasionally yields malignant cells in central lesions. In most cases, central lesions require fiber-optic bronchoscope–guided bronchial washings, brushings, or biopsy. Lymph nodes can be sampled with a bronchoscope (transbronchial needle aspiration) or a mediastinoscope (bronchoscope inserted through an incision above the sternum).

How would you obtain tissue samples if the patient had a peripheral lesion?

Bronchoscopes cannot access peripheral lesions because they do not extend further than the secondary branches of the bronchial tree. Obtain tissue samples using CT-guided transthoracic needle biopsy or video-assisted thoracoscopic surgery (VATS).

What are the different types of bronchogenic carcinoma?

Four histological types account for 95% of lung cancer diagnoses (listed in descending order):

1. Adenocarcinoma (bronchoalveolar carcinoma is an important subtype)
2. Squamous cell carcinoma
3. Large cell carcinoma
4. Small cell carcinoma (oat cell carcinoma is the most common subtype)

> **Adenocarcinoma and hemoptysis**: Hemoptysis is less common because adenocarcinomas are usually peripheral.
> **Small cell carcinomas and hemoptysis**: Small cell carcinomas are usually central, but hemoptysis is less common because small cell carcinomas grow and invade through submucosal tissues.

Bronchoscopy with biopsy reveals a squamous cell carcinoma. Two lymph nodes are positive for malignancy. How is non–small cell lung cancer (NSCLC) treated?

NSCLC responds poorly to chemotherapy alone. Potentially curative surgery is the mainstay of treatment for stage 1 and 2 NSCLC (Table 3-13). Surgery is also an option for a limited number of patients with disease in mediastinal lymph nodes (stage 3A). Treatment of stage 3B and stage 4 NSCLC is primarily palliative (chemotherapy, radiation, and other palliative measures).

> **Stage 3 NSCLC**: To assess whether patient is a candidate for surgery, perform spirometry to evaluate preoperative lung function and refer to a thoracic surgeon.

Why does this patient have hypercalcemia?

Lung cancer can cause a number of paraneoplastic syndromes (Table 3-14). These result from production of biologically active substances by the tumor or in response to the tumor. The most likely cause of hypercalcemia in this patient with squamous cell carcinoma and no bony metastases is production of parathyroid hormone–related peptide.

> **Digital clubbing**: Loss of the normal angle between fingernail and nailbed as a result of subungal soft tissue thickening occurs in 30% of lung cancer patients.

TABLE 3–13 Non Small-Cell Lung Cancer Staging and Treatment

Stage	Spread	Treatment
I	Isolated lesion	Surgery + chemotherapy
II	Hilar node spread	Surgery + chemotherapy and radiation
IIIA	Mediastinal spread, but resectable	Neo-adjuvant chemotherapy and radiation followed by resection
IIIB	Mediastinal spread but unresectable	Palliative care
IV	Metastatic	Palliative care

Note: Adapted from Sabatine M. *Pocket Medicine,* 2nd ed. Lippincott Williams & Wilkins, 2000.

TABLE 3–14 Common Paraneoplastic Syndromes in Lung Cancer

Systemic	Weight Loss, Anorexia
Skin	Digital clubbing Trousseau syndrome (migrating superficial phlebitis)
Endocrine	Hypercalcemia: caused by ectopic PTH-related peptide; most frequent in squamous cell carcinoma. Hyponatremia: caused by ectopic adrenocorticotropic hormone (ACTH) production, which leads to the syndrome of inappropriate antidiuretic hormone (see Chapter 7: Fluids and Electrolytes); most frequently observed in small cell cancer.
Heme	Anemia
Neurological	Lambert-Eaton Myasthenic Syndrome (LEMS): Antibodies against presynaptic calcium-channels lead to decreased acetylcholine release and subsequent weakness. Peripheral neuropathy

What is the most likely cause of hoarseness in this patient with lung cancer?

The most likely cause of hoarseness is compression of the recurrent laryngeal nerve by the tumor (Table 3-15).

Alternative 3.10.1

A non-smoker with no known environmental exposures is diagnosed with lung cancer.

What histologic sub-type is most likely?

Smoking causes approximately 90% of lung cancers. Other important environmental risk factors for lung cancer are asbestos, polycyclic aromatic hydrocarbons, nickel, radon, and arsenic. Bronchoalveolar carcinoma is the most common histologic subtype in patients with no known risk factors.

Alternative 3.10.2

A 75-year-old nonsmoker with a history of asbestos exposure during World War II presents with progressive dyspnea, hemoptysis, and weight loss. CXR demonstrates a large pleural effusion and thickened pleura.

What diagnosis should you suspect?

Malignant mesothelioma is an aggressive cancer that arises from the mesothelial surfaces of the pleural and peritoneal cavities. The most important risk factor is history of asbestos exposure. Cigarette smoking does not increase risk of mesothelioma. Pleural effusion and thickening are the most common radiographic findings. Suspect malignant mesothelioma in a patient with a history of asbestos exposure. Prognosis is dismal.

TABLE 3–15 Syndromes Resulting From Direct Extension of Lung Cancer

Superior vena cava syndrome	Compression of the superior vena cava causes headache, dyspnea, upper extremity and facial swelling, and dilated neck veins. Superior vena cava syndrome is most commonly caused by small cell lung cancer.
Pancoast syndrome	An apical (superior sulcus) lung tumor can compress C8, T1, and T2 cervical nerve roots. This leads to ipsilateral Horner's syndrome (facial ptosis, anhidrosis, miosis), and ipsilateral hand pain and weakness. Evaluate such a tumor with magnetic resonance imaging rather than chest computed tomography imaging to assess the extent of invasion; this syndrome is most commonly caused by squamous cell carcinoma.
Hoarseness	Compression of the recurrent laryngeal nerve is more common with a left-sided tumor and leads to hoarseness.

Alternative 3.10.3

A 64-year-old patient is diagnosed with small cell lung cancer (SCLC).

How does the treatment strategy differ from NSCLC?

SCLC is classified as limited or extensive. Regardless of stage, SCLC is considered metastatic at diagnosis, so surgery is not beneficial. Unlike NSCLC, SCLC is highly responsive to chemotherapy. Limited-stage SCLC is typically treated with a platinum and etoposide regimen plus prophylactic cranial irradiation. Late-stage SCLC is typically treated with irinotecan and etoposide but not radiation. Note that although chemotherapy provides palliative benefit and prolongs survival, it is not curative. SCLC tends to relapse within months despite appropriate treatment.

CASE 3–11 DYSPNEA AND HEMOPTYSIS IN A RECENT IMMIGRANT

A 22-year-old Indian man undergoes CXR for low-grade fever and mild cough. He is in India and has recently been accepted to a graduate program in the United States. He does not smoke cigarettes. CXR shows an ill-defined consolidation in the right upper lobe and enlarged right upper lobe lymph nodes.

What do the CXR findings suggest?

The CXR findings describe a Ghon complex characteristic of primary pulmonary TB infection. Primary TB is often completely asymptomatic. Low-grade fever is the most common early symptom.

The patient's physician recommends that he undergo therapy for active TB. However, the patient does not follow up with his physician in India because he begins to feel better. A few weeks later, he relocates to the United States. Eight months later, he presents to the student health clinic with 3 weeks of dyspnea, hemoptysis, low-grade fever, night sweats, and weight loss. During a screening drive at the university 1 week ago, his HIV test was negative. On physical examination, there are distant hollow breath sounds in the right apex (amphora). What is the most likely diagnosis?

Suspect reactivation TB in a patient with constitutional symptoms and risk factors (Chapter 1: Health Maintenance and Statistics). Hemoptysis and dyspnea are signs of advanced disease.

What is the next step in management?

Obtain a CXR. Nine out of ten cases of reactivation TB involve infiltrates in the apical posterior lung segments. Other common CXR findings of reactivation TB are cavities, air fluid levels, and pleural thickening or effusions.

CXR demonstrates thickened pleura in the right upper lobe and multiple bilateral calcified nodules. What is the next step in diagnosis?

CXR is not particularly sensitive or specific at differentiating active from latent disease. The next step is to obtain three sputum samples. Evaluate the sputum with culture and an acid-fast stain (to detect *M. tuberculosis* bacilli). A positive acid-fast stain or culture indicates active disease. In addition, place the patient in respiratory isolation.

> Sputum culture is more sensitive to indicate active disease, but detection of acid-fast bacilli is more rapid.

Sputum is positive for the presence of acid-fast bacilli. How is active TB treated?

Multidrug therapy for 6 to 12 months is required because of the risk of drug resistance. The recommended initial regimen is a combination of four drugs ("***RIPES***"): **R**ifampin, **I**soniazid (INH), **P**yrazinamide, and **E**thambutol (or streptomycin). If the organism is susceptible to rifampin and INH, discontinue the latter two drugs after 2 months.

> Compliance with therapy is the major determinant of successful treatment.

What baseline studies are recommended prior to starting anti-TB treatment?

Monitor liver enzymes (major toxicity of INH), platelets, and serum creatinine prior to initiating therapy. If ethambutol is chosen, also test visual acuity and red-green discoloration (risk of optic neuritis). INH can cause peripheral neuropathy, so prescribe vitamin B6 to patients with predisposing conditions such as diabetes mellitus, alcoholism, or renal failure.

> Monitoring is not necessary during treatment if baseline labs are normal.

The patient complains that his urine is bright red-orange while on therapy. What is the likely cause of this finding?

This is a common and typically harmless side effect of rifampin that should resolve after the treatment regimen is completed. Advise the patient not to wear contact lenses during treatment because these can be stained red-orange as well.

The patient stops taking his drugs after 3 months of therapy because he is feeling better. He returns to India, so the health department cannot enforce treatment. Six months later, he is admitted to a hospital in India because of headache, confusion, vomiting, and inability to move his right eye laterally (cranial nerve 6 palsy). What is the likely cause of these findings given his history?

The presentation is consistent with TB infection that has spread to the meninges. Perform lumbar puncture to evaluate the cerebrospinal fluid for TB infection. TB infection that has spread hematogenously to other organs is called miliary TB. Common organ systems affected are the lungs, gastrointestinal tract (peritonitis, cholecystitis), adrenals, and spine (Pott's syndrome). A multidrug regimen is also required for miliary TB.

CASE 3–12 PLEURAL EFFUSION

A 72-year-old patient with a 40-pack/year history of smoking is evaluated for mild dyspnea of recent onset. He has also had cough and mild hemoptysis over the last 4 months. Physical examination is significant for dullness to percussion, diminished breath sounds, decreased tactile fremitus, and a friction rub on the right side. Vitals signs are normal. CXR is obtained (Fig. 3-10). PPD is negative, and sputum does not show any acid-fast bacilli.

What is the abnormal finding on the CXR?

The patient has a large pleural effusion (excess fluid in the pleural space). Pleural effusion results from either excess production or impaired removal of pleural fluid.

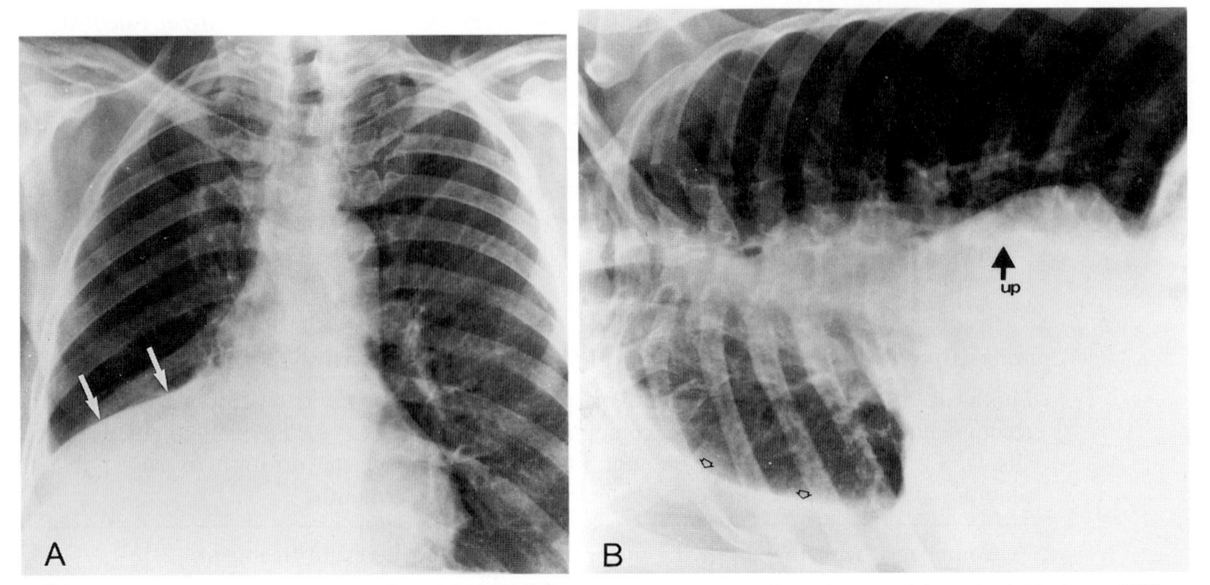

FIGURE 3–10 Chest x-ray of large pleural effusion. From Daffner, RH. *Clinical Radiology: The Essentials*, 3rd ed. Lippincott Williams & Wilkins, 2007.

How much fluid is required to produce this patient's symptoms and CXR findings?

Healthy individuals have <1 mL of fluid between the visceral and parietal pleura. Small effusions are usually only evident on lateral decubitus films. On a lateral decubitus film, small effusions are <1.5 cm, moderate effusions are 1.5 to 4.5 cm thick, and large effusions are >4.5 cm. At least 300 mL of fluid is required to produce the blunted costophrenic angles seen in this patient's upright CXR, and at least 500 mL is required to produce this patient's symptoms.

What kinds of fluid can accumulate in the pleural space?

Four types of fluids can accumulate in the pleural space:

1. Serous fluid (hydrothorax)
2. Blood
3. Chyle
4. Pus (empyema)

What are the causes of a pleural effusion?

Pleural effusions are classified as transudates or exudates:

1. **Transudates** occur when the rate of pleural fluid formation exceeds the rate of lymphatic clearance. Excess fluid can result from increased capillary hydrostatic pressure (e.g., CHF) or decreased plasma oncotic pressure (e.g., cirrhosis or nephrotic syndrome). Because the pleural capillary endothelium is intact, protein content of pleural fluid is low (<3.0 mL).
2. **Exudates** typically exhibit elevated protein content, unlike transudates. There are three major mechanisms of exudate formation. They are:
   (i) Damage to the pleural lining (e.g., bacterial pneumonia, viral infection, collagen vascular disorders, and mesothelioma)
   (ii) Blockage of lymphatic drainage (e.g., metastatic disease)
   (iii) Movement of fluid from the peritoneal space (e.g., chronic pancreatitis, chylous ascites, and peritoneal carcinomatosis)

PE can cause transudates or exudates.

What is the next step in determining the cause of this pleural effusion?

Perform thoracentesis to obtain a sample of pleural fluid for analysis. This patient has a large effusion, so physical exam (dullness to percussion) is sufficient to guide needle placement. Thoracentesis in this patient is also therapeutic, as it will at least temporarily relieve some of his symptoms.

> Insert the needle in the superior border of the rib to avoid damaging the neurovascular bundle.

> Consider ultrasound-guided thoracentesis if the patient is obese or if the effusion is small or loculated.

How can pleural fluid analysis differentiate between a transudate and an exudate?

The fluid is considered an exudate if any of the following are present (Light's criteria):

1. Pleural fluid protein/serum protein (albumin) > 0.5
2. Pleural fluid LDH/serum LDH > 0.6
3. Pleural fluid LDH > 200 international units (IU)

What other lab tests are commonly ordered if pleural fluid analysis demonstrates an exudate?

Consider the following additional pleural fluid analyses if the patient has an exudate: glucose (decreased in bacterial infections), pH (decreased in bacterial infections), Gram stain and culture (may identify pathogen), cell count with differential, amylase (increase in pancreatic effusions), adenosine deaminase activity (increase in effusions due to TB), and cytology (positive in malignancy).

The patient has an exudate; there is no evidence of infection, and cytology is negative. What is the next diagnostic step?

The next step is CT scan. If CT scan is nondiagnostic, consider pleural biopsy because this patient has a high pretest probability of lung cancer despite negative cytology.

CT scan and subsequent work-up confirm the presence of lung cancer. He has repeated symptomatic pleural effusions requiring multiple therapeutic thoracenteses. What measure can you recommend for this patient?

Pleural effusions due to malignancy are often large and recurrent because the underlying cause is difficult to treat. Consider pleurodesis (attaching the two pleural surfaces so no fluid can accumulate between them). Pleurodesis can be achieved surgically or by instillation of chemicals such as talc, bleomycin, or tetracycline/doxycyclin.

Alternative 3.12.1

A patient with known CHF has a small, asymptomatic pleural effusion seen on lateral decubitus but not on upright CXR.

How should you manage this pleural effusion?

Observation is generally recommended for small asymptomatic effusions that occur in the setting of a known cause of transudates like CHF.

Alternative 3.12.2

A patient is admitted to the hospital for a bacterial pneumonia. Antibiotics are started in the emergency department. Lateral decubitus CXR indicates a pleural opacity that does not flow freely.

What is the most likely cause of the pleural effusion?

Pleural effusions that occur in the setting of pneumonia are most likely to be exudates. An exudate that occurs in the setting of pneumonia is called a parapneumonic effusion. Parapneumonic effusions are further categorized as follows:

1. Simple parapneumonic effusion: Initially, damage to pleural lining causes sterile fluid accumulation, so pH, LDH, cell count, and glucose levels are normal. Treatment of the underlying pneumonia usually resolves simple parapneumonic effusions.
2. Complicated parapneumonic effusion: Persistent pleural inflammation causes leakage of bacteria into the pleura. As a result, characteristic biochemical findings develop, such as decreased pH (due to lactate and carbon dioxide production), decreased glucose (because bacteria utilize glucose), and increased LDH (due to increased cell turnover). Cell count usually demonstrates increased neutrophils. Gram stain and culture are often positive. Antibiotics alone are usually insufficient (also require tube drainage)
3. Empyema ("fibrinopurulent stage"): Progressive inflammation leads to fibrin formation, which causes septations and loculations. Lysis of bacteria by neutrophils leads to pus formation. Characteristic biochemical markers may or may not be positive. Treat with antibiotics, tube drainage, and administration of fibrinolytics into the pleural cavity.

What is the next step in management?

The next step is to order a contrast-enhanced chest CT. This test enhances the pleural surface, which helps distinguish an uncomplicated parapneumonic effusion from a complicated parapneumonic effusion with an empyema.

Chest CT shows a loculated parapneumonic effusion with thickened parietal pleura. What is the next step in management?

Any suspected parapneumonic effusion >10 mm requires thoracentesis. "Tap" parapneumonic effusions <10 mm if they are loculated or CT scan shows thickened parietal pleura (because both these findings are suspicious for empyema).

> "Tap": medical slang typically used to describe withdrawal of peritoneal fluid, cerebrospinal fluid, or pleural fluid.

Gross pus is seen during thoracentesis. Analysis of the pleural fluid reveals an exudate with pH 7.18 and glucose 50. Gram stain and culture are negative. What is the next step in management?

The finding of gross pus during thoracentesis is diagnostic of empyema, regardless of other pleural fluid findings. Drain the effusion and administer at least 4 to 6 weeks of broad-spectrum antibiotics. Also, consider administration of fibrinolytic agents into the pleural cavity. If radiologic findings or clinical symptoms do not improve within 7 days, consider VATS. If VATS is unsuccessful, treat with open surgery (thoracotomy).

CASE 3–13 SEVERE HYPOXEMIA IN AN INTENSIVE CARE UNIT PATIENT

A 48-year-old woman is admitted to the intensive care unit for treatment of septic shock. She has a history of pancreatic cancer. Fluids and antibiotics are initiated. Twenty-four hours later, she becomes very dyspneic and tachypneic. Bilateral rales are heard on physical exam. There are no murmurs. Jugular veins are 4 cm. PaO_2 is 100 on 60% FIO_2. $PaCO_2$ is 35. She is intubated and mechanically ventilated. CXR is obtained (Fig. 3-11).

What is the most likely cause of the severe hypoxemia?

The most likely diagnosis acute respiratory distress syndrome (ARDS). ARDS typically presents with rapidly worsening dyspnea and hypoxemia requiring increasingly higher

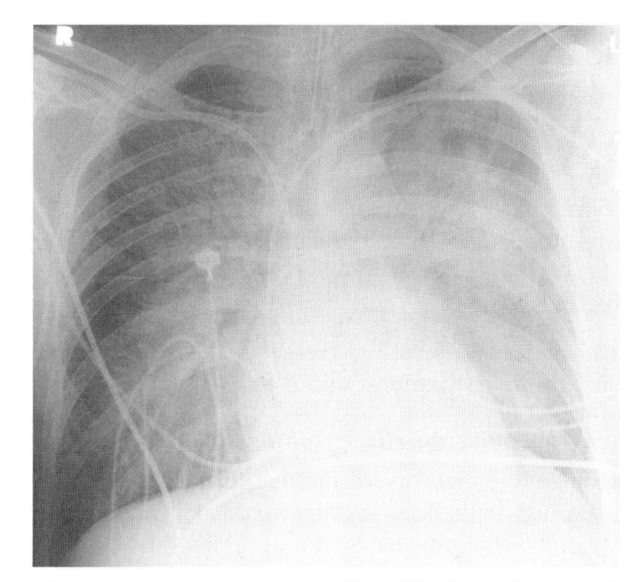

FIGURE 3–11 Acute respiratory distress syndrome. From Daffner, RH. *Clinical Radiology: The Essentials,* 3rd ed. Lippincott Williams & Wilkins, 2007.

concentrations of supplemental oxygen. Symptoms typically occur 24 to 48 hours after an inciting event that injures lung parenchyma. Physical examination usually reveals cyanosis, tachycardia, tachypnea, and diffuse rales. Mechanical ventilation is almost universally required. This patient has all three diagnostic criteria for ARDS:

1. Bilateral fluffy infiltrates on CXR (appearance similar to CHF)
2. Severe hypoxemia ($PaO_2/FIO_2 < 200$)
3. No evidence of increased left atrial pressure (if measured, pulmonary capillary wedge pressure (PCWP) is <18 mm Hg).

What is the most likely cause of ARDS in this patient?

Septic shock is the most common cause of ARDS, particularly among alcoholics. Sepsis causes the release of endotoxins and other microorganism into the blood stream, which can trigger a sequence of events that are toxic to parenchymal cells.

What are other common causes of ARDS?

Common causes of ARDS are "***TIP TABS***"

1. **T**rauma
2. **I**ngestions of drugs
3. **P**neumonia (even in the absence of septic shock)
4. **T**ransfusion of >15 units of blood products
5. **A**spiration of gastric contents, hydrocarbons, or water (drowning).
6. **B**urns
7. **S**eptic shock

How is ARDS treated?

1. Treat the underlying cause (in this case, treat septic shock aggressively).
2. Mechanical ventilation: Administer low tidal volumes to minimize barotrauma. Include positive end expiratory pressure to minimize intrapulmonary blood shunting.
3. Glucocorticoids: The underlying mechanism is inflammation, so glucocorticoids are often administered. Not all studies have shown improved outcomes.

> If PaO_2/FIO_2 is between 200 and 300 but other criteria for ARDS are met, the patient has acute lung injury. Treatment is the same as ARDS.

What is this patient's prognosis?

ARDS carries a 35% to 40% mortality rate. Most patients die from the underlying cause of ARDS and not from respiratory failure.

Alternative 3.13.1

A septic patient in the intensive care unit develops worsening dyspnea and increasing oxygen requirements. He has a history of mitral stenosis. CXR shows bilateral fluffy infiltrates.

How can you determine the etiology of his decline?

Both cardiogenic pulmonary edema due to mitral stenosis and ARDS secondary to sepsis are possible because both share similar clinical and radiographic features during the first several days. Perform echocardiography to document the ejection fraction. If ejection fraction is within normal limits and diastolic function is normal, ARDS is more likely.

Ejection fraction is 30%. What is the next step in the diagnostic evaluation?

The patient has CHF, but concurrent ARDS is also possible. Consider monitoring the PCWP by inserting a Swan-Ganz catheter into the pulmonary artery. The PCWP value is a surrogate marker for left atrial pressure and can help guide fluid administration.

> Swan-Ganz catheterization in the intensive care unit has never been shown to improve mortality, and PCWP is not always a reliable marker of left atrial pressure.

CASE 3–14 SNORING AND DAYTIME SOMNOLENCE

A 55-year-old man presents with a 2-year history of progressively worsening daytime somnolence. He recently crashed his car into a tree because he fell asleep at the wheel during the day. He was terminated from his job because of frequent napping. He does not find the naps refreshing. His wife reports that he snores loudly every night. Past medical history is significant for hypertension controlled with hydrochlorothiazide. On physical examination, he has a low-hanging soft palate. His neck is wide, and his BMI is 33. Vital signs are within normal limits.

What is the most likely cause of his symptoms?

Suspect obstructive sleep apnea (OSA) in a patient with snoring and excessive daytime sleepiness. OSA results from airway obstruction, so look for physical findings of nasal obstruction, a low-hanging soft palate and large uvula, enlarged tonsils or adenoids, and retrognathia or micrognathia. OSA is more common in men. An enlarged neck circumference and obesity are other risk factors for OSA.

What are the complications of OSA?

OSA can cause diminished alertness, HTN, cardiovascular disease, diabetes mellitus, lipid abnormalities, and pulmonary vascular disease.

What testing is indicated to evaluate for OSA in this patient?

Polysomnography is indicated in this patient with a high pretest probability of OSA whose symptoms substantially affect daily activities. Polysomnography monitors sleep stages, respiratory effort, airflow, SaO_2, EKG, body position, and limb movements.

> Consider cheaper tests such as overnight home oximetry in patients with daytime somnolence who have a lower pretest probability of OSA.

Polysomnography documents a number of episodes of oxygen desaturation accompanied by arousals. Respiratory efforts continue during these episodes. The patient is diagnosed with OSA. How do you recommend this patient manage his condition?

The patient should lose weight and avoid alcohol and other sedatives. Nasal CPAP (continuous positive airway pressure) is a noninvasive therapy for OSA. If lifestyle measures and nasal CPAP are ineffective, consider surgery to relieve areas of obstruction.

Alternative 3.14.1

A 50-year-old man presents with fatigue and daytime somnolence. He was fired from his job at the local Dunkin Donuts because he kept falling asleep during the day. His wife mentions that he snores very loudly. Vital signs are temperature 37.2°C, pulse 77 bpm, respirations 8/min, and blood pressure 160/90. SaO_2 is 88% on room air, and BMI is 45.

What additional test is indicated at this time?

Consider the diagnosis of obesity-hypoventilation syndrome in morbidly obese patients with hypoventilation. OSA is a very common coexisting condition, so concurrent symptoms of OSA increase the likelihood of Pickwickian syndrome. The exact mechanism of Pickwickian syndrome is unknown.

> The prototypical obese hypersomnolent man was described in the Charles Dickens novel *The Posthumous Papers of the Pickwick Club.*

What diagnostic test should you order next?

Order an ABG in patients with suspected Pickwickian syndrome. Daytime hypercapnia (increased $PaCO_2$) due to hypoventilation is the diagnostic hallmark of this disorder. Hypoxemia is another common feature (also due to hypoventilation).

ABG shows hypoxemia and hypercapnia. What additional tests should you order?

Order additional tests urgently to screen for other causes of hypoventilation as well as to assess for the presence of complications or coexisting conditions:

1. CBC: because hypoxemia can stimulate excessive erythrocytosis
2. Serum electrolytes, creatine phosphokinase: to screen for other causes of respiratory muscle weakness
3. Thyroid function tests: because hypothyroidism can cause hypoventilation
4. EKG, CXR, and pulmonary function tests: to screen for other underlying heart and lung diseases
5. Polysomnography: to screen for concurrent OSA

How is obesity-hypoventilation syndrome treated?

The most important measure in obesity-related hypoventilation is weight loss. Other measures include phlebotomy (if HCT >65%) and treatment of complicating/coexisting conditions such as OSA.

Alternative 3.14.2

A 25-year-old woman presents with a 2-year history of frequent "sleep attacks" during the day. She finds the naps refreshing. She often has vivid and frightening dreams just as she is falling asleep or waking up. Sometimes, she is unable to move and collapses just as she falls asleep. She undergoes a sleep latency test, which demonstrates three periods of REM-onset sleep.

What is the diagnosis?

Narcolepsy usually begins in the second or third decade. Like OSA, it leads to daytime somnolence. Unlike OSA, patients may have hypnagogic hallucinations (vivid dreams just as the patient is falling asleep or waking up) and cataplexy (sudden episodes of bilateral muscle weakness). Two or more periods of REM-onset sleep during a sleep latency test is diagnostic of narcolepsy.

> Patients with narcolepsy find daytime naps refreshing, whereas patients with OSA do not.

How is narcolepsy treated?

Treat daytime sleepiness with modafinil or other amphetamine-like compounds. Treat cataplexy with γ-hydroxybutyrate. Nonpharmacological measures include scheduled daytime naps, good sleep hygiene, and avoidance of drugs that produce daytime sleepiness.

chapter 4

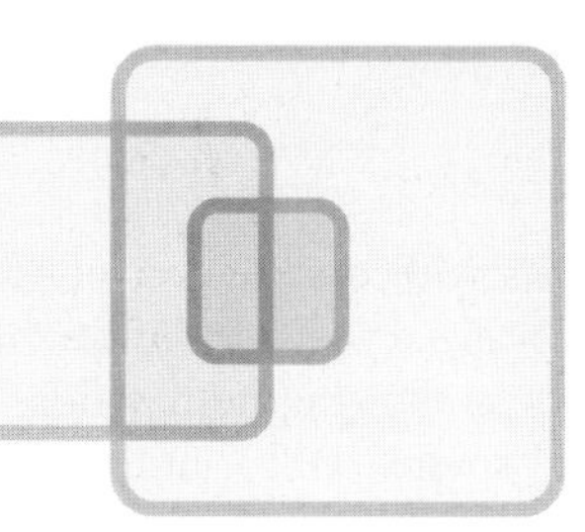

Gastroenterology

CASE 4–1 DIFFICULTY SWALLOWING SOLIDS AND LIQUIDS

A 45-year-old woman presents with a 3-year history of difficulty swallowing (dysphagia) both solids and liquids. She describes the dysphagia as a sensation of food getting stuck substernally a few seconds after she swallows. The dysphagia has gotten worse over the last 12 months, and she reports a 10-lb weight loss this past year. She also complains of substernal burning after meals and occasional regurgitation of food contents. She complains of bad breath (halitosis) despite good oral hygiene. She has taken proton pump inhibitors (PPIs) in the past without any relief.

What are the causes of dysphagia?

1. Oropharyngeal dysphagia presents with a sensation of "food getting stuck" immediately after swallowing. Patients often report coughing or choking after a meal. Symptoms are localized to the cervical region. Causes include oropharyngeal tumor, zenker diverticulum, myasthenia gravis, inflammatory myopathies, and thyrotoxicosis.

2. Esophageal dysphagia presents with a sensation of "food getting stuck" a few seconds after swallowing. Symptoms are localized to the suprasternal notch or substernal region. Dysphagia that begins with difficulty swallowing both solids and liquids suggests a motility disorder (achalasia, diffuse esophageal spasm (DES), nutcracker esophagus, or isolated lower esophageal sphincter (LES) hypertension). Dysphagia that begins with difficulty swallowing solids but not liquids suggests mechanical obstruction (esophageal web, ring, stricture, or tumor).
3. Functional dysphagia has no identified cause after a complete diagnostic evaluation.

> **Dysphagia** = difficulty swallowing
> **Odynophagia** = painful swallowing
> **Globus sensation** = feeling of "lump in throat" even between meals in the absence of dysphagia or odynophagia

What is the most likely cause of this patient's dysphagia?

This patient's symptoms suggest that an esophageal cause is responsible for her symptoms. Dysphagia with both solids and liquids indicates an esophageal motility disorder. Heartburn, regurgitation, halitosis, and weight loss are characteristic symptoms of achalasia (see Fig. 4-1).

What is the pathophysiology of achalasia?

Achalasia is an idiopathic degeneration of myenteric plexus neurons in the distal esophagus. Neurons that cause smooth muscle relaxation are preferentially affected, while those that lead to smooth muscle contraction are spared. As a result, the LES does not adequately relax, and the distal esophagus loses its normal peristaltic function.

What is the next step in diagnosis?

Order a barium swallow (see Fig. 4-2). The classic finding in achalasia is a dilated esophagus that terminates in a beak-like narrowing caused by the persistently contracted LES (see Fig. 4-3). If the barium swallow is positive, confirm the diagnosis with esophageal manometry. Manometry findings of achalasia are increased resting LES pressure, incomplete LES relaxation after swallowing, and aperistalsis in the lower esophagus (Table 4-1).

> **Pseudoachalasia:** Other conditions can cause abnormalities identical to achalasia. Most common among these are malignancies and Chagas' disease. Perform upper endoscopy in all patients with achalasia to rule out malignancy.

> **Upper endoscope:** Also called an esophagogastroduodenoscope (EGD), this scope has a light and a camera at the tip and is used to visualize the esophagus, stomach, and duodenum.

Barium swallow and esophageal manometry confirm the diagnosis of achalasia. There is no evidence of malignancy on endoscopy. How is achalasia treated?

Unfortunately, there is no way to halt neuron degeneration in achalasia. Current therapies all aim to decrease LES pressure.

1. Good surgical candidates: On the basis of patient preference and the availability of physicians with the necessary expertise, perform either pneumatic balloon dilation of the LES or modified Heller myotomy (a surgical procedure that weakens the LES by cutting the muscle fibers). At least half the patients who undergo pneumatic dilation will require another treatment in 5 years. Most patients who undergo Heller myotomy develop gastroesophageal reflux disease (GERD).
2. Poor surgical candidates: These patients can take nitrates and/or calcium channel blockers before meals. If pharmacotherapy fails to control their symptoms, consider injecting botulinum into the LES during endoscopy. Botulinum poisons excitatory acetylcholine-producing neurons.

> Patients with achalasia have an increased risk of esophageal squamous cell carcinoma (SCC), but surveillance EGD is not recommended because it is not cost-effective.

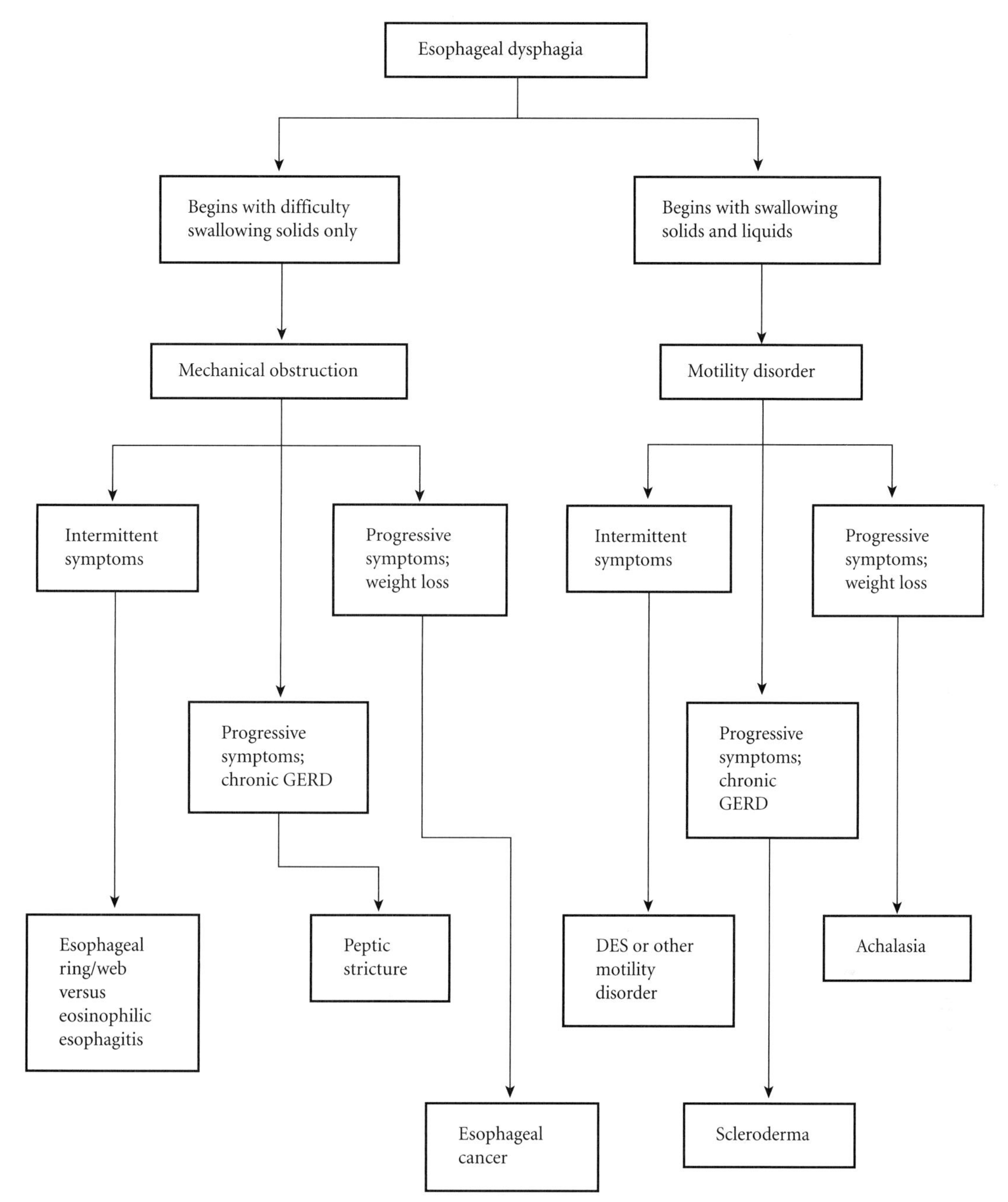

FIGURE 4–1 Causes of esophageal dysphagia.

The patient undergoes pneumatic dilation. Shortly after the procedure, she complains of dyspnea and severe pain in the chest and epigastrium that increases with inspiration and swallowing. Auscultation of the chest reveals a crunching sound (Hamman's crunch). What complication should you suspect?

The most serious complication of pneumatic dilation is esophageal rupture. Suspect an intrathoracic esophageal rupture if a patient develops dyspnea, chest pain, epigastric pain, or back pain that increases with inspiration and swallowing. Common presenting signs are tachycardia, tachypnea, and Hamman's crunch (indicates mediastinal emphysema due to leakage of air from the esophagus to the mediastinum).

> **Cervical perforation** causes neck pain, hoarseness, sternocleidomastoid muscle tenderness, and cervical subcutaneous emphysema (smooth bulging of the skin overlying the neck that crackles on palpation).

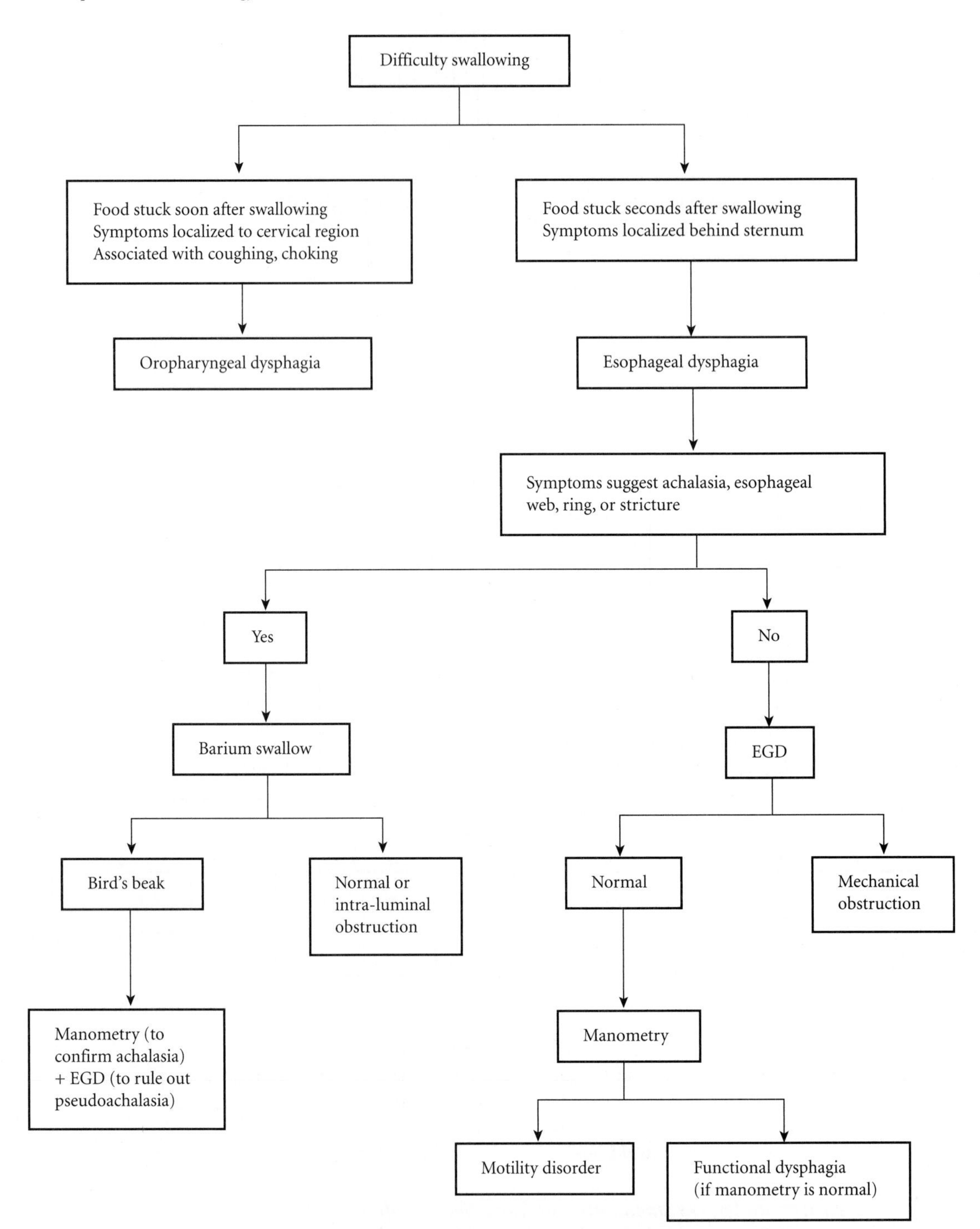

FIGURE 4–2 Diagnostic approach to dysphagia.

What are the next diagnostic steps?

1. Posterior-to-anterior and lateral chest radiograph (CXR): This initial test in suspected esophageal rupture often detects subcutaneous or mediastinal emphysema. CXR may be negative for up to 1 hour after rupture.
2. Contrast esophagography should be obtained if x-rays are positive or negative. In case of positive x-rays, this test confirms the diagnosis. In case of negative x-rays, the test can decrease likelihood of a false-negative x-ray. Use a water-soluble contrast agent (Gastrografin) first because extravasation of a large amount of barium contrast into the mediastinum can

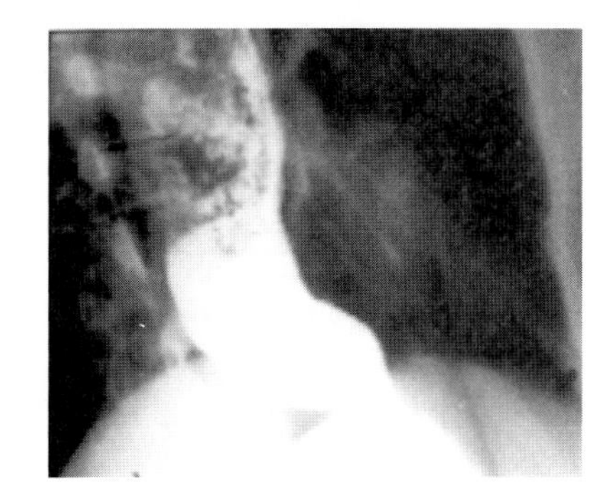

FIGURE 4–3 Barium swallow: achalasia. From Jarrell BE. *NMS Surgery Casebook,* 1st ed. Lippincott Williams & Wilkins, 2003.

cause severe inflammation (mediastinitis). Gastrografin is very sensitive at detecting large perforations, but barium is more sensitive for small perforations. Consider barium to rule out a small perforation if Gastrografin esophagography is negative.

3. CT scan should be used if esophagography is negative because contrast esophagraphy can miss 10% of ruptures. Some centers obtain a CT scan before esophagography.

How is esophageal perforation managed?

1. Medical management comprises no oral intake (nothing per oral (NPO)), total parenteral nutrition, intravenous (IV) broad-spectrum antibiotics, and drainage of fluid collections. This method is indicated only in the subset of patients who are hemodynamically stable and do not have any intrapleural or intraperitoneal contrast extravasation; in addition, the rupture must be diagnosed within 24 hours of the event.
2. Surgery is indicated for all other patients.

This patient with signs of mediastinal emphysema will probably have contrast extravasation and require surgical repair.

Alternative 4.1.1

The patient is 45-year-old woman who presents with intermittent dysphagia to solids and liquids over the last year. She has visited the emergency department three times in the same period for

TABLE 4–1 Manometry Findings in Specific Esophageal Motility Disorders

Disorder	Peristalsis Frequency	Peristalsis Amplitude/Duration	LES
Normal	≥80% of contractions are peristaltic	Mean amplitude 40–160 mm Hg	Resting pressure 10–35 mm Hg above intragastric pressure
Achalasia	Aperistalsis in distal esophagus	Aperistalsis in distal esophagus	Increased resting LES pressure, incomplete relaxation
DES	>30% of distal esophageal contractions are aperistaltic	Frequent multipeaked contraction waves with increased amplitude in distal esophagus	Normal
Nutcracker esophagus	Normal	>30% of distal esophageal contractions with increased amplitude and duration	Normal
Isolated hypertensive LES	Normal	Normal	Increased resting LES pressure

Abbreviations: LES, lower esophageal sphincter; DES, diffuse esophageal spasm.

chest pain, and she has had a negative cardiac evaluation all three times. She undergoes EGD, which does not show any structural abnormalities.

What is the next step in management?

Intermittent dysphagia to both solids and liquids suggests that this patient may have a motility disorder such as DES, nutcracker esophagus, or hypertensive LES. Esophageal motility disorders commonly cause chest pain with negative cardiac and endoscopic findings. The next step in management is esophageal manometry.

More than 30% of distal esophageal contractions on esophageal manometry are nonperistaltic. There are frequent contraction waves with multiple peaks and increased amplitude. Peristaltic contractions are interspersed between waves. LES response is normal. What is the diagnosis?

The manometry findings are diagnostic of DES (see Table 4-1).

> The classic barium swallow radiograph in DES is a "corkscrew pattern" (see Fig. 4-4). This finding is neither sensitive nor specific.

What therapy is recommended?

Many potential therapies may benefit patients with DES, but the ideal therapy and often their mechanism of effect is unknown. Calcium channel blockers and tricyclic antidepressants are generally the initial therapy for DES, nutcracker esophagus, and hypertensive LES. Second-line options are botulinum injection, phosphodiesterase inhibitors, nitrates, and peppermint.

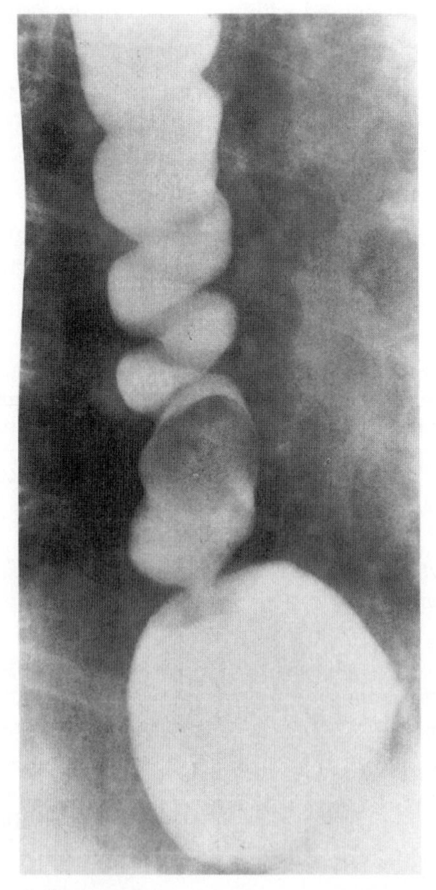

FIGURE 4–4 Barium swallow: diffuse esophageal spasm (corkscrew pattern). From Eisenberg R. *Gastrointestinal Radiology: A Pattern Approach,* 3rd ed. Lippincott Williams & Wilkins, 1990.

CASE 4–2 DIFFICULTY SWALLOWING SOLIDS BUT NOT LIQUIDS

A 50-year-old woman with a history of schizophrenia presents with difficulty swallowing solids but not liquids. She ingested two bottles of drain cleaner 2 months ago. The ingestion required admission to the intensive care unit (ICU). She smokes a pack of cigarettes a day and drinks a six-pack of beer almost every day.

What is the most likely cause of her symptoms?

Ingestion of alkaline agents such as battery fluids, drain cleaners, and other household cleaning products leads to caustic esophageal injury. More than 70% of patients with injuries severe enough to necessitate ICU admission develop dysphagia weeks to months later as a result of esophageal stricture.

> Alkali ingestions damage the esophagus more than acid ingestions. Acid ingestions damage the stomach more than alkali ingestions.

What are other important causes of esophageal stricture?

1. Proximal and mid-esophageal strictures: Common causes are caustic ingestions, "pill-induced" stricture (e.g., alendronate, iron, nonsteroidal anti-inflammatory drugs (NSAIDs)), trauma, and malignancy. Eosinophilic esophagitis is an uncommon but frequently tested condition.
2. Distal esophageal strictures: Most common cause is chronic GERD and Barrett's esophagus (see Case 4–6: Chronic Epigastric Discomfort, Heartburn, and Regurgitation). Collagen vascular diseases are another common cause (see Chapter 9: Rheumatology).

What is the next diagnostic step?

Perform either barium swallow or EGD in patients with suspected stricture. The utility of barium swallow prior to EGD is an area of debate. Consider barium swallow as the initial test for dysphagia when symptoms suggest:

- Achalasia: In older studies, barium swallow was more sensitive.
- Esophageal stricture, web, or ring: EGD may miss subtle narrowing.
- Zenker diverticulum: EGD may be hazardous.

Barium swallow shows an area of intraluminal narrowing. EGD confirms the finding of an esophageal stricture. What is the usual treatment for this complication?

Treat dysphagia due to esophageal stricture with esophageal dilation.

What treatment is the patient likely to have received immediately after her ingestion?

Patients with acute caustic ingestions usually require EGD to assess the degree of injury. If there is only mild mucosal edema and superficial ulcers, the patient can consume a liquid diet and advance to regular foods in 24 to 48 hours. This patient probably had more severe injuries (deep ulcers or necrosis). Such patients maintain fasting and are admitted to the ICU to monitor for life-threatening complications.

> The following are contraindicated immediately after a caustic ingestion:
> 1. **Emetics**: Emesis re-exposes esophagus to caustic agent.
> 2. **Neutralizing agents**: Neutralization causes thermal injury.
> 3. **Nasogastric (NS) intubation**: Induces retching and emesis.

What are important acute life-threatening complications of caustic ingestion?

1. **Esophageal perforation and mediastinitis** present with severe retrosternal or back pain; treatment is emergent surgery.

2. **Gastric perforation and peritonitis** present with abdominal tenderness, rebound, and rigidity; treatment is emergent surgery.
3. **Respiratory distress and shock**: Refer to Chapter 2: Cardiology and Chapter 3: Pulmonary.

The dysphagia resolves with two esophageal dilation treatments. The patient returns 20 years later with a 3-month history of progressive dysphagia. Initially, she had trouble swallowing only solids, but now she has difficulty with liquids as well. She does not have much of an appetite, and she has lost 25 lbs in the last 3 months. What is the suspected diagnosis?

Progressive dysphagia and weight loss are extremely suspicious for esophageal cancer. Caustic alkali injury to the esophagus greatly increases the risk of Squamous cell carcinoma (SCC) of the esophagus 15 to 20 years after the original injury. Major risk factors for SCC in the United States are smoking, alcohol, and achalasia. In other countries, ingestion of betel nuts, extremely hot tea, and nitrosamines are responsible for a significant proportion of esophageal SCC.

> Perform surveillance endoscopy every 1 to 3 years beginning 15 to 20 years after caustic injury to screen for esophageal cancer.

What diagnostic workup is recommended?

Establish the diagnosis using endoscopy with biopsy. If the biopsy is positive, obtain abdominal and chest CT scans to search for distant metastases. If CT detects metastases, the patient has stage 4 disease and the work-up is complete. If CT scans are negative, measure size and invasion of the tumor using endoscopic ultrasound (EUS).

> **EUS**: An ultrasound probe attached to the tip of an upper endoscope or colonoscope helps visualize extraintestinal structures such as pancreas, liver, and lymph nodes. A needle passed through a channel on the endoscope can pierce the stomach or intestine to biopsy any abnormal extraintestinal lesions (fine-needle aspiration).

What is the overall prognosis for patients with SCC of the esophagus?

Overall 5-year survival is only 15% because patients tend to present at later stages. Potentially curative esophagectomy is an option for patients at stage I and stage IIa. For most patients, however, the primary goal of treatment is palliation of pain and dysphagia.

> Symptoms, work-up, and prognosis of esophageal adenocarcinoma and SCC are similar.

Alternative 4.2.1

A 22-year-old man presents with difficulty swallowing solids but not liquids. He has a history of asthma and allergic rhinitis. EGD demonstrates a stricture with concentric rings in the mid esophagus.

What is the most likely diagnosis?

The most likely diagnosis is eosinophilic esophagitis. This uncommon condition is most frequent in boys and young men. The classic finding on EGD is multiple concentric rings in the mid-esophagus that give it the appearance of a trachea. Biopsy demonstrating eosinophil infiltrates is diagnostic. In addition to dilation of the stricture, consider oral fluticasone. Also, consider allergy testing and recommend that the patient avoid any identified allergens.

Alternative 4.2.2

The patient is a 45-year-old woman with a 6-month history of intermittent dysphagia to solids but not liquids. She describes the dysphagia as a sensation of food getting stuck substernally a few seconds after she swallows. She does not have any other symptoms.

What is most likely diagnosis?

Intermittent esophageal dysphagia to solids but not liquids suggests mechanical obstruction due to an esophageal web or ring (Schatzki ring). Esophageal webs typically occur in the upper esophagus and contain squamous epithelium. Esophageal rings typically occur at the gastroesophageal junction and contain both squamous and columnar epithelium.

> **Plummer-Vinson syndrome**: dysphagia due to upper esophageal web + iron deficiency anemia. Recent studies have questioned whether this syndrome truly exists.

Barium swallow shows an area of lower esophageal obstruction. EGD confirms the diagnosis of a lower esophageal ring. How are esophageal webs and rings treated?

Treat esophageal webs and rings with endoscopic dilation. Acid suppression with a PPI may reduce recurrences of both esophageal webs and rings.

CASE 4–3 DYSPHAGIA, COUGH, AND CHOKING AFTER SWALLOWING

A 75-year-old man presents with a 3-month history of coughing and choking immediately after swallowing food and at night. He also reports difficulty swallowing for the past 12 months, and localizes symptoms to his neck. He often has undigested food regurgitate into his mouth hours after eating. He denies any other symptoms. Neurological examination is normal.

What diagnosis should you suspect?

Suspect a Zenker diverticulum in this patient with chronic oropharyngeal dysphagia but no weakness or neurological symptoms. Regurgitation and halitosis are common symptoms. A Zenker diverticulum is an out-pouching of the upper esophageal mucosa in an area of weakness between the lower pharyngeal constrictor and cricopharyngeal muscle. It typically results from increased oropharyngeal pressure due to an abnormal upper esophageal sphincter that resists the passage of food.

> **Aspiration pneumonia**: a common complication of oropharyngeal dysphagia caused by aspiration of gastric contents during coughing or choking.

How do you confirm the diagnosis and treat this condition?

Diagnose this condition using barium swallow. Treatment is surgical or endoscopic esophagomyotomy (to correct the UES dysfunction) and diverticulectomy.

What are other types of esophageal diverticula?

Other esophageal diverticula are midesophageal and epiphrenic diverticula. Most midesophageal and epiphrenic diverticula do not usually require any treatment.

1. **Midesophageal diverticula**: Pulmonary tuberculosis causes mediastinal scarring and hilar adenopathy, which results in diverticula by traction.
2. **Epiphrenic diverticula**: Lower esophageal motility disorders cause out-pouching of the lower esophageal mucosa.

CASE 4–4 CHRONIC EPIGASTRIC DISCOMFORT

A 32-year-old man presents with a 6-month history of burning epigastric pain between meals and at night. Eating and antacids usually resolves his symptoms. He does not have any other medical problems and does not take any medications. He does not smoke or drink alcohol. Vital signs are normal. The attending physician asks you for the differential diagnosis of dyspepsia.

What is dyspepsia?

The term "dyspepsia" refers to chronic and recurrent upper abdominal discomfort. There are three patterns of discomfort:

1. Ulcer or acid-like dyspepsia: burning epigastric pain that is affected by food and may improve with acid-suppressing medications and antacids.
2. Gastroesophageal reflux-like dyspepsia: burning epigastric pain accompanied by heartburn (burning substernal chest pain) and regurgitation; work-up and management differs from other patterns of dyspepsia.
3. Functional dyspepsia (non-ulcer dyspepsia): epigastric fullness, bloating, early satiety, and nausea.

> **Acute abdominal pain**: Pain progressively increases over hours to days.
> **Chronic abdominal pain**: Pain has not changed for months to years.
> **Subacute abdominal pain**: Pain is neither acute nor chronic.

What is the differential diagnosis of dyspepsia?

The most common cause of dyspepsia is functional dyspepsia, followed by peptic ulcer disease (PUD). Other important causes of dyspepsia are:

1. Gastric: gastric cancer and gastritis
2. Biliary: cholelithiasis and cholecystitis
3. Pancreatic: chronic pancreatitis and pancreatic pseudocyst
4. Intestinal: malabsorption, mesenteric ischemia, and irritable bowel syndrome (IBS)

> History and physical do not reliably distinguish functional dyspepsia from PUD.

What cause of dyspepsia do his symptoms suggest?

Burning epigastric pain related to meals suggests that the patient may have PUD. The term "peptic" is a misnomer because peptic ulcers can be duodenal or gastric. This patient's symptoms are typical for duodenal ulcers, which cause pain between meals and improve with food and antacids. Gastric ulcers tend to cause symptoms immediately after meals and are not relieved by food or antacids.

> du**O**denal ulcers are more common in blood type **O** and have l**O**w malignant potential.
> g**A**str**I**c ulcers are more common in blood type **A** and h**I**gh malignant potential.

What causes PUD?

1. ***Helicobacter pylori*** **infection and NSAIDs** are the most common causes of PUD.
2. **Zollinger-Ellison syndrome (ZES)** is rare cause of PUD.
3. **Smoking** may increase the risk of PUD.

> Contrary to popular belief, diet and alcohol are not risk factors for PUD.

How is dyspepsia managed in patients <45 years of age?

First, determine whether the patient has alarm findings for gastric cancer. Obtain EGD if the patient has any of the following alarm findings:

1. Jaundice: Check LFTs.
2. Anemia or gastrointestinal bleeding: Check CBC and fecal occult blood test (FOBT).
3. Protracted vomiting: Check serum electrolytes.

4. Progressive dysphagia or odynophagia
5. Unintentional weight loss
6. Palpable mass or lymphadenopathy

> **Age >45 years:** EGD is indicated in all patients with dyspepsia to rule out cancer.

Lab studies are normal. He does not have any alarm symptoms. What is the next step?

Find out whether the patient smokes cigarettes, drinks alcohol, or takes NSAIDs, and have him discontinue them.

This patient does not have alarm symptoms, does not smoke or drink, and has not recently taken any medications other than antacids. What is the next step?

The next step in management is serology to test for *H. pylori* infection (see Fig. 4-5). If serology is positive, initiate *H. pylori* eradication therapy. There are many regimens to eradicate *H. pylori*. One such regimen is amoxicillin + clarithromycin + PPI for 10 to 14 days. Between 4 and 6 weeks after the patient completes treatment for *H. pylori*, confirm eradication with urea breath test or stool antigen test.

> If initial serology is negative for *H. pylori*, initiate a trial of PPIs.

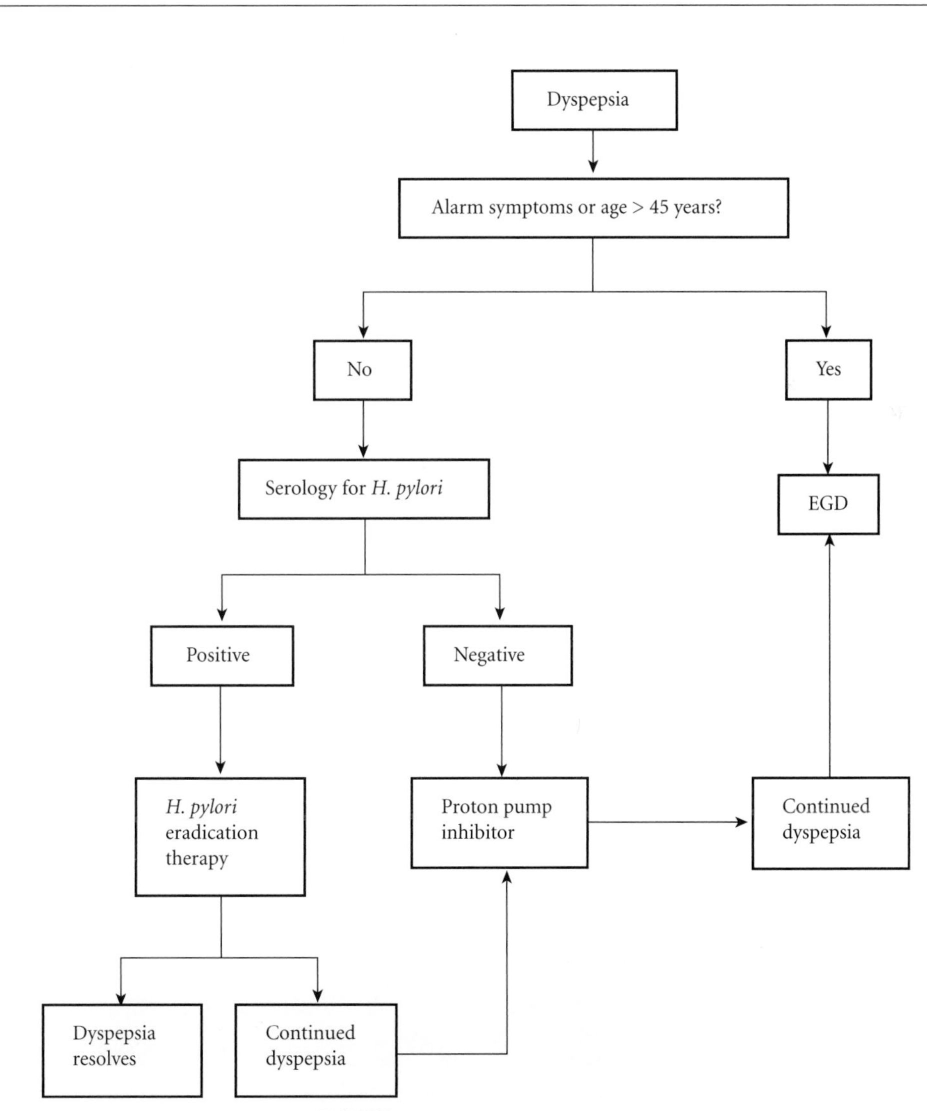

FIGURE 4–5 Workup of dyspepsia.

H. pylori serology is positive. The patient completes a 14-day course of amoxicillin, clarithromycin, and omeprazole. Stool antigen test confirms eradication of H. pylori. The patient remains symptomatic. What is the next step in management?

Initiate a trial of PPIs. If symptoms persist despite 8 weeks of PPIs or recur rapidly after PPI cessation, perform EGD.

The patient responds well to PPIs. Two years later, he presents to the emergency department with a 2-hour history of severe, diffuse abdominal pain. He has been taking ibuprofen for the last 2 weeks. On physical exam, his abdomen is tender with involuntary guarding (rigid abdomen) and rebound tenderness. Vital signs are temperature 37°C, pulse 110 beats per minute (bpm), respirations 20/min, and blood pressure 110/70. What is the most likely cause of his symptoms?

Suspect chemical peritonitis due to ulcer perforation in any patient with a history of PUD who presents signs of a diffuse acute abdomen. Recent NSAID use is the likely cause of perforation in this patient. Perforated peptic ulcer is an emergency because secondary bacterial infection of the peritoneum can lead to septic shock.

> **Acute abdomen (peritonitis)**: acute onset of severe abdominal pain and rebound tenderness; suggests inflammation of an abdominal organ(s) and peritoneum. Many causes of acute abdomen require emergent surgical management.

> The most common laboratory findings in patients with perforated peptic ulcers are leukocytosis and a mildly elevated serum amylase.

What is the next step in diagnosis?

Obtain upright or decubitis abdominal radiographs. Free air under the diaphragm is diagnostic of a perforated ulcer (see Fig. 4-6). If abdominal radiograph is normal but clinical suspicion of perforation is high, obtain abdominal CT scan. If abdominal x-ray or CT scan is positive, evaluate the severity of bleeding with upper GI series (fluoroscopy images obtained after contrast ingestion). Use Gastrografin contrast initially because barium can cause peritonitis if it extravasates into the peritoneum.

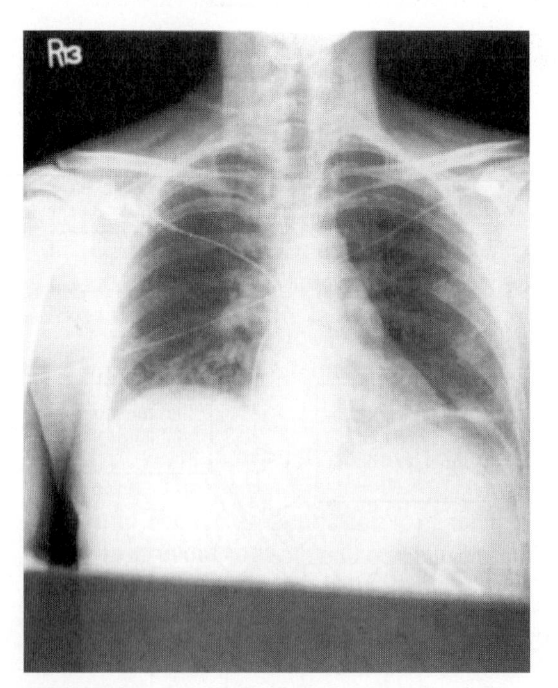

FIGURE 4–6 Abdominal x-ray showing free air under the diaphragm. From Jarrell BE. *NMS Surgery Casebook,* 1st ed. Lippincott Williams & Wilkins, 2003.

Abdominal radiographs show free air under the diaphragm, which confirms the diagnosis of a perforated peptic ulcer. There is no leakage identified on upper GI series. What are the next steps in management?

Medical management is often sufficient for stable patients who present within 12 hours of symptom onset and do not have any leakage documented on upper GI series (i.e., no brisk bleeding). Medical management of perforated peptic ulcer is as follows:

1. Fluids and electrolytes: correct any hypotension with IV normal saline; correct electrolyte imbalances.
2. IV PPIs or H2-blockers
3. NG suction
4. Antibiotics: cover anaerobes, enteric Gram-negative rods, and oral flora with a combination of ampicillin, metronidazole, and a third-generation cephalosporin (or fluoroquinolone).
5. Reassess: Monitor the patient closely in the ICU for deterioration, increased abdominal pain, tenderness, rigidity, or signs of shock (e.g., hypotension, increased pulse or increased temperature); any deterioration is an indication for emergent surgery.

The patient recovers with medical management. Two years later, he presents with a 4-week history of nausea, early satiety, and epigastric fullness after meals. Over the last 7 days, he also reports persistent vomiting after meals. The emesis contains partially digested food contents. He has lost 10 lbs over the past month. Physical examination is significant for a succussion splash over the epigastric area. Vital signs are normal except for a pulse of 110 bpm. Serum potassium is low and bicarbonate is high. What is the most likely complication?

The clinical presentation is consistent with gastric outlet obstruction. Outlet obstruction causes epigastric fullness, nausea, and vomiting after meals, which results in weight loss, dehydration, metabolic alkalosis, and hypokalemia. A succussion splash is sometimes heard over the epigastric area.

What is the next step in management?

Confirm the diagnosis by measuring the quantity of residual gastric contents aspirated during NG suction. A residual volume of 250 to 300 mL establishes the diagnosis. If the residual volume is lower, confirm gastric outlet obstruction with a saline load test.

> **Saline load test:** Administer 750 mL of normal saline into the stomach. Perform NG aspiration 30 minutes later. Retention of $\geq$400 mL indicates a positive test.

270 mL of foul-smelling gastric contents are aspirated, which confirms the diagnosis. What are the next steps in management?

1. Medical management: Initial management is similar to perforated peptic ulcer (fluids and electrolytes, IV PPIs or H2-blockers, antibiotics, and NG suction to decompress bowel).
2. Evaluate nutritional status: After performing initial steps, obtain serum albumin (marker of nutritional status); consider supplemental nutrition if albumin is low.
3. EGD: After 24 to 72 hours of medical management, obtain EGD to define the extent of the obstruction and biopsy to rule out gastric cancer.
4. Endoscopic dilation: If the obstruction does not improve after 5 to 7 days, consider endoscopic dilation.
5. Surgery: If obstruction persists despite dilation, consider surgery.

> **Complications of PUD** (mnemonic: "***POP Blood***"): **P**erforation, **O**bstruction, **P**enetration (ulcer penetrates into other organs like pancreas and causes inflammation of that organ), and **B**leeding (slow or rapid).

Alternative 4.4.1

A 32-year-old man presents with 4 months of burning epigastric pain between meals relieved by food and antacids. He also reports foul-smelling watery diarrhea and steatorrhea. He does not take NSAIDs, smoke cigarettes, or drink alcohol. Serology is negative for *H. pylori.* His symptoms persist despite 8 weeks of daily esomeprazole. He then undergoes EGD, which shows multiple ulcers, one of which is in the jejunum.

What diagnosis should you suspect?

Suspect ZES in the following patients with peptic ulcers:

1. Multiple ulcers refractory to medical therapy
2. Distal duodenal or jejunal ulcers
3. Diarrhea
4. Family history of parathyroid, pituitary, or pancreatic tumors (MEN-1 syndrome)

What causes ZES? How can you confirm the diagnosis?

The cause of ZES is a pancreatic gastrinoma that releases excessive gastrin and stimulates acid hypersecretion. The tumor also inactivates pancreatic enzymes, which leads to malabsorptive diarrhea (foul-smelling watery diarrhea with steatorrhea). See Figure 4-7 for the diagnostic approach to ZES.

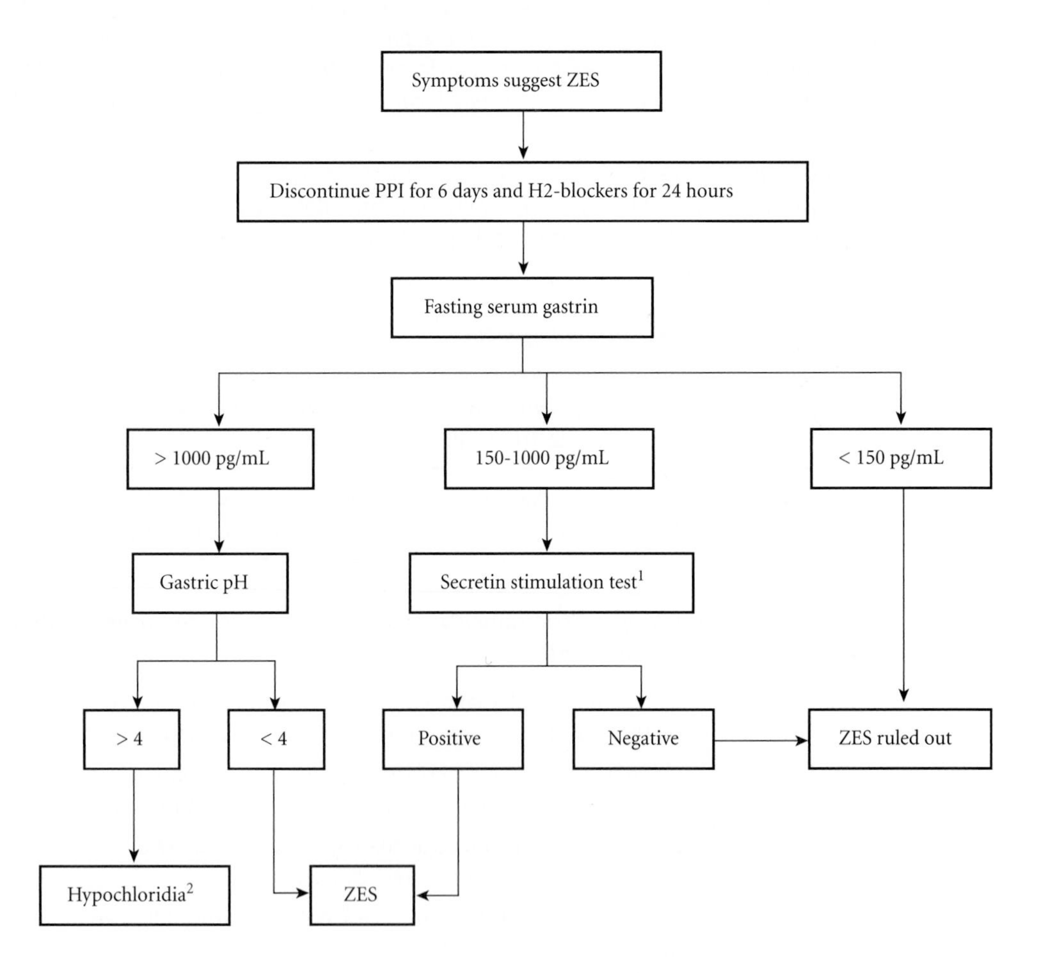

[1]**Secretin stimulation test:** Secretin stimulates a rise in serum gastrin of > 200 pg/mL within 2-30 minutes of administration if the patient has a gastrinoma.

[2]**Hypochloridia:** Conditions like pernicious anemia and atrophic gastritis can result in secondary hypergastrinemia due to hypochloridia

FIGURE 4–7 Diagnostic approach to Zollinger-Ellison syndrome (ZES).

The patient discontinues esomprezole for 1 week. Fasting serum gastrin is 1500 pg/mL and gastric pH is 2.5, which confirms the diagnosis. What are the next steps?

Perform somatostatin receptor scintigraphy (octreotide scan) to localize the tumor and detect liver metastases. If octreotide scan does not localize the primary tumor, perform EUS. Obtain serum PTH, prolactin, FSH, LH, and growth hormone levels to exclude MEN-1 syndrome (refer to Chapter 8: Endocrinology).

How is gastrinoma treated?

1. **Metastases or MEN-1 syndrome**: Medically manage with high-dose PPIs, octreotide, interferon alpha, and chemotherapy (low cure rate).
2. **No metastases and no evidence of MEN-1**: Main treatment is surgery (high cure rate).

Alternative 4.4.2

The patient is a 32-year-old man with 4 weeks of epigastric burning and bloating that sometimes occurs during meals and sometimes between meals. Antacids occasionally relieve symptoms. He drinks at least a six-pack of beer every day. He takes aspirin every day because he heard it is "good for the heart." He sometimes notices blood when he vomits after heavy drinking.

What is the next step in management?

This patient has dyspepsia and an alarm symptom (GI bleeding). The next step in management is EGD.

On endoscopy, the stomach appears diffusely inflamed. There are subepithelial hemorrhages, petechiae, and erosions. Biopsy reveals numerous neutrophil infiltrates. There is no ulcer or mass suggestive of gastric cancer. What is the diagnosis?

The patient has endoscopic findings of gastritis (injury and inflammation of the gastric mucosa). Erosions, petechiae, hemorrhage, and neutrophil infiltrates indicate that the patient has acute gastritis. Acute gastritis often presents with dyspepsia and/or upper GI bleeding. Unlike acute gastritis, chronic gastritis is associated with mononuclear infiltrates and is typically asymptomatic.

Gastropathy: epithelial cell damage and injury but no inflammation.
Gastritis: epithelial cell damage and injury with inflammation.

What risk factors does this patient have for acute gastritis?

Both alcohol and NSAIDs can damage the gastric mucosa, and these agents are likely to be the inciting causes in this patient (Table 4-2). Treatment is to discontinue the offending agents and to take acid-suppressing drugs (PPIs or H2-blockers) for symptomatic relief. Also, consider testing for *H. pylori* and administer eradication therapy if the test is positive.

Alternative 4.4.3

The patient is a 32-year-old male who complains of epigastric pain, fullness, bloating, early satiety, and nausea occurring over the last 12 months. He does not have any diarrhea or alarm findings. Physical examination and vital signs are normal. Serology is negative for *H. pylori.* Daily esomeprazole only partially relieves his symptoms. EGD is normal. Serum electrolytes, LFTs, and CBC are all normal.

What is the diagnosis?

Patients with dyspepsia in the absence of any identifiable structural cause are classified as having functional dyspepsia, a diagnosis of exclusion. Symptoms must be present for at least 3 months to make this diagnosis. No drug consistently improves symptoms. The recommended strategy for patients with functional dyspepsia is acknowledgement that their symptoms are real and reassurance that the disorder is not life threatening.

TABLE 4-2 Etiologies of Gastritis/Gastropathy

Major causes of acute gastritis (erosive, hemorrhagic gastritis)	**Chemical injury (NSAIDs, alcohol, bile acids):** Treatment is to discontinue offending agent and take oral H2-blockers or PPIs for symptomatic relief. **Mucosal hypoxia (stress gastritis due to trauma, burns, or sepsis):** Prevent by administering oral H2-blockers (not PPIs) to all critically ill patients. Early initiation of enteral feeding also reduces the risk of stress gastritis. If clinically significant bleeding develops, treat with intravenous H2-blockers or PPIs. **Portal hypertension:** Reduce recurrences of bleeding with propanolol or nadolol. If these are unsuccessful, consider TIPS.
Major causes of chronic gastritis (nonerosive gastritis)	***H. pylori*:** Almost 50% of the population has chronic *H. pylori* infection with gastritis, but only 15% of patients with chronic gastritis develop peptic ulcers. *H. pylori* ulcers often cause dyspepsia whereas *H. pylori* gastritis rarely causes dyspepsia. Chronic *H. pylori* gastritis increases the risk of gastric adenocarcinoma and gastric lymphoma. **Pernicious anemia:** Autoimmune destruction of parietal cells by antiparietal antibodies leads to achloridia and vitamin B12 malabsorption. Achloridia stimulates hypergastrinemia, which leads to gastritis. Pernicious anemia increases risk of gastric adenocarcinoma and carcinoid, so perform EGD with biopsy at the time of diagnosis.
Uncommon causes of gastritis	**Infections:** Bacterial infection is rare but can cause life-threatening necrotizing gastritis that requires emergent surgery. Immunosuppressed patients may develop viral or fungal gastritis. **Granulomatous gastritis:** Tuberculosis, syphilis, sarcoidosis, and Crohn's disease can cause gastritis with granulomatous inflammation. **Eosinophilic gastritis:** Gastritis due to idiopathic eosinophilic infiltration responds to corticosteroids. **Lymphocytic gastritis:** There is no effective therapy for gastritis due to idiopathic lymphocytic infiltration. **Menetrier's disease:** Idiopathic condition where patients develop giant, thickened gastric folds, which leads to dyspepsia and protein malabsorption (manifests with diarrhea and anasarca). Treatment is directed at symptoms.

Abbreviations: EGD, esophagogastroduodenoscope; NSAIDs, nonsteroidal anti-inflammatory drugs; PPI, proton pump inhibitors; TIPS, transjugular intrahepatic portosystemic shunt.

CASE 4–5 CHRONIC EPIGASTRIC DISCOMFORT AND WEIGHT LOSS

A 50-year-old woman presents with a 3-month history of progressively worsening dyspepsia and anorexia. The symptoms were initially provoked by eating food but are now constantly present. She has unintentionally lost 15 lbs in the last 3 months. Physical examination is significant for an enlarged periumbilical lymph node (Sister Mary Joseph node) as well as an enlarged left supraclavicular lymph node (Virchow node). Stool is guaiac-positive.

What is the most likely finding on endoscopy?

Unintentional weight loss is an alarm symptom for gastric cancer in patients with dyspepsia. The likelihood of gastric cancer is very high in this patient with other suspicious signs including constant symptoms, GI bleeding, an enlarged periumbilical lymph node, and an enlarged left supraclavicular lymph node (Table 4-3).

> Early gastric cancer is usually asymptomatic, so most patients already have advanced disease at the time of diagnosis.

Endoscopy with biopsy confirms the diagnosis of gastric adenocarcinoma. What tests should you order to stage gastric adenocarcinoma?

TABLE 4–3 Physical Signs of Gastric Adenocarcinoma

Physical signs of lymphatic spread	1. Sister Mary Joseph node: enlarged periumbilical lymph node 2. Virchow node: enlarged left supraclavicular lymph node
Physical signs of peritoneal spread	1. Krukenberg tumor: enlarging ovarian mass 2. Blumer's shelf: mass in rectal cul-de-sac 3. Ascites: due to peritoneal carcinomatosis
Physical signs of intestinal spread	1. Gastrocolic fistula: feces in emesis or undigested material in stool
Paraneoplastic signs (not specific for gastric cancer)	1. Leser-Trelat sign: diffuse seborrheic keratoses 2. Acanthosis nigricans: hyperpigmented, velvety patches on skin folds 3. Trousseau syndrome: migrating thrombophlebitis

Order abdominal and chest CT scans to detect distant metastases. If CT scan detects liver lesions, consider laparoscopic biopsy to verify whether or not they are metastatic lesions. Many centers use EUS to define tumor size and nodal involvement.

Gastric adenocarcinoma morphologies:

1. **Superficially spreading**: Early gastric cancer is confined to mucosa or submucosa. Prognosis is excellent.
2. **Linitis plastica**: Diffuse, full thickness extension leads to a rigid, atonic "leather bottle" appearance. Prognosis is dismal.
3. **Polypoid**
4. **Ulcerating**

What are the risk factors for gastric adenocarcinoma?

Established risk factors for gastric adenocarcinoma are:

1. Diet with high N-nitroso and salt intake and low vitamin C and β-carotene intake
2. Chronic gastritis due to *H. pylori* infection and pernicious anemia
3. Surgery: Partial gastric resection increases risk of cancer after approximately 15 years.
4. Smoking
5. Blood type A

The association between gastric ulcer and gastric cancer is controversial. The current recommendation is to biopsy any gastric ulcer to detect early gastric cancer.

Chronic *H. pylori* infection is implicated in 35% to 90% of gastric cancers but <1% of patients with chronic *H. pylori* infection develop gastric cancer.

What malignancies can occur in the stomach besides adenocarcinoma?

1. **Gastric lymphoma** is the second most common gastric malignancy after adenocarcinoma. Most gastric lymphomas are non-Hodgkins B-cell lymphomas. More than half arise from mucosa-associated lymphoid tissue. Clinical presentation and EGD appearance are similar to adenocarcinoma, so biopsy is necessary to distinguish between the two. After diagnosis, stage using abdominal CT, chest CT, and EUS.
2. **Gastric carcinoid** is a rare gastric malignancy. Pernicious anemia and MEN-1 are risk factors. Early carcinoids are typically asymptomatic. Carcinoids that metastasize to the liver may release excessive serotonin, leading to carcinoid syndrome. Symptoms of carcinoid syndrome are blushing, tricuspid, or pulmonary stenosis; diarrhea; and bronchospasm. Carcinoids can occur anywhere in the GI tract, so endoscopy is not sufficient to rule out the diagnosis if the patient has symptoms of carcinoid syndrome. Diagnose carcinoid by

documenting elevated urinary 5-HIAA (end-product of serotonin metabolism). If results are equivocal, obtain whole-blood serotonin levels.

3. **Stromal tumors**: Two thirds of GI stromal tumors occur in the stomach. Leiomyomas are benign stromal tumors, and leiomyosarcomas are malignant stromal tumors.

> **Appendix**: This is the most common location of carcinoids (low metastasis rate).
> **Ileum**: Ileal carcinoids have the highest rate of metastasis.

> Approximately 75% of stage 1 mucosa-associated lymphoid tissue lymphomas regress completely with *H. pylori* eradication.

Alternative 4.5.1

The patient is a 70-year-old man with a history of peripheral artery disease and stable angina. He complains of severe upper abdominal cramping approximately 1 hour after meals for the last 6 months. The pain occasionally radiates to his back. The fear of these cramps has caused him to decrease his food intake considerably, and he has lost 15 lbs in the last 3 months. He has smoked a pack of cigarettes every day for the last 40 years. EGD is unremarkable. Serology as well as biopsy does not reveal any evidence of *H. pylori* infection. Serum amylase and lipase are normal. Albumin is low but other LFTs are normal. There is an upper abdominal bruit. There is no tenderness, guarding, or rebound.

What diagnosis should you suspect?

Maintain a high index of suspicion for chronic mesenteric ischemia in any patient with a history of atherosclerosis who complains of food-induced dyspepsia and unintentional weight loss. Symptoms result from mesenteric atherosclerosis ("intestinal angina"). Abdominal examination is typically benign except for an upper abdominal bruit in 50%. Patients may also report nonspecific GI symptoms like nausea, vomiting, diarrhea, and constipation. Negative EGD rules out PUD, gastritis, and gastric cancer. Normal lab tests decrease the likelihood of biliary and pancreatic causes.

> Risk factors for coronary artery disease and chronic mesenteric ischemia are the same.

How is this condition diagnosed and treated?

Perform mesenteric duplex ultrasound to screen for mesenteric atherosclerosis. If the results are equivocal or positive, perform mesenteric angiography to confirm the diagnosis and define the anatomy. Treatment is either surgery or percutaneous transluminal angioplasty (PTA) with or without stent placement.

> No large controlled trials have compared surgery versus PTA versus PTA + stent.

CASE 4–6 CHRONIC EPIGASTRIC DISCOMFORT, HEARTBURN, AND REGURGITATION

A 32-year-old man presents with episodes of burning substernal pain (heartburn), burning epigastric pain (dyspepsia), and regurgitation of acid material into his mouth. The symptoms are worse after a heavy meal and recumbency. He has no other symptoms. He does not take any medications. He smokes a pack of cigarettes every day and drinks a six-pack of beer on the weekends. Vital signs are normal.

What is the most likely diagnosis?

Dyspepsia in the presence of heartburn and regurgitation are characteristic of GERD.

> **Water brash**: hypersalivation in response to reflux (uncommon).

What is the pathophysiology of GERD?

Heartburn and dyspepsia result from esophagitis due to excessive gastric acid in the esophagus. The pathophysiology involves a combination of decreased LES tone (which causes excessive reflux of gastric contents into the esophagus) and esophageal dysmotility (which leads to decreased clearance of gastric contents from the esophagus).

> **Nonerosive GERD:** Most patients with uncomplicated GERD do not have overt esophagitis. Symptoms result from hypersensitivity to physiological amounts of gastric acid.

What are the next steps in management?

The history is typical for uncomplicated GERD. There are two options in such patients:

1. **Step-up approach**: Start with lifestyle measures and antacids as needed. If symptoms persist, add an over-the-counter H2-blocker or PPI to the regimen. Increase the dosage over the next few weeks until symptoms are controlled.
2. **Step-down approach**: Start with lifestyle measures, antacids as needed, and a potent dose of H2-blocker or PPI. Taper down the dose until the lowest dose that controls symptoms is reached.

Perform EGD only if symptoms persist despite therapy or the patient has any of the alarm findings for gastric cancer described earlier.

What lifestyle measures are recommended to decrease symptoms of GERD?

Remember lifestyle measures with the mnemonic "***WASTED***":

1. Weight loss: Obesity is a risk factor for GERD.
2. Alcohol avoidance
3. Salivation: Use chewing gum and lozenges to increase saliva (neutralizes gastric acid).
4. Tobacco: Avoid cigarettes because they increase stress on the sphincter.
5. Elevate the head of the bed.
6. Diet: Avoid fatty foods, chocolate, and peppermint.

The patient's symptoms improve with lifestyle measures and daily PPIs. What is the next step in management?

Discontinue acid-suppressing medications after 8 weeks of successful empiric therapy. If the patient's symptoms do not recur for at least 3 months off medications, the patient can take the acid-suppressing drugs intermittently on an as-needed basis. Otherwise, restart the previously effective regimen.

> **H2-blockers**: Generic name ends with –tidine (e.g., ranitidine).
> **PPIs**: Generic name ends with –prazole (e.g., pantoprazole).

The patient's symptoms recur in 2 weeks. He restarts the previous regimen. Over the next few years, he requires continually increasing frequency and dosages of PPIs to relieve symptoms. What are the complications of long-standing GERD?

Inflammation and repair can lead to:

1. **Peptic stricture**: Suspect peptic stricture if the patient develops esophageal dysphagia to solid foods. Diagnose with barium swallow and/or EGD. Treat with dilation.
2. **Barrett's esophagus**: Chronic GERD can cause replacement of the normal stratified squamous epithelium with columnar epithelium. Although asymptomatic, this metaplastic change greatly increases the risk of esophageal adenocarcinoma. Consider screening endoscopy for all patients with longstanding GERD (see Fig. 4-8).

Reflux of gastric contents into the tracheobronchial tree and lungs can lead to:

1. **Asthma, chronic cough**: Refer to Chapter 3: Pulmonary.

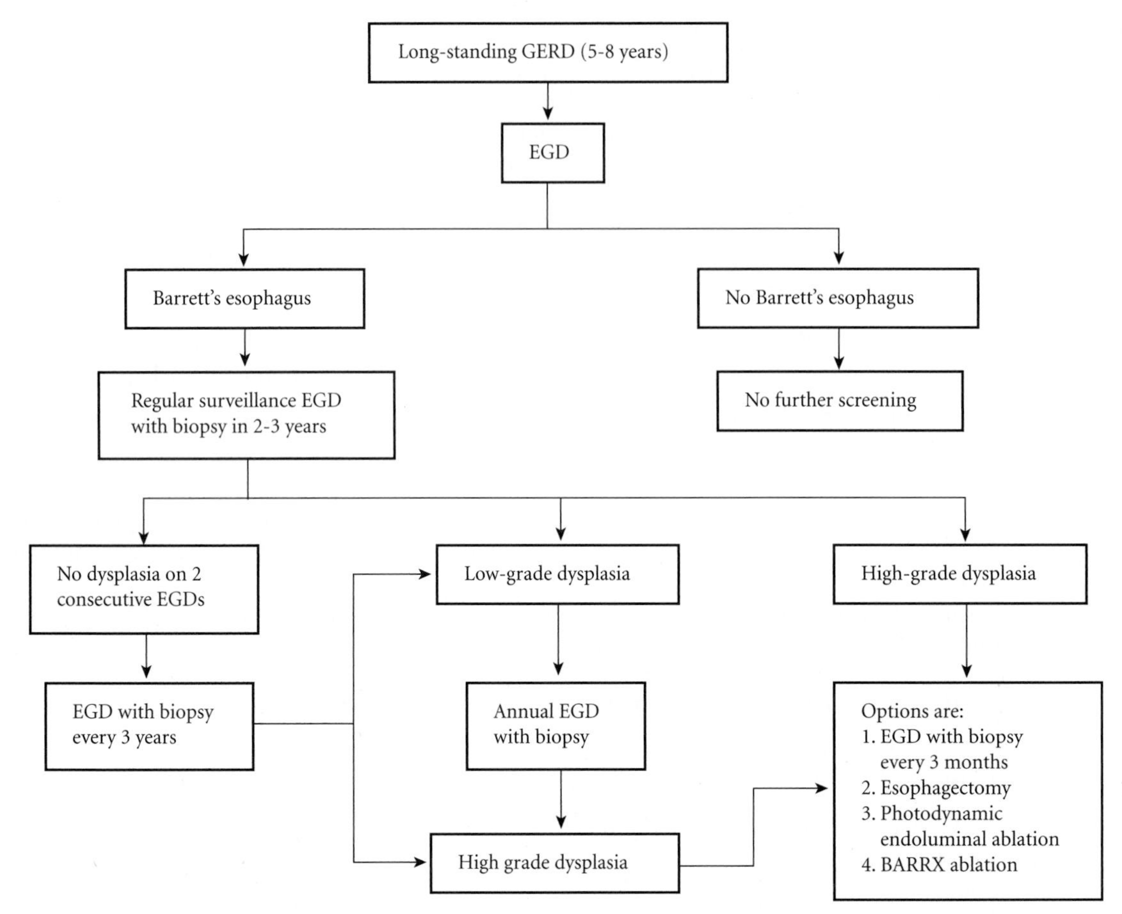

FIGURE 4–8 American College of Gastroenterology recommendations for surveillance endoscopy in patients with Barrett's esophagus.

2. **Aspiration pneumonia**: If GERD is the suspected cause, obtain cytologic aspirates using bronchoscopy. The characteristic finding is lipid-laden macrophages.
3. **Laryngitis**: Suspect laryngitis when a patient with long-standing GERD complains of chronic hoarseness, cough, frequent throat clearing, or sore throat in the absence of infection. Rule out structural causes with a laryngoscope. Treat with a high dose PPI for 12 weeks. If the patient does not respond, evaluate for a pulmonary or allergic cause.
4. **Laryngeal cancer**: SCC may occur in patients with chronic GERD-induced laryngitis. The major risk factors however, are smoking and alcohol.

Complications of long-term PPI use: osteoporosis, pneumonia, *Clostridium difficile* infection, and gastric polyps.

Adding a promotility agent to the acid-suppressing regimen may improve symptoms for some patients with GERD. However, side effects limit their widespread use. Examples are bethanechol, metoclopramide, domperidone, and cisapride (not available in the United States unless GI physician enrolls patient in the compassionate drug program).

The patient undergoes screening endoscopy. There is no columnar metaplasia or dysplasia. The endoscopy report does mention that the patient has a sliding hiatal hernia. What is the significance of this finding?

Type 1 (sliding hiatal hernia) accounts for 95% of hiatal hernias. A wide diaphragm ring allows the gastric cardia (gastroesophageal junction) to herniate upward, which predisposes to GERD. No specific therapy is necessary except control of GERD.

What treatment option exists for patients with refractory symptoms?

Consider antireflux surgery for the following patients with GERD:

1. Persistent esophagitis: Heartburn, regurgitation, or dyspepsia persist despite maximal medical therapy.
2. Persistent complications: Complications persist despite maximal medical therapy.
3. Paraesophageal hiatal hernia (types II, III, and IV): Gastroesophageal junction remains in place, but other parts of stomach herniate through diaphragm ring. Type II requires surgery even if asymptomatic. Types III and IV require surgery if symptomatic.

Preoperative evaluation: Perform manometry (to rule out other causes) and esophageal pH monitoring. Surgery does not benefit patients with visceral hyperalgesia (pH monitoring documents that symptoms occur despite adequate acid control).

BRAVO pH monitor: Implant capsule in esophagus. Capsule collects pH data and transmits data wirelessly to a pager-sized receiver worn by patient.

What surgical procedure is typically performed for refractory GERD?

The most commonly performed surgery for GERD is laparoscopic fundoplication (stomach fundus is sutured around the cardia, and the diaphragm defect is closed).

CASE 4–7 ACUTE ONSET OF DIFFUSE, CRAMPING ABDOMINAL PAIN

A 53-year-old man presents with 12 hours of nausea, vomiting, and cramping abdominal pain. He had an appendectomy 3 months ago. On physical exam, the abdomen is distended, and there are high-pitched bowel sounds. Abdominal percussion demonstrates a low-pitched drum-like sound (tympany). The rectal vault is empty. There are no abdominal masses. Vital signs are temperature 37°C, pulse 110 bpm, respirations 12/min, and blood pressure 100/70.

What diagnosis should you suspect?

Suspect bowel obstruction when a patient presents with acute onset of nausea, vomiting, and diffuse cramping abdominal pain ± obstipation (no passage of gas or feces). Common physical signs of obstruction are abdominal distension, tympany, an empty rectal vault, and high pitched or absent bowel sounds. Distension proximal to the obstruction causes reflex vomiting and decreased absorption, which leads to dehydration, hypokalemia, and metabolic alkalosis.

Proximal versus distal obstruction:

Obstruction proximal to the jejunum: severe nausea and vomiting but minimal abdominal distension because the dilated proximal small intestine acts as a reservoir.

Obstruction distal to jejunum: severe abdominal distension but minimal nausea and vomiting.

Partial versus complete obstruction:

Partial obstruction: Patients can pass gas and may have bowel movements.

Complete obstruction: Classic symptom is complete obstipation; in reality, patients may pass residual gas or stool distal to the obstruction.

What are the next steps in diagnosis?

1. Obstructive series: The initial diagnostic tests to evaluate for obstruction are upright CXR and supine and upright abdominal x-rays. In small bowel obstruction (SBO), abdominal x-rays show multiple air-fluid levels and no air in the colon (see Fig. 4-9). In large bowel obstruction (LBO), the bowel is filled with air and dilated proximal to the obstruction with

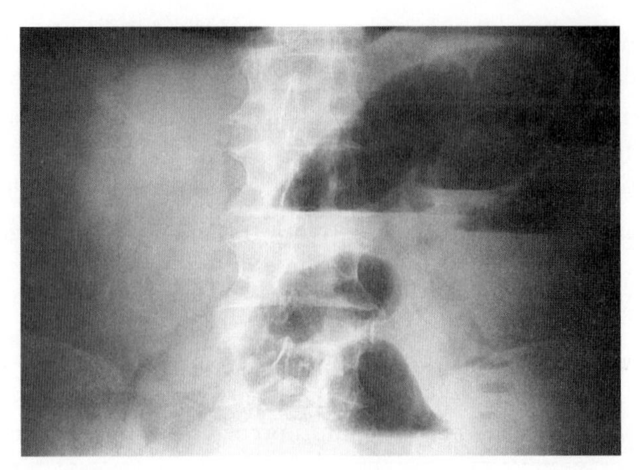

FIGURE 4–9 Abdomen x-ray showing SBO. From Ayala C, Spellberg B. *Boards and Wards*, 3rd ed. Lippincott Williams & Wilkins, 2007.

no air in the distal colon. Upright CXR is obtained to rule out bowel perforation (free air under the diaphragm). If abdominal films are positive, further work-up is unnecessary.

2. CT scan: Order an abdominal CT scan with oral and IV contrast if obstructive series is nondiagnostic.
3. GI series: If both obstructive series and CT scan are nondiagnostic, order an upper or lower GI series with water-soluble contrast depending on whether you suspect SBO or LBO.

> Occasionally, patients with SBO have feculent emesis due to bacterial overgrowth (bacteria ferment and break down food debris).

Abdominal x-ray shows multiple air-fluid levels, dilated loops of small bowel, and no air in the colon, which confirms the diagnosis of SBO. What is the most likely cause of obstruction in this patient?

Three fourths of SBOs result from extrinsic compression by adhesions that form after abdominal surgery (Table 4-4). Postoperative adhesions are the most likely cause in this patient who recently had an appendectomy.

How is SBO treated?

Initial therapy for stable patients is supportive (mnemonic: "***Nine Inch Nails Rock***"):

1. NPO: fasting.
2. IV fluids and electrolytes: Obtain IV access to determine the degree of dehydration by measuring serum electrolytes, hematocrit, and urine output; administer normal saline until the patient is euvolemic and correct electrolyte imbalances.

TABLE 4–4 Etiologies of Bowel Obstruction in Adults

Extrinsic compression	1. **Postoperative adhesions**: Most common cause. 2. **Hernia**: Second most common cause; inguinal hernia always requires surgery. 3. **Volvulus**: Causes LBO more frequently than SBO.
Intrinsic compression	1. **Cancer**: CRC, SI cancers, metastatic melanoma, and metastatic breast cancer. 2. **Radiation enteritis** 3. **Crohn's disease**: Patients may develop strictures, which lead to SBO. 4. **Gallstones**: Gallstones occasionally obstruct the intestines via an enteric-biliary fistula in patients with cholelithiasis or cholecystitis. Abdominal radiograph may show air in the biliary tree (pneumobilia). Surgery is the recommended treatment. 5. **Fecal impaction**: Treat with a mineral oil enema and/or manual disimpaction.

Abbreviation: CRC, colorectal cancer; LBO, large bowel obstruction; SBO, small bowel obstruction; SI, small intestine.

3. **N**G suction: Perform NS suction to prevent further bowel distension.
4. **R**eassess: Frequently reassess the patient for strangulation (signs of acute abdomen or shock), which is an indication for emergent surgery. Some centers also use serial CT scans to detect early signs of bowel ischemia. Serial abdominal films are not helpful.

> **Strangulation**: SBO increases intraluminal pressure, which can cut off blood flow and cause perforation, peritonitis, and septic shock. Closed loop obstruction (lumen occluded at two points) increases the risk of strangulation.

The patient's pain, nausea, and abdominal distension improve over the next 24 hours with fluids and NG suction. NG suction is discontinued. Over the next 4 hours, signs and symptoms of SBO recur. What is the next step in management?

Surgery is indicated for patients who fail medical management (continued symptoms despite 12 to 24 hours of NG suction or prompt recurrence after discontinuing suction).

Alternative 4.7.1

A 53-year man presents with a 12-hour history of cramping abdominal pain. Physical examination is significant for abdominal distension, hyperactive bowel sounds, and an empty rectal vault. Abdominal x-ray is obtained (see Fig. 4-10).

What is the diagnosis?

The abdominal film shows a large, kidney-shaped mass extending into the left upper quadrant ("coffee bean sign"), which is diagnostic of LBO caused by a cecal volvulus. Volvulus is defined as twisting of a segment of bowel on its mesenteric attachment, which can lead to obstruction. The cecum is the most common location of volvulus.

What is the next step in management?

Treatment of cecal volvulus is emergent surgery to untwist (detorse) the volvulus.

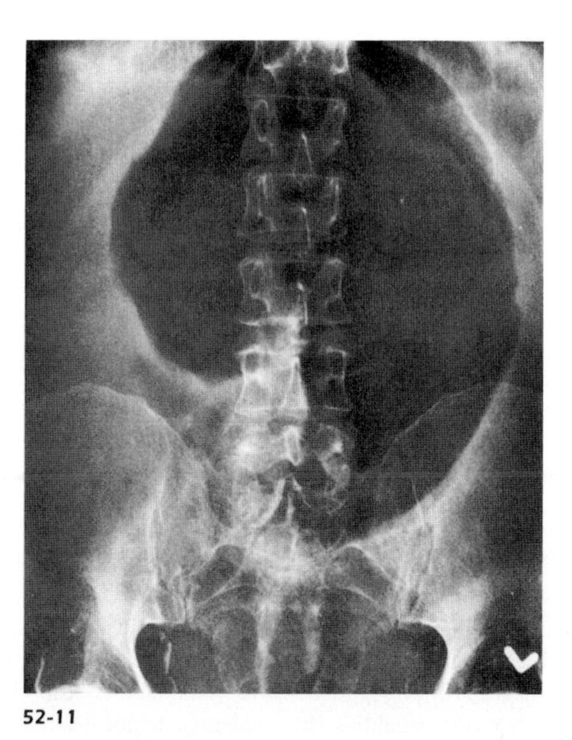

FIGURE 4–10 Abdomen x-ray showing cecal volvulus. From Eisenberg R. *Gastrointestinal Radiology: A Pattern Approach*, 3rd ed. Lippincott Williams & Wilkins, 1990.

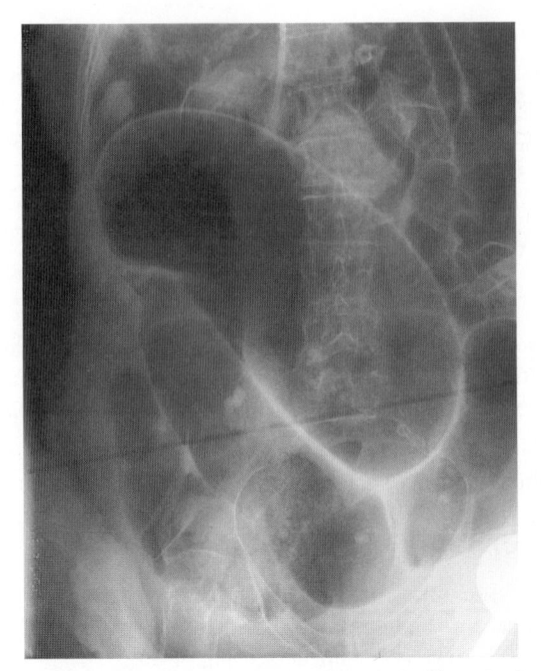

FIGURE 4–11 Abdomen x-ray showing sigmoid volvulus. From Ayala C, Spellberg B. *Boards and Wards*, 3rd ed. Lippincott Williams & Wilkins, 2007.

What diagnosis would be more likely if Figure 4-11 was the patient's abdominal film?

The abdominal x-ray demonstrates a collection of gas extending from the pelvis to the right upper quadrant ("bent inner tube sign"). This finding is characteristic for a sigmoid volvulus, which is the second most common location of volvulus. Sigmoid volvulus is more common in elderly and institutionalized patients. Treatment is to untwist the volvulus with a sigmoidoscope. Surgery is reserved for refractory or recurrent cases.

Alternative 4.7.2

A 65-year-old male with a history of CHF presents with a 6-hour history of nausea, cramping abdominal pain, and diarrhea. He admits to using heroin recently. Physical exam demonstrates abdominal distension, tympany, and hypoactive bowel sounds. Vital signs are temperature 36.8°C, pulse 110 bpm, respirations 25/min, blood pressure 130/80, and SaO_2 91%. Abdominal x-ray is obtained (see Fig. 4-12).

What diagnosis should you suspect?

Although the patient presents with many signs and symptoms of obstruction and abdominal x-ray shows colon dilatation, there is air in the entire GI tract. Also, the patient has hypoactive bowel sounds, which is unusual in bowel obstruction. Suspect acute colonic pseudo-obstruction (Ogilvie's syndrome) as the cause of his symptoms.

> Hyperactive bowel sounds, small bowel air-fluid levels, and lack of air in the distal colon and rectum suggest mechanical obstruction but they may occur in Ogilvie's syndrome as well. Diarrhea is a paradoxical finding in this condition.

What factors predispose this patient to developing Ogilvie's syndrome?

Ogilvie's syndrome results from large bowel paralysis. The pathogenesis is unknown, but most cases occur in older patients with a history of trauma, surgery, underlying medical illnesses (cardiac disease, infection, and neurologic diseases), and retroperitoneal masses (malignancy or hemorrhage). Among patients with risk factors, the risk of Ogilvie's syndrome increases with electrolyte abnormalities (hypokalemia, hypocalcemia, and hypomagnesemia) and certain medications (opiates, epidural analgesics, etc.). This patient has a history of CHF and recently used heroin, which increases the likelihood of developing Ogilvie's syndrome.

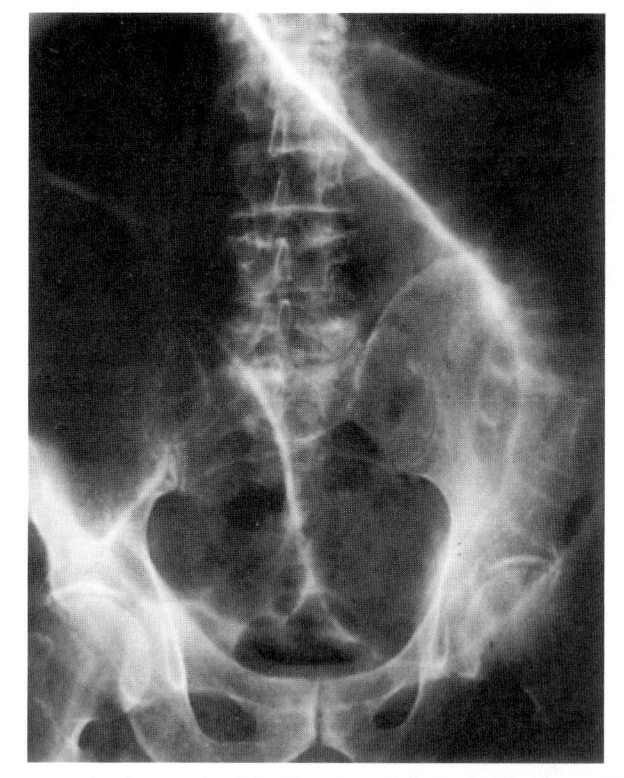

FIGURE 4–12 Abdomen x-ray showing pseudo-obstruction. From Mulholland MW, Lilemoe KD, et al. *Greenfield's Surgery: Scientific Principles and Practice*, 4th ed. Lippincott Williams & Wilkins, 2006.

What is the next step in management?

Obtain a CT scan of the abdomen or lower GI series with water-soluble contrast (contrast enema) to confirm the diagnosis and rule out mechanical obstruction or toxic megacolon.

CT scan of the abdomen does not show any signs of mechanical obstruction or submucosal edema and colon wall thickening characteristic of toxic megacolon. Colon diameter is 7 cm. How should you treat this patient with Ogilvie's syndrome?

Most patients recover with removal of precipitants and supportive measures:

1. Remove precipitants: In this patient, treat the underlying CHF and make sure he does not receive any more narcotics or anticholinergics. Correct electrolyte imbalances.
2. Supportive care: Supportive care involves **N**ine **I**nch **N**ails **R**ock + **R**ectal tube + **P**osition. Make sure the patient is **N**PO and administer **I**V fluids. Place an **N**G tube with suction and a **R**ectal tube with drainage to decompress the bowel. Place the patient in a **P**rone position and periodically move him from side to side to promote gas expulsion. **R**eassess every 12 to 24 hours with serial physical exams and abdominal x-rays.

> **Postoperative ileus**: Paralytic ileus is a physiological response for up to 24 hours after abdominal surgery. Treatment is to remove precipitants, NPO, and IV fluids. If abdominal cramping, distension, or obstipation persist for more than 2 to 5 days, rule out bowel obstruction with abdominal radiograph.

The patient continues to have symptoms 24 hours later despite supportive measures and removal of precipitants. Cecal diameter is now 10 cm. What is the next step in management?

Administer neostigmine (an acetylcholinesterase antagonist) if the patient continues to have symptoms despite 24 hours of conservative therapy or cecal diameter increases to $\geq$10 cm. Symptoms should improve within 30 minutes. Place the patient on a cardiac monitor and have atropine available to administer if the patient develops a symptomatic bradyarrhythmia due to neostigmine.

Two hours after administering neostigmine the patient is still symptomatic. What is the next step in management?

Patients who continue to have symptoms or colon dilation despite neostigmine should undergo colonoscopic decompression. If colonoscopy fails, refer for surgical decompression.

Alternative 4.7.3

The patient is a 65-year-old man presents with a 6-hour history of severe diffuse cramping abdominal pain, nausea, and vomiting. He has a history of atrial fibrillation and peripheral vascular disease. Abdominal examination is benign. Vital signs are temperature 36.8°C, pulse 115 bpm, respirations 25/min, and blood pressure 110/70.

What diagnosis should you suspect?

Maintain a high index of suspicion for acute mesenteric ischemia when patients with risk factors for thrombosis or embolism (hypercoagulable state, atrial fibrillation, atherosclerosis, etc.) present with severe abdominal pain out of proportion to physical exam findings. Although initial findings are benign, patients can develop signs of acute abdomen as ischemia progresses. FOBT may be positive late in the course of the illness.

> Laboratory tests are nonspecific. Common findings include increased white blood cells (WBCs), increased hematocrit (due to dehydration), and metabolic acidosis (due to lactic acidosis).

What are the types of acute mesenteric ischemia?

1. Mesenteric artery embolism: most common cause of acute mesenteric ischemia (due to cardiac embolism to the superior mesenteric artery); onset of symptoms is more sudden and painful than other types.
2. Mesenteric artery thrombosis: due to atherosclerosis.
3. Mesenteric vein thrombosis: associated with hypercoagulable states, portal HTN, malignancy, and trauma.
4. Nonocclusive mesenteric ischemia: due to splanchnic hypoperfusion in patients who are critically ill or have severe atherosclerosis; 25% deny abdominal pain.

What are the next steps in management of patients with suspected mesenteric ischemia?

The initial step is to stabilize the patient and to obtain an obstructive series (to rule out mechanical obstruction). If obstructive series is negative, the next test depends on whether or not the patient has a hypercoagulable state or acute abdomen (see Fig. 4-13).

> Mesenteric angiography is the gold standard for establishing the diagnosis and cause of acute mesenteric ischemia.

Abdominal plain films do not reveal any signs of obstruction. The patient does not have any risk factors for hypercoagulability. He undergoes mesenteric angiogram, which is diagnostic for mesenteric artery embolism. How are the different causes of acute mesenteric ischemia (AMI) treated?

AMI is associated with a high mortality (overall mortality is 70%; after bowel infarction, mortality is >90%). Initial therapy for all types of acute mesenteric ischemia is stabilization, broad-spectrum antibiotics, and NG tube placement. After these initial steps, management strategies for the different types of AMI are as follows:

1. Mesenteric artery embolism: Standard treatment is surgical embolectomy. An alternative to surgery is thrombolytics and papaverine (a vasodilator). After recovery, long-term use of warfarin can prevent recurrence.

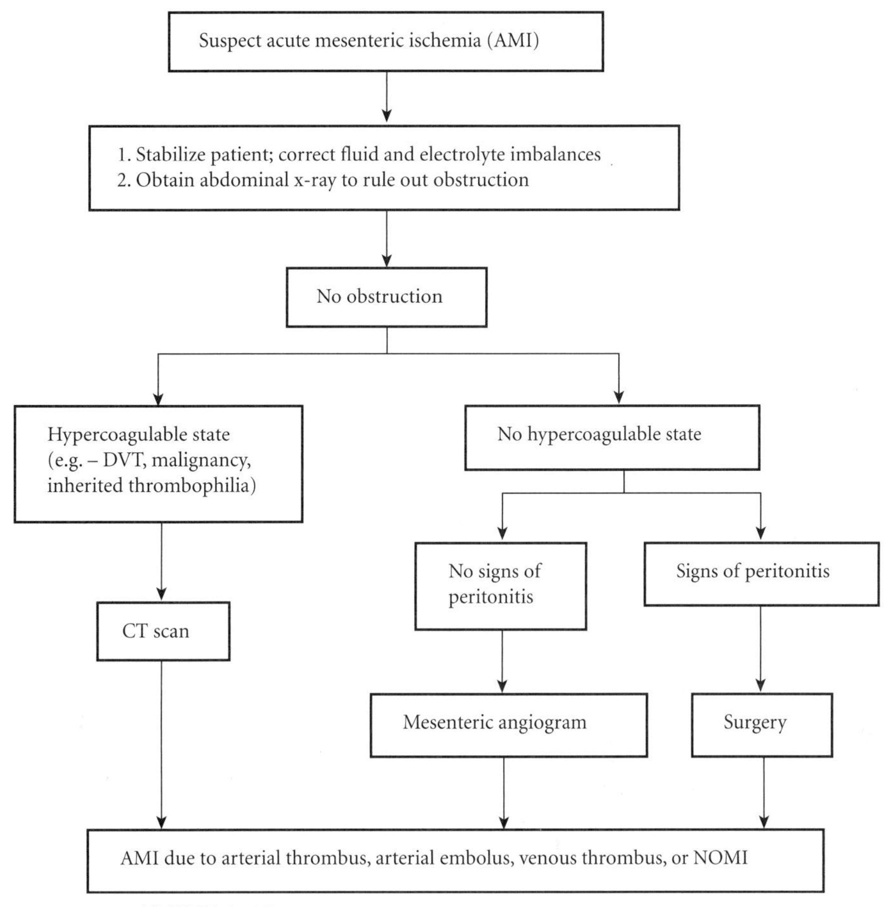

FIGURE 4–13 Algorithm for diagnosis of acute mesenteric ischemia.

2. Mesenteric artery thrombosis: If angiography shows good collateral flow, consider heparin and observation. If collaterals are insufficient, treat with a papaverine drip and emergent surgery. After recovery, long-term use of aspirin can prevent recurrence.
3. Mesenteric vein thrombosis: Treatment is heparin followed by surgery. After recovery, long-term use of warfarin can prevent recurrence.
4. Nonocclusive mesenteric ischemia: Treatment is IV papaverine. Some clinicians also use heparin. After recovery, long-term use of aspirin can prevent recurrence.

Unstable patients with acute abdomen: Surgery is required regardless of the type of AMI; avoid vasopressors because they worsen ischemia.

"Drip": medical slang for continuous infusion.

CASE 4–8 ACUTE LEFT LOWER QUADRANT PAIN

A 75-year-old man presents with 3 days of abdominal pain localized to the left lower quadrant (LLQ) and mild nausea. Past medical history is unremarkable. Physical examination is significant for LLQ tenderness. There is a palpable mass in the LLQ. Stool is guaiac-negative. Vital signs are temperature 38.4°C, pulse 90 bpm, respirations 18/min, and blood pressure 120/80. The only significant laboratory finding is a WBC count of 11,500 cells/cubic mm with a left shift.

What is most likely cause of the patient's current symptoms?

The most common cause of LLQ pain and tenderness in elderly patients is diverticulitis, which results from inflammation of diverticula. Pain is initially mild, so most patients present days rather than hours after symptom onset. Approximately 50% of patients have a palpable mass. Patients often have a low-grade fever and mild leukocytosis.

What are diverticula?

Diverticula are pouches in weak areas of the colon wall near blood vessels. They result from increased intraluminal pressure. Patients with diverticula are termed as having diverticulosis. Diverticulosis may be asymptomatic (detected incidentally on colonoscopy or barium enema) or present with symptoms similar to IBS. Incidence of diverticulosis increases with age. No imaging is recommended to diagnose suspected diverticulosis. Prevent complications of diverticulosis with increased fiber intake.

> Complications of diverticulosis:
>
> 1. **Painless rectal bleeding**: 95% are self-limited, 5% are massive.
> 2. **Diverticulitis**: caused by infection/inflammation of a microperforated diverticulum.

What is the next step in this patient with suspected diverticulitis?

CT scan of the abdomen and pelvis is the preferred test to diagnose diverticulitis. This test can also detect complications of diverticulitis. In addition to CT scan, obtain abdominal and chest radiographs to rule out other causes of abdominal pain. Colonoscopy and barium enema are contraindicated during the initial stages of acute diverticulitis because they can cause perforation.

> **Complications of diverticulitis: POP A** **F**istula (**P**erforation, **O**bstruction, **P**eritonitis, **A**bscess, and **F**istulas).

CT scan confirms uncomplicated diverticulitis. How is this condition treated?

First, triage patients for outpatient versus inpatient management. Criteria for admission are:

1. Elderly patients, immunosuppressed patients, or patients with severe comorbid diseases
2. Patients with signs of acute abdomen, high fever, or WBC count

Admit this elderly patient to the hospital and treat with NPO, IV fluids, and IV antibiotics (clindamycin or metronidazole to cover anaerobes plus a third-generation cephalosporin or fluoroquinolone to cover Gram-negative aerobes). Symptoms should resolve in 2 to 3 days. Surgery is indicated after 72 hours if symptoms or leukocytosis worsens or fails to improve after 72 hours.

> **Outpatient treatment of diverticulitis**: Clear liquids and a 7- to 10-day course of amoxicillin-clavulanate or ciprofloxacin and metronidazole.

Symptoms improve within 2 days. The patient is ready for discharge. What should you recommend after resolution of symptoms?

Recommend colonoscopy 2 to 6 weeks after recovery to evaluate the extent of diverticulitis and to rule out other conditions like cancer. Instruct the patient to consume a high fiber diet to prevent recurrences.

> Some physicians recommend that patients avoid nuts and seeds, which can theoretically lodge in the diverticulum and cause another episode of diverticulitis. There is no convincing evidence to support this recommendation.

What is the risk of recurrence after an episode of diverticulitis treated medically?

Diverticulitis recurs in one third of patients treated medically. Consider elective surgical resection after more than two episodes because recurrences carry a higher risk of complications.

Consider elective surgery after the first attack in the following groups:

1. Diverticulitis patients with complications
2. Immunosuppressed patients
3. Patients <40 years old (controversial)

Two months later, the patient complains that he has been passing air and stool through his penis when he urinates. Occasionally, he passes urine through his rectum. What is the most likely complication?

The patient has developed a fistula between the bladder and the colon (colovesical fistula). Diagnose with sigmoidoscopy followed by barium enema. If these studies are nondiagnostic perform abdomen and pelvis CT scan. Treatment is elective surgery.

Alternative 4.8.1

A 70-year-old man presents with diffuse, cramping LLQ pain. The pain began approximately 24 hours ago. At 16 hours after the onset of pain, he noticed small amounts of bright red blood per rectum (hematochezia) followed by a small amount of bloody diarrhea. Past medical history is significant for peripheral vascular disease and MI 5 years ago. LLQ tenderness is the only abnormal finding on physical examination. Vital signs are normal. The only significant laboratory finding is a WBC count of 11,500 cells/cubic mm with a left shift.

What is the most likely diagnosis?

The most likely diagnosis is acute ischemic colitis, caused by a sudden decrease in blood flow to watershed areas of the colon. Patients are usually elderly and report acute onset of abdominal pain (most commonly in the LLQ) followed by small amounts of hematochezia and bloody diarrhea within 24 hours (Table 4-5). Vital signs are usually normal and mild leukocytosis is the only laboratory abnormality.

What diagnostic tests are indicated?

Consider fecal leukocytes and stool culture to rule out infectious diarrhea. Consider an abdominal plain film to rule out obstruction and perforation. Patients with advanced ischemic colitis may have distension and pneumatosis (intestinal air) on abdominal plain films. CT scan of the abdomen often establishes the diagnosis. Perform colonoscopy only if the etiology is unclear despite history, physical, abdominal film, and CT scan.

Colonoscopy findings in acute ischemic colitis are pale mucosa, petechiae, blue-based ulcers, and bluish hemorrhagic nodules. On barium enema, these hemorrhagic nodules may appear as "thumbprints" (may also be seen in AMI).

Abdominal plain film is nondiagnostic, but CT scan shows segmental thickening of bowel wall indicative of acute ischemic colitis. What treatment is indicated?

Treat supportively with NPO, IV fluids, broad-spectrum IV antibiotics, and an NG tube if the patient has an ileus. Approximately 80% to 90% of patients recover with supportive care alone. Some patients may progress to gangrene and perforation, so frequently reassess for excessive bloody diarrhea or acute abdomen (peritonitis). Clinical deterioration is an indication for surgical management.

TABLE 4-5 Acute Ischemic Colitis Versus Acute Mesenteric Ischemia

	Location of Abdominal Pain	GI Bleeding
Acute ischemic colitis	Lateral (usually left lower quadrant)	Hematochezia and bloody diarrhea
Acute mesenteric ischemia	Periumbilical or diffuse	Occult blood late in course

CASE 4–9 ACUTE RIGHT LOWER QUADRANT PAIN

A 20-year-old woman presents with pain in the right lower quadrant (RLQ). Her symptoms began as periumbilical pain 7 hours ago. She is sexually active and occasionally uses condoms. On physical exam, there is RLQ tenderness and rebound tenderness. Palpation of the LLQ elicits pain in the RLQ (Rovsing sign). Vital signs are temperature 38.4°C, pulse 90 bpm, respirations 20/min, and blood pressure 110/80. Leukocyte count is 11,500 cells/cubic mm. Human chorionic gonadotropin (β-hCG) is negative.

What diagnosis do her symptoms suggest?

Periumbilical pain followed by signs of acute abdomen in the RLQ is the classic presentation of acute appendicitis. Tenderness is most prominent at McBurney's point (two thirds of the distance between the umbilicus and the anterior superior iliac spine). Patients often have nausea, vomiting, constipation, a low-grade fever, and leukocytosis.

> Signs of appendicitis:
>
> **Rovsing sign:** Palpation of LLQ elicits RLQ pain.
> **Psoas sign:** Passive extension of the right hip elicits RLQ pain.
> **Obturator sign:** Internal rotation of the right hip elicits RLQ pain.

> Atypical presentations of appendicitis:
>
> **Pelvic appendix**: Genitourinary symptoms and pain is felt below McBurney's point or in the LLQ; obturator sign is positive.
> **Retrocecal appendix**: Dull ache rather than tenderness is felt in RLQ; Psoas sign is positive.
> **Pregnancy:** Subcostal or periumbilical tenderness is felt because the appendix is displaced.

> Always rule out adnexal causes in females with lower abdominal pain. Obtain β-hCG to rule out pregnancy in all women of childbearing age (Chapter 14: Primary Care Gynecology and Urology).

What is the pathophysiology of appendicitis?

Obstruction of the appendix lumen by lymphoid hyperplasia, a fecalith, foreign body, inflammation, or neoplasm obstructs the flow of blood and lymphatics. Bacteria proliferate in the diseased appendix, leading to appendiceal inflammation. The inflamed, necrotic appendix can perforate (usually after 24 to 48 hours), leading to either diffuse peritonitis or localized abscess formation. Although it can occur at any age, appendicitis is most common between the ages of 10 and 30 years.

β-hCG (pregnancy test) is negative. What is the next step in management?

The next step is emergent appendectomy. Do not delay surgery to perform confirmatory testing if the clinical presentation is characteristic. Try to correct fluid and electrolyte imbalances prior to surgery.

> If the presentation is less obvious, perform CT scan to confirm the diagnosis.

During the operation, a 1.5-cm appendil carcinoid is detected. No adjacent lymph nodes are found. What is the next step in management?

Appendil carcinoids can obstruct the appendiceal lumen and cause appendicitis. Treatment with appendectomy is sufficient. Patients with tumors >2 cm or lymph node involvement should undergo more extensive surgery (right hemicolectomy).

> Approximately 10% to 20% of patients have a normal appendix at surgery, which is acceptable because the risk of perforation outweighs the risk of surgery.

> Diverticulitis in the cecum can present exactly like appendicitis. The diagnosis is clarified by CT scan or during surgery.

Alternative 4.9.1

A 20-year-old woman presents with a 5-day history of RLQ pain, nausea, and vomiting. Physical examination is significant for RLQ tenderness and a palpable abdominal mass. Vital signs are temperature 39°C, pulse 90 bpm, respirations 20/min, and blood pressure 120/80. Leukocyte count is 12,000 cells/cubic mm. β-hCG is negative.

What is the next step in management?

This patient presents with signs of appendicitis that has perforated and formed an abscess (palpable abdominal mass). Surgery is difficult in this setting. At this time, confirm the diagnosis with a CT scan and treat this stable patient medically (NPO, IV fluids, and IV antibiotics). If an abscess is detected, perform percutaneous drainage. Prevent recurrences with elective appendectomy 6 to 8 weeks after recovery.

CASE 4–10 CHRONIC EPISODES OF DIFFUSE, CRAMPY, ABDOMINAL PAIN

A 30-year-old woman presents with episodes of diffuse, cramping, abdominal pain occurring over the last 12 months. The episodes occur about twice a week. The pain is often accompanied by diarrhea, which she defines as frequent loose stools of small to moderate volume. She has noticed mucus in her stool but not blood. The stool is not foul smelling. Sometimes she has constipation rather than diarrhea. During this episode, stool is hard and pellet-shaped. Defecation often improves her abdominal discomfort. She denies anorexia, weight loss, or difficulty swallowing. She does not take any medications. Physical examination and vital signs are normal.

What is the most likely diagnosis?

The patient's symptoms are suggestive of IBS, the most commonly diagnosed GI disorder. Patients present with a variety of GI complaints, but the primary symptoms are chronic abdominal pain and altered bowel habits. Patients may also report abdominal bloating.

> **Rome Criteria for IBS**: Recurrent abdominal pain or discomfort at least 3 days of the month for at least 3 months accompanied by at least two of the following:
>
> **1.** Altered stool appearance
> **2.** Altered stool frequency
> **3.** Symptoms improve with defecation

> Subtypes of IBS are diarrhea-predominant IBS, constipation-predominant IBS, mixed IBS (diarrhea and constipation), and unsubtyped IBS.

What is the next step in management?

This patient's symptoms are consistent with mixed IBS. She does not have any alarm symptoms. Limit diagnostic testing to CBC, serum electrolytes, FOBT ± celiac panel.

What are alarm findings that would warrant further diagnostic testing?

Remember alarm findings that warrant further diagnostic testing with the mnemonic "***DOLLAR***": **D**ysphagia, **O**dynophagia, **L**arge-volume diarrhea, **L**oss of weight, **A**norexia, and decreased **R**BCs (anemia or GI bleeding).

Laboratory testing is normal. Stool is guaiac-negative. How is IBS treated?

1. Education and reassurance: This is the most important intervention in the management of IBS. Acknowledge that the patient's symptoms are real and explain that they are in part caused by visceral hypersensitivity and an imbalance in the brain-gut connection. Reassure her that although there is no simple cure for this chronic condition, IBS does not degenerate into a serious illness or have any effect on mortality.

2. Dietary modification: Consider an empiric trial of lactose avoidance. Avoid excessive caffeine. If bloating is a symptom, avoid foods that increase flatulence. If the patient complains of constipation in the absence of bloating, try to increase fiber intake.
3. Behavioral therapy: Although psychosocial distress does not cause IBS, patients with anxiety, depression, and somatization often perceive symptoms as more severe. Psychotherapy, hypnosis, and biofeedback may benefit motivated patients.
4. Pharmacologic therapy: Consider medications as a short-term adjunctive measure during severe symptom flares. Treat bloating with antispasmodics like dicyclomine. Treat diarrhea with loperamide (use cautiously in this patient with mixed constipation and diarrhea). Tricyclic antidepressants and selective serotonin reuptake inhibitors are an option if the patient also suffers from depression.

Tegaserod: Serotonin-4 agonist improves GI motility and may improve symptoms in constipation-predominant IBS.

Alosetron (serotonin-3 antagonist) has been approved for diarrhea-predominant IBS. Poses risk of ischemic colitis and severe constipation, so consider only for the small subset of patients with intolerable symptoms unresponsive to conventional therapy.

Emerging data suggest altered bacteria in the small intestine play a role in IBS. Treatment with antibiotics and probiotics is a promising new strategy to treat IBS.

CASE 4–11 ACUTE DIARRHEA

A 23-year-old female presents with a 2-day history of diarrhea, nausea, vomiting, and mild abdominal cramps. She describes her stools as watery and unformed occurring three to four times a day. She does not have any abdominal pain, nausea, vomiting, or blood in her stool. She denies recent travel, sick contacts, antibiotic use, or hospitalization. She is a vegan; she has never had sexual intercourse or used IV drugs. She works at home as a software designer. Physical exam and vitals are normal.

What is the differential diagnosis of acute diarrhea?

The number one cause of acute diarrhea is infections (viral > bacterial > parasitic). Other common causes are medications, food intolerance, inflammatory bowel disease, and ischemic colitis (in elderly patients). Carcinoid syndrome and thyrotoxicosis are uncommon etiologies.

What is the next step in management?

Most cases of diarrhea are benign and self-limited. This patient with mild watery diarrhea, nausea, vomiting, and mild abdominal cramping most likely has a viral gastroenteritis. The next step for this stable patient with no concerning findings on history and physical exam is to advise supportive measures such as adequate nutrition, rehydration, and loperamide on an as-needed basis. Avoid dairy products because infectious enteritis often temporarily causes lactose malabsorption.

Diarrhea: ≥3 loose or watery stools per day
Acute diarrhea: duration ≤14 days
Persistent diarrhea: duration 15 to 30 days
Chronic diarrhea: duration >30 days

When are diagnostic tests indicated in patients with acute diarrhea?

Remember the indications for diagnostic testing in patients with acute diarrhea using the mnemonic "***BAD SHIT***":

1. **B**loody stools
2. **A**ge ≥70 years or recent **A**ntibiotic use
3. **D**uration >48 hours
4. **S**evere abdominal pain
5. **H**ypovolemia (or >6 unformed stools/day) or recent **H**ospitalization
6. **I**mmunosuppression
7. **T**emperature >38.5°C

When is empiric antibiotic therapy indicated for patients with acute diarrhea?

Consider empiric therapy with an oral fluoroquinolone after obtaining samples for initial diagnostic tests if the patient has any of the following (mnemonic: "***BaD sHIT***"):

1. **B**loody stools
2. **D**uration >7 days
3. **H**ypovolemia or frequency >8 stools/day
4. **I**mmunosuppression
5. **T**emperature >38.5°C or mild to moderate **T**raveller's diarrhea (refer to Chapter 1: Health Maintenance and Statistics).

The patient returns to the clinic 2 days later. Her diarrhea has worsened and she now has nine watery stools per day. On physical examination, skin turgor is decreased. Temperature is 37°C and heart rate is 90 bpm. Blood pressure is 120/80 supine but falls to 100/60 in the standing position. What is the next step in management?

This patient has had diarrhea for 4 days (>48 hours). She has nine stools per day and signs of hypovolemia (decreased skin turgor and orthostatic hypotension). The next step is to sample stool for occult blood and fecal leukocytes:

1. Negative FOBT and fecal leukocytes: Consider empiric oral fluoroquinolone.
2. Elevated fecal leukocytes: Perform stool culture. Consider empiric oral fluoroquinolone while waiting for the results of the stool culture. If stool culture is positive, tailor antibiotics on the basis of the particular microorganism (Table 4-6).

When should you test a patient for ova and parasites?

Also test for ova and parasites with three separate specimens on consecutive days in the following situations (**O**va & **P**arasites **T**hrive **I**n **B**ad **D**aycare):

1. Waterborne **O**utbreak in community
2. **P**ersistent diarrhea
3. **T**ravel (recent)
4. **I**mmunosuppression
5. **B**loody diarrhea with negative fecal leukocytes
6. **D**aycare center job

Alternative 4.11.1

A 60-year-old woman was hospitalized 5 days ago for treatment of a diabetic foot infection. On the first day in the hospital, clindamycin was initiated. The patient now complains of eight to nine watery stools per day, nausea, vomiting, and abdominal cramps relieved by defecation. On physical examination, skin turgor is decreased. Temperature is 38.6°C. Other vital signs are normal.

TABLE 4–6 Common Infectious Causes of Diarrhea in Immunocompetent Patients

	Organism	First Choice Antibiotic
Bacteria associated with fever and bloody diarrhea (inflammatory diarrhea)	Nontyphoidal salmonella	Usually not indicated
	Campylobacter	Erythromycin (only for severe infection)
	Escherichia coli 0157:H7 (enterohemorrhagic)	Antibiotics contraindicated
	Enteroinvasive *E. coli*	Oral fluoroquinolone
	Yersinia	Oral fluoroquinolone
	Shigella	Oral fluoroquinolone
Bacteria associated with watery diarrhea[a] (noninflammatory diarrhea)	*Vibrio cholerae*	Doxycyclin
	Clostridium perfringens	Not indicated
	Enterotoxigenic *E. coli*	Oral fluoroquinolone
	Staphylococcus aureus	Usually not indicated
	Clostridium difficile	Metronidazole
Parasite associated with fever and bloody diarrhea (inflammatory diarrhea)	*Entamoeba histolytica*	Metronidazole
Parasites associated with watery diarrhea (noninflammatory diarrhea)	Cryptosporidium	Usually not indicated
	Giardia lamblia	Metronidazole
	Cyclospora	Trimethoprim-sulfamethoxazole

[a] Viruses that cause watery diarrhea are Norwalk virus, rotavirus, enterovirus, and adenovirus. No antimicrobial is necessary.

Notes: SBO: voluminous watery diarrhea, periumbilical cramps, bloating, nausea, or vomiting; fecal leucocytes not elevated (noninflammatory diarrhea). LBO: invasion of colon tissue causes fever, and bloody diarrhea, also known as dysentery; fecal leukocytes are elevated (inflammatory diarrhea). Elevated fecal leukocyte levels indicate inflammatory diarrhea or inflammatory bowel disease. Common source of *E. coli* 0157:H7 is undercooked beef; produces symptoms within 2 days due to Shiga-like toxin; antibiotics increase risk of hemolytic uremic syndrome and thrombocytopenia purpura. Shigella symptoms are caused by Shiga toxin; patients often have tenesmus. *Vibrio cholera*: stool often described as voluminous rice water diarrhea. *Staphylococcus aureus* and Norwalk virus produce symptoms hours after consuming contaminated food due to preformed toxin; major presenting symptom is vomiting. *Salmonella typhi* causes typhoid fever (systemic signs, salmon color spots on trunk).

What diagnostic test is indicated in addition to fecal leukocytes and FOBT?

Order an assay for *C. difficile* cytotoxin when a patient presents with acute diarrhea during or shortly after hospitalization or antibiotic administration. *C. difficile* colonizes the gut after antibiotics alter the normal gut flora. The most commonly implicated antibiotics are clindamycin and ampicillin.

Spectrum of *C. difficile* infection:

1. **Asymptomatic**: Most patients are asymptomatic carriers.
2. **Mild diarrhea without colitis**: Second most common presentation is mild watery diarrhea without fever, leukocytosis, or dehydration.
3. **Colitis without pseudomembranes**: Five to 15 watery stools per day, fever, and abdominal cramps are relieved by defecation.
4. **Pseudomembranous colitis**: Symptoms are the same as colitis without pseudomembranes. Patient also has white-yellow plaques on colon mucosa.

Fulminant colitis: Rarely, patients may present with obstruction, toxic megacolon, or perforation.

C. difficile cytotoxin assay is positive. How is C. difficile infection treated?

Discontinue clindamycin and other antibiotics. Correct any fluid and electrolyte imbalances. Avoid loperamide and opiates. Antibiotics are only indicated for patients with symptoms of colitis or persistent diarrhea. This patient with symptoms of colitis should receive a 10- to

14-day course of metronidazole. If symptoms do not resolve with metronidazole, use oral vancomycin. If the patient develops signs of peritonitis, surgical management is indicated.

> Pregnancy is a contraindication to metronidazole. Pregnant patients with *C. difficile* colitis should take oral vancomycin.

> **Prevention of hospital-acquired *C. difficile* infection**: Wear gloves prior to contact with infected patients. Wash hands with soap and water after removing gloves.

CASE 4–12 CHRONIC DIARRHEA

A 24-year-old Caucasian female presents with a 6-month history of diarrhea. She reports three to four watery stools a day. She has not noticed any blood in her stools. She also reports decreased appetite and a 5-lb weight loss. She sometimes takes Imodium (loperamide), which partially controls her symptoms. She tried a trial of lactose avoidance, which failed to control her symptoms. She has not taken any other medications or been hospitalized in the past year. She does not have any other medical problems. Physical examination and vital signs are normal.

What initial workup is indicated for this patient with chronic diarrhea?

History and physical often suggests a possible cause for chronic diarrhea (Table 4-7). Because a specific cause is not apparent in this case, order the following initial tests:

1. CBC and differential: identifies anemia (indicates chronic GI bleeding versus chronic inflammation), leukocytosis (indicates inflammation), and eosinophilia (indicates allergy versus collagen vascular disease versus parasite infection versus eosinophilic gastritis versus cancer).
2. FOBT: identifies GI bleeding.
3. Thyroid function tests: hyperthyroidism can cause chronic diarrhea.
4. Serum electrolytes and LFTs: May identify liver abnormalities or systemic conditions associated with diarrhea such as DM.
5. Total protein and albumin: indicators of general nutritional status.

The only significant laboratory abnormalities are mild iron deficiency anemia and a mildly decreased total protein and albumin. What is the next step in the evaluation?

Order a quantitative stool analysis. The analysis should include stool weight, pH, sodium, potassium, fecal leukocytes, stool occult blood, fecal fat, and a laxative screen.

> **Developing countries**: An empiric trial of metronidazole or oral fluoroquinolone is appropriate prior to stool analysis in countries where parasitic or bacterial causes of diarrhea are highly prevalent.

What stool analysis findings are associated with the different categories of diarrhea?

1. Inflammatory diarrhea: increased fecal leukocytes and guaiac-positive stool.
2. Secretory diarrhea: no abnormal stool analysis findings; normal osmotic gap.
3. Malabsorptive diarrhea: increased osmotic gap and increased fecal fat; stool may or may not be guaiac-positive, and fecal pH is decreased in carbohydrate malabsorption.
4. Osmotic diarrhea: increased osmotic gap; fecal pH is decreased only if osmotic diarrhea is caused by lactose intolerance.

> **Normal fecal fat** is <6 g/day
> **Normal fecal pH** is 5.6.
> **Fecal osmotic gap** (normally <50) $= 290 - 2([\text{fecal sodium}] + [\text{fecal potassium}])$.

TABLE 4–7 Causes of Chronic Diarrhea in Immunocompetent Adults

Inflammatory diarrhea	Classic presentation: Fever, hematochezia, abdominal pain ± pertinent travel history, recent antibiotic use, recent hospitalization, or history of radiation. Causes: 1. Chronic infections 2. Inflammatory bowel disease 3. Radiation enteritis
Secretory diarrhea	Classic presentation: Voluminous diarrhea that does not decrease with fasting. Causes: 1. Laxative abuse 2. Bile salt malabsorption (e.g., after cholecystectomy) 3. Hormonal tumors (VIPoma, carcinoid, medullary thyroid carcinoma, ZES)
Malabsorptive diarrhea	Classic presentation: Voluminous pale, greasy, foul-smelling diarrhea and weight loss despite adequate food intake. Many patients do not present with classic symptoms. Causes: 1. Bacterial overgrowth 2. Small bowel mucosa disorders (celiac sprue, tropical sprue, Whipple's disease) 3. Pancreas insufficiency (chronic pancreatitis, pancreatic carcinoma, cystic fibrosis) 4. Small bowel resection 5. Lymphatic obstruction (intestinal lymphoma, intestinal tuberculosis, carcinoid)
Osmotic diarrhea	Classic presentation: History of fat-free foods, lactulose, antacids, or symptoms worse with dairy products. Causes: 1. Sorbitol (found in fat-free foods) 2. Medications (lactulose, antacids) 3. Lactose intolerance
Motility disorders	Classic presentation: History of systemic disease or prior abdominal surgery Causes: 1. Systemic diseases (diabetes, scleroderma, hyperthyroidism) 2. Abdominal surgery (gastrectomy, gastric vagotomy)
Functional causes	Classic presentation: Abdominal pain relieved by defecation. Stool weight <200 g/day. No weight loss, anemia, gastrointestinal bleeding, or nocturnal diarrhea. Causes: 1. Irritable bowel syndrome 2. Functional diarrhea

Abbreviation: ZES, Zollinger-Ellison syndrome.

Positive findings on stool analysis are osmotic gap 120, steatorrhea, and guaiac-positive stool. Fecal leukocytes are not elevated. Laxative screen is negative. What is the next step in management?

Stool analysis suggests that malabsorption is the cause of this patient's diarrhea. Consider diagnostic testing in the following order:

1. Order H2 breath test (to test for carbohydrate malabsorption), tissue transglutaminase IgA antibody (to test for celiac disease), and stool examination for ova and parasites.
2. If these are negative, perform upper and lower endoscopy with biopsy of both ends of the small intestine. Also consider upper GI series with small bowel follow-through.
3. If small intestine biopsy and upper GI series fail to reveal any small bowel pathology, test for pancreatic insufficiency (refer to Chapter 8: Endocrinology).

> No diagnostic testing is indicated if patients have a known cause for malabsorption such as small intestine resection (causes short bowel syndrome) or cystic fibrosis (causes pancreatic insuffiency).

H2-breath test is positive. Anti-gliadin and anti-endomysial antibodies are elevated. What is the most likely diagnosis?

This patient likely has celiac disease (gluten-sensitive enteropathy). This autoimmune, small-bowel, mucosal abnormality tends to occur more frequently in persons of northern European or Indian ancestry (HLA DQ2 or HLA DQ8). Patients often have coexisting autoimmune conditions such as type 1 DM, autoimmune thyroid disease, and IgA deficiency.

What are the next steps in management?

Confirm the diagnosis of celiac sprue with small-bowel biopsy. Mucosal inflammation, crypt hyperplasia, and villous atrophy are the characteristic findings on biopsy. Patients with a confirmed diagnosis of celiac disease should follow a gluten-free diet (no wheat, rye, or barley). Consider prophylactic pneumococcal vaccine because patients often have hyposplenism. Some physicians perform a repeat biopsy 3 to 4 months after the patient initiates a gluten-free diet to demonstrate resolution of villous atrophy.

What are possible extraintestinal manifestations of celiac sprue?

Remember extraintestinal manifestations of celiac disease (may occur in the absence of diarrhea) using the mnemonic "***A gluten-free diet Demands HI-MAINtenance***":

1. **D**ermatitis herpetiformis: pruritic clusters of vesicles on erythematous, edematous papules on the extremities and trunk (unrelated to herpes virus despite name)
2. **H**yposplenism: absent or decreased spleen function
3. **I**ron deficiency anemia
4. **M**etabolic bone disease: Patients may develop osteoporosis due to secondary hyperparathyroidism and osteomalacia due to vitamin D deficiency.
5. **A**rthritis
6. **I**gA nephropathy and **I**nfertility
7. **N**europsychiatric disease: headache, ataxia, and depression

The patient asks about her long-term prognosis. What should you tell her?

Overall mortality is higher than the general population because celiac disease is associated with a modestly increased risk of non-Hodgkin lymphoma and GI cancers. The effect of a gluten-free diet on the risk of malignancy is not clear.

> **Tropical sprue** is seen in certain tropical countries. Symptoms and small-bowel biopsy findings are often similar to celiac sprue, but the most likely cause is infection. Treatment is tetracycline and folic acid.

Alternative 4.12.1

A 56-year-old white man presents with a 6-month history of abdominal pain and voluminous, greasy, foul-smelling diarrhea. He has lost 10 lbs in the last 6 months. Past medical history is significant for arthritis for the last 6 years that he describes as "migrating from joint to joint." Physical examination is significant for ascites and vertical gaze nystagmus. Serological testing for celiac sprue and stool ova and parasites are negative.

What condition should you suspect?

Suspect Whipple's disease, a rare, small-bowel, mucosal abnormality that affects white males of European ancestry. Symptoms are caused by colonization with *Treponema whipelli* in susceptible individuals. The earliest symptoms are migratory arthralgias. Years later, patients develop malabsorptive diarrhea and weight loss. Patients may have ascites due to hypoproteinemia. Sterile endocarditis and CNS symptoms such as dementia and vertical ataxia may also occur. Confirm diagnosis with small bowel biopsy, which would demonstrate PAS-positive macrophages and villous atrophy. Treat with IV ceftriaxone for 2 weeks followed by TMP/SMX for 1 year.

CASE 4–13 CHRONIC EPISODES OF ABDOMINAL PAIN AND DIARRHEA

A 27-year-old female presents with diarrhea, and mild periumbilical and RLQ cramps. She has had similar episodes over the last 18 months. She has also lost 10 lbs unintentionally over the last 12 months. Temperature is 38.4°C. Other vital signs are normal. Abnormal laboratory findings are mild anemia, mild leukocytosis, and decreased total protein and albumin. Stool analysis is significant for elevated fecal leukocytes and guaiac-positive stool.

What are the next diagnostic steps?

The findings indicate that she has chronic inflammatory diarrhea. The next tests are:

1. Labs: stool culture, ova and parasites, and *C. difficile* assay (TTG)
2. Sigmoidoscopy or colonoscopy with biopsy of colon mucosa

If the above tests do not indicate a specific diagnosis, consider upper GI series with small bowel follow-through (barium swallow).

Stool culture and C. difficile cytotoxin assay are negative. The colonoscopy report mentions that the colon and distal ileum has areas of ulcerations and polypoid mucosa, giving it a "cobblestone appearance." There are many areas of normal mucosa in between diseased segments ("skip lesions"). The rectum is unaffected. Biopsy shows focal areas of ulceration, inflammation, and granulomas. What is the diagnosis?

The endoscopic findings are consistent with inflammatory bowel disease due to Crohn's disease. Symptoms result from idiopathic transmural inflammation. The disease can affect any part of the GI tract from the mouth to the anus, so symptoms are often variable. The most commonly reported symptoms are chronic diarrhea with abdominal pain, fever, weight loss, fatigue, occult bleeding, and fever. Laboratory findings are nonspecific, although patients may have anemia, leukocytosis, and increased CRP.

> **Distribution of Crohn's**: 50% have ileocolitis, 30% have ileitis, and 20% have colitis. Half the patients with colitis do not have any rectal involvement.

> Although colonoscopy with biopsy is the definitive test for Crohn's, barium swallow may demonstrate ulcers, fistulas, or strictures ("string sign").

How is mild Crohn's disease treated?

Initial therapy for mild Crohn's disease is symptomatic. Patients with mild diarrhea should initially take loperamide. Patients with terminal ileum involvement can also take cholestyramine or colestipol to decrease diarrhea secondary to bile acid malabsorption. Patients with ileitis or ileocolitis may have diarrhea as a result of lactose intolerance. Diagnose lactase deficiency with the lactose breath test, and treat this condition by avoiding dairy products and taking calcium supplements.

How would you treat Crohn's disease that is unresponsive to symptomatic therapy?

Therapy for patients with more severe disease or diarrhea unresponsive to symptomatic treatment depends on disease severity and areas of involvement:

1. **Gastroduodenal disease**: An uncommon area of involvement, symptoms are similar to PUD; initial therapy is PPIs, and, if symptoms persist, add prednisone.

2. **Ileal disease**: Many clinicians start with oral mesalamine; other options are antibiotics (ciprofloxacin or metronidazole), prednisone, and budesonide.
3. **Ileocolitis or colitis**: Start with oral sulfasalazine or mesalamine (5-aminosalicylic acid (5-ASA) drugs). If symptoms persist, consider a course of metronidazole. If antibiotics are unsuccessful, treat with prednisone.

In all type of Crohn's disease, immunomodulators are recommended for symptoms refractory to steroids. Surgery is recommended for specific complications or symptoms refractory to medical therapy.

5-ASA drugs: These drugs are inactive when ingested, then they are cleaved by bowel microbes to release active 5-ASA (anti-inflammatory). Mesalamine is used for small bowel and colon involvement (although evidence for its efficacy in small bowel disease is unclear). Sulfasalazine is used only for small bowel involvement (GI side effects often limit its use).

Steroids and immunomodulators: Many patients become steroid-dependent to remain in clinical remission. Immunomodulators can help wean dependent patients off steroids (first-line agents are azothioprine and 6-mercaptopurine). Many physicians start steroids or immunomodulators first if symptoms are severe.

Surgery: Most patients with Crohn's disease eventually require some type of surgery; 10% to 15% of patients have recurrent symptoms each year after surgery. The risk of recurrence is lower in Crohn's colitis than other forms of Crohn's disease.

Maintenance therapy: The best regimen during clinical remission is not clear. Options include 5-ASA drugs, immunomodulators, steroids, and antibiotics.

What are possible long-term complications of Crohn's disease?

Crohn's disease can cause intestinal and nonintestinal complications (Table 4-8). Remember intestinal complications of Crohn's disease with the mnemonic "***Crohn's can AFfect Mouth, Small bowel, Colon, Anus.***"

1. Abscess: Suspect when the patient presents with a tender abdominal mass with fever and leukocytosis. Diagnose with CT scan of the abdomen. Treat with broad-spectrum antibiotics and percutaneous drainage or surgery.

TABLE 4–8 Extraintestinal Complications of Inflammatory Bowel Disease

Eyes	Anterior uveitis: Conjunctival injection and anterior chamber opacity Episcleritis: Episcleral vessel injection with normal appearing sclera
Skin	Erythema nodosum: Erythematous nodular areas, commonly on the shins Pyoderma gangrenosum: Pustular violaceous plaques that may scar
Bones	Peripheral arthritis Ankylosing spondylitis: Much more common in UC Sacroilitis: Presents with prolonged back stiffness in the morning or after rest
Blood	Venous and arterial thromboembolism: Due to hypercoagulable state
Liver and gallbladder	Gallstones: Can occur in ileal Crohn's disease Primary sclerosing cholangitis: Much more common in UC
Lungs	Bronchitis Bronchiectasis Interstitial lung disease

Abbreviation: UC, ulcerative colitis.

2. **F**istula: Asymptomatic patients do not require any treatment. Initial treatment of symptomatic fistulas is immunomodulators. Unfortunately, immunomodulator therapy is not usually successful and most patients require surgery.
3. **M**alabsorption: Enterocolonic fistulas can cause bacterial overgrowth and subsequent malabsorptive diarrhea. Involvement of the terminal ileum can cause bile acid malabsorption and subsequent secretory diarrhea.
4. **S**BO and perforation are caused by acute inflammation and/or strictures from chronic inflammation.
5. **C**olon cancer: Patients should undergo screening colonoscopy 8 years after onset of colitis because Crohn's disease increases the risk of colon cancer.
6. **A**nal discomfort: Perianal discomfort can indicate anal fistula, fissure, or skin tag. Treat with sitz baths and cotton balls to absorb irritating drainage. Severe pain suggests perianal abscess. Treat perianal abscess with incision and drainage.

Alternative 4.13.1

A 27-year-old Caucasian man presents with abdominal pain and bloody diarrhea. He has a 12-month history of similar episodes. Temperature is 38.4°C. Other vital signs are normal. Abnormal laboratory findings are mild anemia and mild leukocytosis. Stool analysis finds elevated fecal leukocytes and guaiac-positive stool. Stool culture, ova and parasites, and *C. difficile* assay are negative. On sigmoidoscopy, the mucosa is erythematous and friable with numerous petechiae, exudates, and pseudopolyps. Colon involvement is continuous. Biopsy reveals crypt abscesses.

What is the diagnosis?

The endoscopy findings are consistent with IBD due to ulcerative colitis (UC). Symptoms result from continuous mucosal inflammation of the colon and rectum. Symptoms vary depending on the extent of inflammation:

1. Mild: Inflammation limited to the rectum and sigmoid causes mild abdominal cramping, mild diarrhea, and rectal bleeding.
2. Moderate: Inflammation extending to the splenic flexure (left-sided colitis) causes mild abdominal cramps, frequent bloody diarrhea, mild anemia, and low-grade fever.
3. Severe: Inflammation that extends beyond the splenic flexure causes severe abdominal cramps, frequent bloody diarrhea, significant anemia, and weight loss with laboratory evidence of malnutrition (decreased serum albumin).

See Table 4-9 for important similarities and differences between UC and Crohn's disease.

How is active UC treated?

Treat mild diarrhea with loperamide. Initial therapy is usually with a topical 5-ASA enema. If symptoms persist despite topical 5-ASA, add the following agents sequentially until symptoms are controlled: topical steroid enemas, oral 5-ASA agents, and systemic steroids. Consider surgery versus immunomodulators for patients with persistent symptoms despite systemic steroids. Surgery is also indicated for specific complications of UC. Surgical colectomy is often curative in UC.

> **Severe disease**: Start with oral and topical 5-ASA drugs ± systemic steroids.

What are possible long-term complications of UC?

Extraintestinal complications are similar to Crohn's disease (see Table 4-8). Remember intestinal complications of UC using the mnemonic "***HOT Colon***" (see Table 4-9):

1. **H**emorrhage: A small percentage of patients have massive hemorrhage requiring colectomy.
2. **O**bstruction: Obstruction in UC is caused by colon strictures from chronic inflammation. Most strictures do not cause obstruction. Evaluate all strictures with colonoscopy and biopsy to rule out malignancy.

TABLE 4-9 Ulcerative Colitis Versus Crohn's Disease

	Crohn's Disease	UC
Age	Bimodal age distribution; first peak between 15 and 40 years, second peak between 50 and 80 years	Same as Crohn's disease
Race	More common in Caucasians, particularly Jewish individuals	Same as Crohn's disease
Gender	Equal incidence in males and females	Same as Crohn's disease
Course	Chronic disorder characterized by episodic flares and remissions	Same as Crohn's disease
Smoking	Smoking increases risk of Crohn's; smoking cessation decreases flares	Smoking decreases the risk of UC; smoking cessation increases flares
Extent of inflammation	Transmural	Usually limited to mucosa
Areas of bowel involved	Can occur anywhere from mouth to anus; 50% of patients have ileocolitis, 30% have ileitis, and 20% have colitis. Half the patients with colon involvement do not have any rectal involvement.	Involves only colorectal area; almost all patients have rectal involvement
Endoscopic findings	Skip lesions, cobblestone mucosa, ulcers	Continuous involvement; friable, erythematous mucosa with petechiae, exudates, pseudopolyps
Key biopsy finding	Granulomas	Crypt abscesses
Antibodies[a]	Usually ANCA-positive	Usually p-ANCA positive
Intestinal complications	Crohn can **AF**fect **M**outh, **S**mall bowel, **C**olon, **A**nus.	**HOT C**olon: risk of colon cancer greater with UC than with Crohn's
Prognosis after surgery	Surgery not usually curative	Surgery often curative

[a] Antibody tests indicated if cause of IBD is unclear despite endoscopy + biopsy.

3. **T**oxic megacolon: Colonic dilation that is caused by mucosal inflammation. Typically presents with bloody diarrhea, abdominal pain, and distension. Patients appear extremely sick with fever, tachycardia, leukocytosis, and anemia ± signs of septic shock. Confirm diagnosis with abdominal x-ray (see Fig. 4-14). Treat with NPO, IV fluids, NG and rectal tube, IV broad-spectrum antibiotics, steroids, position (roll the patient from side to side intermittently), and reassess the patient every 12 hours. Refer for emergent surgery if symptoms continue to worsen or colon diameter continues to increase despite medical therapy. Another indication for surgery is if symptoms improve but colon dilation persists after 3 to 7 days.
4. **C**olon cancer: Perform screening colonoscopy 8 years after onset of colitis unless inflammation is limited to the rectum (distal proctitis).

> ***C. difficile* colitis** is the second most common cause of toxic megacolon after UC. Medical therapy of toxic megacolon due to infectious colitis is NPO, IV fluids, NG and rectal tube, position, discontinuing offending antibiotic, vancomycin ± metronidazole, and reassessment but NOT steroids.

CASE 4–14 HEMATEMESIS

A 45-year-old male with a history of PUD presents to the emergency department with acute onset of hematemesis. He states that he has vomited copious amounts of bright red blood. He

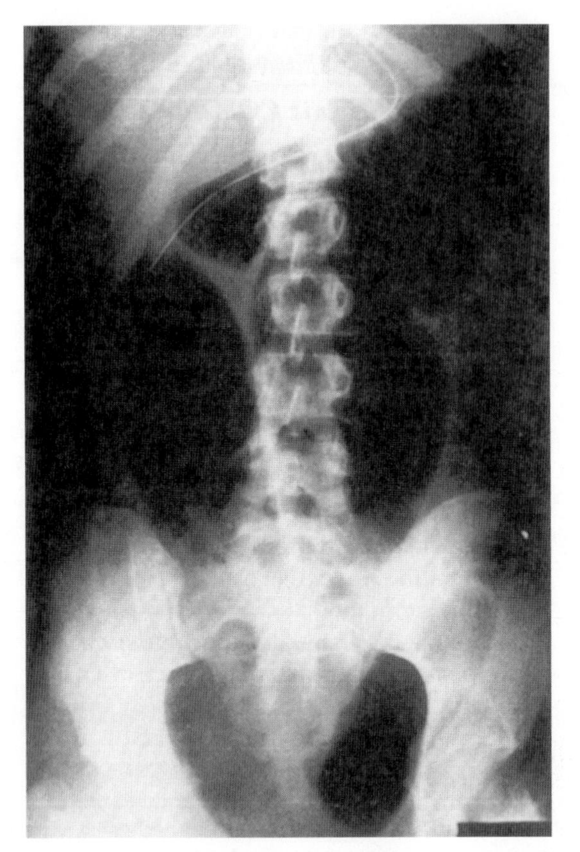

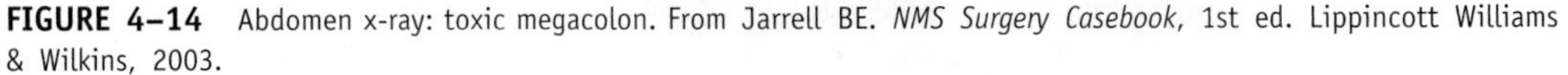

FIGURE 4–14 Abdomen x-ray: toxic megacolon. From Jarrell BE. *NMS Surgery Casebook,* 1st ed. Lippincott Williams & Wilkins, 2003.

does not have any significant past medical history. Vital signs are temperature 37.1°C, pulse 115 bpm, respirations 20/min, and blood pressure 90/60. SaO_2 is 99% on room air.

What are the causes of hematemesis?

Emesis of bright red blood or "coffee-ground" material indicates that the patient's source of bleeding originates in the GI tract above the ligament of Treitz (upper GI bleed). Remember the common etiologies of upper GI bleeding using the mnemonic "***Mallory Got Us Very Alarmed***" (Table 4-10). The most common causes are PUD and gastritis (>50%), followed by variceal bleeding (approximately 15%).

What are the initial steps in the management of this patient with an upper GI bleed?

The first step in the management of any unstable patient with active upper GI bleeding is hemodynamic stabilization. Perform the following initial steps (see Fig. 4-15):

1. Fluids: Place two large-bore peripheral IV lines (18-gauge or larger) or a central line and administer normal saline or lactated ringers.
2. Labs: Draw blood to measure CBC, serum creatinine, coagulation studies (PT, PTT, and INR), serum chemistry, LFTs, type, and cross-match.
3. NG lavage: Aspiration of red blood indicates that the patient has an active brisk upper GI bleed. Aspiration of "coffee-ground" material indicates that the patient has an active but slower upper GI bleed. Clear NG aspirate suggests that bleeding has stopped.
4. Oral or IV PPI: Consider in this patient with a history of PUD.

False-negative aspirate: If a patient has a duodenal bleed but the pylorus is closed, NG aspirate may be clear. Suspect this situation when NG lavage does not yield any bilious (dark green) fluid.

TABLE 4–10 Causes of Upper GI Bleeding

Common causes (Mallory Got Us Very Alarmed)	1. **M**allory Weiss tear 2. **G**astritis and peptic **U**lcers (#1 cause) 3. **V**arices (#2 cause) 4. **A**rteriovenous malformation (more commonly a source of lower GI bleeding)
Uncommon causes	1. **Dieulafoy lesion**: dilated submucosal vessel that erodes the overlying epithelium; appears as a raised nipple on endoscopy. Treatment is endoscopic hemostasis. 2. **Gastric antral vascular ectasia (GAVE)**: idiopathic condition; also known as watermelon stomach because endoscopic appearance is flat, reddish stripes radiating from the pylorus to the antrum. Treatment is endoscopic hemostasis. 3. **Hemobilia**: suspect when a patient with recent liver or gallbladder injury (hepatobiliary procedure or disease) presents with upper GI bleeding, biliary colic, and obstructive jaundice; confirm diagnosis with endoscopic retrograde cholangiopancreatography followed by arteriography to locate the source of the bleeding. Treatment is to correct underlying condition. 4. **Aortoenteric fistula**: fistula from abdominal aorta opens into the small intestine; suspect when a patient with a history of abdominal aortic aneurysm or abdominal aorta graft surgery presents with a small GI bleed. Diagnose quickly with CT scan, endoscopy or enteroscopy because the small bleed is followed by recurrent or massive life-threatening GI bleed hours to weeks later. Treatment is surgical repair. 5. **Upper GI tumors**

History of cirrhosis: Consider octreotide and antibiotics during initial stabilization. Octreotide reduces portal pressure (unclear mechanism). Antibiotics decrease risk of severe nosocomial infection, which is otherwise very high in patients with cirrhosis. IV vasopressin and nitroglycerin is a less effective alternative to octreotide.

History of uremia: Consider desmopressin (DDAVP) during initial stabilization because patients may have platelet dysfunction (mechanism unclear).

Active large volume hematemesis: Electively intubate to prevent aspiration.

The patient receives 2 L of normal saline. Five liters of bright red blood is aspirated. Hematocrit is 31%. Platelets are 100,000/µL and INR is 1.2. LFTs are normal. What is the next step in management?

Hematocrit may take 24 to 72 hours to equilibrate with extravascular fluid, so it is not a reliable indicator of the severity of bleeding. Administer packed red blood cells (PRBCs) to patients with active bleeding regardless of the hematocrit (Table 4-11). If hemodynamic instability persists despite vigorous resuscitation including three units PRBCs, admit the patient to the ICU, administer a single dose of erythromycin, perform urgent EGD, and consult surgery to evaluate if emergent surgery is indicated.

Erythromycin: promotes gastric emptying, which helps clear large clots and thereby improve visualization during EGD (helps shorten endoscopy time).

The patient receives two units of PRBCs and another liter of normal saline. Vital signs are now normal. What is the next step in management?

Once the patient is stable, perform EGD to determine the cause of GI bleeding. Administer a single dose of erythromycin prior to endoscopy to clear large clots.

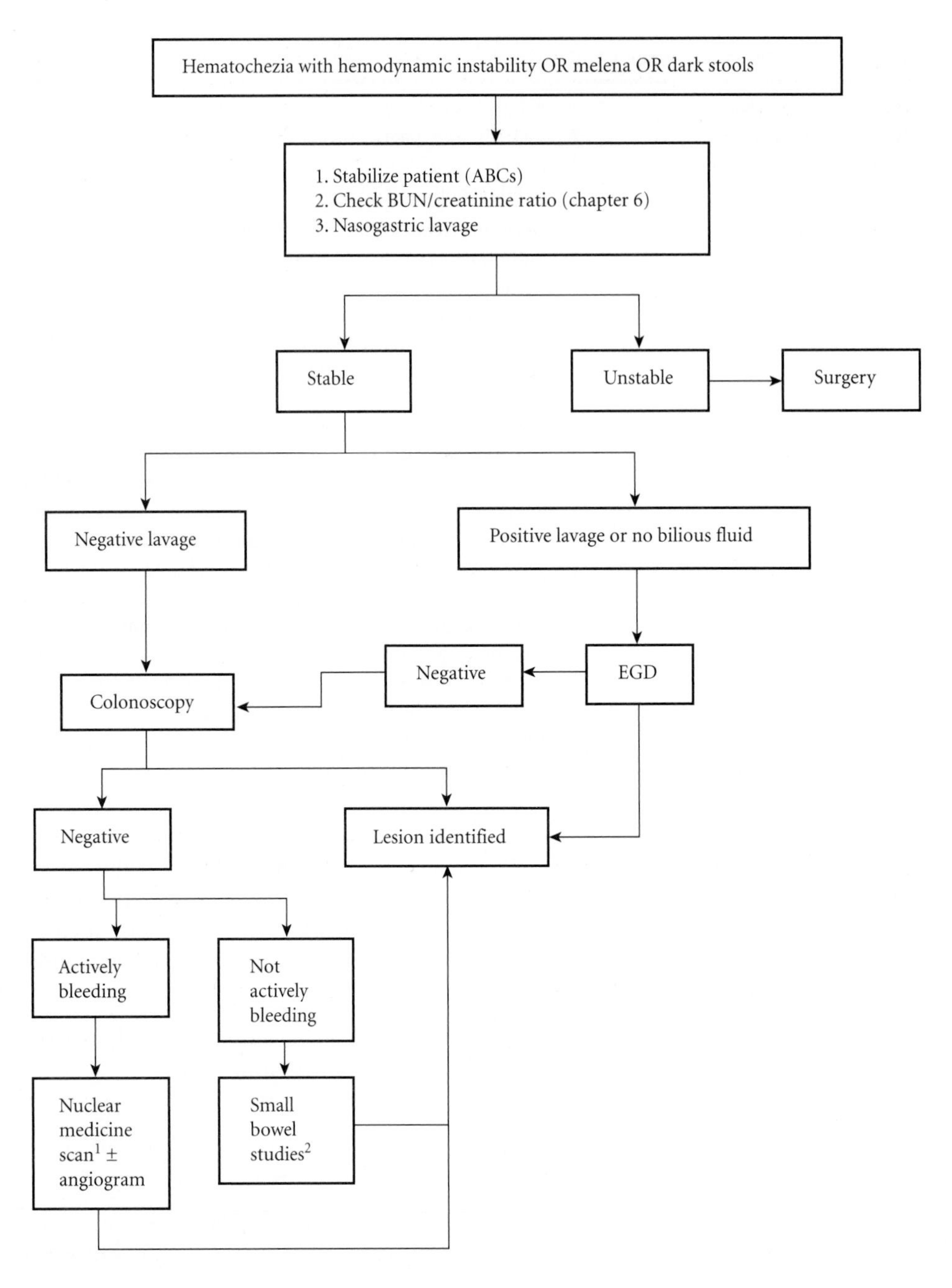

[1]**Nuclear medicine scan (tagged RBC scan):** Inject technetium (Tc), which is taken up by RBCs. Obtain abdominal radiographs over the next 30 mins to observe if Tc-tagged RBCs extravasate outside the intestine.
[2]**Small bowel studies:** enteroclysis, push enteroscopy, or wireless capsule endoscopy.

FIGURE 4–15 Diagnostic approach to severe lower GI bleeding.

EGD detects a duodenal ulcer with a nonbleeding visible vessel. What is the next step?

Actively bleeding ulcers, ulcers with a non-bleeding but visible vessel, and ulcers with adherent clots have a high risk of rebleeding. The next step is endoscopic hemostasis (epinephrine injection and thermocoagulation). An alternative to thermocoagulation is endoscopic endoclip placement.

Indications for surgery:

1. Active bleeding ulcer despite two attempts at endoscopic hemostasis
2. Recurrent bleeding associated with shock or requiring ≥3 units PRBCs per day

TABLE 4–11 Indications for Transfusion in Patients With Upper GI Bleeding

PRBCs[a]	1. Active bleeding 2. HCT ≤30% plus multiple comorbidities or cirrhosis 3. HCT ≤20% in an otherwise healthy patient
Platelets	1. Active bleeding plus platelets <50,000/μL 2. Active bleeding plus recent aspirin use (any platelet level)
FFP[b]	1. Active bleeding and INR >1.5 2. Coagulopathy and INR >1.5 (even if not actively bleeding) 3. Give one unit FFP for every 5 units of PRBCs

Abbreviations: FFP, fresh frozen plasma; HCT, hematocrit; INR, International Normalized Ratio; PRBC, packed red blood cells.
[a] PRBCs: Give blood type O if specific type and cross-match are not available.
[b] FFP: Give type AB if specifically matched FFP are not available.

How would management differ if EGD detected a non-bleeding ulcer with a flat red spot?

Observation for 24 to 48 hours (i.e., no specific endoscopic therapy) is indicated for ulcers with a low risk of rebleeding:

1. Non-bleeding ulcers <2 cm with a clean base
2. Non-bleeding ulcers with a flat red or black spot

What steps are indicated to reduce risk of ulcer rebleeding?

The following steps are indicated after an episode of upper GI bleeding due to PUD to reduce the risk of rebleeding:

1. Avoid NSAIDs: All patients (high and low risk) should avoid NSAIDs.
2. *H. pylori* testing: Test all patients for *H. pylori* and eradicate if detected.
3. Acid lowering therapy: Patients who required endoscopic therapy should take PPIs; other patients should take H2-blockers.

Alternative 4.14.1

A 45-year-old man with a history of cirrhosis due to hepatitis C presents to the emergency department with acute onset of hematemesis. Vital signs are temperature 37.1°C, pulse 115 bpm, respirations 20/min, and blood pressure 90/60. Oxygen saturation is 99% on room air. He receives normal saline, octreotide, and ciprofloxacin. NG aspirate yields 2 L of coffee grounds. Hematocrit is 28%, INR is 1.7, platelets are 100,000/μL. Aspartate aminotransferase and alanine aminotransferase are elevated. He receives PRBCs and fresh-frozen plasma. Vital signs are now stable.

What is the most likely finding on endoscopy?

The most likely finding in this patient with cirrhosis is bleeding varices. Varices are dilated, tortuous blood vessels that develop in the esophagus or stomach as a result of portal hypertension. The most common causes of portal hypertension in the United States are alcoholic liver disease and chronic active hepatitis.

EGD detects an actively bleeding esophageal varix. What is the next step?

Banding and sclerotherapy are the two endoscopic hemostatic procedures commonly used to treat upper GI bleeding due to varices. Most endoscopists prefer sclerotherapy for patients with active bleeding because it is quicker than banding in this situation. Banding is preferred when variceal bleeding has stopped by the time diagnostic endoscopy is performed because risk of rebleeding and other complications are lower.

The patient continues to bleed copiously despite octreotide and endoscopic sclerotherapy of the bleeding varix. What are the next steps in management?

Repeat endoscopy and attempt hemostasis with sclerotherapy, banding, or thermocoagulation. If this is unsuccessful, perform balloon tamponade followed by a transjugular intrahepatic portosystemic shunt (TIPS) procedure. If an experienced interventional radiologist is not available to perform TIPS, refer the patient for emergent surgery.

> **TIPS**: A stent is used to artificially connect the portal and hepatic veins, which decreases portal venous pressure.

> **Balloon tamponade**: An inflated balloon exerts pressure on the bleeding varices, which controls bleeding. Associated with numerous complications, so this is used only as a temporizing measure before TIPS or surgery; always intubate before tamponade.

> **Bleeding gastric varices**: Endoscopic hemostasis is not recommended (high failure rate). Treat with octreotide and balloon tamponade followed by TIPS or surgery.

Alternative 4.14.2

The patient is a 48-year-old man with a history of alcoholism. He presents to the emergency department with acute onset of hematemesis and epigastric pain that radiates to his back. The episode began after a drinking binge that caused him to retch and vomit. Vital signs are stable. Aspartate aminotransferase and alanine aminotransferase are elevated, but other laboratory values are normal. NG aspiration yields a small amount of coffee grounds. During upper endoscopy, the gastroenterologist mentions that the patient has a Mallory Weiss tear.

What is a Mallory Weiss tear?

A Mallory Weiss tear is a partial longitudinal tear at the gastroesophageal junction. If the tear involves a submucosal vessel, the patient can present with GI bleeding. Predisposing factors are heavy alcohol use (which leads to forceful retching and vomiting) and hiatal hernia. Patients may report epigastric and/or back pain.

> Many patients do not present with classic findings, and many patients with a classic history do not have a Mallory Weiss tear.

How are Mallory Weiss tears treated?

Treatment of active bleeding is endoscopic hemostasis. Treatment of non-bleeding vessels or a fresh clot detected at endoscopy is observation for 48 hours. Treatment for all other patients is observation for 24 hours.

> **Boerhaave syndrome**: Full thickness posterolateral esophagus tear caused by forceful retching or vomiting. Symptoms, diagnosis, and treatment are similar to esophageal perforation. Endoscopy is not indicated.

CASE 4–15 RECTAL BLEEDING

A 65-year-old man presents with a 3-day history of painless hematochezia. He has not recently taken any medications. He denies any weight loss. On physical examination, he appears pale. Blood pressure is 110/80 in the supine position and 90/60 in the standing position.

What are the causes of lower GI bleeding?

Remember the common causes of GI bleeding that originates below the ligament of Treitz using the mnemonic "***Anus, Rectal & Colon Cramps Are Disturbing***":

1. Anorectal disorders: hemorrhoids and anal fissures

2. Radiation telangiectasia and proctitis: late complications of abdomen/pelvic radiation
3. Colon cancer and colon polyps
4. Colitis: infectious colitis, ischemic colitis, or IBD
5. Arteriovenous malformation (AVM): incidence increases with age
6. Diverticulosis: number one cause of lower GI bleeding; incidence parallels age (e.g., incidence is 50% in 50-year-olds, 60% in 60-year-olds, 70% in 70-year-olds, and so on)

> "The further you go up, the darker it gets":
> **Hematochezia**: bright red or maroon blood per rectum. Usually caused by rectal or left-sided colon bleeding. Occasionally caused by brisk upper GI bleeding.
> **Melena**: dark, tarry, foul-smelling stool. Usually caused by upper GI bleed. Sometimes caused by small bowel or ascending colon bleed.
> **Occult blood**: guaiac-positive stool detected on FOBT. Source of bleeding can be anywhere along the GI tract.

What is the next step in management?

The first step in management of this patient with orthostatic hypotension is hemodynamic resuscitation. Initial stabilization is similar to upper GI bleeding. Administer IV fluids, obtain labs, and transfuse if necessary (see Table 4-11). If resuscitation is unsuccessful, refer for emergent surgery.

> Rule out an upper GI source of bleeding with NG lavage prior to lower GI evaluation if the patient presents with melena, dark stools, or hemodynamic instability/orthostatic hypotension (see Fig. 4-15).

The patient receives IV fluids. Hematocrit is 20% so he receives PRBCs. Remaining labs are normal. NG lavage yields clear aspirates with bilious fluid. Vital signs are now normal and the patient appears stable. What is the next step in management?

When the patient is stabilized and an upper GI bleed has been excluded, perform colonoscopy to determine the cause of lower GI bleeding (see Fig. 4-15).

Colonoscopy demonstrates several diverticula. A pigmented spot is seen on one of the right-sided diverticula. What is the next step in management?

The patient should consume a high-fiber diet to prevent rebleeding and diverticulitis.

> Most diverticula occur in the left colon, but most bleeding diverticula are in the right colon.

> **Actively bleeding diverticula**: Treat with endoscopic hemostasis or surgery.

Alternative 4.15.1

A 30-year-old man presents to the clinic with anal itching. He has also noticed bright red blood in the toilet bowl and on the toilet paper after defecation. He can palpate a painless lump near his anus when he strains. He does not take any medications. There is no family history of colon cancer. Physical examination and vital signs are normal.

What is the most likely diagnosis?

The most likely cause of this patient's symptoms is a dilated hemorrhoidal vessel ("hemorrhoids"). This common condition typically presents with anal itching and bright red blood on the toilet paper or in the toilet bowl. Some patients may notice a palpable lump on straining (prolapse). Prolonged sitting, straining, and pregnancy are the most common risk factors for hemorrhoids.

How are hemorrhoids classified?

1. **Internal hemorrhoids**: arise superior to the dentate line, and therefore lack sensory innervation. Most symptomatic hemorrhoids are internal. Classified as first degree (bleed but do not protrude), second degree (protrude with defecation but reduce spontaneously), third degree (protrude and require digital reduction), and fourth degree (cannot be reduced).
2. **External hemorrhoids:** arise inferior to the dentate line, and receive sensory innervation. Do not cause symptoms unless thrombosis occurs.
3. **Mixed hemorrhoids**

What is the next step in management?

Perform an anorectal examination, anoscopy, and flexible sigmoidoscopy to detect hemorrhoids as well as exclude other conditions that can cause anorectal discomfort and hematochezia. Prolapsed hemorrhoids appear as purple nodules.

Patients with hematochezia who exhibit the following symptoms require colonoscopy even if anorectal examination and anoscopy detects a hemorrhoid or other anorectal condition:

1. **Dark blood or melena**: Hemorrhoidal bleeding is bright red.
2. **Anemia**: Hemorrhoids rarely cause bleeding severe enough to cause anemia.
3. **Guaiac-positive stools**: This is not a typical finding with hemorrhoids.
4. **High risk of colon cancer**: Age >50 years, history of polyps, early cancer in family.

Anoscopy detects a second-degree internal hemorrhoid as well as an external hemorrhoid. Both are painless to palpation. How is this condition treated?

1. **Conservative therapy**: Initial therapy is conservative. Reduce bleeding with a high-fiber diet and adequate water intake. Treat itching with sitz baths and hydrocortisone cream or suppositories.
2. **Minimally invasive procedures**: Perform if the patient continues to have symptoms despite conservative measures. Band ligation and infrared coagulation are the most frequently utilized procedures. Other procedures include heat or laser coagulation, sclerotherapy, and cryotherapy.
3. **Surgery**: Consider if minimally invasive procedures do not control symptoms.

Do not use hydrocortisone creams and suppositories for longer than 1 week because long-term use can cause contact dermatitis and mucosal atrophy.

The patient's symptoms improve with conservative therapy. He returns 3 months later with a 12-hour hour history of severe anal pain and a palpable lump in the anal area. Anorectal examination reveals a 2-cm, tense, blue nodule. What is the diagnosis?

The patient has a thrombosed external hemorrhoid. Treatment for patients who present within the first 24 hours of symptom onset is clot removal followed by daily sitz baths. If the patient presents after 24 hours of symptom onset, treat conservatively.

Alternative 4.15.2

A 65-year-old man presents with a 2-week history of tearing anal pain during defecation. He has noticed bright red blood in the toilet bowl and on the toilet paper. Physical exam and vital signs are normal.

What is the most likely diagnosis?

Tearing pain during defecation accompanied by bright red blood in the toilet bowl or on the toilet paper are characteristic symptoms of an anal fissure. Risk factors are similar to those of hemorrhoids. The most common location is in the posterior midline.

What is the next step in diagnosis?

Perform anorectal examination and anoscopy to confirm the presence of a fissure. An acute fissure looks like a crack in the epithelium. Chronic fissures result in the development of a skin tag. Also, perform colonoscopy rather than sigmoidoscopy to exclude other causes of hematochezia because this patient is >50 years old (high risk of colon cancer).

> Prior thrombosed external hemorrhoids also appear as a skin tag.

Anorectal examination reveals an anal fissure in the posterior midline. Colonoscopy is negative. How is this condition treated?

Initial therapy is conservative (fiber, sitz baths, topical diltiazem or nitroglycerin). If conservative therapy is unsuccessful, options include botox injection and calcium channel blockers. Surgery is reserved for fissures that persist despite medical therapy.

Alternative 4.15.3

A 30-year-old man presents with hematochezia. He has a history of recurrent nosebleeds that are difficult to control. On physical exam, there are two or three small, purplish macules in the mouth and four or five of these on the fingers. The macules partially blanch when a slide is pressed against them. He has conjunctival pallor. The patient's father had similar lesions as well.

What is the diagnosis?

This patient has the four key features of hereditary hemorrhagic telangiectasia, also known as Osler-Weber-Rendu syndrome:

1. Mucocutaneous telangiectasias: a type of AVM that tends to rupture and bleed.
2. Recurrent epistaxis: earliest symptom that occurs in 90% of patients.
3. GI bleeding: occurs in young adulthood in 25% of patients.
4. Family history.

Patients with this hereditary condition can also have AVMs in the lungs, brain, and liver.

How is this condition diagnosed and treated?

Diagnosis is clinical. Initial treatment of anemia due to GI bleeding is iron supplementation. If iron supplements do not correct the anemia, consider blood transfusion. Consider endoscopic hemostasis if the patient has hematochezia or melena with anemia unresponsive to supplements and transfusion.

> **AVM:** Also known as angiodysplasia or vascular ectasia, these are arteriovenous communications between dilated thin-walled blood vessels. AVMs often do not bleed. Those that do bleed usually present with occult GI bleeding, although sometimes bleeding is acute and massive. No treatment is necessary for asymptomatic AVMs. Treat actively bleeding AVMs with endoscopic hemostasis.

Alternative 4.15.4

An 18-year-old man presents with painless hematochezia. His father was diagnosed with colon cancer at the age of 41 years, and his paternal uncle was diagnosed with colon cancer at the age of 29 years. The patient has never undergone any endoscopic testing in the past. Anorectal examination is normal. Stool is positive for occult blood. Physical exam and vital signs are normal.

What is the next step in management?

This patient with hematochezia is young but has a high risk of colon cancer because of the positive family history of early colon cancer. The next step in management is colonoscopy.

Colonoscopy detects hundreds of adenomatous polyps. What is the diagnosis?

The patient has familial adenomatosis polyposis (FAP), an autosomal dominant condition with variable penetrance. FAP is caused by a mutation in the APC gene (Table 4-12). About one third of patients with FAP have spontaneous mutations in the APC gene, so family history may be negative.

Attenuated FAP: In this less severe variant, few polyps are seen on colonoscopy.

How is this condition managed?

1. Colectomy: Almost all patients develop colon cancer by the age of 45, so prophylactic colectomy is recommended when adenomas >1 cm develop.
2. Upper endoscopy: Perform at diagnosis and then every 3 to 5 years because FAP increases the risk of gastric carcinoma and duodenal ampullary carcinoma. Biopsy any gastric or duodenal polyps. Cyclooxygenase-2 inhibitors may prevent progression of duodenal adenomas, although treatment is usually endoscopic or surgical removal.

TABLE 4–12 Hereditary Syndromes Associated With Increased Colon Cancer Risk

Syndrome	Mutation	Description	Screening Recommendations for Patients With Established Genetic or Clinical Diagnosis
HNPCC (Lynch syndrome)	Mismatch repair gene defect (autosomal dominant)	Family history positive for early right colon cancer. Amsterdam criteria ("**3-2-1**"): colon cancer in at least 3 relatives, 2 generations, and 1 family member before the age of 50.	Screening colonoscopy every 1–2 years beginning at age 20–25 or 10 years before earliest age of diagnosis in a family member (whichever is earlier). Consider upper endoscopy, pelvic exam and endometrial aspirate ± transvaginal ultrasound to screen for ovarian and endometrial cancer, and annual urinalysis after 25 years to screen for renal and ureteral cancer.
FAP	APC gene (autosomal dominant)	Hundreds of adenomatous polyps	Colectomy, upper endoscopy, and thyroid palpation.
Gardner syndrome	APC gene (autosomal dominant)	Variant of FAP associated with soft tissue and bone lesions	Same as FAP.
Turcot syndrome	APC gene (autosomal dominant)	Variant of FAP associated with medulloblastomas	Same as FAP.
Peutz-Jegher syndrome (PJS)	STK-11 gene (autosomal dominant)	Pigmented spots in lips and buccal mucosa, hamartomatous polyps anywhere along GI tract	Colonoscopy, upper endoscopy, and small bowel imaging every 1–2 years beginning at age 18. Perform endoscopic ultrasound beginning at age 25 to screen for pancreatic cancer. Perform mammography in females beginning at age 25.[a]
Juvenile *Polyposis coli* (JPC)	SMAD-4 gene (autosomal dominant)	Presents in childhood with GI bleeding and anemia. Colonoscopy detects >10 hamartomatous polyps.	Consider colonoscopy every 1–2 years starting at age 18. Note that there are no universal screening guidelines.

Abbreviation: FAP, familial adenomatosis polyposis; HNPCC, hereditary nonpolyposis colon cancer

[a] Small bowel studies include upper GI series with small bowel follow-through, enteroclysis, push enteroscopy, and wireless capsule endoscopy.

3. Thyroid palpation: Perform annually because FAP increases thyroid cancer risk.
4. Genetic screening: Screen family members for the patient's APC mutation. Screen any children ≤6 years old with the APC mutation for hepatoblastoma using fetal α-protein and abdominal palpation.

CASE 4–16 MANAGEMENT OF COLON POLYPS AND COLON CANCER

A 50-year-old woman with no family history of colon cancer chooses to undergo screening with sigmoidoscopy. On sigmoidoscopy, two 5-mm polyps are detected.

What is the next step in management?

Remove any polyp detected during colon cancer surveillance and evaluate the histology.

Both polyps have hyperplastic histology. What is the next step in management?

Hyperplastic polyps are not neoplastic. Hyperplastic polyps in the left colon are not associated with increased risk of malignancy. No further therapy is recommended. As with other patients who undergo screening sigmoidoscopy, repeat screening after 5 years.

> **Right-sided hyperplastic polyps**: not neoplastic; increase cancer risk.
> **Hamartomas**: not neoplastic; increase cancer risk when associated with Peutz-Jegher syndrome or juvenile *Polyposis coli.*

The patient reports that she noticed small amounts of bright red blood on her toilet paper and in her toilet bowl 24 hours after sigmoidoscopy. What is the next step?

Patients may observe self-limited GI bleeding for a few days after polypectomy. Unless bleeding persists, no further evaluation is necessary.

Five years later, the patient undergoes screening colonoscopy. Two 0.5-cm polyps are detected in the left colon. There is a stalk between the base of the polyp and the colon mucosa. The polyp is removed. The pathology report states that both polyps are adenomas with tubular histology. What is your recommendation?

Adenomas are considered neoplastic lesions with a risk of progressing to carcinoma. Patients with only one or two small pedunculated adenomas (<1 cm) with tubular histology have the lowest risk of malignant progression. Recommend follow-up colonoscopy in 5 years.

> Adenoma terms:
>
> **Diminutive**: size <5 mm (polyps >1 cm have higher malignant potential).
> **Tubular histology**: >80% of adenomas; lowest malignant potential.
> **Tubulovillous histology**: intermediate malignant potential.
> **Villous histology**: highest malignant potential (**VILL**ous = **VILL**ain).
> **Serrated adenoma**: mixed adenomatous and hyperplastic cells; treat as adenoma.
> **Sessile**: base attached to colon mucosa; high malignant potential if >2 cm (sess**ile** = v**ile**).
> **Pedunculated**: stalk between base and colon wall; lower malignant potential.

Five years later, the patient undergoes colonoscopy. During the evaluation, a 2.5-cm sessile polyp is detected. The physician is unable to remove the entire polyp during the procedure. Histology shows tubular adenoma. What is the next step in management?

Large polyps often require piecemeal resection in two or three sittings. If complete removal is not possible, consider surgical colectomy.

The polyp is completely removed in one sitting. When should this patient next undergo screening for colon cancer?

Recommend follow-up colonoscopy after 3 years if the patient has any of the following: size >1 cm, number ≥3 polyps, villous or tubulovillous histology.

Three years later, she undergoes follow-up colonoscopy. There is a 3-cm pedunculated polyp. The pathology report classifies the histology as a well-differentiated carcinoma limited to the mucosa. Margins are clear. What is the next step in management?

Recommend follow-up in 1 year after polypectomy for patients with carcinoma within the polyp if they match each aspect of the following description: pedunculated polyps containing well-differentiated carcinomas with clear margins and no invasion. Perform surgery if any of these requirements are not met.

> Colon lymphatics do not extend above the muscularis mucosa, so carcinoma limited to the mucosa is unlikely to have spread via lymphatics.

The patient does not show up to her follow-up appointment the following year. She presents 5 years later with a 2-month history of abdominal pain, melena, fatigue, and a 10-lb weight loss. Oh physical examination, she appears pale. If she has colorectal cancer, what is the most likely location based on her symptoms?

Abdominal pain is the most common symptom in both right- and left-sided cancers. However, melena and anemia are more frequent in right-sided colon cancer. The right colon has a large lumen, and right-sided cancers tend to be polypoid or fungating, so obstruction is uncommon.

> **Left colon cancer**: Tends to grow in an annular fashion and constrict the bowel (see Fig. 4-16), so common symptoms are obstruction and change in bowel habits (alternating diarrhea and constipation, pencil-thin stools).
> **Rectal cancer:** Common symptoms are hematochezia and tenesmus.

Colonoscopy reveals a right-sided, poorly differentiated, colon cancer. What are the next steps in management?

The next step in management is preoperative staging with CXR, CT of the abdomen and pelvis, and serum carcinoembryonic antigen (CEA).

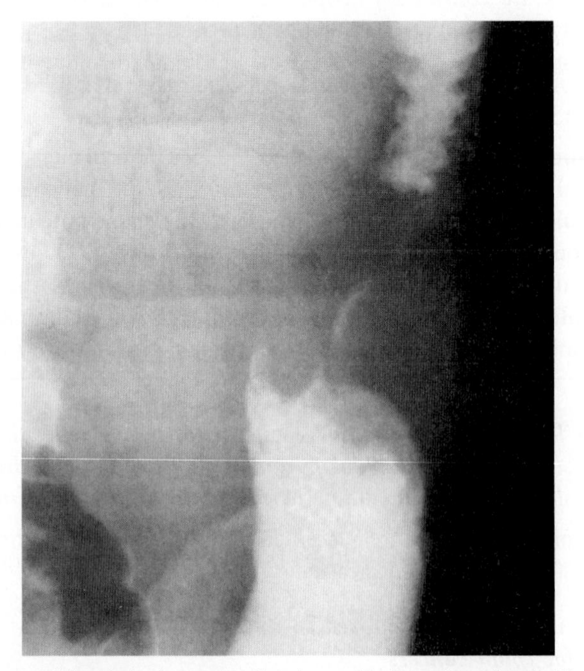

FIGURE 4–16 Barium enema: left-sided colon cancer ("apple core" lesion.) From Jarrell BE. *NMS Surgery Casebook*, 1st ed. Lippincott Williams & Wilkins, 2003.

Rectal cancer: Preoperative staging should also include EUS.

CT scan and CXR do not detect any distant metastases. What is the next step?

The primary therapy for colorectal cancer without any distant metastases is surgery. Perform intraoperative staging during surgery to detect lymphatic invasion. Surgery alone is sufficient in the absence of any lymphatic invasion (stage I and stage II disease). Surgery plus adjuvant (additional) chemotherapy is recommended for node-positive disease (stage III).

Rectal cancer $\geq$ stage II = Radiation and chemotherapy
Colon cancer $\geq$ stage III = Chemotherapy but no radiation

The patient has stage II disease and undergoes surgical resection. What follow-up testing is recommended to detect recurrences in patients with stage II or III disease?

1. History, physical exam, and serum CEA level: every 3 months
2. Annual CT scan of the chest and abdomen
3. Colonoscopy: Perform initial colonoscopy 3 months after surgery if the initial surgery was incomplete, otherwise perform the initial colonoscopy 1 year after resection. Perform follow-up colonoscopies after 3 years. If history, physical, CEA, or CT scan show any abnormalities, perform follow-up colonoscopy earlier.

Serum CEA is not helpful for the initial diagnosis of colorectal cancer. The reason it is obtained preoperatively is to establish a baseline. A rising CEA level after surgery may indicate incomplete removal or recurrence.

Synchronous tumor: polyp or cancer detected at the same time as another cancer.
Metachronous tumor: polyp or cancer detected at least 6 months after initial cancer.

CASE 4–17 PULSATILE ABDOMINAL MASS

A 63-year-old man with a history of HTN and peripheral vascular disease presents for a routine follow-up appointment. He takes hydrochlorothiazide and propanolol. He has a 30-pack/year history of smoking. On physical examination, a pulsatile abdominal mass is palpated just above the level of the umbilicus. Vital signs are normal.

What condition should you suspect?

A pulsatile mass at or above the level of the umbilicus suggests that the patient has an abdominal aortic aneurysm (AAA). Symptoms of AAA are abdominal and back pain. However, AAA is often detected incidentally on abdominal imaging because patients may not have any signs or symptoms. Risk factors for this condition include age, smoking, hypertension, and atherosclerosis.

What is the next step in management?

Perform an abdominal ultrasound to confirm the diagnosis.

Screening for AAA: The USPSTF recommends one-time screening ultrasound for all patients aged 65 to 75 years who have ever smoked.

Ultrasound detects a 4.2-cm AAA. What treatment is recommended at this time?

Aneurysms <6 cm in diameter have a low risk of rupture. The recommended management of an asymptomatic AAA between 4 and 5.4 cm is smoking cessation, CV risk factor control, β-blockers, and monitoring with ultrasound every 6 to 12 months. CT scan is an alternative to ultrasound at some centers.

> **Management of asymptomatic AAA <4 cm:** Monitor with ultrasound every 2 to 3 years; have the patient quit smoking, control CV risk factors, and take β-blockers.

When is elective surgery warranted for AAA?

Consider elective surgery or endoluminal stenting in the following patients:

1. Size > 5.4 cm
2. Rate of growth > 0.5 cm in 6 months
3. Symptomatic AAA (regardless of size or rate of growth)

The patient does not return for his follow-up appointment. He presents to the emergency department 2 years later with severe abdominal pain radiating to the back. Physical exam is significant for a pulsatile abdominal mass above the umbilicus. Blood pressure is 90/60. What is the diagnosis?

The triad of pulsatile abdominal mass, hypotension, and severe abdominal and/or back pain indicates that the patient has a ruptured AAA. Treatment is emergent surgery. When a patient presents with the classic triad, additional confirmatory tests are not needed.

> **Severe abdominal/back pain + pulsatile abdominal mass but no hypotension:** Most likely diagnosis is expanding but unruptured aneurysm; confirm diagnosis with ultrasound and treat with urgent surgery.

CASE 4–18 APPROACH TO CONSTIPATION

A 51-year-old woman presents to the clinic with constipation. She has only had one or two stools/week for the last 6 weeks. She does not have any other symptoms. She had a negative screening colonoscopy in the past year. She does not take any medications. Physical examination, including anorectal examination, is normal. Vital signs are normal.

What is constipation?

Constipation is an extremely common complaint in the general population. Any of the following symptoms can be considered constipation: frequency < 3 stools/week, excessive straining, lumpy or hard stools, incomplete evacuation, or need for digital manipulation to evacuate. Constipation can be idiopathic or due to secondary causes.

What are some common secondary causes of constipation?

1. Medications: opioids, anticholinergics, antacids, calcium channel blockers, and iron
2. GI: IBS, obstruction, pseudo-obstruction, paralytic ileus, and colon cancer
3. Endocrine: hypothyroidism, DM, hypercalcemia, hypokalemia
4. Neurologic: Parkinson's disease, multiple sclerosis

What is the next step in management?

The goal of the history and physical exam is to identify any "red flags" that would suggest a secondary cause. This patient does not have any such red flags for a secondary GI disorder. She does not meet clinical criteria for IBS. She had a colonoscopy last year, which rules out colon cancer. The next step is to advise gradually increasing fiber intake. If symptoms persist, consider milk of magnesium.

> Red flags for a structural GI cause for constipation are cramping abdominal pain, nausea, vomiting, fever, weight loss, and GI bleeding.

The patient returns 3 months later with persistent constipation. She has increased her dietary fiber intake. She has tried milk of magnesia, as well as a number of over-the-counter laxatives without relief. Physical exam and vital signs are normal. What is the next step in management for this patient with chronic constipation?

Order the following inexpensive tests to screen for a secondary cause: FOBT, CBC, thyroid-stimulating hormone, and serum electrolytes. If this patient had not already had a screening colonoscopy last year, colon cancer screening would have been an option if FOBT was positive or all tests were negative.

Laboratory tests are all negative. What are the next steps in management?

Consider using a stimulant such as dulcolax. If the patient continues to have refractory and bothersome symptoms, refer to a gastroenterologist for more specialized testing. These tests can identify patients with pelvic floor dysfunction (which often responds to biofeedback and relaxation training) and slow colonic transit.

What specialized tests are available for patients with constipation?

1. **Anorectal manometry**: Patients with pelvic floor dysfunction may have increased anal sphincter pressure.
2. **Colonic transit test**: Patient swallows a capsule with multiple radio-opaque markers. Serial abdominal radiographs are obtained. In slow colonic transit, the markers are scattered all over the colon and do not pass by day 5. In pelvic floor dysfunction, markers accumulate in the rectum and can get stuck in the rectum.
3. **Balloon expulsion test**: Insert a balloon into the rectum. Normal patients can expel the balloon, but patients with pelvic floor dysfunction cannot.
4. **Defecography**: Thickened barium solution is injected into the rectum. The movement of barium when the patient strains and squeezes the rectum is observed under fluoroscopy to detect rectal prolapse and rectoceles.

chapter 5

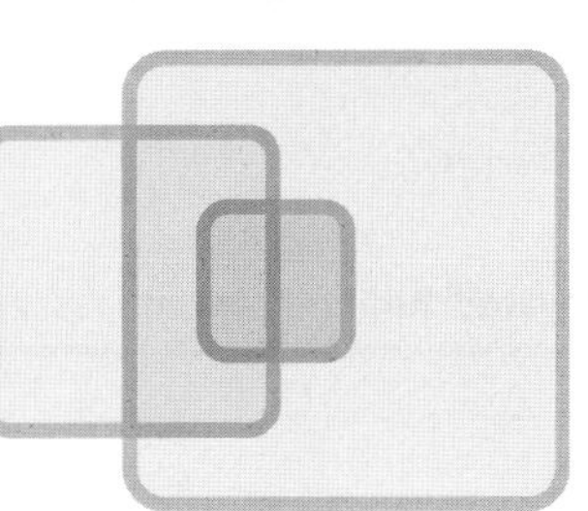

Hepatology and Pancreaticobiliary Disorders

CASE 5–1 APPROACH TO ABNORMAL LIVER FUNCTION TESTS

A 30-year-old woman decides to donate blood. Screening liver function tests (LFTs) are as follows: aspartate amino transaminase (AST) 180, alanine amino transaminase (ALT) 170, γ-glutaryl transpeptidase (GGT) 40 U/L, serum alkaline phosphatase 45 U/L, total bilirubin 1.7 mg/dL. Complete blood count (CBC) is normal. She is completely asymptomatic. There is no family history of liver disease. She does not take any medications or herbal supplements. She occasionally drinks alcohol on social occasions. She denies illegal drug use. Physical exam and vital signs are normal. Body mass index (BMI) is 27.

What are the causes of mildly elevated amino transaminases (AST and ALT <250 U/L)?

Amino transaminases (AST and ALT) are markers of hepatocellular injury. Causes of mildly elevated amino transaminases are listed in (Table 5-1). Approximately 4% of asymptomatic patients with mildly elevated amino transaminases do not have any underlying abnormality (false-positive). A list of laboratory abnormalities in patients with liver disease follows:

1. **LFTs**: Includes amino transaminases (AST and ALT), GGT, alkaline phosphatase, total bilirubin, serum albumin, and prothrombin time (PT).
2. **Amino transaminases**: Markers of hepatocellular injury; ALT is more specific for liver injury but AST is more sensitive. The extent of elevation does not correlate with prognosis.
3. **Alkaline phosphatase**: Marker of cholestasis (extrahepatic or intrahepatic bile duct obstruction). Damage to other organs such as bone, muscle, and heart can also elevate alkaline phosphatase.

TABLE 5–1 Causes of Mildly Elevated Amino Transaminases in Adults

Common hepatocellular causes	1. Alcoholic liver disease 2. Chronic hepatitis B and C infection 3. Nonalcoholic steatohepatitis (NASH) 4. Hereditary hemochromatosis
Uncommon hepatocellular causes	1. Autoimmune hepatitis 2. Wilson's disease 3. α-1-antitrypsin deficiency
Nonhepatic causes	1. Medications or herbal supplements 2. Strenuous exercise 3. Hypothyroidism or hyperthyroidism 4. Celiac sprue 5. Hemolysis 6. Adrenal insufficiency

4. **GGT**: ↑ in GGT correlates with ↑ in alkaline phosphatase. GGT is specific to the liver, so ↑ GGT confirms that the source of ↑ alkaline phosphatase is the liver and not other organs.
5. **Bilirubin**: Both hepatocellular injury and bile duct obstruction can elevate serum bilirubin, so this test does not help distinguish between the two diagnoses. When serum bilirubin is >2 mg/dL, patients become jaundiced (yellow discoloration of skin, mucous membranes, and sclera).
6. **Serum albumin**: The liver produces albumin. Chronic liver disease leads to decreased albumin production and subsequent hypoalbuminemia.
7. **PT**: The liver produces clotting factors. Liver dysfunction can lead to prolonged PT within hours. Vitamin K does not correct the PT.
8. ↑ **Amino transaminases** > ↑ **alkaline phosphatase** indicates hepatocellular injury.
9. ↑ **Alkaline phosphatase** > ↑ **amino transaminases** indicates bile duct obstruction.
10. **Alcoholic liver disease**: Suspect when AST/ALT ratio >2 and GGT >90 U/L. Transaminases are usually <500 U/L.
11. **Wilson's disease**: Suspect when AST/ALT ratio >2.
12. **Amino transaminases > 1000 U/L**: Indicates acute viral hepatitis, medication-induced liver injury, or shock-induced liver injury.
13. **Other possible laboratory abnormalities in patients with liver disease:**
    - Hyponatremia in patients with ascites
    - CBC: Patients with advanced liver disease may have anemia, thrombocytopenia, leukopenia, neutropenia. Patients with alcoholic liver disease may have increased mean red cell volume.

What is the next step in management of this asymptomatic patient with elevated amino transaminases?

No specific clues regarding the underlying cause are evident on history and physical exam, so the next step is to screen for common hepatocellular causes. Order the following tests at this time:

1. Hepatitis B and C serologies: The initial test for chronic hepatitis B infection is hepatitis B surface antigen (HBsAg). The initial test for hepatitis C is hepatitis C antibody.
2. Hemochromatosis screening: Order serum ferritin and transferrin saturation (serum iron/total iron binding capacity).
3. Serum albumin and PT to screen for chronic liver disease (see the list of laboratory abnormalities above).

Viral hepatitis serologies, iron studies, serum albumin, and PT are normal.

What is the next step in management?

Consider a period of alcohol abstinence and weight loss. Recheck serum amino transaminases in 3 to 6 months or sooner if the patient develops symptoms. If amino transaminases are still elevated, obtain right upper quadrant (RUQ) ultrasound to evaluate for nonalcoholic steatohepatitis.

The patient quits alcohol and loses 10 lbs with diet and exercise. Six months later, AST is 200 and ALT is 210 U/L. The patient is still asymptomatic. RUQ ultrasound is unrevealing.

What is the next step in management?

At this stage, order the following tests to screen for nonhepatic as well as uncommon hepatocellular causes of elevated amino transaminases:

1. Serum creatine kinase or aldolase to screen for muscle injury.
2. Thyroid function tests to screen for thyroid disorders.
3. Antiendomyseal and antitissue transglutaminase to screen for celiac sprue.
4. Serum protein electrophoresis (SPEP) to screen for autoimmune hepatitis (AIH).
5. Serum ceruloplasmin to screen for Wilson's disease if patient is <40 years old.
6. α-1 Antitrypsin phenotype.

If these tests are all unrevealing, perform liver biopsy.

> In asymptomatic patients, close observation rather than liver biopsy is sufficient if these tests are all negative and amino transaminases are elevated less than two-fold.

Alternative 5.1.1

An asymptomatic patient has the following pattern of LFTs: AST 30 U/L, ALT 33 U/L, GGT 200 U/L, alkaline phosphatase 400 U/L, albumin 4.0 g/dl, PT 12 seconds.

What do these lab findings indicate?

Elevated alkaline phosphatase with corresponding increase in GGT indicates obstruction of bile flow (cholestasis). Damage to bile ducts within the liver causes intrahepatic cholestasis. Damage or obstruction of bile ducts between the liver and gallbladder or between the gallbladder and small intestine causes extrahepatic cholestasis (Table 5-2).

> ↑ Alkaline phosphatase with normal GGT is normal in third trimester of pregnancy (derived from placenta).

What is the next step in management?

Obtain RUQ ultrasound to assess liver parenchyma and bile ducts. Also consider antimitochondrial antibody (AMA) to screen for primary biliary cirrhosis (PBC) if the patient is a middle-aged woman. If ultrasound demonstrates any liver parenchyma abnormalities,

TABLE 5–2 Hepatobiliary Causes of Elevated Alkaline Phosphatase in Adults

Intrahepatic cholestasis	Drugs (most common drugs are oral contraceptives, steroids, and phenytoin) Primary biliary cirrhosis Intrahepatic cholestasis of pregnancy Atypical: Sometimes conditions that normally cause hepatocellular injury present with a cholestatic pattern of LFTs (alcohol and viral hepatitis, etc.).
Intrahepatic and extrahepatic cholestasis	PSC
Extrahepatic cholestasis	Choledocholithiasis (common bile duct stones) Malignancies of the gallbladder, bile ducts, pancreas, and ampulla.

Abbreviation: LFT, liver function test; PSC, primary sclerosing cholangitis.

perform liver biopsy. If ultrasound detects a dilated bile duct (>6 mm), perform magnetic resonance cholangiopancreatography (MRCP). If MRCP reveals any abnormalities, perform diagnostic endoscopic retrograde cholangiopancreatography (ERCP).

> **Diagnostic ERCP**: Insert the endoscope into the small intestine. Then insert a catheter through the endoscope into the ampulla (cannulation). Inject dye through the catheter into the pancreatic and bile ducts and take x-rays (fluoroscopy) to determine cause of obstruction.

RUQ ultrasound is unrevealing. AMA is negative.

What is the next step in management of this asymptomatic patient?

Observe the patient for 6 months. If alkaline phosphatase is still elevated, perform liver biopsy and MRCP.

> In asymptomatic patients, observation rather than liver biopsy and MRCP is sufficient if alkaline phosphatase is <50% elevated.

Alternative 5.1.2

A physician detects scleral icterus in a 25-year-old asymptomatic male. LFTs are AST 30, ALT 30, alkaline phosphatase 90 U/L, serum albumin 4.5 g/dL, PT 12 seconds, total bilirubin 2.4 mg/dL.

What is the mechanism of bilirubin metabolism?

The mechanism of bilirubin metabolism is as follows:

1. Red blood cell breakdown releases hemoglobin.
2. Hemoglobin travels through the bloodstream to spleen.
3. Macrophages in spleen convert hemoglobin to unconjugated bilirubin (UCB).
4. UCB binds to albumin and travels in bloodstream to liver.
5. Liver converts UCB to conjugated bilirubin (water-soluble).
6. Water-soluble conjugated bilirubin travels to gallbladder and dissolves in bile.
7. Gallbladder excretes bile into intestine.
8. Intestinal bacteria convert conjugated bilirubin to urobilinogen and stercobilin.
9. Stercobilin gives feces its normal dark color.

What are the causes of hyperbilirubinemia in adults?

Three mechanisms cause ↑ UCB with normal conjugated bilirubin:

1. ↑ UCB production due to hemolysis (see Chapter 10: Hematology)
2. ↓ Hepatic UCB uptake due to heart failure and drugs (rifampin, probenecid, etc.)
3. ↓ Liver enzymes needed to conjugated bilirubin due to Gilbert's syndrome

> Hepatocellular damage and intra- and extrahepatic cholestasis can cause elevation in both unconjugated and conjugated bilirubin.

What are the clinical manifestations of hyperbilirubinemia?

1. ↑ **Unconjugated hyperbilirubinemia** binds to tissues, which leads to jaundice.
2. ↑ **Conjugated hyperbilirubinemia** causes dark urine, gray stools, and pruritis.

> **Pruritis**: Mechanism is unknown.
> **Dark urine**: Excess conjugated bilirubin dissolves in urine, giving it a dark color.
> **Gray stool**: Cholestasis causes ↓ excretion of bile into intestines, leading to ↓ stercobilin.

UCB is mildly elevated. Conjugated bilirubin is normal. CBC is normal. Plasma BNP is normal. The patient has not taken any drugs recently. Laboratory findings are consistent over the next 6 months.

What is the most likely diagnosis?

Gilbert's syndrome is the presumptive diagnosis in this asymptomatic patient with persistent and isolated unconjugated hyperbilirubinemia in the absence of hemolysis. Jaundice is usually the only clinical manifestation of this autosomal recessive disorder. The condition is benign, so no further work-up or treatment is necessary.

CASE 5–2 DISORDERS WITH PREDOMINANT TRANSAMINASE ELEVATION

A physician detects scleral icterus in a 40-year-old woman with a history of type 1 diabetes. LFTs are AST 270, ALT 290, GGT 40 U/L, alkaline phosphatase 45 U/L, total bilirubin 2.2 mg/dL. Viral serologies are negative. Iron studies are normal. Elevated amino transaminases persist for 6 months. SPEP reveals polyclonal increase in serum globulins more than twice the upper limit of normal (hypergammaglobulinemia).

What is the most likely diagnosis?

Hypergammaglobulinemia indicates that this patient has AIH. This condition is most common in girls and young women. Patients with AIH often have other coexisting autoimmune disorders such as type 1 diabetes and Hashimoto's thyroiditis.

What is the next step in management?

The next step is to obtain anti-nuclear antibodies (ANA), anti-smooth muscle antibodies (ASMA), and anti-liver kidney muscle antibodies (ALKM). Also, perform liver biopsy to confirm the diagnosis.

Elevated ANA and/or ASMA = type 1 AIH
Elevated ALKM = type 2 AIH

ANA and ASMA levels are elevated. Liver biopsy confirms the diagnosis of AIH. There is no evidence of cirrhosis on biopsy.

How should you treat this patient with AIH?

Treatment is indicated for the following patients with AIH:

1. Liver biopsy shows signs of cirrhosis.
2. Aminotransferases > 500 U/L.
3. Aminotransferases > 250 U/L plus gamma globulins twice upper limit of normal.
4. All children.

First-line therapy for AIH is corticosteroids. If patients do not achieve clinical remission within 3 months, consider adding azathioprine.

Acute hepatitis: ↑ Amino transaminases and positive labs (viral serology, SPEP, etc.) for <6 months.
Acute liver failure: Acute hepatitis with encephalopathy (altered mental status) or coagulopathy (INR >1.5); treatment is urgent liver transplantation.
Chronic hepatitis: ↑ Amino transaminases and (+) liver biopsy findings for >6 months.
Cirrhosis: Chronic hepatitis that progresses to irreversible fibrosis and nodular regeneration; amino transaminases are often normal or only slightly elevated.

The patient is lost to follow-up. She returns to the clinic 3 years later with a chief complaint of increased fatigue over the last few months. On physical exam, the patient has yellow discoloration of the nail bed and sclera (jaundice). Liver edge is palpable 4 cm below the costal margin (hepatomegaly). There are erythematous nodules on the face and trunk. The nodules blanch on palpation and are surrounded by smaller blood vessels (spider nevi). Abdominal inspection reveals dilated blood vessels (caput medusae). AST is 100 U/L and ALT is 80 U/L; alkaline phosphatase is 100 U/L and serum bilirubin is 2.3 g/dL. Liver biopsy shows extensive fibrosis, nodularity, and bridging necrosis.

What is the next step in management?

The patient now has physical signs as well as histological evidence of cirrhosis (Table 5-3). Treatment is directed at controlling complications and treating the underlying cause of cirrhosis, which include (mnemonic: ***Alcohol and Viruses Begin A Really Horrible Disease Named Cirrhosis***):

1. **A**lcoholic liver disease (number one cause in the United States)
2. Chronic **V**iral hepatitis (hepatitis C is the number two cause in the United States)
3. **B**udd Chiari syndrome (hepatic vein thrombosis)
4. **A**IH
5. **R**ight heart failure
6. **H**ereditary (hemochromatosis, Wilson's disease, α-1 anti-trypsin deficiency)
7. **D**rugs (examples are acetaminophen and methotrexate)

TABLE 5–3 Symptoms and Signs of Cirrhosis

SYMPTOMS OF CIRRHOSIS

Constitutional symptoms (fatigue, weakness, anorexia, weight loss) and abdominal pain

SIGNS OF CIRRHOSIS

Skin

- Spider angioma (nevi): Central arteriole is surrounded by smaller vessels radiating outward and is located on the upper half of the body. The lesions are telangiectasias, so they blanch when compressed by a glass slide.
- Palmar erythema: Mottled redness on thenar and hypothenar areas.
- Caput medusae: Portal hypertension causes prominent abdominal wall veins.
- Jaundice

Nails

- Muerhcke nails: Horizontal white bands separated by normal color.
- Terry nails: Proximal two thirds of the nail bed is white and distal one third is normal color.

Fingers

- Clubbing: Angle between nail bed and proximal nail fold >180°. Most common in primary biliary cirrhosis and other biliary causes of cirrhosis.
- Dupuytren's contracture: Thickening and contracture of palmar fascia causes flexion deformity in fingers.

Bones

- Hypertrophic osteoarthropathy: Pain and swelling in long bones.

Breast/genitals

- Gynecomastia
- Testicular atrophy

Abdomen

- Hepatomegaly: Liver edge palpated >3 cm below costal margin.
- Splenomegaly: A palpable spleen tip usually indicates splenomegaly.
- Epigastric murmur: Venous hum that increases with valsalva.

Feet

- Peripheral edema

Note: Palmar erythema, spider angiomata, gynecomastia, and testicular atrophy are caused by altered sex hormone metabolism. Muerhcke and Terry nails are caused by hypoalbuminemia.

8. Nonalcoholic steatohepatitis

9. Cholestasis

When no underlying cause is detected, the disease is classified as cryptogenic cirrhosis.

Initial presentation of cirrhosis is usually one of the following:

1. Nonspecific constitutional symptoms with characteristic physical findings
2. Complication of cirrhosis
3. Incidentally detected on laboratory/imaging tests in an asymptomatic patient

Diagnosis of cirrhosis requires one of the following:

1. Abnormal physical exam signs, laboratory, and imaging findings
2. Liver biopsy

MELD score (Model for End-stage Liver Disease): Predicts patient's likelihood of dying in the next 3 months using total bilirubin, INR, and creatinine.

Liver transplantation: Refer cirrhotic patients for liver transplant evaluation if they develop a complication of cirrhosis or have a MELD score >10. Under the current system, the sickest patients (highest MELD score) receive the highest priority.

Alternative 5.2.1

A 40-year-old man presents to the emergency department for treatment of bruises he received during a brawl with some strangers. There is jaundice on physical examination, so LFTs are obtained. The laboratory values are AST 250 U/L, ALT 100 U/L, alkaline phosphatase 100 U/L, GGT 100 U/L, serum bilirubin 2.2 g/dL, serum albumin 3.4 g/dL, PT 12 seconds. Vital signs are normal.

What is the most likely cause of the jaundice and abnormal LFTs?

The pattern of LFTs is classic for alcoholic hepatitis (see the list of laboratory abnormalities in Case 5-1). Early-stage alcoholic liver hepatitis (fatty liver) is reversible, and prognosis is excellent with abstinence (most important recommendation). Although not all heavy drinkers develop alcoholic liver disease, continued alcohol ingestion assures progression to cirrhosis if the patient already has fatty liver deposits.

The patient continues to drink a six-pack of beer every day. He presents 4 years later with a 3-week history of fatigue and anorexia. Physical exam is significant for jaundice, spider nevi, and palmar erythema. Both parotid glands appear swollen. Vital signs are normal. LFTs are AST 450 U/L, ALT 200 U/L, alkaline phosphatase 100 U/L, GGT 100 U/L, serum bilirubin 2.4 g/dL, serum albumin 2.8 g/dL, PT 20 seconds.

What treatment options exist for patients with alcoholic (Laennec) cirrhosis?

Corticosteroids reduce mortality in patients with severe alcoholic cirrhosis. Severe alcoholic cirrhosis is defined as discriminant function >32. Discriminant function is calculated with serum bilirubin and PT values in the following equation: Discriminant function = 4.6 × (patient PT − control PT) + serum bilirubin

Parotid gland enlargement is a sign of Laennec cirrhosis but not other types of cirrhosis.

Patients who do not abstain from alcohol for at least 6 months are not considered candidates for liver transplantation.

Nonalcoholic steatohepatitis: Liver biopsy findings are identical to alcoholic hepatitis despite negligible alcohol consumption. Risk factors are obesity, hyperlipidemia, and diabetes. Prevent progression to cirrhosis by controlling risk factors.

Alternative 5.2.2

A 30-year-old man presents to the clinic with a 7-day history of fatigue, anorexia, pruritis, and dark-colored urine. He also reports light gray stools. He recently returned from a trip to Mexico. He has not taken any medications recently. Physical exam is significant for yellow discoloration of nail beds and scleral icterus (jaundice). Temperature is 38.4°C. Other vital signs are normal. LFTs are AST 1200 U/L, ALT 1600 U/L, alkaline phosphatase 150 U/L, GGT 70 U/L, serum bilirubin 2.4 g/dL, serum albumin 3.5 g/dL, PT 25 seconds.

What is the most likely diagnosis?

Aminotransferase values >1000 U/L indicate medication-induced liver injury, acute viral hepatitis, or shock (ischemic hepatitis) (see the list of laboratory abnormalities in Case 5-1). This patient has not recently taken any medications and does not have any signs of shock, so the most likely cause is acute viral hepatitis.

Serum IgM anti-hepatitis A virus (HAV) is positive; hepatitis B serologies and hepatitis C antibodies are negative.

What is the diagnosis?

The patient has hepatitis A virus (HAV) infection. HAV spreads via the fecal–oral route and is commonly acquired by consuming contaminated food and water. This condition is infrequent in the United States, but it is common in many developing countries such as Mexico. Patients typically develop symptoms within 15 to 30 days of exposure.

Serum IgM HAV: Positive as soon as symptoms begin and usually disappears in 3 to 6 months. Sometimes, serum IgM can stay positive for a prolonged period, so positive IgM HAV does not always indicate acute infection.
Serum IgG HAV: Appears after a month of illness and persists for decades.

What treatment is recommended?

Treatment is supportive because the illness is usually acute and self-limited. Patients do not progress to chronic hepatitis or cirrhosis.

Hepatitis E virus (HEV): Rare in the United States, so a diagnostic test (IgM HEV) is not routinely available. Spread via the fecal-oral route. Infection is acute and self-limiting **except** in pregnant women (10% to 20% mortality from acute liver failure).

The patient lives with his wife and stepmother. None of them have been vaccinated against HAV.

Is any therapy recommended to prevent HAV in close personal contacts?

Administer a single dose of HAV immunoglobulin (passive prophylaxis) as well as HAV vaccine (active prophylaxis) to close household and sexual contacts.

Consider HAV immunoglobulin but not HAV vaccine for persons who have had infrequent contact with the patient. Administer immunoglobulin no later than 2 weeks after the last known exposure.

Postexposure prophylaxis is not necessary for people who have received at least one dose of HAV vaccine at least 1 month prior to exposure.

Alternative 5.2.3

A 30-year-old man presents to the clinic for a routine physical. On examination, the physician detects scleral icterus and yellow nail beds. LFTs are AST 1200 U/L, ALT 1600 U/L, alkaline phosphatase 150 U/L, GGT 70 U/L, serum bilirubin 2.4 g/dL, serum albumin 3.5 g/dL, PT 12 seconds, International Normalized Ratio (INR) 1.0. Hepatitis virus serologies are HCV antibody (–), HBsAg (+), HbcAb IgM (+), and HBsAb (–).

What is the diagnosis?

The patient has acute hepatitis B virus infection (Table 5-4). He is among the 30% of patients with acute HBV who develop jaundice (the other 70% are asymptomatic). Less than 1% of patients develop acute liver failure. Most patients who develop acute liver failure have coexisting hepatitis D virus infection or other comorbid liver diseases.

> **Hepatitis D virus**: Infection is benign unless superimposed with HBV infection. Diagnose with anti-hepatitis D virus antibodies.

How is HBV transmitted?

There are three modes of transmission:

1. **Vertical transmission**: Transmission from mother to baby during the perinatal period is the major mode of infection in developing countries.
2. **Unprotected sexual intercourse**: Major mode of transmission in developed countries.
3. **Exposure to infected blood**: Sharing needles, razors, toothbrushes, or chewing gum are possible modes of exposure to infected blood. Such horizontal transmission is common in developing countries.

There is no evidence for any other coexisting liver diseases on further testing.

What treatment is recommended for this patient with acute infection?

No antiviral therapy is indicated in the absence of coexisting liver disease or acute liver failure because 95% of patients infected during adulthood do not progress to chronic hepatitis. Monitor HBV serologies and LFTs over the next 3 to 6 months.

TABLE 5-4 Hepatitis B Serology

	HBsAg[a]	HbsAb[b]	HbcAb[c]	HbeAg[d]
Acute infection	Positive	Negative	IgM	Positive
Window period	Negative	Negative	IgM	Negative
Chronic infection (infectious)	Positive	Negative	IgG	Positive
Chronic infection (not infectious)	Positive	Negative	IgG	Negative
Recovery	Negative	Negative	IgG	Negative
Immunization	Negative	Positive	Negative	Negative

Abbreviations: HBV, hepatitis B virus; Ig, immunoglobulin.

Note: HBV DNA assay: Levels of HBV DNA detected by PCR and other tests are used mainly to determine whether the patient is a candidate for antiviral therapy.

[a] Hepatitis B surface antigen (HBsAg): Appears before onset of symptoms and indicates HBV infection. If the patient recovers, HBsAg becomes negative in 4–6 months. If the patient develops chronic hepatitis, HBsAg remains positive.

[b] Hepatitis B surface antibody (HBsAb): HbsAb appears shortly after HBsAg disappears and persists for life. Presence of HbsAb indicates either complete recovery or prior immunization. Chronic carriers do not form HBsAb.

[c] Hepatitis B core antibody (HBcAb): IgM HBcAb appears during initial infection. Its main purpose is to remain positive during the "window period" after HBsAg disappears and before HBsAb appears. After acute infection, IgM HBcAb disappears and IgG HBcAb appears. IgG HBcAb remains positive in both chronic infection and completely recovered patients.

[d] Hepatitis B e antigen (HBeAg): Marker of HBV infectiousness and replication. HBeAg appears during acute infection. It disappears if the patient recovers. When HBeAg disappears, anti-HBe antibody appears, indicating decreased viral replication. HBeAg persists in some chronically infected patients, which indicates continued viral replication and infectivity.

The patient admits to sharing needles with a male friend while using intravenous (IV) drugs. The male friend recently immigrated to the United States from China. He has the following serologies: HCV Ab (–), HBsAg (+), HbcAb IgG (+), HBsAb (–), and HBeAg (+). HBV DNA is 25,000 IU/ml. AST is 150 and ALT is 220 U/L.

What is the diagnosis?

The partner has chronic HBV infection and is infective (see Table 5-4); he is the most likely source of infection. It is possible he acquired the infection via perinatal transmission from his mother because 90% of patients who acquire HBV as neonates progress to chronic infection.

> Chronic HBV increases the risk of developing polyarteritis nodosa.

What therapy is recommended for the male friend?

Many hepatologists would recommend antiviral therapy for this patient. Antiviral options include interferon-alfa, lamivudine, adefovir, and entecavir. Deciding when to treat HBV and which agent to use is an area of active investigation and debate. Some general indications for treatment are:

1. No signs of cirrhosis: Consider treatment if HBV DNA >20,000 IU/mL and ALT is greater than twice the upper limit of normal.
2. Compensated cirrhosis: Treat if HBV DNA >2000 IU/mL.
3. Decompensated cirrhosis: Treat if patient has any detectable HBV DNA.

The patient often shares razors with his roommate. The roommate is asymptomatic. Physical exam and vital signs are normal. CBC and LFTs are normal. Viral serologies are HCVAb (–), HBsAg (–), HBcAb (-), HBsAb (+), and HBeAg (–).

How should you interpret these serologies?

Negative HBsAg indicates no current infection. Negative HBcAb indicates no past history of infection. Positive HBsAb indicates immunity against HBV. The serologies indicate prior immunization (see Table 5-4).

Six months later, the original patient's serologies are HBsAg (–), IgG HBcAb (+), HBsAb (+), and HBeAg (–).

What is the next step in management?

The patient has recovered from HBV infection and has developed immunity against repeat infection (see Table 5-4). No further therapy is necessary.

The patient has had unprotected sexual intercourse with one woman over the last 7 to 8 months. Her amino transaminases are ALT 190 and AST 160 U/L. Sclera are icteric. Viral serologies are HCVAb (+), HBsAg (–), HBcAb (–), HBsAb (+), and HBeAg (–).

What is the diagnosis?

The female sexual partner does not have HBV infection because of prior immunization, but she does have HCV infection. The major mode of HCV transmission is infected blood. Perinatal transmission and transmission through unprotected sex can occur, but the risk is lower than with HBV. Acute infection is usually asymptomatic. Unlike HBV, approximately 80% of patients with HCV develop chronic hepatitis.

> **Lichen planus**: Shiny, flat, violaceous, polygonal papules ± white lacelike striae can occur on skin, nails, and mucosal surfaces such as the mouth and genitalia. Lichen planus is more common in patients with HCV infection. First-line therapy is topical steroids.

What is the next step in management for the sexual partner?

Confirm the diagnosis with HCV RNA testing. If HCV RNA is positive, obtain liver biopsy to assess the chronicity and severity of disease.

> Chronic hepatitis C increases the risk of developing cryoglobulinemia (suspect if patient develops purpura, arthralgias, or Raynaud's phenomenon).

PCR for HCV RNA confirms the diagnosis of HCV infection, and liver biopsy indicates that the patient has chronic hepatitis.

How is chronic HCV treated?

First-line therapy for chronic HCV infection is pegylated-interferon alfa plus ribavarin.

> Treatment of acute HCV is controversial, and there is currently no drug approved by the United States Food and Drug Administration for this indication. Many hepatologists advocate an interferon-based regimen because of the high risk of progressing to chronic hepatitis.

Alternative 5.2.4

A 40-year-old man presents to the clinic with a 2-month history of fatigue and weakness. He has had diabetes for the last 2 years. His uncle died of liver disease in his 50s. Physical exam is significant for jaundice, spider nevi, palmar erythema, and skin hyperpigmentation. LFTs are ALT 300 U/L, AST 280 U/L, serum bilirubin 2.4 mg/dL, alkaline phosphatase 99 g/dL, serum albumin 2.8 g/dL, PT 18 seconds.

What is the most likely cause of cirrhosis?

Skin hyperpigmentation, diabetes, and cirrhosis are the classic triad of hereditary hemochromatosis ("bronze diabetes"). This autosomal recessive condition is caused by a mutation in the HFE gene that leads to increased intestinal iron absorption. Clinical manifestations are caused by excessive iron deposition in liver (leads to cirrhosis), skin (leads to skin hyperpigmentation), pancreas (leads to diabetes), heart (leads to dilated cardiomyopathy), joints (leads to arthritis), and other organs.

What diagnostic tests are indicated?

Obtain serum iron, total iron binding capacity, and serum ferritin. If serum iron/TIBC (transferrin saturation) is >0.45 and serum ferritin is elevated, perform genetic testing and liver biopsy to confirm the diagnosis.

> First-degree relatives of hereditary hemochromatosis patients are usually screened with iron studies and genetic testing. As a result, 75% of patients are asymptomatic at diagnosis.

How is hereditary hemochromatosis treated?

Both symptomatic and asymptomatic patients should undergo repeated phlebotomy (blood removal) to remove excess iron.

Alternative 5.2.5

A 20-year-old woman presents to the clinic for a medical evaluation required for entry into the US Air Force. The physician detects scleral icterus and yellow nail beds. AST is 180 U/L, ALT is 90 U/L, alkaline phosphatase is 90 U/L, GGT is 32 U/L, serum albumin is 4 g/dl, and PT is 14 seconds. Viral hepatitis serologies are all negative. Iron studies are normal. Ceruloplasmin is 13 mg/dL. Her father and a paternal aunt died of liver disease in their 40s.

What is the diagnosis?

The patient with a family history of liver disease, AST > ALT, and decreased ceruloplasmin (<20 mg/dL) most probably has Wilson's disease. Patients with this autosomal recessive condition have defective biliary excretion of copper. Clinical manifestations result from deposition of excess copper in the liver, brain, eyes, and other organs.

Liver: Clinical findings range from asymptomatic increase in amino transaminases to acute liver failure to cirrhosis.
Brain: Clinical findings range from asymptomatic to psychiatric abnormalities to Parkinsonian symptoms (due to basal ganglia deposits).
Eye: Copper deposits form a golden-brown band near the limbus (Kayser-Fleischer ring).

What are the next diagnostic steps?

Perform a slit-lamp examination (to detect Kayser-Fleischer rings) and measure 24-hour urinary copper excretion (increased in Wilson's disease). Perform liver biopsy if diagnostic tests are inconclusive.

In practice, the diagnosis of Wilson's disease is challenging because ceruloplasmin levels are often normal and Kayser-Fleishcer rings are often absent.

How is Wilson's disease treated?

First-line therapy is lifelong copper chelation using penicillamine or trientene. Add zinc to the regimen if the patient does not respond adequately to first-line agents. Zinc can also be used as monotherapy for patients who cannot tolerate first-line medications.

Screen all first-degree relatives with LFTs and serum ceruloplasmin.

Alternative 5.2.6

A 35-year-old woman with a history of polycythemia vera presents with a 2-month history of fatigue and vague discomfort in the RUQ. Physical examination is significant for scleral icterus and hepatomegaly. LFTs are AST 140 U/L, AST 120 U/L, GGT 100 U/L, alkaline phosphatase 100 g/dl, total bilirubin 2.4 g/dL, serum albumin 3.0 g/dL, PT 20 seconds. There is no history of alcohol use. Serologies for viral and nonviral causes of liver disease are negative. RUQ ultrasound shows occlusion of the hepatic vein.

What is the diagnosis?

The patient has Budd-Chiari syndrome (thrombosis of the hepatic vein or inferior vena cava). This uncommon cause of cirrhosis usually occurs in young women with a history of myeloproliferative disorders like polycythemia vera or hypercoagulable states such as pregnancy, oral contraceptive pill use, and inherited thrombophilia. LFTs are usually abnormal but nonspecific. The initial diagnostic test is RUQ ultrasound. If ultrasound is negative but index of suspicion is high, order magnetic resonance imaging (MRI) angiogram. Confirm the diagnosis with venography (invasive gold standard).

How is Budd-Chiari syndrome treated?

Treat the underlying cause if possible. Other treatment options prior to transplant are medical (anticoagulation, thrombolytics), radiologic (hepatic angioplasty, stenting, and transjugular intrahepatic portosystemic shunt (TIPS)), and surgical shunting. The specific treatment depends on patient preference and physician expertise.

Alternative 5.2.7

A 25-year-old woman is brought to the emergency room by her roommate after she told the roommate that she ingested a large amount of acetaminophen in a suicide attempt. The patient recently broke up with her boyfriend. She thinks she ingested about two bottles approximately 5 hours ago. Physical exam and vital signs are normal.

How does acetaminophen cause liver damage?

Liver metabolism of acetaminophen produces NAPQ1, which is hepatotoxic. Normally, NAPQ1 binds to hepatic glutathione and is converted to harmless byproducts. However, large

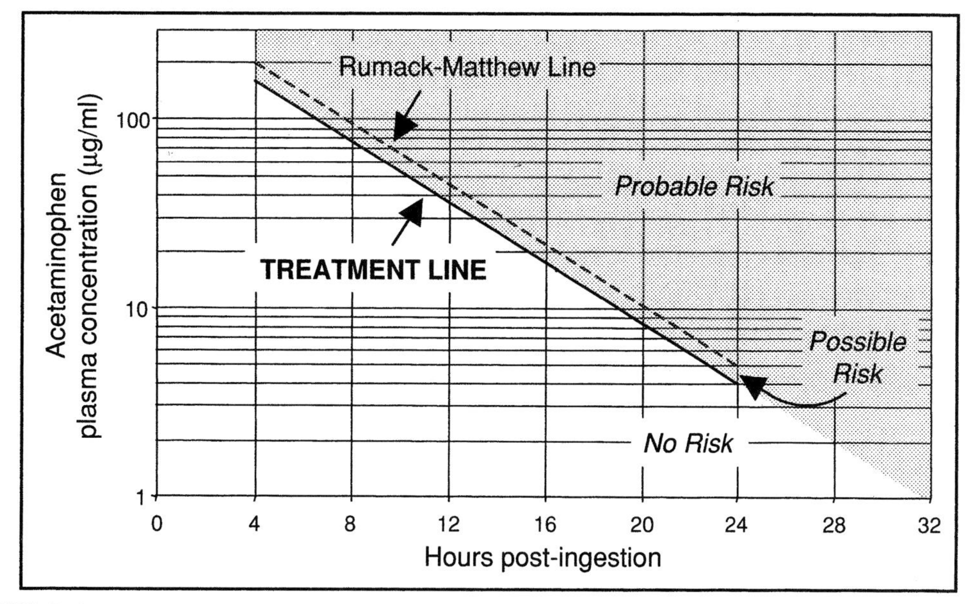

FIGURE 5-1 Rumack-Mathew nomogram. From Sabatine M. *Pocket Medicine,* 3rd ed. Lippincott Williams & Wilkins, 2008.

doses of acetaminophen deplete hepatic glutathione stores, leaving excess NAPQ1 free to cause oxidative injury to hepatocytes.

What are the clinical manifestations of untreated acetaminophen overdose?

0 to 24 hours: Patient is asymptomatic or reports nonspecific symptoms (nausea, vomiting, malaise, etc.). Laboratory findings are normal.

24 to 72 hours: Initially, patient improves clinically but amino transaminases begin to rise. Later, patient develops hepatomegaly and RUQ pain.

48 to 96 hours: Amino transaminases peak (often >10,000 U/L), and patients develop signs of acute liver failure (encephalopathy and INR >1.5). One fourth of patients develop acute renal failure as well (rising BUN and creatinine).

What is the next step in management?

Measure serum acetaminophen concentration and estimate whether she has ingested a toxic dose using the Rumack-Mathew nomogram (Fig. 5-1). If the dose is above the level indicating possible risk, administer N-acetylcysteine to prevent acute liver failure. Also, obtain a toxicology screen to determine if she has ingested any other substances and measure baseline LFTs, serum electrolytes, and urinalysis.

N-acetylcysteine: Binds to NAPQ1 and also increases glutathione stores. In patients with hepatocyte injury, N-acetylcysteine acts as an antioxidant. No patient has died when N-acetylcysteine was administered within 10 hours of ingestion.
Activated charcoal: Administer if the patient presents within 4 hours of ingestion.

Alcoholism: Alcoholics have a lower threshold for acetaminophen toxicity.

CASE 5-3 DISORDERS WITH CHOLESTATIC LIVER FUNCTION TESTS

A 40-year-old woman presents with a 3-month history of fatigue and itching. She has a history of type 1 diabetes. She does not take any medications. Physical examination is significant for scleral icterus and skin hyperpigmentation. Vital signs are normal. LFTs are AST 30 U/L, ALT 35 U/L, alkaline phosphatase 400 U/L, GGT 200 U/L, PT 15 seconds, serum albumin 4.1 g/dl, and total bilirubin 2.3 g/dL. AMA is positive. Extrahepatic bile ducts are not dilated.

What is the diagnosis?

Cholestatic pattern of LFTs and positive AMA indicate that the patient has PBC. The pathophysiology involves autoimmune (T lymphocyte–mediated) destruction of intrahepatic bile ducts. Retained bile acids cause liver inflammation (hepatitis) that eventually progresses to cirrhosis. Most patients are asymptomatic at diagnosis. Among symptomatic patients, the most common presenting complaints are fatigue and pruritis. Some patients may report RUQ discomfort. Jaundice is a late finding in PBC.

False-positive AMA: Confirm PBC with liver biopsy because false-positive AMA can occur.
Autoimmune cholangitis: Negative AMA but histological features of PBC appear on liver biopsy. Also referred to as AIH/PBC overlap syndrome.
ANA: 70% of PBC patients are positive for ANA. Some of these patients may have histological findings of both PBC and AIH.

PBC epidemiology: 90% of symptomatic patients are middle-aged women.

Liver biopsy confirms the diagnosis.

What other conditions are associated with PBC?

Remember conditions associated with PBC using the mnemonic "***ABCD***":

1. **A**utoimmune disorders: Approximately 50% of patients have symptoms of Sjögren's syndrome, and 10% have CREST syndrome (see Chapter 9: Rheumatology). Patients also have increased incidence of other autoimmune disorders such as type 1 diabetes mellitus and rheumatoid arthritis.
2. **B**ones: 25% of patients develop osteoporosis; 10% develop inflammatory arthritis of the peripheral joints (PBC arthritis).
3. **C**ardiovascular: 50% of patients have hyperlipidemia, often with xanthomas.
4. **D**ermatologic: Some patients have skin hyperpigmentation similar to hemochromatosis.

How is PBC managed?

1. Treatment of underlying disease: Ursodeoxycholic acid is the only therapy that delays progression to end-stage liver disease. This medication decreases endogenous bile acids by unknown mechanisms.
2. Treatment of cholestatic symptoms (pruritis, fat malabsorption, etc.) and associated conditions.

First-line treatments for pruritis are bile acid–binding resins (cholestyramine and colestipol).

Intractable osteoporosis or pruritis are potential indications for liver transplant even if the patient does not have complications of cirrhosis or a high MELD score.

Alternative 5.3.1

The patient is a 40-year-old man with ulcerative colitis. He presents to the clinic with a 2-month history of fatigue and pruritis. LFTs detect a cholestatic pattern. AMA is negative. RUQ ultrasound shows nonspecific intra- and extrahepatic bile duct dilatation, so he undergoes ERCP. ERCP shares multifocal strictures and dilation of the intra- and extrahepatic bile ducts.

What is the diagnosis?

ERCP shows multifocal strictures and dilation of the intra- and extrahepatic bile ducts, which is diagnostic of primary sclerosing cholangitis (PSC). The cause is unknown, but progressive damage to bile ducts eventually leads to cirrhosis. Like PBC, most patients are asymptomatic at diagnosis and among symptomatic patients, fatigue and pruritis are the most common presenting complaints. Jaundice is a late finding. No therapy reverses the underlying disease process other than liver transplantation. Medical therapy is aimed at relief of cholestatic symptoms.

> Most patients with PSC have underlying ulcerative colitis.

> ERCP usually confirms the diagnosis, but liver biopsy helps assess disease chronicity and severity. Liver biopsy sometimes shows small bile ducts replaced by connective tissue in an "onion skin pattern," which is specific for PSC. Note that false-negative liver biopsy is possible (because biopsy can sample an unaffected area of liver).

MELD score is >10. The patient is placed on the wait list for a liver transplant. During a follow-up appointment 2 years later, he reports increasing pruritis unresponsive to cholestyramine, dark urine, and light gray stools over the last 4 weeks. Physical examination reveals jaundice. He is afebrile.

What is the next step in management?

PSC increases the risk of developing cholangiocarcinoma (Table 5-5). Suspect this complication when a patient with PSC develops worsening cholestasis or when ERCP identifies a

TABLE 5–5 Cholangiocarcinoma Versus Gallbladder Cancer

COMMON FEATURES:

Initially asymptomatic with cholestatic LFTs. As the tumor grows, patients develop anorexia, weight loss, painless jaundice, and other signs of cholestasis. Palpable gallbladder (Courvoisier sign) is an uncommon sign of advanced disease. Prognosis is dismal.

DISTINGUISHING FEATURES:

	Cholangiocarcinoma	**Gallbladder cancer**
Location	Bile duct cancer. Two thirds of cases arise at confluence of hepatic ducts (Klatskin tumor), and one fourth arise in distal extrahepatic bile duct; the remaining cases are intrahepatic.	Gallbladder cancer
Persistent, dull RUQ pain	Late symptom	Early symptom
Risk factors	1. Choledochal cysts 2. PSC	1. Gallstones 2. Mirizzi syndrome 3. Porcelain gallbladder

MANAGEMENT OF RISK FACTORS:

Choledochal cysts: Bile duct cysts are usually asymptomatic and detected incidentally on ultrasound. Large cysts cause cholestasis. Diagnose with ultrasound and ERCP/MRCP. Surgically excise cysts to prevent cancer.

Gallstones: Refer to Case 5-6.

Mirizzi's syndrome: A large stone in the cystic duct extrinsically compresses the common hepatic duct. Secondary inflammation can present with signs of bile duct infection (cholangitis). Ultrasound and ERCP differentiates Mirizzi's syndrome from cholangitis. Remove gallbladder and cystic duct to prevent cancer.

Porcelain gallbladder: Chronic gallbladder inflammation (chronic cholecystitis) causes gallbladder calcification. Usually asymptomatic and detected incidentally on abdominal radiograph. Confirm diagnosis with CT scan or ultrasound. Remove gallbladder to prevent cancer.

Abbreviation: CT, computed tomography; ERCP, endoscopic retrograde cholangiopancreatography; MRCP, magnetic resonance cholangiopancreatography; RUQ, right upper quadrant.

dominant stricture. The first step is to perform RUQ ultrasound to confirm bile duct dilation, localize the site of obstruction, and exclude gallstones. Then perform ERCP to obtain brushings or biopsy. Also order the tumor markers carbohydrate antigen (CA 19-9) and carcinoembryonic antigen (CEA) (often elevated in cholangiocarcinoma). If ERCP is unsuccessful at establishing or ruling out the diagnosis, consider either percutaneous transhepatic cholangiogram with biopsy, CT-guided biopsy, or endoscopic ultrasound with fine-needle aspiration.

CA 19-9 and CEA are normal. ERCP detects a dominant stricture, but brushings obtained during ERCP rule out cholangiocarcinoma.

What is the next step in management?

Therapeutic ERCP (balloon dilation or stent placement) can decrease cholestatic symptoms in patients with PSC and a dominant stricture by allowing bile drainage.

Therapeutic ERCP:

1. Stent placement to assist bile drainage.
2. Balloon dilation to assist bile drainage and passage of gallstones.
3. Ampullary sphincterotomy with an electrified wire to assist passage of gallstones.
4. Basket insertion to remove gallstones.

Alternative 5.3.2

A 25-year-old man presents to the clinic with a 3-month history of fatigue. He emigrated from the Republic of Congo 6 years ago. Physical examination is significant for hepatomegaly. LFTs are AST 30 U/L, ALT 28 U/L, GGT 100 U/L, alkaline phosphatase 170 U/L, total bilirubin 1.2 g/dL, PT 12 seconds, albumin 3.5 g/dL. CBC shows increased eosinophils. AMA is negative. Imaging shows portal fibrosis but the liver parenchyma itself does not appear cirrhotic. Bile ducts are not dilated.

What diagnosis should you suspect?

Although rare in the United States, hepatic schistosomiasis is a common cause of portal hypertension in sub-Saharan Africa and many other tropical countries. The infectious form of this parasite lives in freshwater, which is the major vehicle of infection. Initial infection is often asymptomatic, but the parasite eggs can lodge in the portal vasculature and cause a granulomatous reaction and fibrosis over the next 5 to 15 years, leading to signs of portal hypertension. The liver parenchyma is unaffected, so patients do not have histological findings of cirrhosis. LFTs are normal or show mild elevation in alkaline phosphatase and GGT.

Swimmer's itch: Patients may report a pruritic papular rash approximately 24 hours after infection at the site of larva entry. Symptoms usually resolve within 1 week.
Katayama fever: A few patients develop fevers, chills, and myalgia with peripheral eosinophilia 4 to 8 weeks after infection. Symptoms usually resolve within a few weeks.

How do you diagnose and treat schistosomiasis?

Confirm the diagnosis using stool microscopy to detect parasite eggs ± rectal biopsy and ELISA antibody tests. Treat with praziquantel.

CASE 5–4 COMPLICATIONS OF CIRRHOSIS

A 45-year-old man presents to the clinic with a 3-week history of abdominal swelling. He has a history of alcoholic cirrhosis. He drinks five to six 12-oz beers every day. The patient has jaundice, spider nevi, and palmar erythema. The abdomen is distended, and palpation demonstrates flank dullness that shifts when the patient rotates. Both feet are swollen (peripheral edema).

What is the next step in management?

Perform a 24-hour urine collection and measure urine sodium. Urine sodium >78 mEq indicates noncompliance with dietary sodium restrictions. Urine sodium <78 mEq indicates true diuretic-resistant ascites. Treat diuretic-resistant ascites with repeated, large-volume paracentesis or TIPS. Without liver transplant, mortality is very high in cirrhotic patients with diuretic-resistant ascites.

> Measure cell count and differential of peritoneal fluid to exclude peritoneal fluid infection in patients with recurrent ascites.

The patient's 24-hour urine sodium is 150 mEq. After careful counseling, he restricts sodium intake and his ascites improves. Three months later, he has a recurrent episode of tense ascites. Temperature is 38.6°C. Leukocyte count of peritoneal fluid is 780/μL with 60% PMNs.

What is the next step in management?

Leukocyte count >500/μL indicates peritoneal inflammation (peritonitis), and PMN >250/μL indicates bacterial infection of the peritoneal fluid. The next step in management is to order peritoneal fluid protein, glucose, lactate dehydrogenase (LDH), and bacterial culture as well as culture of blood and urine. These tests help distinguish between spontaneous bacterial peritonitis (SBP) and secondary bacterial peritonitis (Table 5-7). Then initiate empiric antibiotic therapy for SBP with cefotaxime or another third-generation cephalosporin.

> Although a tender abdomen is the hallmark of peritonitis, patients with ascites often do not report this classic finding.

> Patients with alcoholic cirrhosis often have low-grade fever, abdominal pain, and peritoneal fluid leukocyte count >500/μL but PMNs are not >250/μL unless the patient has bacterial peritonitis.

> Suspect bacterial peritonitis in any patient with ascites due to cirrhosis who has fever, abdominal pain, or sudden, unexplained altered mental status.

Peritoneal fluid glucose is 80 mg/dL, AFTP is 0.8 g/dL, and LDH is 80 U/L. Culture of peritoneal fluid grows *Escherichia coli.*

What are the next steps in management?

The patient has SBP. The next step is to tailor antibiotic therapy. Also administer IV albumin on day 3 (may improve survival). Patients who have had one or more episodes of SBP should take an oral quinolone or trimethoprim/sulfamethopyrazine after recovery to prevent further episodes.

TABLE 5–7 Spontaneous Bacterial Peritonitis Versus Secondary Bacterial Peritonitis

	Spontaneous bacterial peritonitis	Secondary bacterial peritonitis
Cause	Primary bacterial infection of ascitic fluid	Secondary bacterial infection of ascitic fluid due to bowel perforation or intra-abdominal abscess
AFTP	<1 g/dL	<1 g/dL
Glucose	<50 mg/dL	<50 mg/dL
LDH	<225 U/L	<255 U/L
Culture	One organism	Multiple organisms
Treatment	Antibiotics	Antibiotics + surgery

Abbreviation: LDH, lactate dehydrogenase.

Organisms responsible for SBP:

1. **Gram-negative rods (70%)**: *E. coli* is the number one organism and *Klebsiella* is number two organism overall.
2. **Gram-positive cocci (30%)**: *Streptococcus pneumoniae* is the number three organism overall.

The patient follows up in clinic 5 days after discharge. He has been unable to urinate for the last 3 days. He has not taken NSAIDs or any other nephrotoxic drugs recently. Blood pressure is 95/65. Baseline creatinine in the hospital was 1.3 mg/dL. Current creatinine is 4 mg/dL. Urine sodium is 8 mEq/L. Analysis of urine sediment does not indicate any specific cause. He receives 2 L of normal saline, but blood pressure does not increase.

What is the most likely cause of his symptoms?

Suspect hepatorenal syndrome when a patient with end-stage liver disease develops acute renal failure (rapidly rising creatinine over days or weeks) that does not respond to volume repletion. A recent infection like SBP is often the precipitating cause. Urine sodium is <10 mEq and kidney parenchyma is normal because this is a prerenal cause of acute renal failure. To make this diagnosis, you must first rule out other causes of acute renal failure (see Chapter 6: Nephrology).

How is hepatorenal syndrome treated?

Prognosis is dismal without liver transplantation. If the patient is a candidate for liver transplant, treat with hemodialysis. If the patient is not a liver transplant candidate, consider midodrine and octreotide (not very effective, but commonly used because currently there is little else to offer in this situation).

Alternative 5.4.1

The patient is a 50-year-old man with a history of cirrhosis secondary to HCV infection. He has a history of ascites that is well controlled with dietary sodium restriction, spironolactone, and furosemide. Over the last couple of months he has had difficulty sleeping. His wife brings him to the clinic for a follow-up appointment. She complains that he seems increasingly confused. Physical exam is significant for muscle wasting, spider nevi, and caput medusae. His breath smells musty (fetor hepaticus). His hands flap when his arm is held outstretched with the palm dorsiflexed (asterixis). LFTs are AST 90 U/L, ALT 90 U/L, GGT 30 U/L, alkaline phosphatase 60 g/dL, total bilirubin 1.6 g/dL, PT 22 seconds, serum albumin 3.2 g/dL, serum potassium is 3.2 mEq/L.

What is the most likely cause of his symptoms?

The patient most likely has hepatic encephalopathy, which can present with a spectrum of neurological and psychiatric abnormalities in patients with advanced liver disease. Symptoms can range from subclinical to severe cognitive impairment and coma. Onset can be acute (precipitated by infection or electrolyte/metabolic abnormality) or gradual. Sleep derangements (insomnia or hypersomnia) are a common early feature. As encephalopathy worsens, patients develop signs such as fetor hepaticus, asterixis, and hypo- or hyperactive reflexes.

What causes hepatic encephalopathy in patients with cirrhosis?

Decreased metabolic function of the liver leads to numerous metabolic derangements that contribute to development of this complication. Decreased metabolism of ammonia is the most clearly defined abnormality.

What is the next step in management?

The characteristic signs, symptoms, and laboratory evidence of decreased hepatic synthetic function (decreased albumin, increased PT) are sufficient to establish the diagnosis of hepatic encephalopathy. CT scan of the head is only indicated if the diagnosis is in question.

How is hepatic encephalopathy treated?

1. **First-line therapy**: Administer lactulose and correct any underlying infections, hypovolemia, electrolyte, or metabolic abnormalities (in this case, hypokalemia).
2. **Second-line therapy**: If mental status does not improve within 48 hours, consider ornithine-aspartate (increases hepatic ammonia metabolism) or sodium benzoate (increases ammonia excretion).
3. **Chronic therapy**: After the acute episode of HE resolves, continue lactulose.

> Neomycin and other antibiotics are commonly used as second-line agents for hepatic encephalopathy, but evidence for their effectiveness is lacking.

> **Lactulose**: Gut flora metabolize lactulose (a disaccharide) to short-chain fatty acids. Short-chain fatty acids reduce colon pH. Lower colon pH prevents ammonium metabolism to ammonia, which leads to trapping of ammonium in the gut.

Alternative 5.4.2

A 50-year-old man with cirrhosis secondary to PSC presents to the clinic with a 2-month history of progressive dyspnea. Symptoms are worse in the upright position and improve somewhat on recumbency (platypnea). Physical exam is significant for spider nevi and palmar erythema. Heart and lung exam are normal. The patient is afebrile. Oxygen saturation is 89%, heart rate is 105 beats/min, and respirations are 25/min. CXR shows nonspecific interstitial infiltrates. The only abnormal findings on spirometry are decreased DLCO (carbon monoxide diffusion capacity) and elevated A-a gradient.

What complication should you suspect?

Suspect hepatopulmonary syndrome (HPS) when patients with cirrhosis develop dyspnea of uncertain origin. The pattern of dyspnea is usually platypnea, and common spirometry findings are decreased DLCO and increased A-a gradient.

> **HPS triad**: cirrhosis, increased A-a gradient, and intrapulmonary vascular dilatations.

What is the next step in management?

Perform contrast-enhanced echocardiogram to detect intrapulmonary vascular dilatations, which would confirm the diagnosis. The only treatment of benefit for HPS is liver transplantation.

> Other pulmonary complications of cirrhosis:
> 1. **Hepatic hydrothorax**: Excess ascitic fluid causes right pleural effusion.
> 2. **Portopulmonary hypertension**: Portal hypertension causes pulmonary hypertension.

> Remember complications of cirrhosis with the mnemonic "***ERAS Boldly Determines The Housestaff Placements***" (**E**ncephalopathy, hepato**R**enal syndrome, **A**scites, **S**BP, **B**leeding varices, **D**iabetes, portal vein **T**hrombosis, **H**epatocellular carcinoma (HCC), **P**ulmonary complications).

What routine tests are indicated in all patients with cirrhosis?

1. **Blood tests**: Measure LFTs, CBC, and serum electrolytes every 3 to 4 months in all patients with cirrhosis.
2. **Upper endoscopy**: All patients with cirrhosis should undergo upper endoscopy. If endoscopy detects large varices, treat with nonselective β-blockers (propanalol or nadolol) to prevent variceal hemorrhage (primary prophylaxis).

3. **Serum alpha feto protein (AFP) and abdominal ultrasound**: Use serum AFP and ultrasound to screen the following patients with cirrhosis for HCC every 6 to 12 months:
   - Cirrhosis due to viral hepatitis, alcohol, hemochromatosis, and PBC.
   - Any patient on the wait list for liver transplantation (limited HCC raises priority for transplant whereas extensive HCC excludes the patient from transplant eligibility).

CASE 5–5 INCIDENTALLY DETECTED LIVER LESIONS

Routine ultrasound surveillance for HCC in a patient with alcoholic cirrhosis detects a 0.8-cm solid lesion. Serum AFP is 5 ng/mL.

What is the next step in management?

Repeat ultrasound and serum AFP in 3 to 6 months. If there is no growth, revert to routine HCC surveillance (every 6 to 12 months). Otherwise, obtain two of the following dynamic tests: helical CT scan, MRI with contrast, or ultrasound with contrast.

> **Lesion >1 cm**: Don't wait 3 to 6 months to obtain follow-up dynamic imaging.

> **AFP**: Suspect HCC when a patient with liver disease has a rising AFP level (normal < 10 ng/mL). Test is not sensitive (40% of patients with HCC have normal AFP) or specific (AFP is also elevated in germ cell tumors).

Three months later, the lesion size is 1.3 cm. AFP is 5 ng/mL. Helical CT scan and MRI with gadolinium contrast demonstrate a hypervascular lesion with washout during the portal venous phase.

What is the diagnosis?

The radiographic description is characteristic of HCC (hepatoma). HCC is the most common primary liver malignancy. Most patients are asymptomatic except for signs of chronic liver disease. Advanced lesions may cause dyspepsia, anorexia, weight loss, or a palpable mass in the upper abdomen.

> **Lesion 1 to 2 cm**: Characteristic findings of HCC are required on at least two dynamic studies for diagnosis. If dynamic imaging findings are ambiguous, perform liver biopsy.
> **Lesion >2 cm**: Characteristic findings of HCC are required on at least one dynamic study or AFP >200 ng/mL for diagnosis. If neither of these is present, perform liver biopsy.
> **Liver biopsy**: Only perform biopsy if diagnosis of HCC is ambiguous because of the risk of tumor spreading along the needle's path.

> HCC risk factors:
> 1. Cirrhosis (most important risk factor)
> 2. Chronic viral hepatitis and hemochromatosis (increased risk independent of cirrhosis)
> 3. High aflatoxin intake (found in corn, peanuts, and soybeans)

What treatment options exist for HCC?

1. **Partial hepatectomy**: Only patients with a solitary lesion confined to a single lobe of the liver and no portal hypertension are candidates for hepatectomy.
2. **Liver transplant**: Patients who are not candidates for hepatectomy because of severe liver disease but meet Milan criteria are candidates for potentially curative transplant.
3. **Other**: Radiofrequency ablation, transarterial chemoembolization, and percutaneous ethanol injection are options for patients who are not candidates for hepatectomy or liver transplant.

Milan criteria: one lesion ≤5 cm or up to three lesions all ≤3 cm with no distant spread.

Overall prognosis of HCC is dismal because most patients are diagnosed late and do not meet criteria for resection or transplant. Median survival after diagnosis is 6 to 20 months.

Alternative 5.5.1

A 35-year-old woman is involved in a motor vehicle crash. Ultrasound examination of her abdomen incidentally detects a 3-cm, well-demarcated, hyperechoic (solid) liver lesion. She does not have any known medical conditions. She does not take any medications. CBC, serum electrolytes, and LFTs are normal.

What are the causes of solid liver lesions in otherwise healthy young women?

The differential diagnosis of solid liver lesions with no evidence of HCC or liver metastases includes cavernous hemangioma, hepatic adenoma, and focal nodular hyperplasia (FNH). All three lesions are usually asymptomatic. Occasionally, a large lesion can cause vague RUQ or epigastric pain. Sometimes, ultrasound is sufficient to make the diagnosis. Most patients require CT scan, MRI, and/or technetium-labeled red blood cell scan to establish the diagnosis and rule out malignancy (Table 5-8).

Buzzword for FNH: "Central stellate scar" on CT scan or MRI.
Technetium-labeled scan: Hemangioma and FNH show uptake; hepatic adenoma does not.

Alternative 5.5.2

A 40-year-old woman is involved in a motor vehicle crash. Ultrasound examination of the abdomen incidentally detects a hypoechoic (cystic) lesion. She does not have any other medical conditions.

What is the diagnostic work-up of cystic liver lesions?

Ultrasound can distinguish between the various causes of cystic liver lesions. If ultrasound is nondiagnostic, perform CT scan or MRI.

Solid lesion: hyperechoic (brighter than surrounding tissue) on ultrasound.
Cystic lesion: hypoechoic (darker than surrounding tissue) on ultrasound.

TABLE 5-8 Incidentally Detected Nonmalignant Solid Liver Lesions

	Hepatic Hemangioma	Hepatic Adenoma	Focal Nodular Hyperplasia
Epidemiology	Most common in young women	Most common in young women	Most common in young women
Risk factors	OCPs and pregnancy may ↑ risk (association is debatable)	OCPs, steroids, and pregnancy (due to ↑ endogenous steroids)	Osler-Weber Rendu syndrome and hepatic hemangioma
Management	No treatment unless symptomatic; cannot make clear recommendation regarding OCPs and pregnancy	Discontinue OCPs and advise against pregnancy; surgically resect large (>5 cm) or symptomatic adenomas	No treatment necessary

Abbreviation: OCP, oral contraceptive pills.

What is the differential diagnosis of asymptomatic cystic liver lesions?

1. **Simple cyst**: This is the most common cystic liver lesion (more common in women than men). No treatment is required unless the patient reports symptoms (indication for surgery). Monitor large asymptomatic cysts (≥4 cm) with ultrasound. If the cyst grows over time, consider an alternative diagnosis (cystadenoma, cystadenocarcinoma).
2. **Cystadenoma**: This is a rare tumor that is malignant in 15% of patients. Treatment is complete surgical resection of the cyst (enucleation).
3. **Cystadenocarcinoma**: This lesion typically arises from malignant transformation of cystadenoma in elderly patients. Treatment is liver resection.
4. **Echinococcal cyst**: This lesion is caused by parasitic infection with *Echinococcus granulosus* or *Echinococcus multilocularis.* Use ELISA to confirm imaging diagnosis with serology for antibodies. Treatment is surgery or the PAIR procedure (puncture, aspirate, inject normal saline (NS) or ethanol, and reaspirate) followed by albendazole or mebendazole.
5. **Polycystic liver disease**: This disease usually occurs in patients with polycystic kidney disease. Patients have multiple liver cysts. Kidney cysts tend to cause renal failure and are the main determinant of overall prognosis, whereas liver cysts are generally benign and require no further treatment.

> **PAIR procedure**: **P**uncture, **A**spirate, **I**nject NS or ethanol, and **R**easpirate.

> Some patients with these conditions have RUQ or epigastric pain/discomfort.

CASE 5–6 RUQ PAIN

A 45-year-old woman presents with a 2-week history of RUQ pain. The pain begins an hour after eating a heavy meal, increases in intensity over an hour, and then resolves over the next couple of hours. She describes the pain as constant and dull discomfort that radiates to the right shoulder and scapula. She does not have any other medical conditions. Physical examination and vital signs are normal.

What is the most likely diagnosis?

This patient's symptoms are the classic description of biliary colic due to symptomatic gallstones (cholelithiasis). Symptoms occur when the gallbladder contracts after a fatty meal, which pushes stones to the gallbladder outlet and causes obstruction to bile flow. Physical exam and vital signs are typically normal. Uncomplicated cholelithiasis should not cause any laboratory abnormalities.

> **Types of gallstones**: cholesterol gallstones (yellow-green), pigment gallstones (brown-black), and mixed gallstones (majority of gallstones contain pigment and cholesterol).

What are risk factors for cholelithiasis?

1. Risk factors for cholesterol gallstones are the **2 Cs**, and **2 Ds**, **1 E**, and **5 Fs**: **C**rohn's, **C**irrhosis, **D**iabetes, **D**rugs (clofibrate, ceftriaxone, and octreotide), **E**strogen and oral contraceptive pills, **F**emale, **F**at (obesity), **F**ertile (pregnancy), age >**F**orty, and **F**amily history (increased risk in Native Americans).
2. Risk factors for pigment gallstones are hemolysis and alcoholic cirrhosis.

What is the next step in management?

Order RUQ ultrasound. If ultrasound shows gallstones in a patient with biliary colic, refer for cholecystectomy (surgical removal of gallbladder) to prevent complications.

Asymptomatic gallstones: Gallstones are often incidentally detected in asymptomatic patients. There is a low risk of complications, so no treatment is recommended.
Gallstones and atypical symptoms: Ultrasound may detect gallstones in patients who report symptoms of dyspepsia rather than biliary colic. First rule out other causes of dyspepsia (see Chapter 4: Gastroenterology). If no other cause is found, treat with ursodeoxycholic acid to dissolve gallstones.
Biliary colic but no gallstones: Ultrasound can miss extremely small stones (microlithiasis) or sludge. The next step is to perform upper endoscopy with endoscopic ultrasound. During the procedure, also collect bile for microscopic analysis. If endoscopic ultrasound and/or bile microscopy detect sludge or microlithiasis, perform cholecystectomy.

What are possible complications of cholelithiasis?

1. Cholecystitis (gallbladder and cystic duct inflammation)
2. Choledocholithiasis (gallstones travel to common bile duct (CBD))
3. Cholangitis (CBD infection)
4. Gallstone pancreatitis (gallstones travel to ampulla of Vater and obstruct flow of pancreatic fluids)
5. Gallstone ileus (gallstones enter intestine via a fistula and cause obstruction)

Alternative 5.6.1

A 50-year-old woman presents with a 2-week history of biliary colic. Physical examination is significant for scleral icterus. LFTs reveal a cholestatic pattern. Ultrasound shows gallstones as well as CBD dilation.

What is the most likely cause of her symptoms?

Both gallstones and CBD stones can cause biliary colic, but the additional findings of jaundice and biliary dilation on ultrasound suggest that her symptoms are due to CBD stones (choledocholithiasis).

Choledocholithiasis is often asymptomatic with normal laboratory values for years. CBD dilation on ultrasound is usually the only indication in asymptomatic patients.

What is the next step in management?

Perform diagnostic ERCP to confirm the diagnosis (Fig. 5-3) and therapeutic ERCP to remove the CBD stone once identified. Patients with choledocholithiasis should also undergo elective cholecystectomy to prevent more stones from entering the CBD.

Primary CBD stones: 5% of CBD stones originate in the CBD, so cholecystectomy does not offer complete protection against future choledocholithiasis.
Secondary CBD stones: 95% of CBD stones originate in gallbladder and travel to the CBD.

Unlike cholelithiasis, even asymptomatic patients require removal of CBD stones to prevent ascending cholangitis and gallstone pancreatitis.

Alternative 5.6.2

A 50-year-old man presents with a 2-month history of biliary colic episodes. Past history is significant for cholecystectomy 1 year ago for symptomatic gallstones. Ultrasound shows a dilated CBD, but ERCP does not demonstrate any CBD stones. LFTs obtained during two of his symptomatic episodes showed mildly elevated AST, ALT, GGT, and alkaline phosphatase. LFTs are

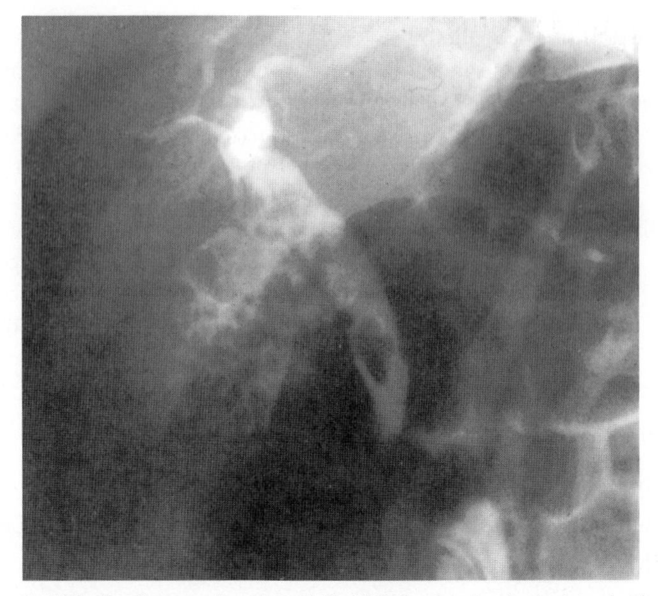

FIGURE 5–3 Diagnostic ERCP of gallstones. From Jarrell B. *NMS Surgery Casebook,* 1st ed. Lippincott Williams & Wilkins, 2003.

normal between episodes. He does not have any diarrhea or constipation. Physical exam and vital signs have been normal during every evaluation.

What diagnosis should you suspect?

Suspect biliary dyskinesia in patients with biliary colic and dilated CBD but no evidence of gallbladder or CBD stones. This condition is also called biliary sphincter of Oddi (SOD) dysfunction because it results from stenosis or spasm of the SOD (located at the opening of the CBD and the ampulla of Vater into the duodenum). LFTs are often transiently elevated during symptomatic episodes.

What are the next diagnostic steps?

Perform fatty meal ultrasonography or biliary scintigraphy (measures rate of radionuclide flow from CBD into the duodenum). If any of these tests are positive or if symptoms persist despite negative testing, perform SOD manometry (gold standard for diagnosis). Treatment is endoscopic sphincterotomy.

What test would you perform first if the patient did not have a history of cholecystectomy?

If there is no history of cholecystectomy, the first diagnostic step is hepatobiliary iminodiacetic acid (HIDA) scan. The test is positive for biliary SOD if the rate of radionuclide emptying by the gallbladder (ejection fraction) is $<40\%$. Treatment is cholecystectomy $\pm$ endoscopic sphincterotomy.

CASE 5–7 FEVER AND RUQ PAIN

A 67-year-old man presents to the emergency department with a 9-hour history of severe and persistent epigastric and RUQ pain that radiates to his right shoulder and scapula. He also reports nausea and anorexia. He has had past episodes of biliary colic that resolved in a couple of hours. He has a history of diabetes. RUQ is tender to palpation with guarding and rebound. Palpation of the RUQ during deep inspiration causes the patient to stop breathing for a second because of increased tenderness (Murphy's sign). Vital signs are temperature 38.7°C, pulse 115 bpm, respirations 25/min, blood pressure 120/80. Oxygen saturation is 99% on room air. Significant laboratory findings are leukocytosis with a left shift and mildly elevated amino transaminases and amylase.

What is the most likely diagnosis?

Suspect acute cholecystitis when a patient presents with fever and RUQ pain that persists for >4 hours. Physical exam usually demonstrates RUQ rebound, tenderness, guarding, and a positive Murphy's sign. Patients are frequently tachycardic and tachypneic. The most common laboratory abnormality is leukocytosis with a left shift.

> **Amylase and lipase**: Amylase is sometimes mildly elevated but, unlike acute pancreatitis, lipase is normal.
>
> **LFTs**: Amino transaminases are sometimes mildly elevated but, unlike cholangitis, alkaline phosphatase and GGT should be normal because there is no bile duct obstruction.

What is the next step in management?

Order RUQ ultrasound to confirm the diagnosis. Ultrasound findings include gallstones, gallbladder wall thickening, and edema with pericholecystic fluid ("double wall sign"). Patients will also have a positive sonographic Murphy's sign (palpation of gallbladder with ultrasound probe during inspiration causes inspiratory arrest).

> **HIDA scan**: Perform if ultrasound is inconclusive. In acute cholecystitis, radionuclide flows from the liver to the biliary tree but does not enter the gallbladder because edema and thickening obstructs the cystic duct.

Ultrasound confirms cholecystitis (Fig. 5-4). How is this condition managed?

1. Supportive care: Order IV fluids, nothing by mouth (nothing per oral (NPO), and NG suction (if the patient is vomiting). Control pain with intramuscular NSAIDs such as ketorolac.
2. Antibiotics: Even though cholecystitis is inflammation of the gallbladder and not infection, administer antibiotics to prevent secondary infection.
3. Cholecystectomy: Perform electively after 24 to 48 hours to prevent future cholecystitis.

Four hours after admission, the nurse notices that the patient appears confused. His urine output has dropped. Abdomen is diffusely tender. Vital signs are temperature 39°C, pulse 120 bpm, respirations 22/min, and blood pressure 90/60. Oxygen saturation is 98% on room air.

What is the next step in management?

With altered mental status, oliguria, fever, and hypotension, this patient is in septic shock. Suspect a life-threatening complication of cholecystitis such as gallbladder gangrene (i.e., necrosis) or perforation. These complications are more common in elderly patients with diabetes. Treatment is emergent surgery.

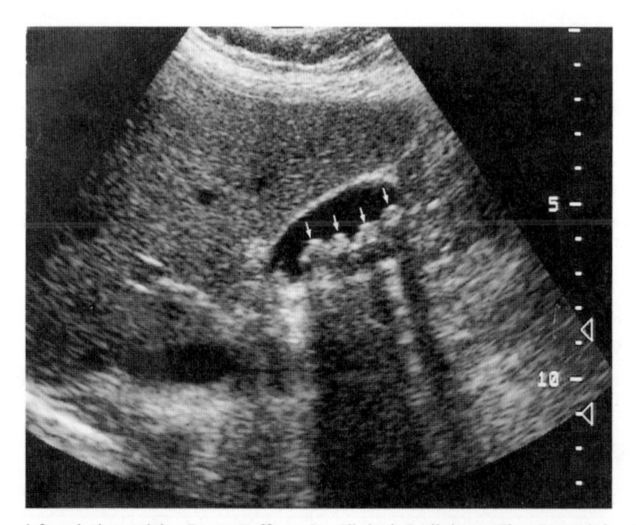

FIGURE 5–4 Ultrasound for cholecystitis. From Daffner R. *Clinical Radiology: The Essentials*, 3rd ed. Lippincott Williams & Wilkins, 2007.

Acalculous cholecystitis: Critically ill patients often develop acute cholecystitis without gallstones. Clinical presentation is similar to gallstone (calculous) cholecystitis, except that patients may also have jaundice and a palpable RUQ mass. Treatment is broad-spectrum IV antibiotics and emergent cholecystectomy because risk of gangrene and perforation is high. If the patient is too ill for surgery, perform percutaneous cholecystostomy to enable gallbladder drainage.

Emphysematous cholecystitis: Suspect secondary infection with a gas-forming organism if ultrasound detects gas bubbles in the gallbladder or if RUQ palpation detects crepitus. Treatment is emergent cholecystectomy because most patients progress to gangrene or perforation.

Alternative 5.7.1

A 48-year-old woman with a history of asymptomatic gallstones presents with an 8-hour history of RUQ pain. There is jaundice on exam. Murphy's sign is negative. Vital signs are temperature 38.8°C, pulse 120 bpm, respirations 25/min, and blood pressure 125/80. Significant laboratory findings are leukocytosis with a left shift, mildly elevated amylase, and cholestatic LFTs.

What is the most likely diagnosis?

Fever, RUQ pain, and jaundice are the classic signs of acute ascending cholangitis (Charcot's triad). Like cholecystitis, patients have leukocytosis with a left shift ± mildly elevated amylase. Unlike cholecystitis, LFTs reveal a cholestatic pattern because the infection is in the CBD.

What are risk factors for cholangitis?

1. **Biliary obstruction**: Stones, strictures, or pancreatic/biliary tumors obstruct the biliary tree, which increases biliary pressure and promotes migration of bacteria from portal to biliary circulation.
2. **Mechanical barrier disruption**: ERCP or biliary surgery can disrupt the mechanical barrier provided by the SOD, which allows bacteria to enter the biliary tree.
3. **Foreign body**: Gallstones and stents can act as a nidus for bacterial growth.

What are the next diagnostic steps?

Order ultrasound (detects gallstones and biliary dilation). Then perform diagnostic ERCP to confirm the diagnosis.

MRCP is a noninvasive alternative to ERCP (uses MRI to visualize biliary and pancreatic ducts). Consider MRCP rather than ERCP if the patient with suspected cholangitis does not have Charcot's triad or ultrasound findings are ambiguous.

Percutaneous transhepatic cholangiography is indicated if ERCP cannot establish the diagnosis. Locate bile ducts using fluoroscopy and inject contrast percutaneously into the ducts.

Diagnostic ERCP confirms the diagnosis of cholangitis.

How is this condition treated?

Treat with supportive care and broad-spectrum antibiotics to cover enteric Gram-negative bacteria and enterococci (e.g., ampicillin and gentamycin). Fever and abdominal pain should improve within 24 hours. After clinical improvement, perform therapeutic ERCP (sphincterotomy and stone extraction ± stent placement) on an elective basis.

Reynold's pentad: Charcot's triad with hypotension and altered mental status. Indicates severe (suppurative) cholangitis. Requires urgent rather than elective therapeutic ERCP.

Twenty-four hours later, the patient appears confused. Physical exam is significant for RUQ tenderness and jaundice. Vital signs are temperature 39.2°C, pulse 120 bpm, respirations 25/min, and blood pressure 90/60.

What is the next step in management?

Patients with persistent fever, abdominal pain, or signs of septic shock (Reynold's pentad) despite supportive care and antibiotics require urgent therapeutic ERCP. If ERCP is unsuccessful, percutaneously insert a cholecystostomy tube (T-tube) to decompress the biliary tree.

The patient recovers after ERCP but returns 1 week later with fever, chills, malaise, and RUQ pain. Physical exam is significant for jaundice and RUQ tenderness. CBC demonstrates leukocytosis. LFTs reveal a cholestatic pattern. Murphy's sign is negative. Ultrasound demonstrates a well-demarcated, hypoechoic lesion in the right lobe of the liver that the radiologist interprets as a possible liver abscess.

What is the next step in management?

Contiguous spread of bacteria from the biliary tree to the liver to form a pyogenic liver abscess is a potentially life-threatening complication. Fever and RUQ pain are the most common symptoms. Patients may have jaundice and nonspecific symptoms like nausea, vomiting, anorexia, and malaise. CBC usually shows leukocytosis. LFTs may or may not be elevated (elevated alkaline phosphatase is the most common abnormality). Ultrasound usually establishes the diagnosis. If ultrasound is equivocal, confirm the diagnosis with CT scan. Treatment is broad-spectrum IV antibiotics and percutaneous ultrasound or CT-guided aspiration and catheter drainage of the abscess. Tailor antibiotics when culture results of the abscess fluid are available.

> 50% of patients do not have RUQ pain or jaundice.

> **Sources of bacteria in pyogenic liver abscess**: contiguous spread from biliary tree to liver (number one source), contiguous spread from peritonitis (number two source), and hematogenous spread.

Alternative 5.7.2

A 30-year-old man presents with a 2-week history of fever and RUQ pain. He does not have any other medical conditions. He has never had any surgery or invasive procedures. He recently moved to the United States from Mexico. RUQ is tender to palpation. There is no jaundice or Murphy's sign. Temperature is 38.7°C. Other vital signs are normal. CBC shows leukocytosis. Alkaline phosphatase is mildly elevated. Ultrasound shows a possible abscess in the right lobe of the liver. CT scan confirms the diagnosis of liver abscess.

What is the next step in management?

This recent young male immigrant with no prior medical history is more likely to have an amebic liver abscess than a pyogenic liver abscess. Amebic liver abscess results from infection by the parasite *Entamoeba histolytica*, which is endemic to many developing countries. Infection is transmitted via fecal–oral contact and is far more common in men for unclear reasons. Imaging findings do not reliably distinguish between pyogenic and amebic liver abscess, so the next step is serology for *E. histolytica* antibodies. Also initiate empiric therapy with IV metronidazole. Avoid aspirating a suspected amebic liver abscess if possible because the needle can rupture the cyst and cause hematogenous spread. However, if the patient deteriorates despite treatment with metronidazole, perform aspiration with CT or ultrasound guidance to reduce infection load and to rule out pyogenic liver abscess.

> **False-negative serology**: Antibodies are often negative in the first 7 days of infection.
> **False-positive serology**: Patients with past infection can have positive antibodies.

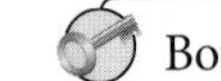

Both pyogenic and amebic liver abscess are more frequent in the right lobe.

CASE 5–8 ACUTE EPIGASTRIC PAIN

A 60-year-old alcoholic man presents with a 12-hour history of severe epigastric pain radiating to the back, nausea, and vomiting. Pain is somewhat better when he leans forward. He drank a 24-pack of beer 2 days ago. He does not take any medications. Physical exam is significant for abdominal distension, decreased bowel sounds, and epigastric tenderness with guarding. Vital signs are temperature 38.1°C, pulse 110 bpm, respirations 27/min, and blood pressure 130/85.

What is the most likely diagnosis?

Acute, steady, epigastric pain radiating to the back with nausea and vomiting is highly suggestive of acute pancreatitis, particularly in an alcoholic with a recent binge-drinking episode. Patients may report that pain improves on leaning forward. Physical findings vary depending on the severity of illness. Possible findings are abdominal distension, decreased bowel sounds, and epigastric tenderness with guarding. Vital signs may show tachycardia, tachypnea, and a low-grade fever.

Some patients have diffuse/RUQ pain rather than the classic epigastric pain.

What are the causes of acute pancreatitis in adults?

Remember the causes of acute pancreatitis using the mnemonic "***BAD SHIT***":

1. **B**iliary (gallstones): number one cause in women
2. **A**lcohol: number one cause in men
3. **D**rugs: ***"Drugs SAVE TIA"*** (thiazide and loop **D**iuretics, **S**ulfonamides, **A**nti-inflammatory drugs including NSAIDs and 5-ASA drugs, **V**alproic acid, **E**strogen, **T**amoxifen, **I**mmunosuppressants like **A**zathioprine, **A**IDS drugs)
4. **S**corpion bite: common in Trinidad but not in the United States
5. **H**ypertriglyceridemia and **H**ypercalcemia
6. **I**diopathic (number three cause) and **I**nfectious (viruses such as mumps and coxsackievirus), and **I**atrogenic (postoperative, post-ERCP)
7. **T**rauma

Pancreas divisum: Dorsal and ventral portions of embryonic pancreas do not fuse, resulting into two pancreatic ductal systems. This is a common anatomic variant in humans, and its association with pancreatitis is controversial.

What are the next diagnostic steps?

Base the diagnosis of acute pancreatitis on a combination of clinical, laboratory, and radiologic findings. Order the following initial tests in hemodynamically stable patients:

1. **Serum amylase and lipase**: Serum amylase and lipase levels are usually more than three to five times the upper limit of normal in acute pancreatitis. Elevated lipase is more sensitive and specific for acute pancreatitis than amylase (increased in many other conditions).
2. **Abdominal radiograph**: The main utility of abdominal radiograph is to exclude other causes of abdominal pain such as obstruction and perforation. Patients with severe acute pancreatitis may have the sentinel loop sign (localized ileus of a segment of small intestine) and colon cutoff sign (increased air in transverse colon, decreased air distal to splenic flexure).
3. **CBC, serum electrolytes, LFTs, and LDH**: Abnormal LFTs suggest a biliary cause. Elevated calcium suggests hypercalcemia as the cause. The other tests do not aid in diagnosis, but

TABLE 5-9: Ranson's Criteria for Acute Pancreatitis Prognosis

At Admission ("A Good LAW")	At 48 Hours ("Can BOB Have Flu?")	Prognosis
• **A**ge > 55 years • **G**lucose > 200 mg/dL • **L**DH > 350 U/L • **A**ST > 250 U/L • **W**BC > 16,000/cubic mm	**Electrolytes:** • **C**alcium < 8 mg/dL • **B**UN ↑ > 8 mg/dL **Arterial blood gas:** • Pa**O**$_2$ < 60 mm Hg • **B**ase deficit > 4 mEq/L **Complete blood count:** • **H**ematocrit ↓ > 10% • **F**luid sequestration > 6 L	**1–3 criteria:** • Mild pancreatitis **>3 criteria:** • Severe pancreatitis (high mortality)

Abbreviations: BUN, blood urea nitrogen; WBC, whole blood count.

they are included in scoring systems that estimate disease severity such as Acute Physiology and Chronic Health Evaluation (APACHE) II and Ranson's (Table 5-9).

> The level of amylase and lipase elevation is not indicative of disease severity.

> **Signs of hemorrhagic pancreatitis**: hypovolemic shock, Grey-Turner's sign (flank ecchymoses) and Cullen's sign (periumbilical ecchymosis).
> **CT scan with contrast**: Most accurate test for detecting acute pancreatitis and its complications. Do not order this test initially unless the patient has signs of intraabdominal hemorrhage.

Serum amylase is 400 U/L, and serum lipase is 900 U/L. LFTs are normal. WBC count is 17,000. There is no evidence of obstruction or perforation on abdominal radiograph.

What additional test is indicated at this time?

Order abdominal ultrasound to evaluate for gallstones and CBD dilation (suggests gallstone pancreatitis).

> Laboratory findings in alcohol versus gallstone pancreatitis:
> **1.** ALT >150 U/L suggests gallstone pancreatitis.
> **2.** Lipase/amylase ratio >2 suggests alcohol-induced pancreatitis.

There are no gallstones or CBD dilation on ultrasound.

What is the next step?

The patient has clinical and laboratory evidence of acute alcohol-induced pancreatitis. He does not have signs of severe pancreatitis. Management is supportive (NPO, IV fluids, NG suction if the patient is vomiting, opioid analgesics, and reassess).

> **Classic teaching**: Morphine increases SOD spasm, so use meperidine instead.
> **Current guidelines**: There is no evidence that morphine increases SOD spasm. Avoid meperidine because it poses an increased risk of seizures, myoclonus, and tremors.

> **Gallstone pancreatitis**: In addition to supportive care, initial management includes early ERCP if the patient has signs of jaundice or cholangitis.

The patient reports increased abdominal pain 48 hours later. Abdomen is tender to palpation with rebound and guarding. Vital signs are temperature 38.3°C, pulse 120 bpm, respirations 25/min, and blood pressure 110/80. He has sequestered approximately 7 L of fluid (fluids administered – fluids lost in urine, stool, etc.). Base deficit is 5 mEq/L.

What is the next step in management?

Obtain a CT scan of the abdomen with contrast if the patient does not improve or worsens despite initial supportive care. Also, transfer this patient to the intensive care unit regardless of CT scan findings because he has more than three of Ranson's criteria, which is associated with a high mortality (age >55 years, admission WBC count >16,000, fluid sequestration >6 L at 48 hours, and base deficit >4 mEq/L at 48 hours).

CT scan confirms the diagnosis of acute pancreatitis. The report also mentions approximately 40% necrosis of the pancreas.

What is the next step in management?

Acute pancreatitis causes pancreatic enzyme activation and leakage. These enzymes can digest pancreatic parenchyma and cause necrotizing pancreatitis. Initiate IV imipenem if the patient has >30% pancreatic necrosis to prevent secondary pancreatic infection. Also continue supportive care. Patients with necrotizing pancreatitis often require large volumes of IV fluids.

> **<30% necrosis**: Continue supportive care; do not initiate antibiotics.

One week later, the patient continues to report persistent abdominal pain despite IV imipenem and supportive care. Temperature is 38.9°C, pulse 120 bpm, respirations 28/min, blood pressure 110/80.

What is the next step in management?

Patients who do not improve despite 7 days of antibiotics and supportive care require percutaneous CT-guided fine-needle aspiration of the necrotic material. Perform Gram stain and culture of the aspirated material to evaluate whether it is infected. Infected pancreatic necrosis requires surgical debridement (necrosectomy).

> Some surgeons prefer continued supportive care and antibiotics rather than necrosectomy if the patient with infected pancreatic necrosis is stable.

Gram stain and culture of the necrotic material is negative (sterile pancreatic necrosis). Imipenem and supportive care are continued for 4 weeks. The patient improves and is discharged. He is asymptomatic during a follow-up visit 3 weeks later. Vital signs are normal. Figure 5-5 is the follow-up CT scan at 3 weeks.

What is the diagnosis?

The CT scan shows a pancreatic pseudocyst (a collection of fluid in the lesser sac of the abdomen). Approximately 10% of patients develop pseudocysts within 2 to 3 weeks of an episode of acute pancreatitis. These cysts develop from liquefaction of the necrotic pancreatic material. Unlike true cystic lesions of the pancreas, pseudocysts are lined by granulation tissue and not epithelial tissue.

How are pancreatic pseudocysts managed?

Most pseudocysts resolve spontaneously and do not require any specific treatment. Consider resection or drainage if the patient develops uncontrollable symptoms (abdominal pain) or complications. Important complications include:

1. **Pseudocyst infection**: Suspect if the patient develops fever. CT scan will show an abscess in the region of the pseudocyst.
2. **Pseudocyst rupture**: Suspect if the patient develops ascites or pleural effusion with increased amylase in ascitic or pleural fluid.

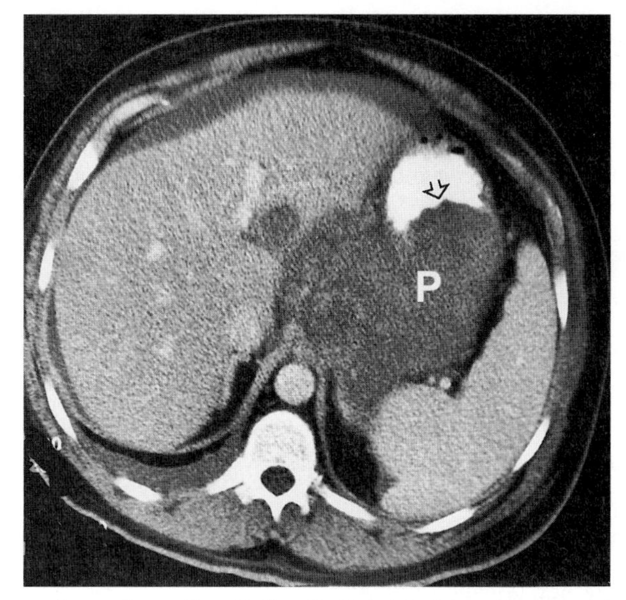

FIGURE 5–5 CT of pancreatic pseudocyst. From Daffner R. *Clinical Radiology: The Essentials*, 3rd ed. Lippincott Williams & Wilkins, 2007.

3. **Pseudoaneurysm**: Digestion of an adjacent blood vessel by pancreatic enzymes in the pseudocyst. Suspect if the pseudocyst expands or the patient has unexplained GI bleeding (or decreased hematocrit). Confirm diagnosis with spiral CT scan, MRI, or mesenteric angiography. Treat with embolization prior to drainage.

Three drainage options: surgery, endoscopy, and percutaneous catheter drainage. ERCP findings (perform prior to drainage) and local expertise determines which technique to use. Pseudoaneurysm is a contraindication to endoscopic drainage.

Cyst in lesser sac with no history of pancreatitis: Suspect cystic pancreatic neoplasm. Consider tumor markers (CEA, CA 19-9) and endoscopic ultrasound with fine-needle aspiration to examine cystic fluid. Differentiation between cystic lesions is challenging.

Remember complications of acute pancreatitis with the mnemonic "***New Pancreatitis Has Cruel Complications***": pancreatic **N**ecrosis (sterile or infected), pancreatic **P**seudocyst ($\pm$abscess, rupture, pseudoaneurysm), **H**emorrhagic pancreatitis, **C**holangitis (if the patient has gallstone pancreatitis), and **C**hronic pancreatitis.

CASE 5–9 CHRONIC EPIGASTRIC PAIN

A 54-year-old man presents with a 12-month history of severe epigastric pain radiating to the back. The pain occurs in episodes that last for 7 to 8 days and are followed by 1 to 2 pain-free months. Past history is significant for alcoholism and acute pancreatitis. He smokes two packs of cigarettes a day. Physical exam and vital signs are normal. CBC, serum electrolytes, LFTs, amylase and lipase are all normal.

What diagnosis should you suspect?

Suspect chronic pancreatitis when a patient presents with chronic epigastric pain radiating to the back, particularly if the patient has a history of alcoholism. Pain is sometimes associated with nausea and vomiting. Laboratory findings including amylase and lipase are all normal (occasionally amylase and lipase are mildly elevated).

> Pain does not radiate to the back in 50% of patients. Even in the absence of back pain, a history of alcoholism and the above pattern of symptoms would make chronic pancreatitis and not other causes of dyspepsia the most likely diagnosis.

What are the causes of chronic pancreatitis in adults?

1. Alcohol (number one cause): occurs in 5% to 10% of chronic alcoholics.
2. Idiopathic (number two cause).
3. Obstruction of pancreatic duct by gallstones (number three cause) and strictures.
4. Hereditary: Autosomal dominant mutation accounts for a small percentage of cases.
5. Autoimmune disorders such as systemic lupus erythematosus and primary hyperparathyroidism.
6. Tropical pancreatitis: number one cause in south India; cause is unknown.

What is the next diagnostic step?

Order a CT scan of the abdomen to establish the diagnosis and rule out pseudocysts and pancreatic malignancies. The characteristic findings on CT scan are pancreatic calcifications ± pancreatic duct dilation (Fig. 5-6). If CT scan is nondiagnostic, perform ERCP (gold standard for diagnosis). The characteristic ERCP findings are dilated side duct branches and beading of the main duct in a "chain of lakes" pattern.

> **False-negative ERCP**: Possible in early chronic pancreatitis. Consider endoscopic ultrasound and/or pancreatic function tests if ERCP is normal despite severe pain.

> **Abdominal x-ray**: Detects pancreatic calcifications but low sensitivity (30%).

CT scan demonstrates pancreatic calcifications.

What is the natural history of chronic pancreatitis?

The presenting complaint is usually abdominal pain that is initially episodic but progresses to constant, unrelenting pain. Later in the course, progressive damage to the pancreatic islet cells leads to insulin-dependent diabetes mellitus (endocrine dysfunction). After the disease

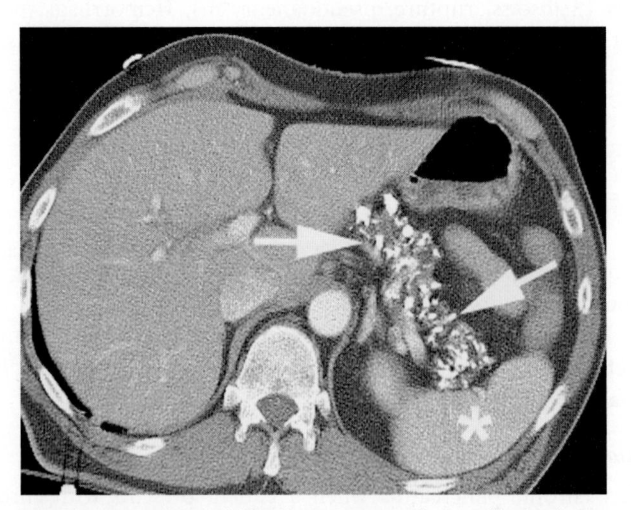

FIGURE 5–6 CT scan of chronic pancreatitis (calcifications ± pancreatic duct dilations). From Daffner R. *Clinical Radiology: The Essentials*, 3rd ed. Lippincott Williams & Wilkins, 2007.

disrupts approximately 90% of pancreatic function, patients do not secrete sufficient digestive enzymes and therefore develop malabsorptive diarrhea and vitamin A, D, E, and K deficiency (exocrine dysfunction).

What are common complications of chronic pancreatitis?

Remember complications of chronic pancreatitis with the acronym "***SOAP***": **S**plenic vein thrombosis, **O**bstruction of CBD or duodenum, **A**scites or pleural effusion, and **P**seudocyst.

1. **Splenic vein thrombosis**: Pancreatic inflammation can affect the nearby splenic vein and cause thrombosis. Suspect this complication if the patient develops bleeding gastric varices and splenomegaly. Treatment is splenectomy.
2. **CBD obstruction**: Suspect if the patient develops jaundice and cholestatic pattern of LFTs. Diagnose with ERCP. Treat with therapeutic ERCP. If obstruction persists, consider surgery (choledochoenterostomy).
3. **Duodenal obstruction**: Suspect if the patient develops postprandial pain and early satiety. Diagnose with upper endoscopy or upper GI series. Treatment is often surgery (gastrojejunostomy).
4. **Pancreatic ascites and pleural effusions**: Ascites or effusions sometimes occur in the absence of pseudocyst due to ductal disruption. Treat with aspiration, diuretics, and octreotide. If symptoms persist, consider surgery.
5. **Pancreatic pseudocyst**: Unlike acute pancreatitis, the mechanism is pancreatic duct disruption. Management is similar to that of a pseudocyst that occurs in the setting of acute pancreatitis.

How is chronic pancreatitis treated?

The main goal of therapy is pain control. Approach this goal in a stepwise fashion:

1. **Conservative measures**: First attempt to control pain with NSAIDs and lifestyle measures (quit alcohol and eat small, low-fat meals). If unsuccessful, attempt an 8-week trial of pancreatic enzymes + H2-blockers.
2. **Analgesics**: If pain does not respond to the above measures, admit the patient during a painful episode, keep him NPO, and administer a short course of narcotic analgesics, amitriptyline, and an NSAID. This approach often breaks the cycle of pain.
3. **Narcotics versus invasive therapy**: If the patient continues to have refractory pain, discuss the risks of narcotic addiction versus invasive therapies and base the next step on the outcome of this discussion. Invasive therapies include therapeutic ERCP, extracorporeal shock wave lithotripsy, celiac nerve block, and surgery.

Steatorrhea: Treat with decreased fat intake, pancreatic enzymes, and vitamins.

When fibrosis completely "burns out" the pancreas, the pain spontaneously resolves. However, this process can take years or may never occur at all.

The patient stops drinking alcohol and begins to eat small meals. He is able to control his symptoms with NSAIDs, pancreatic enzymes, H2-blockers, and intermittent narcotic analgesics. Ten years later, he reports increased abdominal pain and anorexia. He has unintentionally lost 10 lbs in the last 2 months. He has noticed bluish-black discoloration in his left leg that disappeared, and now he has similar lesions on his right arm (migratory thrombophlebitis or Trousseau syndrome). Physical examination is significant for jaundice.

What is the most likely cause of his symptoms?

Smoking and chronic pancreatitis are associated with an increased risk of pancreatic adenocarcinoma. Suspect pancreatic adenocarcinoma when patients report increased abdominal pain, weight loss, anorexia, or jaundice. Jaundice is more common if the lesion is in the head of the pancreas.

Migratory thrombophlebitis: This condition is associated with lung and pancreatic cancer.
Courvoisier's sign: Painless, palpable gallbladder is a late finding in some patients.
Virchow node: Enlarged left supraclavicular node can indicate abdominal cancer, lung cancer, breast cancer, lymphoma, or infection.

Pancreatic adenocarcinoma (exocrine pancreas tumor): also called pancreatic cancer because it accounts for 95% of pancreatic malignancies.
Neuroendocrine tumors (endocrine pancreas tumors): include gastrinoma (ZES), insulinoma, glucagonoma, somatostatinoma, and VIPoma (see Chapter 8: Endocrinology); these tumors account for 5% of pancreas malignancies.

What are risk factors for pancreatic cancer?

1. Cigarette smoking (number one risk factor)
2. Chronic pancreatitis
3. Diabetes mellitus
4. Partial gastrectomy (15 to 20 years later)

The role of other agents such as diet, coffee, and alcohol is less clear.

How can you confirm your suspicion of pancreatic cancer?

1. Order LFTs and CA 19-9 (levels often increase in pancreatic cancer).
2. Obtain abdominal ultrasound (first imaging test in patient with jaundice).

If patient is not jaundiced, the first test for suspected pancreatic cancer is abdominal CT scan.

LFTs reveal a cholestatic pattern of elevation. CA 19-9 is elevated. Ultrasound detects a solid mass lesion in the head of the pancreas.

What is the next step in management?

Pancreatic mass on ultrasound or CT scan is considered diagnostic of pancreatic cancer, particularly when CA 19-9 is also elevated. The next step is helical CT angiography to assess the degree of tumor invasion. This test helps determine whether or not the tumor is amenable to surgical resection (Whipple procedure). Most patients present at an advanced stage and are not candidates for curative surgery. In such patients, palliation is the most important goal of therapy.

No mass lesion on CT scan or ultrasound: The next step in management is ERCP. If ERCP identifies a mass (diagnostic of cancer), the next step is helical CT angiography.

Helical CT angiography: helical CT plus IV contrast (angiography).

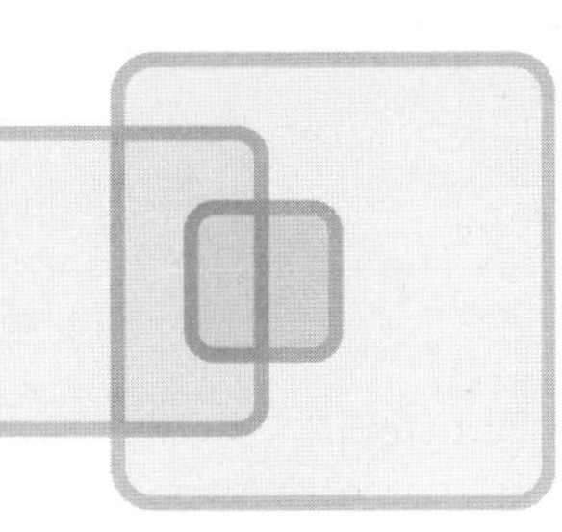

chapter 6

Nephrology

CASE 6–1 DYSURIA, URGENCY, AND FREQUENCY

A 35-year-old woman presents to the clinic with a 2-day history of painful burning urination (dysuria), frequency, and urgency. She does not have any discharge or pain during intercourse (dyspareunia). Physical exam is significant for suprapubic tenderness. There is no CVA tenderness. She has been in a monogamous relationship with her husband for the last 10 years. Vital signs are normal.

What is the most likely diagnosis?

Dysuria, frequency, urgency, and suprapubic tenderness are the characteristic clinical manifestations of bladder inflammation (cystitis) due to a urinary tract infection (UTI). UTIs are more common in women because they have a shorter urethra than men. They occur when fecal flora colonize the vagina and spread upward into the urinary tract.

> **Uncomplicated patients**: young, healthy, non-pregnant females.
> **Complicated patients**: all others (males, elderly, pregnant, comorbidities, etc.).

What are the risk factors for UTIs in adults?

Remember risk factors for UTIs with the mnemonic "***Sex, Sperm, & Sugar make Stacy & Betsy PP Constantly***":

1. **Sex**: Intercourse pushes vaginal contents upward into the urinary tract.
2. **Sperm**icide-containing contraceptives.
3. **Sugar** (diabetes) weakens immune system and predisposes to neurogenic bladder.
4. Urinary **Stas**is: Causes include incomplete voiding, neurogenic bladder, and obstruction (due to nephrolithiasis, benign prostatic hypertrophy (BPH), etc.).
5. **B**edridden (Immobility) and **B**owel incontinence.

6. **P**regnancy.
7. **P**ast episodes.
8. **C**atheter (indwelling urinary catheter).

> **Specific risk factors in men:** anal intercourse and lack of circumcision.

What is the next step in management?

Empiric therapy without further diagnostic work-up is indicated for this uncomplicated patient with all of the characteristic symptoms. First-line treatment is a 3-day course of trimethroprim/sulfamethoxazole (TMP-SMX). If the patient's symptoms are severe (affects daily routine) or she lives in an area with high TMP/SMX resistance, consider a 3-day course of an oral fluoroquinolone. Also prescribe phenazopyridine (urinary analgesic) if the patient reports severe dysuria. If symptoms persist despite antibiotics, treat her as a complicated patient.

> Uncomplicated UTI microbiology:
>
> **Gram-positive cocci:** *Staphylococcus saprophyticus* (number two cause), enterococcus.
>
> **Gram-negative rods:** Enterobacteriaceae such as *Escherichia coli* (number one cause), klebsiella, and proteus.
>
> **Note:** *E. coli* accounts for 80% to 85% of UTIs, whereas *S. saprophyticus* accounts for 10% to 15% of UTIs.

> A 7-day course of nitrofurantoin is an alternative to a 3-day course of oral fluoroquinolone.

What would have been the next steps in management if the patient did not have characteristic symptoms?

Confirm the diagnosis using urinalysis (Table 6-1) prior to initiating antibiotics. First, evaluate the urine dipstick. Positive leukocyte esterase (indicates pyuria) ± positive nitrite (detects enterobacteriaceae) is diagnostic. If leukocyte esterase is negative but the patient has symptoms suggestive of a UTI, evaluate the unspun urine sample for white blood cells (WBCs); >10 WBCs per high-powered field indicates pyuria and is diagnostic. Treatment is as described earlier.

> Urethritis due to a sexually transmitted disease can cause dysuria. Patients with UTI often have hematuria, whereas those with sexually transmitted disease generally do not. Include pelvic exam in the diagnostic evaluation if the patient reports any of the **4Ds**:
>
> 1. **D**yspareunia
> 2. **D**ysuria in her partner
> 3. Vaginal **D**ischarge, odor, or pruritus
> 4. **D**uration: Symptom onset is gradual (weeks)

What would have been the next steps in management if the patient was complicated?

1. First, obtain urinalysis and urine culture (with Gram stain and antibiotic susceptibility pattern).
2. If urinalysis indicates the patient has a UTI, treat with a 7-day course of an oral fluoroquinolone; tailor antibiotics if urine culture detects an organism resistant to fluoroquinolones.
3. If symptoms do not resolve despite 24 to 48 hours of treatment with appropriate antibiotics (culture and susceptibility confirmed), repeat urine culture. Also, consider renal ultrasound or computed tomography (CT) scan to identify any urinary tract abnormalities that would predispose the patient to UTIs.

TABLE 6–1 Urinalysis and Normal Values

COLLECTION

Obtain a mid-stream specimen. Within 30 minutes, centrifuge the specimen to obtain supernatant and sediment. Perform gross inspection and chemical analysis of the supernatant and microscopic analysis of the sediment.

GROSS INSPECTION OF SUPERNATANT (color and clarity): Normally light yellow and clear.
CHEMICAL ANALYSIS (urine dipstick)

pH	Can range from 4.5–8, but typically between 5.5 and 6.5
Specific gravity	1.002–1.03
Protein	Negative to trace
Glucose	Negative
Blood	Negative
Ketones	Negative
Nitrite	Negative
Leukocyte esterase	Negative

MICROSCOPIC ANALYSIS OF SEDIMENT

Red blood cells	0–2/HPF
White blood cells	0–2/HPF
Red blood cell casts	0/HPF

Abbreviation: HPF, high-powered field.

Interstitial cystitis: Consider this diagnosis if a patient has recurrent UTI symptoms but laboratory tests do not show any evidence of infection.

Positive culture (bacteriuria): Traditional criterion is $\geq 10^5$ colony forming units (CFU)/mL; however, some patients may have as low as 10^2 CFU/mL.

Asymptomatic bacteriuria: Do not treat unless the patient is pregnant or the patient will soon undergo a urological surgery/procedure.

Pregnant patients: Treat symptomatic and asymptomatic bacteriuria with a 3 to 7 day course of oral nitrofurantoin, amoxicillin, or cephalexin; avoid fluoroquinolones, which can cause fetal arthropathy.

The patient's symptoms improve with a 3-day course of TMP/SMX. Over the next 2 years, she has six more UTIs, all of which respond to TMP/SMX. What strategies are generally recommended to prevent recurrences?

Remember strategies to decrease UTI recurrences with the mnemonic "***Taking Juice Can Avoid Infections***":

1. **T**opical estrogen: Prevents recurrences in post-menopausal women.
2. Cranberry **J**uice
3. **C**ontraceptives: Avoid spermicides and diaphragms.
4. **A**ntibiotics: Consider continuous or postcoital antibiotics if the patient has two or more UTIs every 6 months or three or more UTIs every 12 months that markedly alter daily routine.
5. Decreased **I**ntercourse: Abstinence decreases the frequency of UTIs; many physicians also recommend urinating soon after intercourse (unclear benefit).

Classification of recurrent UTIs:

1. **Relapse**: Symptoms recur within 2 weeks of treatment, and urine culture identifies the same strain.
2. **Re-infection**: Symptoms recur within 2 weeks, but urine culture identifies a different strain OR symptoms recur after 2 weeks (same or different strain on urine culture).

Men with recurrent UTIs: Evaluate the patient for prostatitis (see Chapter 14: Primary Care Gynecology and Urology).

Alternative 6.1.1

A 50-year-old man undergoes hematopoietic stem cell transplantation for treatment of acute myelogenous leukemia. Before transplantation, he received high-dose cyclophosphamide and busulfan. Two days after the procedure, he presents with dysuria, urgency, frequency, and suprapubic pain. His urine is bright red with blood clots. Vital signs are normal.

What diagnosis should you suspect?

Suspect a severe type of cystitis called hemorrhagic cystitis when a patient with one of the following risk factors presents with symptoms of cystitis, hematuria, and/or blood clots:

1. Immunocompromised (increased risk of infections such as BK polyoma virus, etc.)
2. Pelvic radiation
3. Chemotherapy with cyclophosphamide, ifosfamide, or busulfan (bladder toxins)

Bone marrow transplantation poses a very high risk because patients are immunosuppressed, and they usually receive high dose cyclophosphamide and busulfan.

What is the next diagnostic step?

In addition to urinalysis and urine culture, order viral cultures and a complete blood count. Also, perform cystoscopy with biopsy to confirm the diagnosis.

Urinalysis demonstrates pyuria and hematuria. Cultures are negative. Complete blood count shows pancytopenia. Cystoscopy with biopsy confirms the diagnosis.

How is hemorrhagic cystitis treated?

Initial therapy for stable patients is to increase fluid intake. If symptoms do not resolve, options include:

1. Administer hyperbaric oxygen (only in stable patients).
2. Perform cystoscopy with clot extraction and/or intravesical administration of agents such as alum, formalin, prostaglandin, or estrogen.
3. Surgery is indicated if there are signs of hypovolemic shock due to severe hemorrhage.

Note: No method is superior to any other in this list.

Use one of the following to prevent hemorrhagic cystitis when using a bladder toxin such as cyclophosphamide:

1. **Mesna**: An additional benefit is decreased future risk of bladder cancer due to cyclophosphamide.
2. **Suprahydration**: Normal saline plus furosemide maintains increased urine output.
3. **Continuous bladder irrigation**

CASE 6–2 FEVER AND FLANK PAIN

A 35-year-old woman presents to the emergency department with a 2-day history of fever, flank pain, nausea, and vomiting. She also complains of frequency, urgency, dysuria, and suprapubic pain for the last 4 days. She has no other medical conditions. Physical exam is significant for right costovertebral angle (CVA) tenderness. Vital signs are temperature 38.4°C, pulse 115 bpm, respirations 18/min, and blood pressure 118/75.

What diagnosis should you suspect?

Fever, flank pain, and CVA tenderness are highly suggestive of acute upper UTI (acute pyelonephritis). The source of infection is usually ascending infection from the lower urinary tract, so patients often report symptoms of cystitis as well (frequency, urgency, dysuria, and suprapubic pain).

> **Uncomplicated patients**: young, healthy, non-pregnant females.
> **Complicated patients**: anyone else.

What is the next step in management?

The most important initial test is urinalysis and urine culture. Positive leukocyte esterase and/or nitrite tests are an indication for empiric antibiotics. Urinalysis may also demonstrate white cell casts (localizes infection to the kidney if present) and hematuria. If urinalysis is positive, obtain complete blood count (typically shows leukocytosis with a left shift) and a pregnancy test (if the patient is a premenopausal woman).

Leukocyte esterase and nitrite are positive. β-hCG (pregnancy test) is negative. Complete blood count is significant for leukocytosis with a left shift.

Which patients with pyelonephritis require hospitalization?

Outpatient therapy is indicated only for uncomplicated patients who are likely to be compliant and do not appear extremely ill (able to tolerate oral intake, fever <39°C, pain not very severe, and no signs of septic shock). All other patients require hospitalization.

> Order blood culture if you decide to hospitalize the patient.

This young, non-pregnant female with no other medical conditions appears to have good social support at home. She is able to tolerate oral intake. The physician decides to treat the patient as an outpatient.

What empiric antibiotics are indicated?

Initiate a 10- to 14-day course of an oral fluoroquinolone. Tailor antibiotics later on the basis of Gram stain and culture results. For instance, if the Gram stain shows Gram-negative bacilli susceptible to TMP-SMX, you can switch to this agent. If Gram stain shows Gram-positive cocci, add amoxicillin to the regimen to cover enterococcus.

> Microbiology of pyelonephritis is similar to cystitis.

What empiric agents are recommended for hospitalized patients?

Initially, treat the patient with IV antibiotics. First-line therapy for uncomplicated patients is ceftriaxone. If the Gram stain shows Gram-positive cocci, switch to ampicillin and gentamycin or piperacillin-tazobactam to cover enterococcus. When the patient improves clinically and can tolerate oral intake (should occur within 24 to 48 hours), switch to oral antibiotics (oral fluoroquinolone or TMP/SMX depending on susceptibility pattern). As with outpatients, total duration of therapy is usually 10 to 14 days.

When is imaging indicated for patients with pyelonephritis?

Most uncomplicated patients with pyelonephritis do not require any imaging tests. Remember indications for CT scan or renal ultrasound (perform ultrasound first; obtain CT if ultrasound shows renal enlargement) with the mnemonic "***Complicated Pyelonephritis Requires Cat Scan***":

1. **C**omplicated patients (anyone who is not a young, healthy, non-pregnant female)
2. **P**ersistent fever despite 72 hours of antibiotics
3. **R**ecurrence of symptoms in <2 weeks
4. **C**ulture demonstrates pseudomonas
5. **S**tones (paroxysmal flank pain or stones identified incidentally on radiographs)

> The goal of imaging is to rule out "***AOA***":
> 1. **A**bscess (perinephric or intrarenal)
> 2. **O**bstruction (e.g., renal stones, tumors)
> 3. **A**natomic abnormality that predisposes to pyelonephritis (e.g., vesicoureteral reflux, neurogenic bladder, polycystic kidney disease (PKD)

Alternative 6.2.1

A 65-year-old man with type 2 diabetes presents with right flank pain and fever. Physical exam is significant for right CVA tenderness. Leukocyte esterase and nitrite are positive. Complete blood count shows leukocytosis with a left shift. CT scan shows a wedge-shaped hypodense collection in the right kidney.

What is the diagnosis?

The CT scan shows a collection in the right kidney consistent with renal abscess. Most cases occur as a complication of pyelonephritis in patients with a predisposing condition (obstruction, an anatomic abnormality, or diabetes). Occasionally, patients develop renal abscess through hematogenous spread. Clinical presentation is similar to pyelonephritis.

> **Ascending infection** causes renal abscess in medulla.
> **Hematogenous spread** causes renal abscess in cortex.

How are renal abscesses treated?

1. Drainage: If the patient has an identifiable obstruction or anatomic abnormality, drain surgically. Otherwise, percutaneous drainage under CT or ultrasound guidance is sufficient. This patient with diabetes is likely to have neurogenic bladder, so surgical drainage is preferable.
2. Antibiotics: If you identify the abscess during initial presentation (as is the case with this patient), treat empirically with an IV aminoglycoside for 10 to 14 days plus a fluoroquinolone for a few weeks. If you identify the abscess later, continue antibiotics initiated for treatment of pyelonephritis. Tailor antibiotics on the basis of blood and abscess fluid culture.

What are other important complications of pyelonephritis?

1. **Perinephric abscess**: This infection of fat surrounding the kidney has a clinical presentation similar to uncomplicated pyelonephritis, except that patients can have flank erythema and a palpable flank mass. Risk factors, diagnosis and treatment are similar to renal abscess.
2. **Emphysematous pyelonephritis**: This severe infection of the renal parenchyma is caused by gas-producing organisms. Approximately 90% of cases occur in diabetics. Clinical presentation is similar to uncomplicated pyelonephritis, but CT scan shows gas bubbles. Treat with antibiotics and percutaneous drainage. Patients with perirenal extension or bilateral infection require surgery (partial nephrectomy).
3. **Urosepsis**: This is an infection that spreads to the bloodstream. In some patients, urosepsis can progress to septic shock.

CASE 6–3 ACUTE ONSET OF COLICKY (PAROXYSMAL) FLANK PAIN

A 45-year-old man presents with an 8-hour history of intense pain in the right flank. The pain waxes and wanes in severity. Over the last hour, the pain has begun to radiate to the right groin. He noticed blood in his urine a couple of hours ago. This is his first such episode. Vital signs are temperature 37.1°C, pulse 110 bpm, respirations 21/min, blood pressure 140/85, and oxygen saturation 100% on room air. Urine dipstick is positive for blood. Urine nitrite and leukocyte esterase are negative.

What is the most likely diagnosis?

Renal colic (acute paroxysms of flank pain) and hematuria (gross or microscopic) is the classic description for ureteral obstruction by a kidney stone (nephrolithiasis). Upper ureter obstruction causes flank pain. As the stone migrates down to the lower ureter, the pain radiates to the ipsilateral groin. When the stone enters the bladder and urethra, the patient may report dysuria and urgency. Patients may also report nausea and vomiting.

> Some patients report mild discomfort and not renal colic; 10% of patients do not have hematuria.

> **Types of kidney stones:** calcium stones (80% to 85%), uric acid stones (10%), struvite stones (5% to 10%), cystine stones (<1%).

What is the next diagnostic step?

The test of choice to confirm suspected nephrolithiasis is helical (spiral) CT scan of the abdomen without contrast. Many institutions also perform KUB (abdominal radiograph that includes the kidney, ureter, and bladder). KUB detects calcium, struvite, and cystine stones because they are radiopaque.

Note: KUB does not detect **U**ric acid stones because they are radiol**U**cent.

> **Intravenous pyelogram (IVP):** Inject IV contrast and obtain KUB. This test is more sensitive and specific than KUB alone, and it can detect all four types of stones. CT scan is usually preferred to IVP because CT is more accurate and does not use contrast.
>
> **Pregnant patients:** Avoid CT scan because of radiation exposure. The first diagnostic test is renal and pelvic ultrasound. If initial tests are negative, order transvaginal ultrasound. If ultrasound tests are negative but the patient has persistent suspicious symptoms, order IVP.

CT scan confirms the presence of two to three stones in the lower ureter, all <3 mm. KUB detects the stones as well (radioopaque).

What are the next steps in management?

Most stones <5 mm pass spontaneously, so initial therapy is conservative. Administer IV fluids and analgesics (opiates or IV nonsteroidal anti-inflammatory drugs (NSAIDs) such as ketorolac). Then discharge the patient and instruct him to drink plenty of fluids at home. Also ask him to strain his urine and bring any stones and gravel that pass for analysis.

> Indications for hospitalization and urgent urology consult in patients with nephrolithiasis (mnemonic: "***Stones Are Inside, Ouch!***"):
>
> 1. **S**evere pain unresponsive to analgesics
> 2. Acute postrenal failure/**A**nuria (due to obstruction)
> 3. **I**nfection of the urinary tract (fever, positive leukocyte esterase and nitrite)
> 4. **O**ral intake not tolerated

How would you manage stones that do not pass spontaneously?

If the stone does not pass within a few days (more common if size >5 mm), refer the patient to an urologist. The surgeon's first-line management of persistent stones depends on the size and location:

1. **Proximal ureter stones**: Extracorporeal shock wave lithotripsy (ESWL) if stone <10 mm, intracorporeal lithotripsy (with laser) if stone >10 mm.
2. **Mid-ureter stones**: intracorporeal lithotripsy (with laser).
3. **Distal ureter stones**: ESWL or intracorporeal lithotripsy.

> **ESWL**: Locate stone using ultrasound. Then pass shock waves from outside the body to break the stone. This method is not indicated for cystine stones.
> **Intracorporeal lithotripsy**: Pass ureteroscope close to the stone. Then use laser, basket with grasper, pneumatic, or electrical device at the tip of the scope to break/remove the stone.
> **Percutaneous nephrolithotomy**: This is usually second-line treatment if ESWL and/or intracorporeal lithotripsy is unsuccessful (exception: this is the first-line treatment for struvite stones).

The patient spontaneously passes three stones.

In addition to analysis of the stones, what work-up is recommended?

Patients with a family history of nephrolithiasis, multiple stones, or recurrent stones should undergo a complete evaluation to search for risk factors. Order the following tests in this patient with multiple stones:

1. Serum chemistries and serum uric acid
2. Urinalysis
3. Obtain 24-hour urine collection 2 to 3 months after the acute episode (measure urine volume, pH, and excretion of calcium, uric acid, citrate, oxalate, sodium, and creatinine).

> **Single uncomplicated kidney stone**: Follow-up recommendations are less clear; some physicians advocate a complete evaluation, whereas others recommend a limited evaluation.

> **Urine calcium/creatinine**: Ratio >0.3 indicates hypercalciuria. This measure is less accurate but more convenient than 24-hour urine collection.

Analysis of the stones indicates he had calcium phosphate stones.

What are the risk factors for calcium stones?

Risk factors for calcium stones are elevated urine calcium and oxalic acid, decreased urine citrate, and medullary sponge kidney:

1. **Causes of increased urine calcium (hypercalciuria):**
    - Hypercalcemia: causes secondary hypercalciuria (Chapter 8: Endocrinology)
    - Idiopathic hypercalciuria (stable serum Ca, increased urine Ca excretion)
2. **Causes of increased urine oxalic acid (increased risk of calcium oxalate stones):**
    - Severe malabsorption (Crohn's, bowel resection)
    - Excessive vitamin C
3. **Causes of decreased urine citrate:**
    - Chronic metabolic acidosis (diarrhea, carbonic anhydrase inhibitors)
    - Type 1 RTA (stable anion gap metabolic acidosis yet urine pH >5.5)

4. **Medullary sponge kidney**: Cystic dilation of collecting tubules is an idiopathic, asymptomatic condition usually detected incidentally on imaging. Patients have increased risk of calcium stones and UTIs, but otherwise the condition is benign.

> Citrate in urine normally binds calcium and prevents stone formation. Metabolic acidosis promotes citrate reabsorption.

Metabolic work-up is significant for elevated urine calcium. Serum calcium and all other labs are normal.

How can you prevent stone recurrence?

The evaluation indicates that the patient has idiopathic hypercalciuria. Prevent recurrent calcium stones in patients with increased urine calcium by prescribing thiazide diuretics and increased fluid intake.

> Increased fluid intake helps prevent recurrence of all four types of kidney stones.

> Preventing recurrent calcium stones in patients with other 24-hour urine abnormalities:
> **Increased uric acid**: Decreased protein (purine) intake and weight loss only if urine pH <6.0.
> **Decreased citrate**: Consider potassium citrate or potassium bicarbonate only if urine pH <6.0.
> **Increased oxalate**: Increased calcium (binds oxalate) and decreased oxalate intake only if urine calcium is not elevated.

Alternative 6.3.1

A patient with no past medical history presents with renal colic, hematuria, and urine pH of 4.8. CT scan identifies a 4-mm stone in the upper ureter. KUB is negative. He receives IV fluids and ketorolac and is discharged home. Twenty-four hours later, he passes a stone. Serum uric acid is elevated, and stone analysis reveals that he had a uric acid stone.

What are risk factors for uric acid stones?

Remember risk factors for uric acid stones with the mnemonic "***Gout Can Create Most Dreadful Colic***":

1. **G**out: This is a risk factor because of increased uric acid production or decreased excretion.
2. **C**ancer: Dying cells release uric acid.
3. **C**hemotherapy: Dying cells release uric acid.
4. **M**yeloproliferative disorders: Dying cells release uric acid.
5. **D**iabetes: This is a risk factor because it predisposes to acidic urine.
6. **C**hronic diarrhea: This is a risk factor because it predisposes to acidic urine.

> Excess uric acid also predisposes to calcium stones.

> Most uric acid stones occur in patients with no known risk factors, although metabolic evaluation often demonstrates abnormalities similar to primary gout such as elevated serum uric acid, decreased uric acid excretion, and low urine pH (<5.5).

How would you prevent recurrent uric acid stones in this patient?

Prevent recurrent stones with increased fluid intake (decreases urine uric acid concentration) and potassium citrate or potassium bicarbonate (maintains alkaline urine). If the patient has recurrent uric acid stones despite fluids and alkali, add allopurinol (prevents uric acid production) to the regimen.

Alternative 6.3.2

An 18-year-old man presents with a 10-hour history of renal colic. His father and a paternal uncle have a history of nephrolithiasis. Urinalysis is significant for hematuria and hexagonal crystals. CT scan and KUB demonstrate a 2-mm stone in the right upper ureter.

What is the most likely composition of this stone?

Positive family history and hexagonal crystals indicate that this patient has a cystine stone (Table 6-2). Cystine stones form in patients with a rare autosomal recessive disorder called hereditary cystinuria.

The patient receives fluids and ketorolac and is discharged home. He passes the stone 36 hours later. Stone analysis confirms the presence of a cystine stone. A 24-hour urine collection reveals increased urinary cystine.

What is the recommended therapy to prevent recurrence?

First-line therapy is increased fluid intake and urine alkalinization with potassium citrate or potassium bicarbonate. If the patient continues to have recurrent stones, consider cystine-binding drugs like tiopronin or penicillamine.

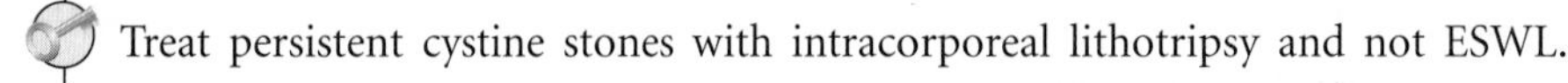

Treat persistent cystine stones with intracorporeal lithotripsy and not ESWL.

TABLE 6-2 Comparison of Different Types of Renal Stones

	Calcium	Uric Acid	Cystine	Struvite
Gender	Male > Female	Male > Female	Male > Female	Female > Male
Causes[a]	Increased urine calcium and oxalic acid, decreased urine citrate, and medullary sponge kidney	**G**out **C**an **C**reate **M**ost **D**readful **C**olic	Hereditary cystinuria (autosomal recessive)	Urinary tract infection with urease-producing bacteria
Urine pH[b]	5.5–7.0	<5.5	5.5–7.0	>7.0
Urine crystals	Calcium oxalate stones are needle-shaped or square envelope shape	Yellow-brown diamond or barrel shape	Hexagonal	Coffin-lid shape
KUB	Radiopaque	Radiolucent	Radiopaque	Radiopaque
Treatment	Fluids and analgesics; ESWL or intracorporeal lithotripsy if persistent.	Fluids and analgesics; ESWL or intracorporeal lithotripsy if persistent.	Fluids and analgesics; intracorporeal lithotripsy if persistent (not ESWL).	Percutaneous nephrolithotomy; antibiotics and potassium citrate if fragments persist.
Prophylaxis to prevent recurrences[a]	Thiazides (if increased urine calcium)	Allopurinol (if refractory to increased fluid intake and alkali)	Tiopronin or penicillamine (if refractory to increased fluid intake and alkali)	Treat urinary tract infections aggressively

Abbreviations: ESWL, extracorporeal shock wave lithotripsy; KUB, kidneys, ureter, bladder radiograph.

[a] Decreased fluid intake is a risk factor for all four types of stones, so increased fluid intake is recommended in all patients to prevent recurrences.

[b] In normal subjects, urine pH is usually 5.5–6.5.

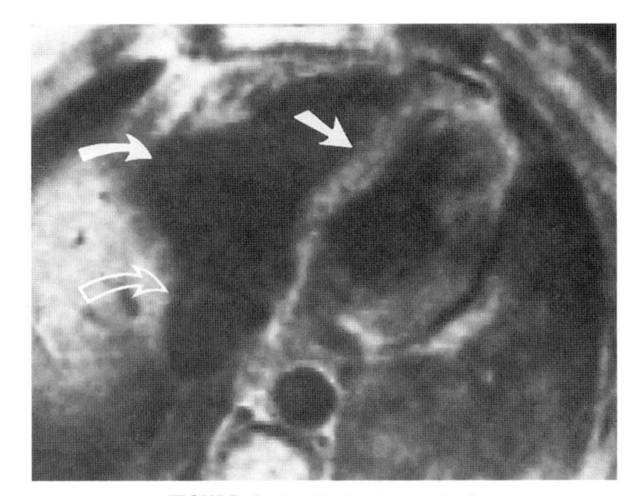

FIGURE 6–1 CT: Staghorn calculi.

Alternative 6.3.3

A 40-year-old woman presents to the clinic with mild flank pain. Past history is significant for UTIs. Urinalysis is significant for hematuria, urine pH of 7.6, positive leukocyte esterase and nitrite, and coffin lid–shaped crystals. Figure 6-1 is the patient's CT scan. Vital signs are normal.

What do the imaging findings demonstrate?

The CT scan and KUB demonstrate staghorn calculi (i.e., the calculi (stone) has an appearance like the horns of a deer;). These large stones involve the renal pelvis and at least two calyces and usually contain magnesium ammonium phosphate (struvite). Occasionally, staghorn calculi arise from calcium oxalate or calcium phosphate stones.

What causes struvite stones?

Struvite stones result from UTI due to urease-producing bacteria such as proteus (number one cause), klebsiella, and *Ureaplasma urealyticum* but not *E. coli* (do not produce urease). Urease breaks down urea to form ammonium; ammonium leads to an alkaline urine (pH > 7.0) and combines with magnesium phosphate to form struvite stones (also called infection stones, urease stones, or triple phosphate stones). Struvite stones tend to grow rapidly (weeks to months) into staghorn calculi.

How are struvite stones managed?

Medical management is usually insufficient. First-line treatment is percutaneous nephrolithotomy. If stone fragments persist 8 weeks later, administer antibiotics and potassium citrate (see Table 6-2).

> Percutaneous nephrolithotomy is recommended even for asymptomatic patients because untreated staghorn calculi can progress to septic shock and chronic renal failure.

CASE 6–4 FLANK PAIN AND HYPERTENSION IN A MIDDLE-AGED PATIENT

A 40-year-old woman presents with a 4-week history of flank pain. Past history is significant for UTIs. Her father and paternal grandfather died of kidney disease in their 50s. Blood pressure is 160/100. Other vital signs are normal. Urinalysis is significant for hematuria.

What diagnosis should you suspect?

Suspect adult polycystic kidney disease (PKD) (APKD) in this patient with chronic flank pain, hypertension, and a family history of renal failure in late adulthood. This autosomal dominant condition results from a mutation in the PKD-1 or PKD-2 gene.

> **Autosomal recessive PKD**: more severe than APKD; presents at birth or infancy.
> **Acquired PKD**: develops secondary to scarring in patients with end-stage renal disease (ESRD).

What are the clinical manifestations of APKD?

Patients are typically asymptomatic until adulthood. As cysts grow in size, they can cause any of the following renal manifestations:

1. **Hematuria**: Due to rupture of a cyst into urinary tract.
2. **Acute flank pain**: Results from cyst infection or hemorrhage into a cyst. APKD also predisposes to uric acid stones and pyelonephritis, which cause acute flank pain.
3. **Chronic flank/abdominal pain**: Enlarged kidney stretches renal capsule.
4. **Hypertension**: Enlarged cysts cause areas of renal ischemia. Renal ischemia activates increased renin release, which leads to hypertension.
5. **Renal insufficiency**: Most patients develop ESRD in their 50s or 60s.

APKD can also cause a number of extrarenal manifestations:

6. **Cerebral aneurysms**: May be asymptomatic or cause focal neurological deficits. The most dreaded risk is rupture with subsequent subarachnoid or intracerebral hemorrhage.
7. **Heart valve abnormalities**: Usually not clinically significant.
8. **Liver cysts**: Typically asymptomatic; sometimes, liver cysts can get infected.
9. **Diverticulosis**

What is the next diagnostic step?

The next step is to perform renal ultrasound or CT scan. The presence of multiple kidney cysts (bilateral or unilateral) confirms the diagnosis. Imaging may also detect enlarged kidneys.

Renal ultrasound confirms the diagnosis. How is APKD managed?

There is currently no specific therapy for APKD. Management involves prevention and treatment of complications:

1. **Intractable flank/abdominal pain**: Consider surgical drainage for patients with severe pain unresponsive to opioid analgesics.
2. **Nephrolithiasis and pyelonephritis**: Refer to Cases 6-2 and 6-3.
3. **Hypertension**: Attempt to maintain blood pressure $\leq$120/80. Angiotensin-converting enzyme (ACE) inhibitors are the first-line antihypertensives in patients with APKD.
4. **Cerebral aneurysm**: Perform CT angiography or magnetic resonance angiography to screen for cerebral aneurysms in the following patients:
   - All symptomatic patients (focal neurological deficits)
   - Asymptomatic patients with family history of ruptured aneurysm
   - Asymptomatic patients who require anticoagulation
5. **Infected liver/kidney cysts**: Suspect if a patient develops fever and flank pain or RUQ pain. Diagnose with CT scan. Treat with surgical drainage and antimicrobial drugs.
6. **Renal insufficiency**: Refer to Case 6-5.

> APKD does not increase the risk of polycystic ovarian syndrome.

> Flank pain results from a ***SICC*** kidney (kidney **S**tones, **I**nfection, **C**ysts, or **C**ancer).

Alternative 6.4.1

A 40-year-old woman is involved in a motor vehicle accident. CT scan incidentally detects two cysts in the right kidney. The cysts are fluid-filled with thin walls and regular margins.

What is the next step in management?

The description is characteristic of simple renal cysts, which may be unilateral or bilateral. Simple cysts are the most common kidney mass. These benign lesions are usually detected incidentally. No further work-up is necessary. Most cysts are asymptomatic. Occasionally they cause flank/abdominal pain (treat with acetaminophen or NSAIDs), infection (treat with antimicrobials and drainage), or hypertension (treat with ACE inhibitors).

> If there are any uncharacteristic findings on CT or ultrasound (thickened walls, irregular margins, contrast enhancement), order magnetic resonance imaging with contrast to rule out malignancy. Suspicious lesions on magnetic resonance imaging require surgical consultation.

CASE 6–5 ACUTE ELEVATION IN BLOOD UREA NITROGEN AND SERUM CREATININE

A 60-year-old woman presents to her primary care physician with chronic knee pain. She has a history of diabetes and hypertension. Medications include insulin and enalapril. Her physician recommends an ice pack. She presents 1 week later for a follow-up appointment. The ice pack was not helpful, so she has been taking increasing amounts of naproxen for pain relief. Physical exam is significant for 2+ lower extremity pitting edema. Vital signs are normal. Abnormal serum chemistries are potassium 5.2 mEq/L, blood urea nitrogen (BUN) 74 mg/dL, and serum creatinine 3.2 mg/dL. Last week, BUN and serum creatinine were 27 mg/dL and 2.0 mg/dL, respectively; 3 months ago, BUN and serum creatinine were 25 mg/dL and 2.0 mg/dL, respectively.

What do elevated BUN and serum creatinine indicate?

Elevated serum creatinine and BUN indicate reduced glomerular filtration rate (GFR). Of the two, serum creatinine is more helpful because BUN can increase independent of GFR in patients with increased dietary protein intake and increased catabolism (steroids, surgery, infection, etc.). A slow increase in serum creatinine over months or years indicates chronic renal insufficiency (CRI), also called chronic kidney disease (CKD). A rapid increase in serum creatinine $\geq$0.5 mg/dL in $\leq$2 weeks indicates acute renal failure (ARF). This patient has ARF superimposed on underlying CKD.

> Research criteria for ARF:
>
> **All patients**: Serum creatinine increases by $\geq$0.5 mg/dL in $\leq$2 weeks.
> **Baseline creatinine >2.5 mg/dL**: Serum creatinine increases by $\geq$20% in $\leq$2 weeks.

> Increased serum creatinine occurs after >50% of nephrons are destroyed.

What are the clinical manifestations of acute and chronic renal failure?

Many patients present with asymptomatic azotemia. Others may present with any of the signs, symptoms, or laboratory abnormalities of uremia (Table 6-3).

> **Azotemia**: elevated BUN and serum creatinine.
> **Uremia**: azotemia + signs and symptoms due to nitrogenous waste accumulation. Initial clinical manifestations are often nonspecific (nausea, vomiting, fatigue, etc.). Uremia is more common in CRI but can occur in ARF as well.

What are the causes of ARF?

There are three broad categories of ARF (Table 6-4):

TABLE 6-3 Clinical Manifestations of Uremia

General	1. **Fatigue:** A major cause of fatigue is *anemia*. Renal failure leads to anemia because the kidney cannot produce sufficient erythropoietin. 2. **Uremic fetor:** Toxic metabolites give breath ammonia-like smell.
Neuro	1. **Encephalopathy:** Toxic metabolites enter the central nervous system and lead to asterixis and altered mental status. 2. **Peripheral neuropathy:** Pain and paresthesia in lower extremities; mechanism is unclear.
ENT	1. **Red eye:** Mechanism is unclear. 2. **Nosebleeds:** Uremia leads to *thrombocytopenia*.
CV	1. **Uremic pericarditis:** Signs and symptoms of pericarditis are present but there is no characteristic diffuse ST elevation on EKG; cause is unclear. 2. **Arrhythmias:** Because of electrolyte and acid–base disturbances. 3. **Pre-existing heart failure and hypertension worsen:** The kidney cannot excrete sufficient fluid.
Lungs	1. **Pulmonary edema:** The kidney cannot excrete sufficient fluid.
Gastrointestinal	1. **Nausea, vomiting, anorexia:** Cause is unclear but symptoms can lead to malnutrition (*hypoalbuminemia*). 2. **Occult gastrointestinal bleeding:** Another cause of *anemia* in renal failure, toxic metabolites cause erosive gastritis and colitis; uremia also leads to *thrombocytopenia* (increased risk of mucosal bleeding).
Skin	1. **Uremic frost:** Sweat contains excess urea; when sweat evaporates, a powdery white residue remains on skin. 2. **Pruritis:** The kidney cannot remove excess calcium phosphate, which deposits on skin and leads to itching. 3. **Hyperpigmentation and velvety skin**
Extremities	1. **Peripheral edema:** The kidney cannot excrete sufficient fluid.
MSK pain	1. **Muscle cramps:** The kidney cannot excrete normal potassium load, which leads to *hyperkalemia* (responsible for muscle cramps). 2. **Renal osteodystrophy:** The kidney cannot hydroxylate vitamin D. Decreased hydroxylated vitamin D leads to decreased calcium absorption from the gastrointestinal tract. *Hypocalcemia* activates secondary hyperparathyroidism, which leads to bone resorption and *hyperphosphatemia*.
Endocrine	1. **Impotence and infertility:** Production of sex hormone is decreased. 2. **Glucose control:** Kidney clearance of insulin is decreased, so hyperglycemia normalizes in diabetics; however, diabetics have increased risk of hypoglycemic episodes.
Acid–base	1. ***Anion gap metabolic acidosis*:** The kidney cannot regulate metabolic acid–base balance so lactic acid, phosphate, etc., accumulate.

Abbreviation: MSK, musculoskeletal.

Note: Laboratory abnormalities are italicized (anemia, hypoalbuminemia, thrombocytopenia, hyperkalemia, hypocalcemia, hyperphosphatemia, anion gap metabolic acidosis).

1. Prerenal failure (60% to 70%): caused by decreased blood flow to the kidney.
2. Intrinsic renal failure (25% to 40%): caused by damage to the renal parenchyma.
3. Postrenal failure (5% to 10%): caused by obstruction of the urinary outflow tract.

Intrinsic renal failure is categorized on the basis of primary site of injury:

1. **Acute tubular necrosis (85%)**: renal tubule damage.
2. **Acute interstitial nephritis (10%)**: immune-mediated renal interstitial damage.
3. **Acute glomerulonephritis (5%)**: glomerular damage (refer to Case 6-5)
4. **Microvascular ARF (uncommon)**

TABLE 6-4 Major Causes of Acute Renal Failure

PRERENAL FAILURE	
Hypovolemia	Hemorrhage, third spacing (pancreatitis, burns, etc.), vomiting, diarrhea, or decreased fluid intake
Systemic vasodilation	Septic shock, general anesthesia
Decreased cardiac output	Congestive heart failure
Renal vasoconstriction	Hepatorenal syndrome and contrast dyes
Macrovascular disease	RAS, malignant hypertension, emboli (from atherosclerosis, cholesterol, endocarditis)
Drugs	• **N**SAIDs: prostaglandin (a vasodilator) inhibition • **A**CE inhibitors/ARBs: angiotensin II (a vasoconstrictor) inhibition. Vasodilation in the setting of hypovolemia or RAS can decrease renal perfusion. • **T**acrolimus, **C**yclosporine: cause renal vasoconstriction • **D**iuretics: cause hypovolemia
ACUTE TUBULAR NECROSIS	
Ischemia	Progression of prerenal disease
Toxins	• Pigments: myoglobinuria (secondary to rhabdomyolysis), hemoglobinuria (secondary to hemolysis) • Drugs: **A**minoglycosides, **C**isplatin, **A**mphotericin • Contrast dyes • Proteins (e.g., light-chain proteins in multiple myeloma) • Crystals (most commonly uric acid crystals)
ACUTE INTERSTITIAL NEPHRITIS (acronym to remember causes is *A(a)I(i)N*)	
Allergy to drug	Most common drugs are **P**enicillins, **A**llopurinol, **C**ephalosporins, **C**iprofloxacin, **R**ifampin, **S**ulfonamides such as TMP/SMX, **N**SAIDs.
Autoimmune disorders	Systemic lupus erythematosus, etc.
Infection	Bacterial or viral
Infiltration	Sarcoidosis, etc.
Neoplasms	
MICROVASCULAR ARF: TTP/HUS, HELLP syndrome, vasculitis	
ACUTE GLOMERULONEPHRITIS: Discussed in Case 7.	
POSTRENAL FAILURE: BPH, prostate and cervical cancers, neurogenic bladder (bladder nerve damage due to diabetes, spinal cord injury, etc., causes loss of voluntary voiding)	

Abbreviations: ACE, angiotensin-converting enzyme; AIN, acute interstitial nephritis; ARB, angiotensin receptor blocker; ARF, acute renal failure; ATN, acute tubular necrosis; BPH, benign prostatic hyperplasia; HELLP, obstetric complication (hemolytic anemia, elevated liver enzymes, and low platelet count); HUS, hemolytic uremic syndrome; NSAID, nonsteroidal anti-inflammatory drug; RAS, renal artery stenosis; TMP/SMX, trimethroprim/sulfamethoxazole; TTP, thrombotic thrombocytopenic purpura.

Notes:

1. Contrast dyes can cause prerenal failure or ATN.
2. NSAIDs can cause prerenal failure or AIN.
3. Cephalosporins, TMP/SMX can cause AIN or false-positive increased serum creatinine.
4. Drug mnemonics:

- Prerenal failure: *"**NAT** **C**ole **D**ied **PRE**maturely."*
- ATN: *"**Aminoglycosides** **C**ause **A**TN."*
- AIN: *"**P**enicillin **A**llergies **C**an **C**ause **R**eally **S**evere **N**ephritis."*

What is the next diagnostic step?

Order the following tests to determine the category of renal failure (Table 6-5):

1. **Blood**: complete blood count, culture, and chemistries.
2. **Urine**: urinalysis, osmolality, sodium, fractional sodium excretion (FeNa), and creatinine.

TABLE 6–5 Laboratory Findings in ARF

URINE AND SERUM LABS

	Prerenal ARF	Intrinsic ARF	Postrenal ARF
Urine osmolality	>500 mOsm/kg	<500 mOsm/kg	<500 mOsm/kg
FeNa	<1%	>1%	<1% (early) >1% (few days)
Urine sodium	<20 mEq/L	>20 mEq/L	<20 mEq/L (early) >20 mEq/L (few days)
Urine volume	Oliguria	Oliguria or normal	Oliguria or anuria
Serum BUN/creatinine	>20	<20	<20

Abbreviations: BUN, blood urea nitrogen; FeNa, fractional sodium excretion.
Notes:
1. **Urine volume**: Normal, 400 mL/day; oliguria, 100–400 mL/day; anuria, <100 mL/day.
2. **Complete blood count**: Thrombocytopenia and hemolytic anemia are seen in TTP/HUS and HELLP syndrome, and increased eosinophils are seen in AIN.
3. **Acute glomerulonephritis, contrast-induced ATN**: FeNa is often <1%.

URINE DIPSTICK

Type of ARF	Dipstick Protein	Dipstick Blood	Specific Gravity
Prerenal	–	–	>1.02
ATN[a]	Trace	–	1.01–1.02
AIN	+	+	1.01–1.02
Glomerulonephritis	++	++	1.01–1.02
Postrenal	–	–	

URINE SEDIMENT

Benign sediment: Normal patients; prerenal and postrenal ARF.

Hyaline casts: Nonspecific, clear, cylindrical casts made up of Tamm-Horsfall protein.

Granular casts: Nonspecific marker of kidney damage.

Muddy brown casts: Coarse, granular, pigmented, cigar-shaped casts indicate ATN.

Broad or waxy casts: Wide casts with cracked edges indicate advanced ATN.

Pigment casts: Reddish gold casts indicate myoglobinuria or hemoglobinuria.

Fatty casts: Hyaline casts with yellow fat globules that appear as a "Maltese cross" under polarized light indicate nephrotic syndrome.

WBC casts: Casts with WBCs indicate inflammation (pyelonephritis, AIN, GN).

RBC casts: Casts with RBCs indicate glomerulonephritis.

Dysmorphic RBCs: Indicate glomerulonephritis; also seen in TTP/HUS.

Hansel's stain: Stains eosinophils bright red; positive stain indicates AIN.

Abbreviations: GN, glomerulonephritis; RBC, red blood cells; WBC, white blood cells.
[a] **ATN due to rhabdomyolysis**: Urine may be red, but supernatant and sediment are clear. Urine dipstick is positive for blood in 50% of cases, but no RBCs are found on sediment analysis. Key laboratory finding is increased creatinine kinase. **ATN due to hemolysis**: Urine may be red and supernatant is red, but sediment is clear. Urine dipstick is positive for blood, but no RBCs are found on sediment analysis.

3. **Bladder catheterization**: Suspect postrenal obstruction if a large volume of urine flows on inserting the catheter. This maneuver is also therapeutic.

A large volume of urine does not flow upon insertion of the bladder catheter. Complete blood count is within normal limits. Urine osmolality is 700 mOsm/kg, urine sodium is 12 mEq/L,

FeNa is 0.6%, serum BUN/creatinine is 23. Urine output is 10 mL/hour (240 mL/day). Urine dipstick findings are specific gravity 1.025 and no protein or blood. Urine sediment reveals few hyaline casts. Hansel's stain is negative.

What is the cause of ARF?

The laboratory findings indicate that the patient has prerenal ARF (see Table 6-5). The kidneys reabsorb sodium and water as if in response to volume depletion, so urine osmolality and specific gravity are high while FeNa and urine sodium are low. Also, BUN is reabsorbed out of proportion to decrease in GFR, so the ratio is high (>20).

What are the next steps in management?

General measures in all types of ARF are as follows:

1. Fluids and electrolytes: Correct any imbalances if present.
2. Nephrotoxins: Discontinue nephrotoxic agents.
3. Nutrition: Provide adequate calories; restrict protein and potassium.
4. Infection: Minimize indwelling lines and catheters to decrease infection risk.

This patient with pitting edema and oliguria should receive loop diuretics. Also, administer Kayexalate to treat hyperkalemia. Eliminate the offending agent, which in this case is the recently initiated NSAID. Do not discontinue the ACE inhibitor at this time because it improves mortality in patients with hypertension and diabetes, and renal function was stable on the ACE inhibitor prior to initiating ibuprofen.

Fluid imbalances:

Volume depletion: Suspect if the patient has hypotension/orthostatic hypotension, tachycardia, dry mucous membranes, and weight loss. Treat with normal saline.
Volume overload: Suspect if the patient has weight gain, peripheral/pulmonary edema, or urine output <1mL/kg per hour. Treat with loop diuretics such as furosemide (lasix).

Electrolyte imbalances in ARF:

Hyperkalemia and metabolic acidosis: Most common electrolyte abnormalities.
Hypo- or hypernatremia: Also common abnormalities.

What are the indications for urgent dialysis?

Urgent dialysis is indicated in the following settings ("***AEIOU***"):

1. **A**cidosis (metabolic): pH remains <7.1 despite treatment.
2. **E**lectrolytes: Hyperkalemia or sodium imbalances persist despite treatment.
3. **I**ntoxication with a dialyzable toxin (lithium, methanol, or ethylene glycol).
4. **O**verload of volume (peripheral or pulmonary edema) refractory to diuretics.
5. **U**remic pericarditis, encephalopathy, or bleeding.

Alternative 6.5.1

A 57-year-old woman with insulin-dependent type 2 diabetes presents to her primary care physician with acute onset of left lower quadrant pain. She undergoes CT scan with iodinated contrast (an ionic contrast agent) to rule out diverticulitis. Baseline BUN and serum creatinine are 25 mg/dL and 2.0 mg/dL, respectively. BUN and serum creatinine 5 hours later are 30 mg/dL and 3.5 mg/dL. Vital signs are normal. A large volume of urine does not flow upon insertion of a bladder catheter. Complete blood count is normal. Urine osmolality is 200 mOsm/kg, urine sodium is 25 mEq/L, FeNa is 0.6%, and serum BUN/creatinine is 8.5. Urine output is 40 mL/hour. Urine dipstick findings are specific gravity 1.012, trace protein, and no blood. Urine sediment reveals few granular casts. Hansel's stain is negative.

What is the cause of ARF?

This patient has intrinsic ARF (see Table 6-5). The most likely cause is ATN from the contrast agent. Contrast nephropathy can cause nonoliguric ARF within 12 to 24 hours of administration, particularly in patients with underlying chronic renal failure like this patient.

How is intrinsic renal failure treated?

As with other types of ARF, monitor for and treat any fluid and electrolyte imbalances, discontinue nephrotoxins, provide adequate nutrition, and minimize infection risk. Most patients with contrast nephropathy recover in 3 to 5 days.

> Measures to prevent contrast nephropathy if baseline creatinine is $\geq$1.5:
> 1. IV normal saline and N-acetylcysteine before and after contrast administration.
> 2. Avoid high osmolality ionic contrast (use nonionic agents such as gadolinium instead).

Alternative 6.5.2

A 28-year-old fireman is brought to the hospital after being rescued from the rubble of a collapsed building. On exam, mucous membranes are dry. Vital signs are temperature 37.5°C, blood pressure 98/60, pulse 120 bpm, respirations 25/min. Abnormal serum chemistries are potassium 5.9 mEq/L, BUN 80 mg/dL, creatinine 6.0 mg/dL, bicarbonate 18 mg/dL, and calcium 6.5 mg/dL. A large volume of urine does not flow upon insertion of a bladder catheter. Complete blood count is normal. Urine osmolality is 150 mOsm/kg, urine sodium is 30 mEq/L, FeNa is 3%. Urine output is 6 mL/hour (140 ml/day). Urine is red. Urine dipstick findings are specific gravity 1.013, trace protein, and 2+ blood. Urine sediment and supernatant are clear. Sediment analysis reveals reddish gold as well as muddy brown casts but no red blood cells (RBCs).

What is the cause of ARF?

The patient has intrinsic renal failure due to ATN. The cause of ATN is rhabdomyolysis (see Table 6-5). Crush injuries cause skeletal muscle breakdown (rhabdomyolysis). Muscle breakdown leads to release of myoglobin, potassium, uric acid, and phosphate from cells. Myoglobin spills into urine and causes ATN.

> Not all cases of rhabdomyolysis result in ARF.
> Patients with advanced ARF due to rhabdomyolysis may not have myoglobinuria.

What are the major causes of rhabdomyolysis in adults?

1. **Trauma**: crush injuries, burns, electrical shock, surgery, excessive physical exertion, and coma (local muscle compression).
2. **High fever**: malignant hyperthermia, neuroleptic malignant syndrome.
3. **Toxins/drugs**: alcohol, lovastatin, etc.

What fluid and electrolyte abnormalities commonly occur in rhabdomyolysis?

1. **Hyperkalemia, hyperphosphatemia, hyperuricemia**
2. **Metabolic acidosis**: because cells release phosphate and uric acid.
3. **Hypocalcemia**: because phosphate binds to calcium.
4. **Hypovolemia**: because plasma water gets sequestered in injured myocytes.

What are the next steps in management?

1. Order creatinine kinase: increased creatinine kinase confirms the diagnosis.
2. Fluids: Administer normal saline to all patients with rhabdomyolysis (even if normovolemic) to stimulate diuresis. Patients often require a large volume of fluids. If urine output is not sufficient, consider mannitol to stimulate diuresis.

3. Correct any electrolyte imbalances, particularly hyperkalemia. Provide adequate nutrition and minimize infection risk. Remember indications for urgent dialysis.

> **Hypercalcemia**: may develop after ARF resolves because the kidney produces increased vitamin D.

Alternative 6.5.3

A 48-year-old woman with hypertension and osteoarthritis presents to the clinic with fever and malaise. She recently completed a course of amoxicillin for streptococcal pharyngitis. Two weeks ago, she started taking lisinopril. She also takes ibuprofen off and on to control symptoms of arthritis. Physical exam is significant for a rash. Temperature is 38.4°C, pulse 70 bpm, blood pressure 120/80, respirations 12/min. Abnormal serum chemistries are BUN 26 mg/dL and serum creatinine 2.5 mg/dL. Complete blood count is significant for increased eosinophils. Urine osmolality is 110 mOsm/kg, urine sodium is 40 mEq/L, FeNa is 2%. Urine dipstick findings are specific gravity 1.011, 1+ protein, and 1+ blood. Sediment analysis reveals hyaline casts. Hansel's stain is positive.

What is the cause of ARF?

This patient has a number of risk factors for ARF. Lisinopril and ibuprofen can cause prerenal failure. Streptococcal infection, amoxicillin, and ibuprofen can cause acute interstitial nephritis (AIN) (see Table 6-4). Fever, rash, and laboratory findings indicate that the cause of ARF is AIN (see Table 6-5).

> **Classic triad of AIN**: Fever, rash, and eosinophilia/eosinophiluria. Only 10% of AIN presents with classic triad. Triad is most common in penicillin-induced AIN.

What is the next step in management?

This patient does not appear to have any fluid and electrolyte imbalances, so the next step is to discontinue offending medications (amoxicillin and ibuprofen). Most patients will recover in 3 to 5 days.

Amoxicillin and ibuprofen are discontinued. Three days later, creatinine is 2.8 mg/dL.

What is the next step in management?

If azotemia persists or increases after 3 to 5 days in patients with suspected AIN, perform renal biopsy to confirm the diagnosis. If biopsy confirms AIN, consider treatment with oral or IV steroids.

> **NSAID-induced AIN**: Studies have not shown any benefit from steroids.

Alternative 6.5.4

A 60-year-old, previously healthy man presents with a chief complaint of difficulty with urination. He has not been able to urinate in the last 48 hours. He does not take any medications. On physical exam, the bladder feels distended. Vitals signs are normal. Serum chemistries are significant for BUN 30 mg/dL and serum creatinine 2.7 mg/dL. A large volume of urine flows on insertion of a bladder catheter.

What is the next step in management?

ARF is most likely caused by postrenal obstruction in this patient with anuria, distended bladder, and withdrawal of copious urine on bladder catheterization. The next step is to confirm the diagnosis with renal ultrasound, which should demonstrate hydronephrosis. If ultrasound confirms the diagnosis, identify and treat the underlying cause. If ultrasound is not diagnostic, obtain urine and serum labs to rule out prerenal and intrinsic ARF. As with all other types of

ARF, correct any fluid or electrolyte imbalances, discontinue nephrotoxins, provide adequate nutrition, and minimize infection risk. Remember the indications for urgent dialysis ("***AEIOU***").

CASE 6–6 AN ASYMPTOMATIC PATIENT WITH REDDISH-BROWN URINE

A 60-year-old patient reports that he noticed his urine was reddish-brown yesterday and the day before. He is otherwise asymptomatic. He does not take any medications. He has a 30-pack/year history of smoking. Physical exam and vital signs are normal.

What is the next step in management?

Red, brown, or pink urine suggests the patient has increased RBCs in his urine (hematuria). However, myoglobin, hemoglobin, and other pigments can also cause red, brown, or pink urine (Fig. 6-2). The next step in management is urinalysis. Examine the color of the supernatant and sediment, check the urine dipstick and assess for the presence of RBCs on sediment microscopy (see Fig. 6-2).

Microscopic hematuria: Urine is clear; $\geq$3 RBCs/high-powered field (HPF) on urinalysis.
Gross hematuria: Urine is pink, red, or brown. Urinalysis detects $\geq$3 RBCs/HPF.
Pseudohematuria: Urine is pink, red, or brown, but sediment is clear with <3 RBCs/HPF.

Urine dipstick: sensitive but not specific for hematuria.

Urine sediment is red and microscopy detects 10 RBCs/HPF.

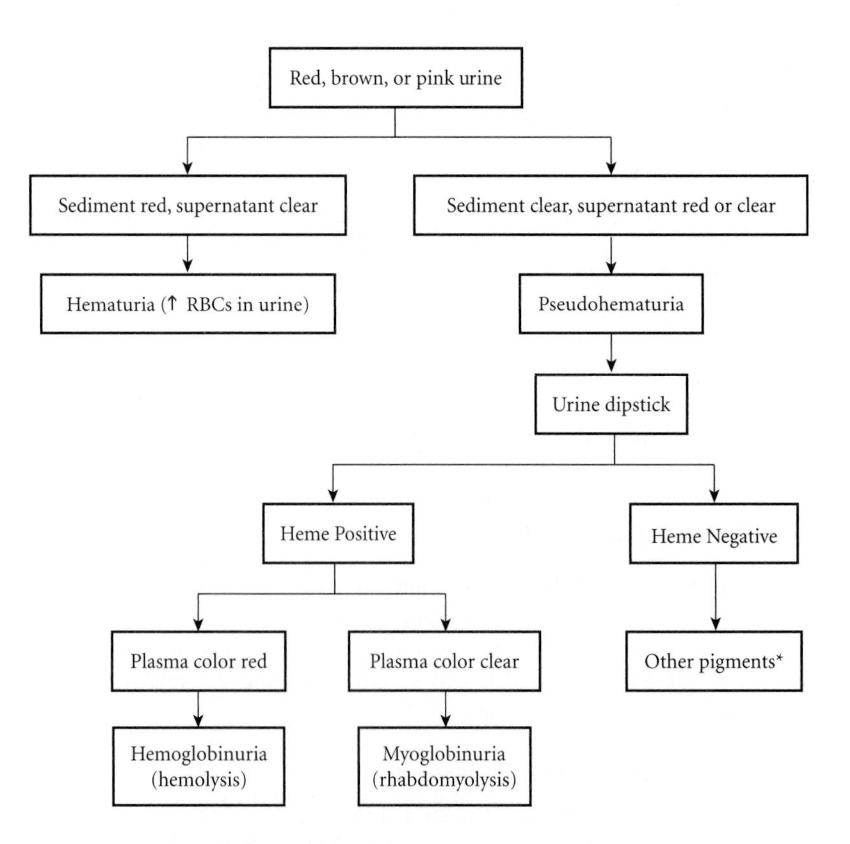

* Other pigments responsible for pseudohematuria are medications (rifampin, phenytoin, phenolphthalein laxatives), foods (beetroot, blackberries, excess vitamin C intake), and porphyrins (porphyria).

FIGURE 6–2 Approach to patients with red, brown or pink urine.

TABLE 6–6 Key Features of Major Urological Cancers

KIDNEY CANCERS	
Epidemiology	Major kidney cancers are RCC (80%–85%) and renal transitional cell carcinoma (10%).
Origin	• RCC originates in the renal cortex • Renal transitional cell carcinoma originates in renal pelvis
Clinical presentation	• Most common initial presentation is painless hematuria (transient or persistent). • <10% of patients present with the classic triad (hematuria, flank pain, palpable abdominal or flank mass). • Advanced disease can present with fever, weight loss, anemia of chronic disease, and paraneoplastic syndromes (hypercalcemia (ectopic PTH), polycythemia (ectopic EPO), Cushing syndrome (ectopic cortisol)).
Diagnostic tests	First test is renal ultrasound or CT scan of the abdomen. If imaging suggests RCC or renal transitional cell carcinoma, perform nephrectomy or partial nephrectomy to confirm the diagnosis histologically.
Screening for RCC	Screening ultrasound or CT scan is recommended only for the following: • Patients with Von Hippel Lindau syndrome or tuberous sclerosis. • Young patients with end-stage renal disease on dialysis for >3 years. • Patients with family history of RCC or personal history of radiation.
BLADDER CANCER	
Epidemiology	Bladder cancer is more common than kidney cancer. 90% of bladder cancer cases are transitional cell carcinomas; 10% of cases are squamous cell carcinoma and adenocarcinoma.
Clinical presentation	• Most common initial presentation is painless hematuria (transient or persistent). • Second most frequent finding is chronic urinary frequency, urgency, and dysuria. • Advanced disease can present with abdominal or flank pain and constitutional symptoms (fever, weight loss, etc.).
Diagnostic tests	Key diagnostic test is cystoscopy with biopsy.

Abbreviations: CT, computed tomography; EPO, erythropoietin; PTH, parathyroid hormone; RCC, renal cell carcinoma.
Note: Patients with renal and bladder cancer tend to present at a late stage so overall prognosis is poor.

What is the differential diagnosis of hematuria?

1. Kidneys:
   - Parenchymal disease (glomerulonephropathy or interstitial nephritis): Suspect glomerulonephropathy if urinalysis detects proteinuria, RBC casts, or dysmorphic RBCs; suspect interstitial nephritis if urinalysis detects pyuria and mild proteinuria.
   - Kidney infection (pyelonephritis, renal and perinephric abscess)
   - Kidney stones
   - Kidney cysts
   - Renal papillary necrosis
2. Bladder: lower UTI (cystitis) and hemorrhagic cystitis.
3. Prostate: prostate cancer (rare), BPH, and prostatitis.
4. Urinary tract cancers (kidney or bladder) (Table 6-6)
5. Bleeding disorders or anticoagulants (e.g., warfarin)
6. Trauma or strenuous exercise are benign, transient causes of hematuria.

Patients on chronic anticoagulation: Do not assume hematuria is due to warfarin without excluding other causes first.

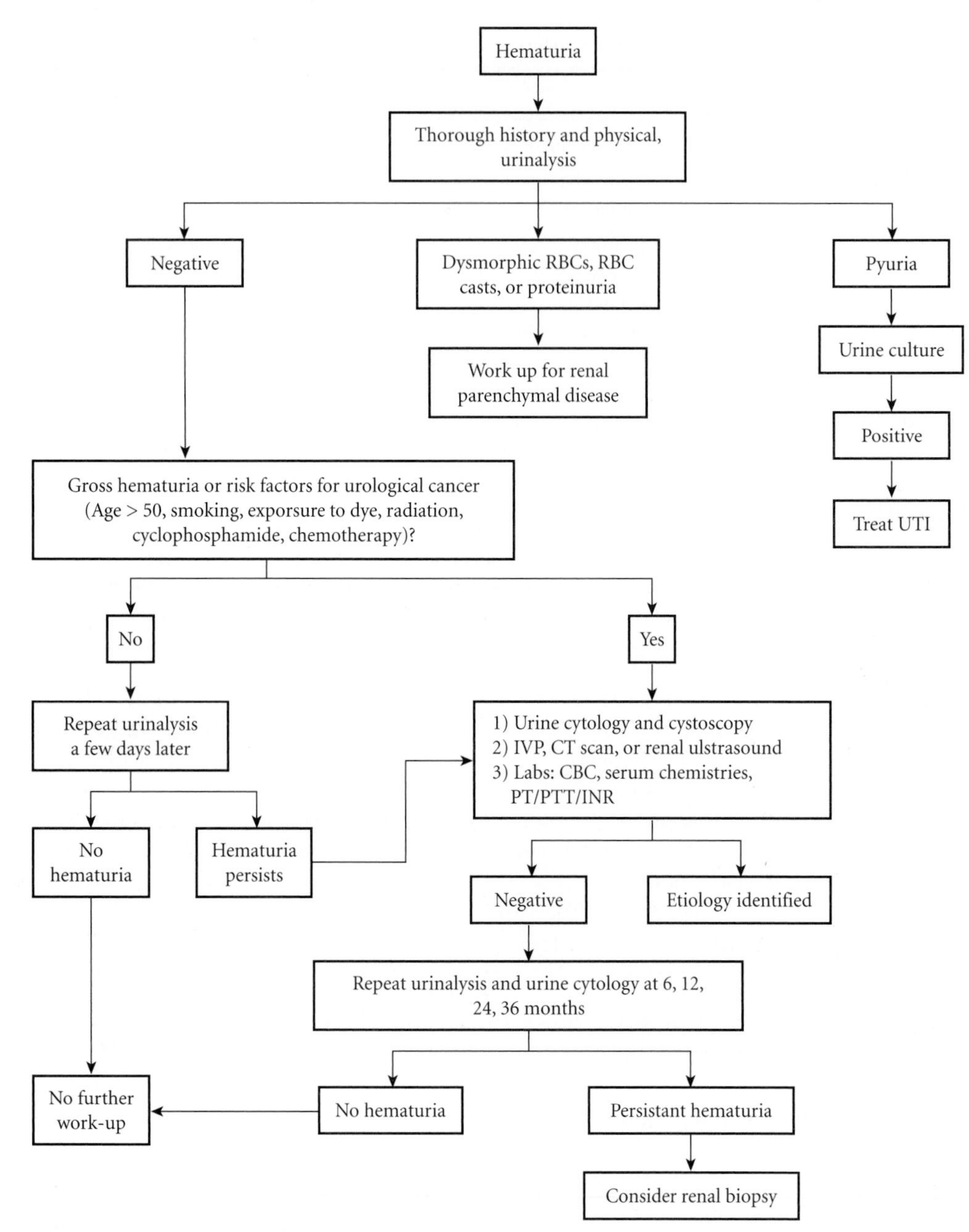

FIGURE 6–3 Approach to patients with hematuria.

Urine dipstick is negative for protein. No RBC casts, dysmorphic RBCs, or WBCs are evident on urine microscopy.

What is the next step in management?

A thorough diagnostic evaluation is indicated in the following patients with asymptomatic hematuria and no identifiable cause on urinalysis (Fig. 6-3):

1. All patients with gross hematuria
2. Gross or microscopic hematuria in patients any risk factor for a urological cancer

Risk factors for urinary tract cancers:

1. Age > 50 years
2. Cigarette smoking
3. Chemicals: exposure to aromatic amines or benzenes (used in dye industry)
4. History of radiation therapy or chemotherapy with cyclophosphamide/ifosfamide

Alternative 6.6.1

Urinalysis in a 33-year-old asymptomatic woman incidentally detects positive urine dipstick for heme and 5 RBCs/HPF. There is no pyuria, proteinuria, RBC casts, or dysmorphic RBCs. Her urine is clear, and she ran a marathon the day before. Past medical history is noncontributory. Physical exam and vital signs are normal.

What is the next step in management?

This asymptomatic patient does not have gross hematuria or risk factors for urological cancers. Urinalysis does not indicate any specific causes. The most likely diagnosis is exercise-induced hematuria. The next step is to repeat the urinalysis a few days later to determine whether hematuria is transient or persistent. If hematuria persists on follow-up examination, perform a full diagnostic work-up. On the other hand, if there is no hematuria on follow-up, further work-up is unnecessary (Fig. 6-3).

Menstrual blood: can cause false-positive hematuria in women.

Cystoscopy for persistent hematuria but no risk factors for urological cancer: Some physicians recommend cystoscopy only if urine cytology is suspicious, whereas others recommend cystoscopy regardless of cytology.

Causes of other urine colors (rare):

1. **White urine**: pyuria, phosphate crystals
2. **Green urine**: medications (amitriptyline, methylene blue, propofol)
3. **Black urine**: ochronosis or malignancy

Ochronosis (hereditary alkaptonuria): This autosomal recessive defect in homogentisic acid oxidase leads to excess tyrosine and phenylanine byproduct deposits in skin, cartilage, and eyes. Clinical manifestations include black urine or earwax, skin pigmentation, arthritis, and grey-brown spot in sclera. Treatment is to avoid foods that contain phenylalanine or tyrosine.

CASE 6–7 REDDISH-BROWN URINE, HYPERTENSION, AND EDEMA

An 18-year-old man presents with a 2-day history of reddish-brown urine. He was diagnosed with streptococcal pharyngitis 2 weeks ago (treated with amoxicillin). Physical exam is significant for 2+ bilateral peripheral edema. Blood pressure is 160/100. Other vital signs are normal. Urine dipstick detects 3+ blood and 1+ protein. Urine sediment reveals 12 RBCs/HPF, RBC casts, and dysmorphic RBCs.

What is the diagnosis?

Hematuria, proteinuria, dysmorphic RBCs, and RBC casts indicate glomerular injury (glomerulonephropathy). There are two clinical patterns of glomerular injury:

1. **Nephritic (glomerular inflammation)**: Inflammation of <50% of glomeruli leads to focal nephritis. More extensive inflammation leads to nephritic syndrome.
2. **Nephrotic (increased permeability but no inflammation)**: Proteinuria and lipiduria but no RBC casts or dysmorphic RBCs. Severe damage leads to nephrotic syndrome.

Focal nephritis: gross or microscopic hematuria, RBC casts, dysmorphic RBCs, 1+ proteinuria.
Nephritic syndrome: focal nephritis plus hypertension, edema, and renal insufficiency; can cause CRI and ARF. Mnemonic is "***PHAROH***" (**P**roteinuria, **H**ematuria, **A**zotemia, **R**BCs (RBC casts and dysmorphic RBCs), **O**liguria, and **H**ypertension).
Nephrotic syndrome: >3.5 g/day of proteinuria leads to hypoalbuminemia, edema (due to sodium retention), hyperlipidemia (liver's response to decreased oncotic pressure), fatty casts (due to lipiduria), hypercoagulable state (decreased clotting cascade

proteins), and increased infections (decreased immunoglobulin proteins). Can cause CRI; infrequently causes ARF.

Urine dipstick protein: trace = 50 to 150 mg/day, 1+ = 150 to 500 mg/day, 2+ = 500 to 2000 mg/day, 3+ = 2 to 5 g/day, 4+ = >5 g/day.

What is the next diagnostic step?

Obtain serum chemistries (to determine if the patient has azotemia) and 24-hour urine collection (to quantify the level of protein excretion).

Renal ultrasound: Consider this test if the patient has azotemia and baseline chemistries are not available. Renal scarring indicates underlying CRI.

BUN and serum creatinine are 28 mg/dL and 2.8 mg/dL, respectively. Protein excretion is 200 mg/day. There is no scarring on renal ultrasound.

What is the next step?

This patient has acute glomerulonephritis with laboratory evidence of ARF. Obtain the following battery of serum tests to rapidly determine the cause of glomerulonephritis: serum complement, antistreptolysin O (ASO) titer, anti-nuclear antibody and anti-dsDNA, anti-neutrophilic cytoplasmic antibodies (ANCA), anti-glomerular basement membrane (anti-GBM), cryoglobulins, hepatitis B and C serologies, and blood cultures if febrile (Table 6-7). If serology is negative or nonspecific, perform renal biopsy.

TABLE 6–7 Major Causes of Focal and Diffuse Glomerulonephritis in Adults

	Disorder	Possible Serology Findings
Systemic causes associated with decreased complement	Type III or IV lupus nephropathy	(+) ANA or anti-dsDNA
	Cryoglobulinemia[a]	(+) HCV serology (90%), increased cryoglobulins
	Endocarditis	(+) Blood cultures
	Shunt nephritis[b]	(+) Blood cultures
Primary renal disorders associated with decreased complement	Postinfectious GN	(+) ASO titer
Systemic causes associated with normal complement	Wegener's disease[c]	(+) c-ANCA >>(+) p-ANCA
	Microscopic polyangiitis[c]	(+) p-ANCA >>(+) c-ANCA
	Churg-Strauss syndrome[c]	(+) p-ANCA >>(+) c-ANCA
	Polyarteritis nodosa[c]	(+) Hepatitis B serology (occasionally)
	Goodpasture's syndrome	(+) Anti-GBM antibodies
Primary renal disorders associated with normal complement (serology negative)		
IgA nephropathy (Berger's disease)		
Benign familial hematuria (thin basement membrane disease)		
Hereditary nephritis (Alport's syndrome)		
Idiopathic RPGN		

Abbreviations: ANA, anti-nuclear antibody; ANCA, anti-neutrophilic cytoplasmic antibody; ASO, antistreptolysin O; GBM, glomerular basement membrane; HCV, hepatitis C virus; RPGN, rapidly progressive GN.

[a] First-line therapy is to treat underlying HCV infection.

[b] Shunt nephritis is caused by antibodies that develop in response to chronic infection of a surgically placed shunt (e.g., ventriculoatrial shunt). Treatment is antibiotics and removal of the shunt.

[c] Vasculitides.

Asymptomatic nephritis and no azotemia: First obtain serum complement (disorders with immune complex deposition cause decreased complement). Then obtain serologies on the basis of complement levels and clinical manifestations. Order renal biopsy if serologies are not diagnostic or the patient develops azotemia.

Complement levels are decreased. ASO titer is positive.

What is the diagnosis?

The patient has postinfectious glomerulonephritis (PIGN). Streptococcus is the most common infection associated with PIGN (occurs approximately 10 days after infection). Most cases are self-limiting, so limit treatment to close monitoring of serum chemistries and correction of fluid and electrolyte abnormalities. Obtain renal biopsy only if the patient's symptoms persist.

Alternative 6.7.1

A 33-year-old man presents to the clinic with gross hematuria. About 5 days ago, he had a fever, runny nose, and sore throat. He is currently asymptomatic. There is no family history of hematuria or renal failure. Physical exam and vital signs are normal. Urinalysis demonstrates dysmorphic RBCs, RBC casts, and trace proteinuria. Serum chemistries are normal. Serum complement and other serologies are normal. Hematuria persists 1 week later.

What is the most likely diagnosis?

The most common glomerulonephropathies associated with persistent asymptomatic hematuria in adults are IgA nephropathy, benign familial hematuria, and Alport's syndrome. This patient with negative family history and gross hematuria 5 days after an upper respiratory infection most likely has IgA nephropathy.

Benign familial hematuria: Suspect if microscopic hematuria and 50% of first-degree relatives have microscopic hematuria (autosomal dominant condition).
Alport's syndrome: Suspect if family history of renal failure with or without deafness.

IgA nephropathy versus PIGN: IgA nephropathy occurs approximately 5 days after upper respiratory infection, and PIGN occurs approximately 10 days after upper respiratory infection. Serum complement and ASO are normal in IgA nephropathy.

How is asymptomatic glomerular hematuria managed?

IgA nephropathy and benign familial hematuria are typically benign (focal nephritis), so limit management of these conditions to close monitoring of blood pressure, serum chemistries, and urine protein. Obtain renal biopsy only if the patient develops signs of nephritic syndrome.

Alport's syndrome: Obtain skin biopsy if the patient has suggestive features.

Alternative 6.7.2

A 40-year-old man presents with clinical manifestations and urinalysis indicative of acute glomerulonephritis. BUN and serum creatinine are 33 mg/dL and 3.5 mg/dL. Serum complement level is normal. C-ANCA is positive.

What does positive ANCA indicate?

A number of conditions can cause positive ANCA, such as:

1. Vasculitides (Wegener's disease, Churg-Strauss syndrome, microscopic polyangiitis)
2. Connective tissue disorders (systemic lupus erythematosus (SLE), Sjögren's, rheumatoid arthritis, etc.)
3. Inflammatory bowel disease

> **Wegener's disease**: Among ANCA-positive patients, 90% are c-ANCA (10% are p-ANCA).
> **Other disorders**: Among ANCA-positive patients, the majority are p-ANCA.

What is the next step in management?

Obtain renal biopsy in ANCA-positive patients to determine the cause of acute glomerulonephritis. Renal biopsy also helps assess disease severity.

> **Negative ANCA** does not rule out vasculitis (need biopsy if vasculitis suspected).

Renal biopsy demonstrates vasculitis, granulomas, and areas of necrosis, which is diagnostic of Wegener's disease. The biopsy also notes numerous "crescents."

What is the significance of this finding?

The presence of glomerular crescents indicates rapidly progressing glomerulonephritis (RPGN). RPGN typically occurs in normal complement disorders. Systemic causes like Wegener's pose a much higher risk for RPGN than renal-limited causes like IgA nephropathy (see Table 6-7). Patients with RPGN progress to end-stage renal failure and death within weeks to months if left untreated.

> **<50% crescents**: Prognosis is good with treatment.
> **>80% crescents**: Prognosis is poor even with treatment.

How is Wegener's disease treated?

Treat ANCA-positive vasculitides (Wegener's, microscopic polyangitis, Churg-Strauss syndrome) with prednisone and cyclophosphamide. Untreated, these disorders are fatal (particularly when associated with crescents).

What other organ systems can Wegener's disease affect?

Wegener's disease most commonly affects the kidneys and respiratory tract. Respiratory manifestations include dyspnea (due to subglottic stenosis), saddle-nose deformity (due to nasal cartilage inflammation), and hemoptysis (due to vascular lung granulomas). Other frequently affected organ systems include the eye (proptosis and double-vision due to retro-orbital pseudotumor), skin (ulcers and purpura), and peripheral nerves (mononeuritis multiplex).

> Disorders associated with glomerulonephritis and lung infiltrates:
> 1. **Wegener's disease**
> 2. **Churg-Strauss syndrome** (refer to Chapter 3: Pulmonary)
> 3. **Goodpasture's syndrome**: Classic presentation is glomerulonephritis and pulmonary hemorrhage. Associated with (+) anti-GBM and not (+) ANCA. Treat with prednisone, cyclophosphamide, and plasmapheresis.

Alternative 6.7.3

A 45-year-old man presents with clinical manifestations and urinalysis consistent with acute glomerulonephritis. Past history is significant for 10-lb weight loss due to episodes of diffuse abdominal pain after meals (intestinal angina). There are red, non-blanchable, reticulated lesions on his legs (livedo reticularis). Serum creatinine is 2.8 mg/dL, and BUN is 28 mg/dL. Serum complement is normal. The only significant serology finding is (+) HBsAg.

What diagnosis should you suspect?

Suspect polyarteritis nodosa (PAN) in this patient with acute glomerulonephritis and (+) HBsAg. This ANCA-negative vasculitis can affect a number of organ systems besides the kidney including the abdomen (microaneurysms cause intestinal angina), skin (purpura, tender nodules, livedo reticularis), eyes (scleritis), and peripheral nerves (peripheral neuropathy). PAN does not usually affect the lungs though.

Hepatitis B: responsible for only small percentage of PAN (most cases are idiopathic).

How can you establish the diagnosis?

First obtain a mesenteric angiogram to screen for microaneurysms. If there are no microaneurysms, confirm the diagnosis with renal biopsy. If angiography detects aneurysms, consider biopsy of another affected organ to confirm the diagnosis (because renal biopsy can cause aneurysm rupture).

Mesenteric angiography demonstrates microaneurysms. Colorectal biopsy confirms the diagnosis.

How is PAN treated?

First-line treatment is prednisone. Add cyclophosphamide if prednisone does not induce remission.

All forms of vasculitis often present initially with nonspecific constitutional symptoms (fever, weight loss, etc.) and increased ESR (nonspecific marker of inflammation).

CASE 6–8 BILATERAL PEDAL AND PERIORBITAL EDEMA

A 54-year-old man presents with a 3-week history of bilateral pedal edema. He does not have any dyspnea or chest pain. Medical history is significant for poorly controlled type 2 diabetes. He last visited a physician 1 year ago. At that time, urinalysis detected trace protein and serum creatinine was 2.0 mg/dL. He is not compliant with losartan and insulin. He does not smoke or drink alcohol. On physical exam, there is periorbital and bilateral pitting pedal edema. Vital signs are normal.

What is the most likely cause of this patient's edema?

The major causes of bilateral pitting edema are heart failure, cirrhosis, drugs, and nephrotic syndrome. This patient with diabetes and periorbital edema most likely has nephrotic syndrome. Lack of dyspnea or abnormal lung findings makes heart failure unlikely. Cirrhosis is less likely in this non-drinker with no ascites. He does not take any drugs associated with pedal edema (e.g., calcium channel blockers).

Non-pitting edema: Suspect lymphatic obstruction or hypothyroidism.

What are the causes of nephrotic syndrome?

Diabetes mellitus is the number one cause of nephrotic syndrome among adults in the United States. Other important causes include SLE, HIV, neoplasms (such as multiple myeloma), drugs (most commonly NSAIDs), and amyloidosis. Many cases are idiopathic (Table 6-8).

Serum lipid, serum albumin, and 24-hour urine protein are obtained, which confirm the diagnosis of nephrotic syndrome.

What are the next diagnostic steps?

Obtain serum chemistry (to assess BUN, serum creatinine, and glucose), HbA1c (to measure glucose control), and an ophthalmology evaluation (to evaluate for diabetic retinopathy). If the evaluation indicates stable CRI and poorly controlled diabetes, no further diagnostic work-up is necessary. If diabetes appears well controlled (no retinopathy, HbA1c <7) or if the patient has signs of ARF, obtain renal biopsy to rule out other causes.

Random urine protein/creatinine: Ratio >0.15 indicates proteinuria. This ratio is an accurate and less cumbersome alternative to 24-hour urine collection (Fig. 6-4).

TABLE 6–8 Major Causes of Nephrotic Syndrome in Adults

Renal Biopsy	Differential Diagnosis
Minimal change	1. Idiopathic minimal change disease 2. NSAIDs 3. Hodgkin's disease
Kimmelstein-Wilson nodules	Pathognomic for diabetes mellitus
FSGS	1. Idiopathic FSGS 2. HIV 3. Intravenous heroin 4. Type II lupus nephropathy
MN	1. Idiopathic MN 2. Infections (syphilis, malaria) 3. Drugs: Penicillamine, Probenecid, gold 4. Type V lupus nephropathy
MPGN	1. Idiopathic MPGN 2. Hepatitis C virus
Green birefringence with Congo red stain	Amyloidosis
Immunoglobulin light chains	Multiple myeloma

Abbreviations: FSGS, focal segmental glomerulosclerosis; MN, membranous glomerulonephritis; MPGN, membranoproliferative glomerulonephritis.
Note: The majority of minimal change, FSGS, MN, MPGN are idiopathic.

Serum creatinine is 2.3 g/dl. HbA1c is 9%. Ophthalmology evaluation shows evidence of diabetic retinopathy.

In addition to treating the underlying diabetes, what management strategies are recommended for all patients with CKD?

1. **Monitor GFR and nutritional status**: Monitor GFR using serum creatinine, Cockcroft-Gault equation, and Modification of Diet in Renal Disease (MDRD) equation (equations take into account age, weight, race, and gender). Monitor nutritional status using anthropometric measurements and plasma proteins (serum albumin, pre-albumin, and transferrin).
2. **Blood pressure**: Maintain pressure <130/80. First-line antihypertensives are ACE inhibitors/ARBs. If these are insufficient, add loop diuretics to the regimen.
3. **Lipids**: Treat hyperlipidemia with a statin drug if low-density lipoprotein cholesterol >100 mg/dL.
4. **Diet**: Restrict protein intake to 0.7 to 0.8 g/kg. Restrict dietary potassium, phosphate, and magnesium. Take calcium and vitamin D supplements to prevent renal osteodystrophy.
5. **Treat symptoms and laboratory abnormalities associated with CRI/uremia**:
   - Fluids and electrolytes: Correct hypovolemia with normal saline. Correct volume overload (edema) with loop diuretics and sodium restriction. Correct electrolyte and acid–base abnormalities (hyperkalemia, hyperphosphatemia, hypocalcemia, and metabolic acidosis).
   - Anemia: Maintain hemoglobin between 11 to 13 mg/dL using erythropoietin or darbapoietin.

Major causes of ESRD in the United States: diabetes (28%), hypertension (24%), glomerulonephritis (21%), idiopathic (20%).

When are dialysis/renal transplant indicated for patients with CRI?

Refer patients for renal transplant evaluation when GFR <30 mL/min. Because the demand for organs exceeds supply, many patients require maintenance dialysis while on the transplant wait list. ***AEIOU*** are absolute indications for urgent dialysis. Relative indications for maintenance dialysis are:

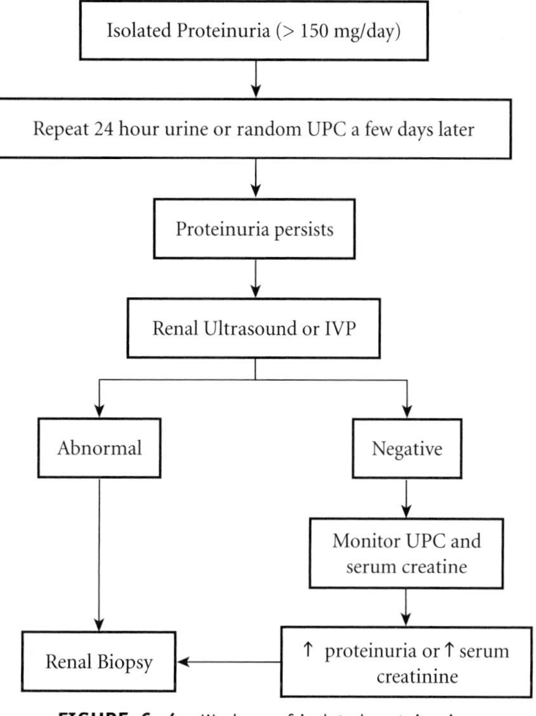

FIGURE 6–4 Work-up of isolated proteinuria.

1. Serum creatinine >10 mg/dL and BUN >100 mg/dL
2. GFR <15 to 20 mL/min
3. Chronic malnutrition

Over the next 2 years, the patient's GFR continues to decline. The nephrologist decides to place the patient on the transplant wait list and institute maintenance dialysis.

What are the different types of dialysis?

1. **Traditional hemodialysis**: Tubes deliver the patient's blood to a machine (dialyzer) outside the body. The dialyzer has two compartments separated by a semipermeable membrane. One compartment contains the patient's blood, and the other contains dialysate fluid. Waste products and excess free water in the blood diffuse across the membrane into the dialysate (ultrafiltration). Tubes return the purified blood to the body. The dialysate is discarded. Typically performed three times a week in 3- to 4-hour sessions.
2. **Peritoneal dialysis**: Dialysate is instilled into the peritoneum. The peritoneal membrane acts as a natural semipermeable membrane. Either the patient or a machine removes the old dialysate and instills fresh dialysate at least once a day. Peritoneal dialysis is more convenient than hemodialysis but carries a risk of complications like peritonitis and abdominal or inguinal hernia.
3. **Hemofiltration**: Tubes deliver blood to a machine with a highly porous semipermeable membrane, so lots of water and solutes enter the other compartment (there is no dialysate). Desired solutes and water are added to the remaining blood, which is returned to the body. Performed slowly and continuously for 12 to 24 hours daily. Main use is for ARF patients in the intensive care unit setting.
4. **Hemodiafiltration**: hemodialysis + hemofiltration.

Hemodialysis/hemofiltration access: Initially, obtain blood through a central venous catheter (temporary access). In the long term, first-line access is a surgically created arteriovenous fistula in the nondominant arm. If the fistula fails or cannot be created, second-line access is an arteriovenous graft (Gore-Tex connects artery and vein).
Peritoneal dialysis access: surgically placed catheter (runs from peritoneum to navel).

Thirty minutes after the first hemodialysis session begins, the patient complains of chest pain, back pain, nausea, and vomiting. Vital signs are normal.

What is the most likely cause of his symptoms? What is the next step in management?

The patient has "first use syndrome (type B)," a complement-mediated reaction to the semi-permeable membrane that can occur 15 to 30 minutes after the first hemodialysis session begins. Chest pain, back pain, nausea, vomiting, and hypotension are the most common symptoms. Continue hemodialysis unless the patient is hemodynamically unstable or develops signs of anaphylaxis (rare). Use the same dialyzer for subsequent hemodialysis sessions. Symptoms recur less frequently during subsequent sessions.

> **First use syndrome (type A)**: Occurs <5 minutes after the first session begins. This type is more severe but far less common than type B. Stop the session immediately and treat symptoms. Pretreat with antihistamines and/or steroids during subsequent sessions.

Alternative 6.8.1

The patient is a 20-year-old man with clinical manifestations and laboratory evidence of nephrotic syndrome. Blood glucose is normal. Renal biopsy shows minimal changes. There is no history of NSAID use. Physical exam and vital signs are normal.

What is the next step in management?

The patient has idiopathic minimal change disease, which accounts for 10% to 15% of nephrotic syndrome in adults. Treat with a course of high-dose oral steroids. Most patients recover fully without any complications.

> Minimal change disease accounts for 90% of nephrotic syndrome in children.

Alternative 6.8.2

A 67-year-old man with multiple myeloma presents with clinical manifestations of nephrotic syndrome. In addition to edema, physical exam is significant for a thickened, waxy tongue (macroglossia). Blood glucose is normal. When the renal biopsy sample is stained with Congo red stain and examined under polarized light, there is green birefringence.

What is the diagnosis?

The patient has amyloidosis. In this condition, low molecular weight proteins deposit on the tissues of multiple organs. There are two main categories of amyloidosis:

1. **Primary amyloidosis**: Plasma cell dyscrasia that often occurs with multiple myeloma (this patient). Tissue deposits are light-chain immunoglobulins.
2. **Secondary amyloidosis**: Secondary to chronic inflammatory diseases like rheumatoid arthritis. Tissue deposits are serum amyloid A (acute phase reactant).

> Minor categories of amyloidosis:
> 1. **Familial amyloidosis**: Many different mutations can cause amyloidosis.
> 2. **Hemodialysis-related amyloidosis**: β-2 microglobulin deposits in bones and joints.
> 3. **Senile amyloidosis**: Transthyretin deposits in myocardium, etc., but not the kidney.

> Primary amyloidosis and secondary amyloidosis can affect any organ system. Most common are heart (restrictive cardiomyopathy) and skin (waxy thickening, ecchymoses, and periorbital purpura).

TABLE 6–9 Types of Renal Disease in Systemic Lupus Erythematosus

	Renal Biopsy	Clinical Manifestations
Class I	Minimal mesangial deposits	Asymptomatic
Class II	Focal segmental mesangial deposits	Isolated microscopic hematuria, proteinuria
Class III	Focal glomerulonephritis	Variable
Class IV	Diffuse glomerulonephritis	Nephritic ± nephrotic syndrome and ARF (most common and most severe form)
Class V	Membranous GN	Nephrotic syndrome but no azotemia
Class VI	Advanced sclerosis	End-stage renal disease

How is primary amyloidosis treated?

Treat the underlying plasma cell dyscrasia (refer to Chapter 10: Hematology). In the case of secondary amyloidosis, treat the underlying inflammatory disorder. Most patients with renal amyloidosis progress to ESRD and require dialysis/kidney transplant.

Alternative 6.8.3

The patient is a 36-year-old woman with clinical features of nephrotic syndrome. Past history is significant for fatigue and joint pain. Physical examination is significant for areas of alopecia and an erythematous rash across the nose and cheeks (malar rash).

What is the most likely diagnosis?

The clinical picture is consistent with SLE. Renal biopsy is always indicated to determine the class of lupus nephropathy (Table 6-9).

Renal biopsy indicates the patient has stage III disease.

How is lupus nephritis treated?

1. **Class I and II disease**: No specific treatment.
2. **Other classes**: Optimal therapy uncertain (usually includes corticosteroids + another immunosuppressant); also, treat CKD as described earlier.

> **Repeat renal biopsy**: Obtain if serum creatinine rises, proteinuria does not decrease, or active sediment persists (RBC casts, dysmorphic RBCs).

CASE 6–9 CHRONIC AZOTEMIA WITHOUT NEPHROTIC SYNDROME OR GLOMERULONEPHRITIS

Serum creatinine of a 46-year-old woman is incidentally found to be 3.0 mg/dL. Urinalysis is normal. Review of prior records indicates serum creatinine was 2.8 mg/dL 6 months earlier. She has a history of chronic headaches for which she takes high doses of aspirin and ibuprofen. Physical exam and vital signs are normal. CT scan without contrast is significant for renal papillary necrosis.

What is the most likely cause of this patient's CRI?

The most likely diagnosis is chronic interstitial nephritis due to chronic NSAID use (analgesic nephropathy). Chronic interstitial nephritis leads to CRI with nonspecific urinalysis (normal, mild pyuria, or mild proteinuria) ± renal papillary necrosis. Treatment is to discontinue NSAIDs to prevent progression to ESRD.

What are other common causes of chronic interstitial nephritis?

1. Chronic urinary tract obstruction (ruled out by CT scan or ultrasound)
2. APKD (ruled out by CT scan or ultrasound)
3. Hypertensive nephrosclerosis (ruled out if normotensive and no history of hypertension)

Renal papillary necrosis: Differential diagnosis includes NSAIDs, diabetes, urinary tract obstruction, and sickle cell anemia/trait.

chapter 7

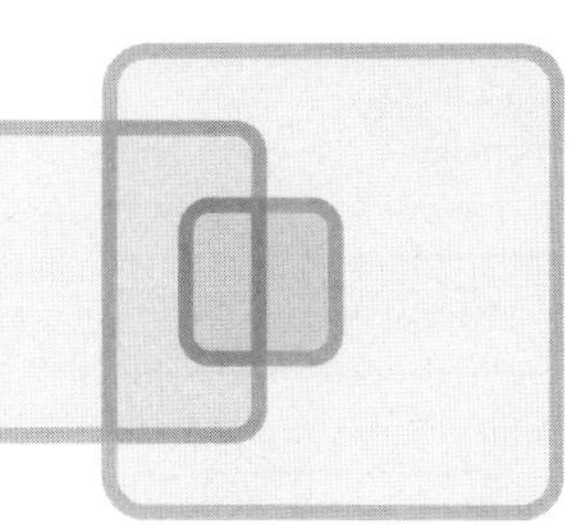

Fluids, Electrolytes, and Acid–Base Disorders

CASE 7–1 ELEVATED ANION GAP METABOLIC ACIDOSIS

A 25-year-old man is brought to the emergency department for evaluation of altered mental status. There is no known past medical history or any history of trauma. The patient responds to verbal commands with slurred, incomprehensible speech. He does respond to pain and moves his eyes spontaneously. Vital signs are temperature 37.8°C, pulse 110 bpm, respirations 28/min, and blood pressure 155/90. Serum chemistries are sodium 139, potassium 4.0, chloride 102, HCO_3 11, blood urea nitrogen (BUN) 15, Cr 0.8, and glucose 110. Arterial blood gas values are pH 7.19, pCO_2 24, PO_2 95.

What is the acid–base abnormality?

A pH <7.35 indicates that this patient has an acidosis. HCO_3 <22 indicates that this is a metabolic acidosis. On the basis of the following calculations, the respiratory compensation is appropriate, which indicates that this patient has a simple metabolic acidosis (Fig. 7-1):

$$\text{Decrease in } HCO_3 = 24 - 11 = 13$$
$$\text{Expected decrease in } PCO_2 = 13 \times 1.2 = 15.6 \approx 16$$
$$\text{Therefore, expected } PCO_2 \text{ value} = 40 - 16 = 24.$$

Kussmaul breathing: Rapid, deep, and labored breathing (hyperventilation) causes respiratory alkalosis (decreased PCO_2) to compensate for metabolic acidosis.

What causes metabolic acidosis?

1. Increased acid production (e.g., ketoacidosis, lactic acidosis)
2. Decreased acid excretion (e.g., uremia)
3. Increased bicarbonate excretion (e.g., diarrhea)

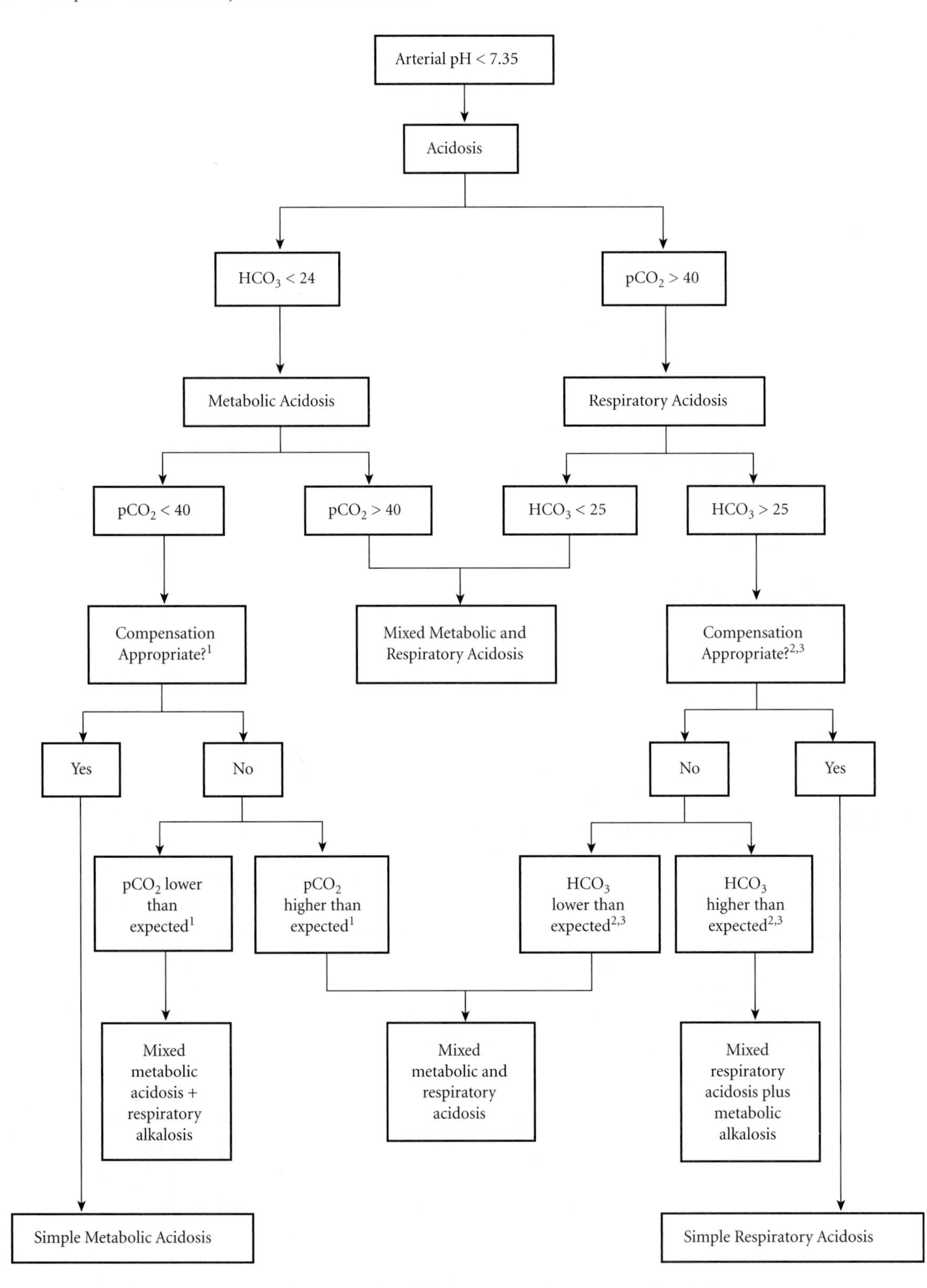

[1] = Metabolic acidosis: For every 1 mEq/L ↓ in HCO_3, pCO_2 ↓ by 1.2 mm Hg.
[2] = Acute respiratory acidosis: For every 10 mm Hg ↑ in pCO_2, HCO_3 ↑ by 1 mm Hg.
[3] = Chronic respiratory acidosis: For every 10 mmg Hg ↑ in pCO_2, HCO_3 ↑ 3.5 mm Hg.

FIGURE 7–1 Approach to acidosis.

What is the next step in determining the cause of this patient's metabolic acidosis?

Step 1: Calculate the anion gap (AG). AG = serum sodium – (serum chloride + serum bicarbonate). The AG represents the unmeasured plasma anions. Normal AG is 3 to 11. With an AG of 26, this patient has an elevated AG.

Step 2: Calculate the gap-gap (delta gap) and HCO_3 gap if the patient has an elevated AG. Delta gap = patient's anion gap – 12 (this patient's delta gap is 14). HCO_3 gap is 25 – patient's HCO_3 (this patient's HCO_3 gap is 14).

Step 3: Calculate delta gap/HCO_3 gap. The value should be 1 to 2 (this patient's value is 1). If the value is <1, suspect a combined non-gap and gap acidosis. If the value is >2, suspect a concurrent metabolic alkalosis.

What are the causes of elevated AG metabolic acidosis?

1. Acidoses (diabetic ketoacidosis (DKA), alcoholic ketoacidosis (AKA), lactic acidosis)
2. Ingestions (mainly methanol, ethylene glycol, salicylic acid)
3. Renal failure (uremia)

DKA is unlikely in this patient with normal glucose levels; uremia is unlikely in the absence of azotemia.

"***MUDPILES***" (**M**ethanol, **U**remia, **D**KA, **P**araldehyde, **I**ron and **I**soniazid, **L**actid acidosis, **E**tOH ketoacidosis, **E**thylene glycol, **S**alicylate).

Methanol and ethylene glycol: Found in antifreeze and other industrial solvents.

What diagnostic tests are indicated at this point to determine the cause of the elevated AG metabolic acidosis?

Order the following tests:

1. Serum ketones and blood alcohol levels (to rule out AKA)
2. Serum lactate (to rule out lactic acidosis)
3. Serum levels of methanol, ethylene glycol, and salicylic acid. Methanol and ethylene glycol tests take a long time to return, so in the acute setting suspect ingestion of these substances if plasma osmolal gap is >10.
4. Urine toxicology screen and urinalysis

Plasma osmolal gap = measured plasma osmolality – calculated plasma osmolality
Calculated plasma osmolality = $(2 \times Na) + (glucose/18) + (BUN/2.8) + (ethanol/4.6)$

Serum ketones, alcohol, and salicylic acid are negative. Urinalysis and urine toxicology screen are negative. Lactate is within normal limits. Plasma osmolal gap is 25. The physician suspects methanol or ethanol ingestion.

What are the clinical manifestations of ingesting these substances?

1. **Stage 1**: Central nervous system (CNS): Patient appears inebriated but does not smell of alcohol.
2. **Stage 2**: Cardiopulmonary: Hypertension, tachycardia, etc.
3. **Stage 3**: Renal failure: Azotemia ± Ca oxalate urine crystals after 24 to 72 hours.

If left untreated, patients usually die from renal or cardiac failure.

Methanol: Patients often develop blurry vision ± scotoma and scintillations during stage 2 that progresses to blindness unless treated promptly.
Ethylene glycol: Converted to oxalate in the body. Oxalate can bind to calcium and cause hypocalcemia during stage 2 or stage 3.

How are suspected ingestions of methanol or ethylene glycol treated?

1. **ABCs**: Secure the patient's airway, breathing, and circulation first.
2. **Sodium bicarbonate**
3. **Fomepizole**: Inhibits alcohol dehydrogenase. If unavailable, administer ethanol. Also administer folic acid, thiamine, and pyridoxine along with fomepizole.
4. **Hemodialysis**: Administering fomepizole can eliminate the need for hemodialysis only if the patient is asymptomatic with normal serum creatinine and serum pH >7.3. This symptomatic patient with profound metabolic acidosis should undergo hemodialysis.

> Gastric decontamination (ipecac, gastric lavage, activated charcoal) is not indicated for methanol and ethylene glycol ingestions.

Alternative 7.1.1

A 25-year-old woman presents to the emergency department with fatigue, anorexia, nausea, vomiting, and diffuse abdominal pain. Her symptoms began about 5 days ago after a urinary tract infection. She has a history of type 1 diabetes mellitus. On physical exam, there is decreased skin turgor, and her oropharynx is dry. Breaths are deep and labored (Kussmaul respirations). She is oriented to person but not to place and time. Vital signs are temperature 37.4°C, pulse 112 bpm, respirations 29/min, and blood pressure 95/70. Serum chemistries are sodium 130, potassium 4.0, chloride 102, HCO_3 14, BUN 25, Cr 2.0, and glucose 400. Serum ketones are elevated and urine ketones are 3+. Arterial blood gas values are pH 7.28, pCO_2 28, PO_2 95.

What is the diagnosis?

This patient has the diagnostic triad of DKA:

1. Hyperglycemia (usually, serum glucose >250 mg/dL but <800 mg/dL)
2. AG metabolic acidosis
3. Increased serum and/or urine ketones

> DKA almost always occurs in type 1 diabetics; it is rare in type 2 diabetes mellitus.

What causes DKA?

DKA usually results from a stressful precipitant in patients with type 1 diabetes (and occasionally in patients with type 2 diabetes). Stress stimulates increased secretion of glucagon, cortisol, and catecholamines. Increased glucagon inhibits insulin (which leads to hyperglycemia) and stimulates gluconeogenesis (which leads to increased ketoacid production and subsequent AG metabolic acidosis). The most common precipitants are:

1. Infection (40%): Urinary tract infection is the most common infection associated with DKA.
2. Nonadherence with insulin therapy (25%)
3. Initial presentation of diabetes (15%)
4. Others: trauma, surgery, myocardial infarct, etc.

> Ketoacids in DKA are β-hydroxybutyrate (75%) and acetoacetate (25%). Urine dipstick for ketones (nitroprusside test) does not detect β-hydroxybutyrate.

What are the clinical manifestations of DKA besides the classic triad?

Symptoms:

1. **Polyuria and polydipsia**: These most common initial symptoms of DKA occur because hyperglycemia causes osmotic diuresis.
2. **Altered mental status**: This occurs when serum glucose is >300 mOsm/kg.
3. **Nausea, vomiting, and abdominal pain**: These also occur frequently in DKA.

Signs:

1. **Hypovolemia**: Polyuria, vomiting, and anorexia lead to decreased skin turgor, dry oropharynx, weight loss, tachycardia, and hypotension.
2. **Fruity breath**: This sign is caused by increased exhaled acetone.

Electrolyte abnormalities:

1. **Sodium**: Hyperglycemia causes water to move out of cells, so serum sodium is low. To correct for this, add 1.6 to the measured serum sodium for every 100 mg/dL of glucose >100 mg/dL. For example, in this patient, corrected serum sodium is $130 + (3 \times 1.6) = 130 + 4.8 \approx 135$ mEq/L.
2. **Potassium and phosphate**: Osmotic diuresis leads to potassium and phosphate loss. However, measured serum potassium and phosphate are normal to high because insulin deficiency drives them out of cells into serum.
3. **BUN and serum creatinine**: These may be elevated because of hypovolemia.

> **Amylase and lipase**: often elevated in DKA (does not indicate pancreatitis).

How is DKA managed?

1. Fluids, insulin (regular intravenous (IV) insulin), and K^+ replacement comprise the cornerstone of management (Fig. 7-2).
2. HCO_3: This is not indicated unless pH is <7.0 after the initial hour of hydration.
3. Phosphate: Administer half of the K^+ as potassium phosphate if PO_4 low (<1.0).
4. Magnesium: Give oral magnesium if Mg low (<1.8 mg/dL).

Alternative 7.1.2

A 58-year-old man is brought to the emergency department for evaluation of altered mental status. He was found lying on a sidewalk. Physical exam is significant for spider angioma and palmar erythema. His breath has a fruity odor. Vital signs are temperature 37.4°C, pulse 112 bpm, respirations 29/min, and blood pressure 95/70. Laboratory evaluation indicates simple metabolic acidosis with elevated AG. Urine dipstick detects 2+ ketones. Blood glucose is 80 mg/dL. Urine toxicology screen is pending.

What diagnosis should you suspect?

Suspect AKA in this patient with AG metabolic acidosis and ketosis but no hyperglycemia. Physical signs of cirrhosis increase the likelihood of this diagnosis.

> **Suspected AKA/DKA but negative nitroprusside test**: Directly measure β-hydroxybutyrate or add a few drops of hydrogen peroxide to urine specimen and repeat nitroprusside test (peroxide converts β-hydroxybutyrate to acetoacetate).

> For unknown reasons, some patients with AKA have mild hyperglycemia (<250 mg/dL).

Urine toxicology screen is positive for alcohol.

How is AKA treated?

Treat with normal saline and 5% dextrose (D5NS). Give all suspected alcoholics thiamine before administering a solution containing glucose to avoid precipitating Wernicke-Korsakoff syndrome (damage to mammillary bodies in brain).

> **Wernicke syndrome**: Suspect if patient has triad of "*ACE*": **A**taxia, **C**onfusion, and **E**ye signs (gaze palsy, nystagmus). Reversible with thiamine.
> **Korsakoff syndrome**: Suspect if patient has anterograde and retrograde amnesia ± confabulation. Usually irreversible.

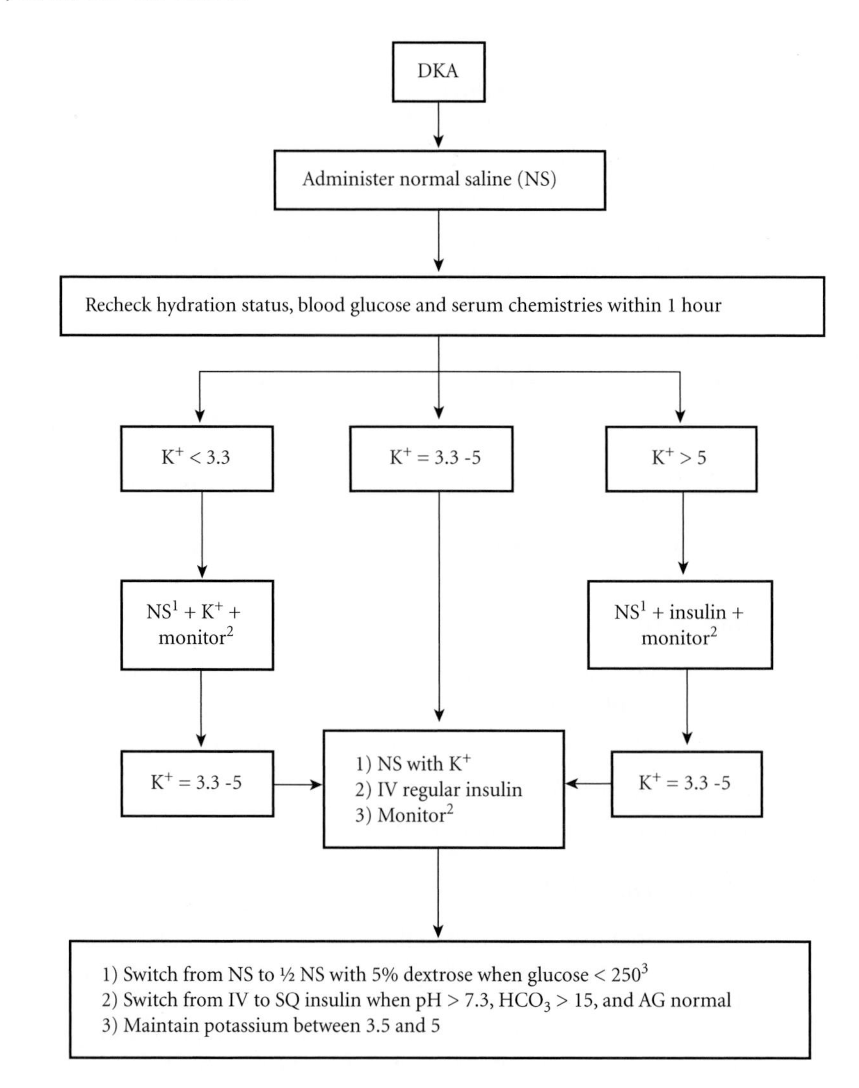

[1] If blood pressure normal and corrected sodium normal-high, switch to ½ NS.
[2] Monitor blood glucose every 1-2 hours and serum chemistries every 2-6 hours.
If blood pressure is normal and corrected sodium normal-high, switch to ½ NS.
[3] Give dextrose because lowering glucose to < 200 mg/dL can cause cerebral edema.

FIGURE 7–2 Management of diabetic ketoacidosis (DKA).

> As in DKA, HCO_3 is not indicated unless pH is <7.

Mental status and metabolic acidosis improve with D5NS. Eight hours later, the patient complains of palpitations and nausea. Physical exam is significant for hand tremor. Vital signs are normal.

What is the next step in management?

Alcoholics may experience mild withdrawal symptoms such as tremulations, palpitations, anxiety, and gastrointestinal (GI) disturbances 6 to 36 hours after alcohol cessation. Treat with oral benzodiazepines to prevent seizures or progression to severe withdrawal. Use a short-acting agent such as lorazepam or oxazepam in this patient with underlying cirrhosis. Use long-acting agents such as diazepam or chlordiazepoxide in patients without underlying cirrhosis.

> **Clinical Institute Withdrawal Assessment (CIWA) scale:** A score >8 on this questionnaire indicates that the patient is in withdrawal.

> **Generalized tonic-clonic seizures (rum fits)**: These can occur 6 to 48 hours after alcohol cessation in an alcoholic.

The patient is discharged from the hospital. He is brought to the emergency department 2 months later with altered mental status. His brother mentions that he quit drinking 3 days ago. The paramedic states that the patient mentioned "seeing cockroaches everywhere" in the ambulance. He is oriented to person but not to place and time. On physical exam, he is sweating profusely. Vital signs are temperature 38.3°C, pulse 120 bpm, blood pressure 160/100, respirations 28/min.

What is the most likely cause of his symptoms?

The patient is most likely in severe withdrawal (delirium tremens), associated with a 5% mortality rate. Delirium tremens typically occurs 2 to 4 days after untreated alcohol cessation and is characterized by delirium with visual or tactile hallucinations, low-grade fever, hypertension, and diaphoresis.

> **Alcoholic hallucinosis**: Visual hallucinations can occur 12 to 48 hours after alcohol cessation. The patient is not delirious. This condition is less life-threatening than delirium tremens.

How is delirium tremens treated?

1. **ABCs first**: Administer oxygen and place two large-bore IVs. Administer D5NS (remember to give thiamine before any solution containing glucose).
2. **Sedation**: Administer IV diazepam every 5 to 10 minutes until the patient is calm but awake (use IV lorazepam if you suspect that the patient has cirrhosis). If IV access is not possible, use intramuscular lorazepam. Patients are rarely refractory to benzodiazepines and require phenobarbital or propofol.
3. **Position**: Place in a lateral decubitus position to protect patient and caregivers.
4. **Monitoring**: Admit all patients with delirium tremens to the intensive care unit. Place the patient on a cardiac monitor because arrhythmias are the most common cause of death.
5. **Electrolytes**: Correct electrolyte or nutritional abnormalities (folic acid, multivitamin).

CASE 7–2 NORMAL ANION GAP METABOLIC ACIDOSIS

An 18-year-old woman is found to have the following serum chemistries during routine examination: sodium 132, potassium 2.9, chloride 110, bicarbonate 15, BUN 20, creatinine 1.0, glucose 100. PCO_2 is 29 and pH is 7.3. Physical exam and vital signs are normal.

What is the acid–base abnormality?

This patient with pH <7.4 and decreased HCO_3 has a metabolic acidosis. Respiratory compensation is appropriate, so this is a simple metabolic acidosis. AG is 7, so the patient has a normal AG metabolic acidosis. Normal AG metabolic acidosis is also called hyperchloremic metabolic acidosis because increased chloride replaces the loss of HCO_3.

What are the major causes of normal AG metabolic acidosis?

1. GI bicarbonate loss: diarrhea (number one cause), ureterosigmoidostomy, GI fistulas
2. Renal tubular acidosis (RTA): All three types (1, 2, and 4).

In addition to taking a thorough history, how can you distinguish GI losses from RTA?

Obtain urine pH and urine electrolytes:

1. Urine pH: Suspect a GI cause if pH <5.5 and RTA if pH >5.5 (does not always apply).

2. Urine AG: GI losses cause increased NH_4^+ excretion, which leads to negative urine AG (appropriate response). On the other hand, positive urine AG suggests RTA.
3. Urine potassium: Levels <25 mEq/L indicate a GI cause (appropriate response to hypokalemia). Higher values in the setting of hypokalemia suggest RTA.

> **Toluene ingestion (glue sniffing)**: Acid–base and urine findings are similar to GI losses.

Urine pH is 5.2, urine AG is –3, urine potassium is 15 mEq/L. She runs varsity cross-country at her university. Body mass index (BMI) is 16. She does not sniff glue. She admits that she often uses laxatives to lose weight.

What cause of diarrhea should you suspect?

Suspect factitious diarrhea due to chronic laxative abuse. Laxative abuse is one method used by patients with anorexia nervosa to induce weight loss. Test for bisacodyl (stool turns purple-blue on adding alkali) and magnesium (increased serum magnesium).

> A large volume of diarrhea is needed to produce normal AG metabolic acidosis and hypokalemia.

> **Anorexia nervosa:** Suspect if BMI <17.5 and few or no menstrual periods.

Serum magnesium is mildly elevated.

What are the next steps in management?

The first step is to correct hypokalemia and dehydration, if present. Then, consider bicarbonate only if pH <7.0. After correcting fluid and electrolyte abnormalities, refer this patient for psychotherapy or cognitive behavioral therapy.

Alternative 7.2.1

A 60-year-old man complains of polyuria and polydipsia. The only abnormal serum chemistries are potassium 2.9 and HCO_3 12. Further work-up indicates he has a normal AG metabolic acidosis. Urine pH is 5.8, urine AG is positive, and urine potassium is 30. The physician suspects RTA.

What are the different types of RTA and their causes?

1. **Type 1 RTA**: Due to decreased H^+ secretion in the distal tubule. The most common cause in adults is an autoimmune disorder like Sjogren's.
2. **Type 2 RTA**: Due to decreased proximal tubule HCO_3 reabsorption. The most common causes in adults are multiple myeloma and carbonic anhydrase inhibitors.
3. **Type 4 RTA**: Hypoaldosteronism.

What is the next step in management?

Type 4 RTA is unlikely because serum potassium is low, not high (Table 7-1). The first step is to correct hypokalemia. Then, distinguish between type 1 and type 2 RTA by measuring

TABLE 7–1 Key Laboratory Findings in Renal Tubular Acidosis

	Serum HCO_3 (mEq/L)	Serum K^+ (mEq/L)	Urine pH
Type 1	<10	↓	>5.3
Type 2	10–20	↓	Variable
Type 4	>17	↑	<5.3

urine pH and urine HCO_3 after a bicarbonate infusion. Response to HCO_3 infusion in type 2 RTA is urine pH >7.5 and fractional HCO_3 excretion >15% to 20%. Urine pH remains stable in type 1 RTA, and $FeHCO_3$ is <3%.

Bicarbonate infusion in a patient with hypokalemia can precipitate cardiac arrhythmias.

1. **Type 1 RTA:** Leads to decreased urine citrate, which predisposes to calcium stones.
2. **Type 2 RTA:** If proximal tubule dysfunction is generalized (Fanconi syndrome), patients may have polyuria, polydipsia, osteomalacia, increased urine PO_4, uric acid, and glucose (leads to decreased serum PO_4 and uric acid but serum glucose is normal).

In addition to treating the underlying cause, how are type 1 and type 2 RTA treated?

1. **Type 1 RTA**: Correct acidosis with bicarbonate. Administer potassium citrate if the patient has hypokalemia or develops calcium stones.
2. **Type 2 RTA**: Treat acidosis with bicarbonate and potassium citrate. If serum bicarbonate does not normalize despite large doses, administer thiazide diuretics. If the patient has hypophosphatemia, treat with phosphate and vitamin D to prevent osteomalacia.

CASE 7–3 METABOLIC ALKALOSIS

An 18-year-old woman is found to have the following serum chemistries: Na 139, K 2.8, chloride 95, HCO_3 30, BUN 15, Cr 0.9, glucose 96. Arterial blood gases are pH 7.5, pCO_2 44, and PO_2 98. Vital signs are temperature 37.2°C, pulse 90 bpm, respirations 12/min, and blood pressure 98/70.

What is the acid–base abnormality?

The pH of 7.5 indicates she has an alkalosis. HCO_3 >25 indicates that this is a metabolic alkalosis (Fig. 7-3). On the basis of the following calculations, respiratory compensation is appropriate, which indicates that she has a simple metabolic alkalosis:

$$\text{Expected increase in } pCO_2 = 6 \times 0.7 = 4.2 \approx 4$$
$$\text{Therefore, expected } pCO_2 \text{ value} = 40 + 4 = 44.$$

What are the major causes of metabolic alkalosis?

Saline-responsive: usually associated with volume depletion and hypokalemia.

1. **Vomiting or nasogastric suction**: Patients lose gastric HCl and KCl, which leads to metabolic alkalosis, hypokalemia, and hypochloremia.
2. **Voluminous diarrhea**: Diarrhea usually causes metabolic acidosis, but voluminous chloride-rich diarrhea due to a villous adenoma of the colon can cause alkalosis (exact mechanism unclear).
3. **Loop and thiazide diuretics**: These agents cause increased excretion of HCO_3-poor fluid, so serum HCO_3 concentration increases ("contraction alkalosis") (Table 7-2).

Saline-resistant: often associated with volume overload (edema).

1. **Hyperaldosteronism**: Leads to increased H^+ and K^+ secretion with increased Na^+ and H2O reabsorption. Net result is metabolic alkalosis, hypokalemia, and hypertension.
2. **Exogenous alkali (milk-alkali syndrome)**: Excess HCO_3, citrate, or calcium.
3. **Severe hypokalemia**: Drives H+ into intracellular compartment.
4. **Bartter's and Gitelman's syndromes**: Electrolyte abnormalities in these rare genetic disorders are similar to loop diuretics and thiazide diuretics, respectively (see Table 7-2).

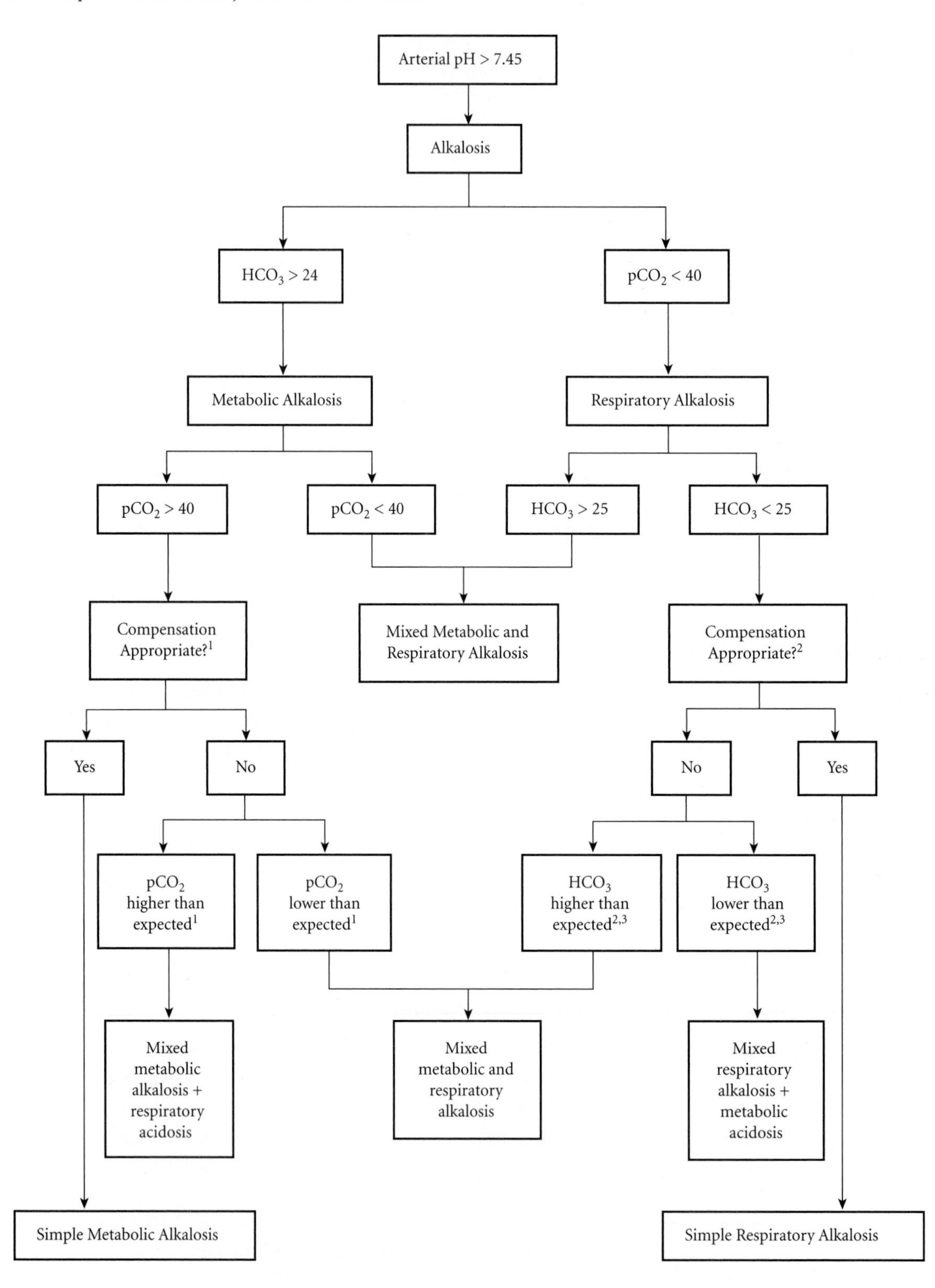

[1] = Metabolic alkalosis: For every 1 mEq/L ↑ in HCO_3, pCO_2 ↑ by 0.7 mm Hg.

[2] = Respiratory alkalosis: For every 10 mm Hg ↓ in pCO_2, HCO_3 ↓ by 2 mEq/L.

FIGURE 7–3 Approach to alkalosis.

TABLE 7–2 Effects of Diuretics

Class	Mechanism	Specific Drugs	Acid–Base Effects	Serum Electrolytes[a]	Other Possible Side Effects
Carbonic anhydrase inhibitors	Inhibits carbonic anhydrase in PCT, which prevents bicarbonate reabsorption	Acetazolamide	Normal AG metabolic acidosis	↓ ***K^+***	Contraindicated in cirrhosis because it worsens encephalopathy
Osmotic diuretics	Increases tubule osmolality, which leads to ↓ fluid reabsorption	Mannitol	Metabolic acidosis (in renal failure patients)	↑ Na with high doses	Hypovolemia with high doses; contraindicated in heart and renal failure
Loop diuretics	Inhibit $Na^+/K^+/2Cl^-$ cotransporter in ascending limb of loop of Henle and early DCT	Furosemide, torsemide, bumetanide, and ethacrynic acid	Metabolic alkalosis	↓ ***Ca^+***, ***K^+***, and Mg^{+2}	Ototoxicity, hypovolemia
Thiazide diuretics	Inhibit Na^+/Cl^- cotransporter in DCT and early cortical collecting tubule	HCTZ	Metabolic alkalosis	↑ ***Ca^{+2}*** and ***uric acid***, ↓ ***K^+*** and Mg^{+2}	Hyperglycemia and hyperlipidemia *("Hyper**GLUC**": ↑ **G**lucose, **L**ipid, **U**ric acid, and **C**alcium)*
K^+-Sparing diuretics	Competitive aldosterone antagonist in late DCT and collecting duct	Spironolactone and eplerenone	Normal AG metabolic acidosis	↑ ***K^+***	Gynecomastia and amenorrhea
K+ sparing diuretics (other type)	Inhibit Na^+ channel in late DCT and collecting duct	Amiloride and triamterene	Normal AG metabolic acidosis	↑ ***K^+***	GI disturbances

Abbreviations: AG, anion gap; DCT, distal convoluted tubule; ECF, extracellular fluid; GI, gastrointestinal; HCTZ, hydrochlorothiazide; PCT, proximal convoluted tubule.
[a] All diuretics prevent sodium reabsorption, which leads to ↑ urine NaCl (↓ serum NaCl).

Common causes of increased citrate are massive blood transfusion (citrate is added to stored blood products to chelate Ca^{2+}) and hemodialysis (citrate is used for anticoagulation if heparin is contraindicated).

The history and physical examination the intern obtains is unrevealing.

What test can you use to differentiate between saline-resistant and saline-responsive metabolic alkalosis?

Obtain spot urine chloride (U_{Cl}). U_{Cl} is <20 mEq/L in saline-responsive metabolic alkalosis and >20 in saline-resistant metabolic alkalosis.

Saline-responsive metabolic alkalosis: U_{Cl} is low as a result of volume contraction and chloride loss in GI secretions.

Is there an exception to the rule regarding urine chloride (U_{Cl})?

U_{Cl} is >20 in patients with metabolic alkalosis due to loop or thiazide diuretics (or concurrent diuretics and another cause of saline-responsive metabolic alkalosis). Consider testing for serum diuretic levels if a hypovolemic patient has U_{Cl} >20.

Urine chloride is 8 mEq/L.

How is saline-responsive metabolic alkalosis treated?

In addition to treating the underlying cause, administer normal saline (to correct hypovolemia) and KCl (to correct hypokalemia, chloride depletion, and alkalosis).

How would treatment of metabolic alkalosis differ in patients with edema (saline-resistant metabolic alkalosis or cirrhosis, heart failure, nephrotic syndrome, etc.)?

Treat the underlying cause and administer KCl. If alkalosis persists, consider acetazolamide when serum K^+ is near normal (see Table 7-2). If KCl and acetazolamide do not correct the alkalosis, consider hydrochloric acid. Normal saline is contraindicated.

Bartter and Gitelman: Treatment is lifelong nonsteroidal anti-inflammatory drugs (NSAIDs), spironolactone, K^+ and Mg^{2+} supplements.

The senior resident notices that the patient's tooth enamel is eroded and the back of her hands are scarred.

What diagnosis should you suspect?

The patient's signs raise suspicion for bulimia nervosa. Patients with bulimia binge on large amounts of food and then purge (vomit) to avoid gaining weight. Chronic exposure to gastric HCl causes erosion of tooth enamel. Patients often push their fingers to the back of the throat to induce vomiting, which scars the back of their hands. Unlike in anorexia, BMI is often normal. Anorexia and bulimia may co-exist in the same patient, and psychiatric treatment of both conditions is similar (psychotherapy or cognitive behavioral therapy).

CASE 7–4 RESPIRATORY AND MIXED ACID–BASE DISORDERS

A 45-year-old woman with a history of major depression is brought to the emergency department 2 hours after she ingested approximately 60 pills of aspirin (salicylate). Vitals signs are temperature 38.4°C, pulse 110 bpm, respirations 30/min, and blood pressure 110/80. Abnormal serum chemistries are potassium 2.8 and HCO_3 15. Na is 136 and chloride is 102. Arterial blood gases are pH 7.28, pCO_2 21, and PO_2 98.

What is the acid–base abnormality?

The patient with pH <7.3 has an acidosis. HCO_3 <15 indicates she has a metabolic acidosis. AG is 136 − (102 + 15) = 19. The expected decrease in pCO2 is 9 × 1.2 = 10.8 ≈ 11. Therefore, the expected pCO_2 is 29. This patient's pCO_2 of 21 indicates that she has a mixed AG metabolic acidosis and respiratory alkalosis.

> Early after ingestion, salicylates directly stimulate the respiratory center, which leads to hyperventilation (respiratory alkalosis). Later, lactic acid and ketoacids accumulate, which leads to metabolic acidosis.

> **Signs of salicylate overdose**: fever, tachycardia, and tachypnea.
> **Symptoms of salicylate overdose**: GI disturbances, tinnitus, and altered mental status.

Serum salicylates are 80 mg/dL.

How is salicylate overdose managed?

1. **ABCs**: First, stabilize the patient.
2. **Activated charcoal (gastric decontamination)**: Administer if the patient presents within 4 hours of ingestion.
3. **Electrolytes**: Administer HCO_3 to all patients. Administer glucose if the patient has altered mental status (aspirin overdose can decrease glucose levels in the CNS even if serum glucose is normal). Correct any other electrolyte abnormalities (particularly hypokalemia, which occurs frequently).

The patient's mental status deteriorates despite aggressive treatment.

What is the next step in management?

Consider hemodialysis for the following patients with salicylate overdose ("***DARE 100***"):

1. **D**eterioration despite aggressive treatment (this patient)
2. **A**ltered mental status (this patient)
3. **R**enal insufficiency
4. **E**dema (pulmonary or cerebral)
5. Salicylate level >**100** mg/dL

Alternative 7.4.1

A 25-year-old man is brought by paramedics to the emergency department for evaluation of altered mental status. He is a suspected drug trafficker who swallowed two bags of an unknown substance 1 hour ago after being chased by the police. Physical examination is significant for decreased bowel sounds and pinpoint pupils (miosis). Vital signs are temperature 37.4°C, pulse 80 bpm, respirations 8/min, blood pressure 100/70, and oxygen saturation 90% on 2 L. Fingerstick glucose is normal. Arterial blood gas values are pH 7.3, PCO_2 50, PO_2 90. Serum electrolytes are pending.

What is the most likely cause of his symptoms? What is the most likely acid–base abnormality?

Remember the classic clinical manifestations of opiate overdose with the mnemonic ***RAMBo***: decreased **R**espiratory rate, **A**ltered mental status, **M**iosis, and decreased **B**owel sounds. Decreased respiratory rate (hypoventilation) leads to simple respiratory acidosis, which is suggested by the combination of pH <7.4 and pCO_2 >45.

> Hyperventilation (tachypnea) causes respiratory alkalosis.
> Hypoventilation causes respiratory acidosis.

What is the next step in management?

Continue supplemental oxygen and administer IV naloxone (opiate antagonist).

> Opiate intoxication is a clinical diagnosis. Do not wait for toxicology screen to treat.

The patient's respiratory rate increases and his mental status improves with naloxone. Six hours later, the patient appears agitated. He complains of nausea, abdominal cramping, and diarrhea. Physical exam is significant for increased bowel sounds, goosebumps (piloerection), and dilated pupils (mydriasis). He yawns every 2 to 3 minutes. Abnormal vital signs are blood pressure 150/90 and pulse 110 bpm.

What is the cause of his symptoms?

The patient has signs and symptoms of opiate withdrawal (agitation, GI symptoms, increased bowel sounds, dilated pupils, yawning, and piloerection). Withdrawal is typically not life threatening except when it is triggered by overtreatment with an opioid antagonist (possibility in this patient).

What is the next step in management?

Administer clonidine every hour until hypertension and tachycardia resolve. Patients with cardiovascular disease and elderly patients may also require a benzodiazepine.

What are other important causes of respiratory acidosis (hypoventilation)?

1. **CNS**: brainstem injury (see Chapter 12: Neurology)
2. **Neuromuscular**: myasthenia gravis (Chapter 12: Neurology)
3. **Respiratory muscle fatigue**: severe asthma exacerbation, obesity-hypoventilation syndrome (see Chapter 3: Pulmonary).
4. **Pulmonary disorders**: chronic obstructive pulmonary disease (COPD) and other causes of airway obstruction (see Chapter 3: Pulmonary).
5. **Drugs**: narcotics, clonidine, sedative-hypnotics, etc.

> **Sedative-hypnotics**: benzodiazepines and barbiturates; flumazenil is often administered to reverse benzodiazepine intoxication.

CASE 7–5 HYPONATREMIA

A 65-year-old man who has just moved to the area presents for his first clinic visit. Prior records indicate that serum sodium was 129 mEq/L and serum creatinine was 2.1 last week. Remaining serum electrolytes are normal. Vital signs are currently normal.

What does serum sodium generally indicate?

Serum sodium is a marker of water balance in the body. It does not give any information regarding volume status.

What are the initial steps in determining the cause of hyponatremia?

In addition to obtaining a detailed history, the initial step in determining the cause of hyponatremia is physical examination to determine volume status and measurement of serum osmolarity (Table 7-3 and Fig. 7-4).

> **Hypervolemia**: weight gain, pedal or pulmonary edema, ascites, or elevated jugular vein distension.
> **Hypovolemia**: weight loss, decreased skin turgor, dry oropharynx, orthostatic hypotension, and increased BUN/creatinine.

TABLE 7–3 Causes of Hyponatremia

HYPERTONIC

1. **Hyperglycemia or mannitol:** Glucose and mannitol are osmotically active solutes that increased serum osmolarity. ↑ Osmolality pulls H_2O out of cells, which dilutes ECF.

ISOTONIC

1. **Isotonic glycine:** Isotonic non-sodium-containing fluid that is often used to irrigate the bladder or prostate during urological or gynecological surgery.
2. **Pseudohyponatremia:** ↑↑ Proteins (e.g., multiple myeloma) or ↑↑ lipids reduce fraction of plasma that is water and sodium.

HYPOTONIC

Hypovolemic

1. **Renal fluid loss (diuretics, sodium losing nephropathy, renal artery stenosis):**
2. **Nonrenal fluid loss (GI losses, severe burns, third spacing, etc.):** In both renal and nonrenal fluid loss, hypovolemia activates ADH, which stimulates the kidneys to reabsorb water but not sodium.

Euvolemic (*"TAPAS"*)

1. **HypoThyroidism:** Exact mechanism is unclear.
2. **Adrenal insufficiency:** Two reasons for hyponatremia: ↓ aldosterone leads to ↓ Na reabsorption and ↓ K secretion; ↓ cortisol removes hypothalamic CRH inhibition (↑ CRH stimulates ↑ ADH release).
3. **Primary polydipsia:** Drinking large quantities of water dilutes ECF. Suspect after ingestion of anti-psychotics (schizophrenics) and MDMA ("ecstasy"), because they cause dry mouth. ADH level is appropriately low in these patients.
4. **Alcoholism ("beer potomania") and malnourishment ("tea and toast syndrome")[2]:** Beer contains very little sodium or solutes. Without sufficient solutes, the osmolarity is not sufficient to excrete free water.
5. **SIADH:** Inappropriate ADH release causes water reabsorption. Water retention stimulates diuresis of urine rich in sodium and uric acid.

Hypervolemic

1. **Cirrhosis, congestive heart failure, nephrotic syndrome:** Patients have ↑ ECF but carotid sinus baroreceptors sense ↓ plasma volume (↓ effective arterial volume), which stimulates ADH release.
2. **Advanced renal failure:** Kidneys cannot dilute or concentrate fluid. Patients develop hyponatremia if they consume more free water than they can excrete.

Abbreviations: ADH, antidiuretic hormone (also called vasopressin or arginine vasopressin (aVP)); CRH, corticotropin-releasing hormone; SIADH, syndrome of inappropriate antidiuretic hormone.

It is often difficult to distinguish hypovolemia from euvolemia because mildly hypovolemic patients frequently do not have specific signs.

Serum osmolarity = 2 × (Na + glucose + urea).
Normal serum osmolarity is 280-295.

Past records indicate that he has a history of congestive heart failure and early chronic renal insufficiency. On physical exam, there is bilateral pedal edema. Serum osmolarity is 270.

What is the next step in management?

The patient has hypotonic hypervolemic hyponatremia (see Table 7-3). Both renal failure and congestive heart failure can cause hyponatremia. The next step is to obtain urine sodium (U_{Na}) (see Fig. 7-4).

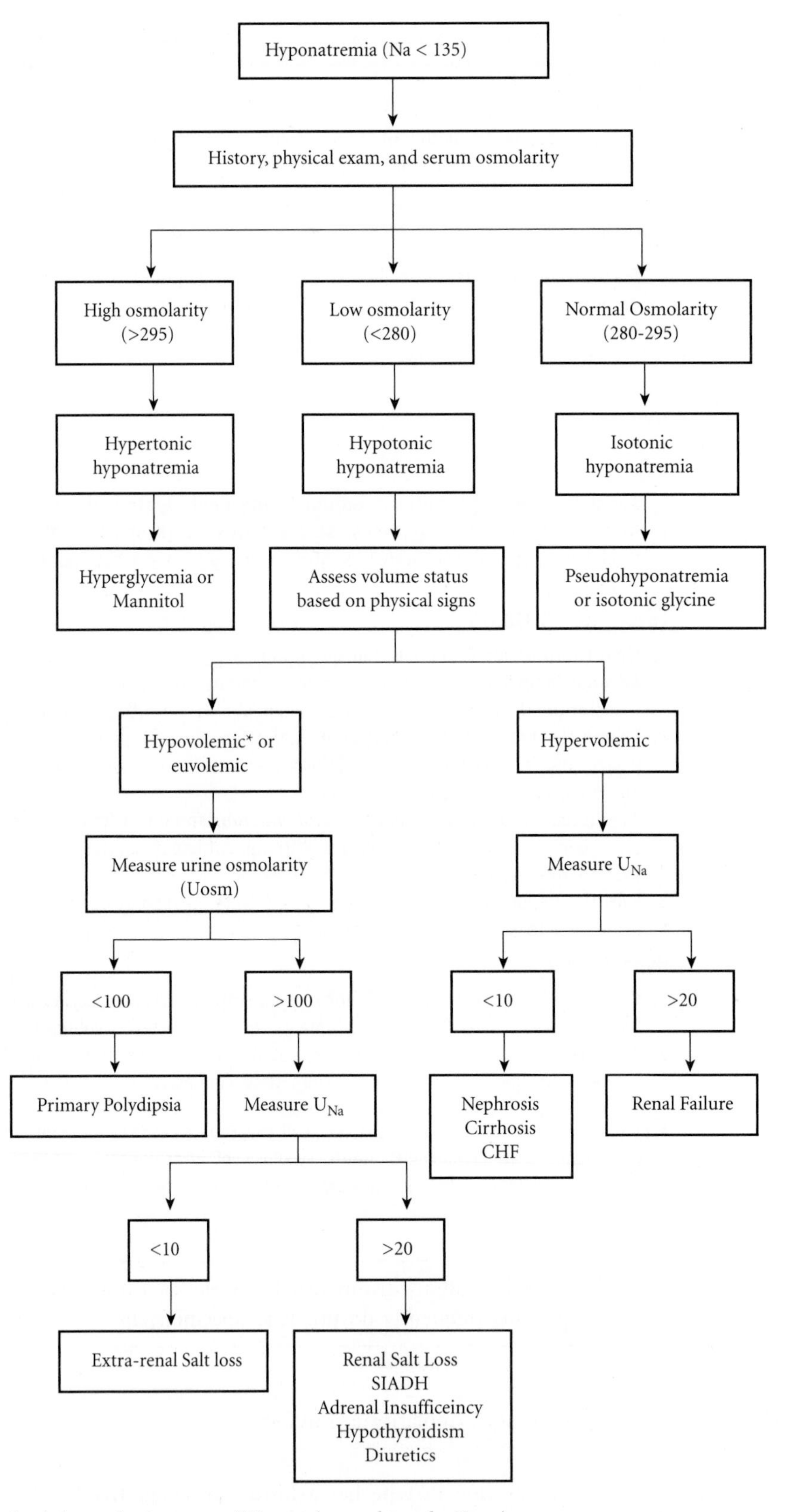

* If patient is obviously hypovolemic, measure UNa next (no need to order Uosm)

FIGURE 7–4 Workup of hyponatremia.

U_{Na} is 10, which indicates that heart failure rather than renal failure is responsible for his symptoms.

How is hypervolemic hyponatremia treated?

Treat hypervolemic hyponatremia with fluid and sodium restriction. If hyponatremia persists, administer loop diuretics.

> Hyponatremia is an independent risk factor for complications and death in patients with cirrhosis or heart failure.

> **Vasopressin** (antidiuretic hormone (ADH)) **receptor antagonists**: currently under investigation for treatment of chronic hypervolemic or euvolemic hyponatremia.

Two months later, the patient is admitted for treatment of acute decompensated heart failure. He receives furosemide. On hospital day 1, sodium is 132 mEq/L. On hospital day 2, serum electrolytes are sodium 129, potassium 2.9, chloride 98, HCO_3 40, BUN 20, creatinine 1.3, glucose 105. Serum osmolarity is 173. On admission the patient had 2+ peripheral edema, but currently there is no edema. Blood pressure is 100/80.

What is the most likely cause of hyponatremia?

Absence of edema indicates that the patient is currently either euvolemic or hypovolemic. The history of loop diuretic administration along with concurrent hypokalemia and metabolic alkalosis ("contraction alkalosis") strongly suggest renal fluid losses due to furosemide. Most clinicians would treat such patients without any further work-up. If the diagnosis were not as obvious, the next step would be to obtain urine osmolarity followed by U_{Na} (see Table 7-6).

> **Hypotonic euvolemic hyponatremia**: U_{Na} is usually >30.

> Other causes of renal fluid loss–mediated hyponatremia:
> 1. **Renal artery stenosis**: Suspect if decreased serum K^+ and hypertension are present.
> 2. **Salt-wasting nephropathy (autosomal polycystic kidney disease, chronic pyelonephritis)**: Suspect if increased serum K^+ is present.

How should you treat this patient's hyponatremia?

Treat asymptomatic hypovolemic hyponatremia with normal saline (volume repletion removes the stimulus for ADH release). Raise serum sodium ≤0.5/hour, because overly rapid correction can cause central pontine myelinolysis.

> **Central pontine myelinolysis**: Presents with confusion, horizontal gaze paralysis, and spastic quadriplegia 48 to 72 hours after overly rapid sodium correction. Magnetic resonance imaging confirms diagnosis. This condition is often fatal, and there is no cure for survivors.

During rounds the next day, you realize that the furosemide dose was increased and no fluids were administered. Serum sodium is 114. The patient is not oriented to person, place, or time.

What is the next step in management?

Mild hyponatremia is usually asymptomatic. However, a rapid decrease in serum sodium to levels <120 can cause GI or CNS symptoms (altered mental status, seizures, and coma). Treat any acutely symptomatic patient with hypertonic saline at a rate that increases serum sodium ≤2 mEq/L per hour. When symptoms resolve or serum sodium >120, switch to normal saline at a rate that increases serum sodium ≤0.5 mEq/L per hour.

Pathophysiology: Hyponatremia → water enters brain cells → cerebral edema → neurologic symptoms.

Advanced renal failure: Consider hemodialysis if fluid and salt restriction does not correct sodium <120.

Alternative 7.5.1

A 65-year-old woman is admitted to the hospital after a suicidal gesture. She has a history of hypertension, COPD, and major depression. Medications are metoprolol, inhaled albuterol/ipratropium, and paroxetine. She has a 30-pack/year smoking history. Physical exam is normal. Blood pressure is 160/90 and serum sodium is 122. She is admitted to the medical ward for stabilization of medical issues prior to psychiatric hospitalization. The intern orders serum osmolarity, U_{Na}, and serum uric acid. He administers normal saline and increases the metoprolol dose. The next day, blood pressure is 129/80 and serum sodium is 118. Serum osmolarity is 270, urine osmolarity is 450, U_{Na} is 42, and serum uric acid is low.

What is the most likely cause of hyponatremia?

Suspect the syndrome of inappropriate antidiuretic hormone (SIADH) in patients with hypotonic euvolemic hyponatremia, urine osmolarity >serum osmolarity, and U_{Na} >30. Serum uric acid is often low, but acid–base balance is normal. Fluid administration worsens hyponatremia.

What are the major causes of SIADH?

1. **CNS**: stroke, head injury or CNS infection
2. **Pulmonary**: small cell lung cancer or lung infections
3. **Major surgery**: abdominal, thoracic, or pituitary surgery
4. **Drugs**: "*Drugs Can Cause SIADH*" (**D**DAVP or vasopressin, **C**arbamazepine, **C**yclophosphamide, **S**elective serotonin reuptake inhibitors)

What is the next step in management?

SIADH is a diagnosis of exclusion. The first step is to rule out other causes of euvolemic hyponatremia associated with urine osmolarity >100 (hypothyroidism and adrenal insufficiency).

Serum thyrotropin and serum cortisol are normal. What is the next step in management?

Obtain head and chest CT scan to rule out CNS and pulmonary causes of SIADH. If these are normal, the most likely cause of SIADH is paroxetine (a selective serotonin reuptake inhibitor).

Head and chest CT are normal.

How is SIADH treated?

1. First-line therapy is to correct the underlying cause and restrict fluid.
2. If the patient is symptomatic or if hyponatremia persists, consider salt therapy (hypertonic saline ± loop diuretics).
3. If the patient cannot tolerate (or does not respond to) fluid restriction and salt therapy, consider demeclocycline (induces diabetes insipidus (DI)) or urea.

Reset osmostat: In this rare variant of SIADH, patients have a lower threshold for ADH release. Serum sodium is chronically low but stable (approximately 125 to 130). No treatment is indicated.

> Summary of hyponatremia therapy:
> **Hypovolemic hyponatremia**: normal saline
> **Hypervolemic hyponatremia**: fluid and salt restriction ± loop diuretics
> **SIADH**: fluid restriction ± hypertonic saline, loop diuretics
> **Primary polydipsia**: fluid restriction
> **Hyperglycemia, adrenal insufficiency, and hypothyroidism**: treat underlying cause
> **Reset osmostat and pseudohyponatremia**: no treatment
> **Symptomatic patients**: hypertonic saline (increase Na ≤2 mEq/L per hour)

CASE 7–6 HYPERNATREMIA AND MAINTENANCE FLUIDS

A 45-year-old man presents with a 2-month history of polyuria and polydipsia. Past history is unremarkable. Physical exam and vital signs are normal. Fingerstick glucose is normal. Serum sodium is 148 mEq/L. Other serum chemistries are normal.

What are the clinical manifestations of hypernatremia?

Most patients are asymptomatic. However, hypernatremia can cause neurological symptoms ranging from lethargy and weakness to seizures and coma.

> **Pathophysiology**: Hypernatremia (increased serum osmolarity) → water moves from brain cells to extracellular fluid → decreased brain volume → rupture of intracerebral veins → neurologic symptoms.

In addition to taking a detailed history, what is the next step in determining the cause of this patient's hypernatremia?

The first step is to assess the patient's volume status. On the basis of physical exam findings, this patient is clinically euvolemic. The next step is to measure urine osmolarity (Fig. 7-5). Urine osmolarity is 350 mosm/L.

What is the most likely diagnosis? What is the next step in management?

DI is the most likely diagnosis in this patient with polyuria, polydipsia, mild hypernatremia, and dilute urine. The next step is to confirm the diagnosis using the water deprivation test (Fig. 7-6).

> **Polyuria**: >3 L of urine output/day. Major causes are diabetes mellitus, DI, diuretics, primary polydipsia.

Four hours later, urine osmolarity is 200 and serum osmolarity is 295.

What is the next diagnostic step?

Urine that is more dilute than serum despite water deprivation confirms the diagnosis of DI. There are two types of DI (see Table 7-4). To determine which type of DI is responsible for this patient's symptoms, administer exogenous ADH in the form of desmopressin (dDAVP) or vasopressin:

1. **Central DI**: There is a defect in ADH production. Exogenous ADH causes increased renal free water reabsorption, which leads to increased urine osmolarity.
2. **Nephrogenic DI**: There is a defect in ADH responsiveness. Exogenous ADH has no effect on urine osmolarity.

How are central and nephrogenic DI treated?

The primary treatment goal is to reduce urine output (see Table 7-4). A secondary goal is to correct serum sodium with 5% dextrose in free water (D5W). Note that patients compensate

Hypovolemia hypernatremia (loss of fluid that is more dilute than serum)
1) **GI fluid losses:** Osmotic diarrhea (e.g. – lactulose-induced).
2) **Renal fluid losses:** Osmotic diuresis (due to hyperglycemia, mannitol, or urea).
3) **Other fluid losses:** Diaphoresis, respiratory losses

Euvolemic hypernatremia
1) **Diabetes insipidus:** ↓ ADH secretion (central DI) or action (nephrogenic DI).
2) **Severe exercise or seizures:** Causes glycogen in cells to break down into osmotically active solutes. These solutes pull water into cells. Hypernatremia usually resolves within 5-15 minutes of exertion.

Hypervolemic hypernatremia (least frequent)
1) **Iatrogenic:** Administration of excessive hypertonic saline-containing solutions (e.g. – $NaHCO_3$ for treatment of metabolic acidosis, artificial nutrition).
2) **Hyperaldosteronism:** ↑ cortisol → ↓ CRH → ↓ ADH → hypernatremia. Also, ↑ aldosterone → ↑ Na and water reabsorption → hypervolemia.

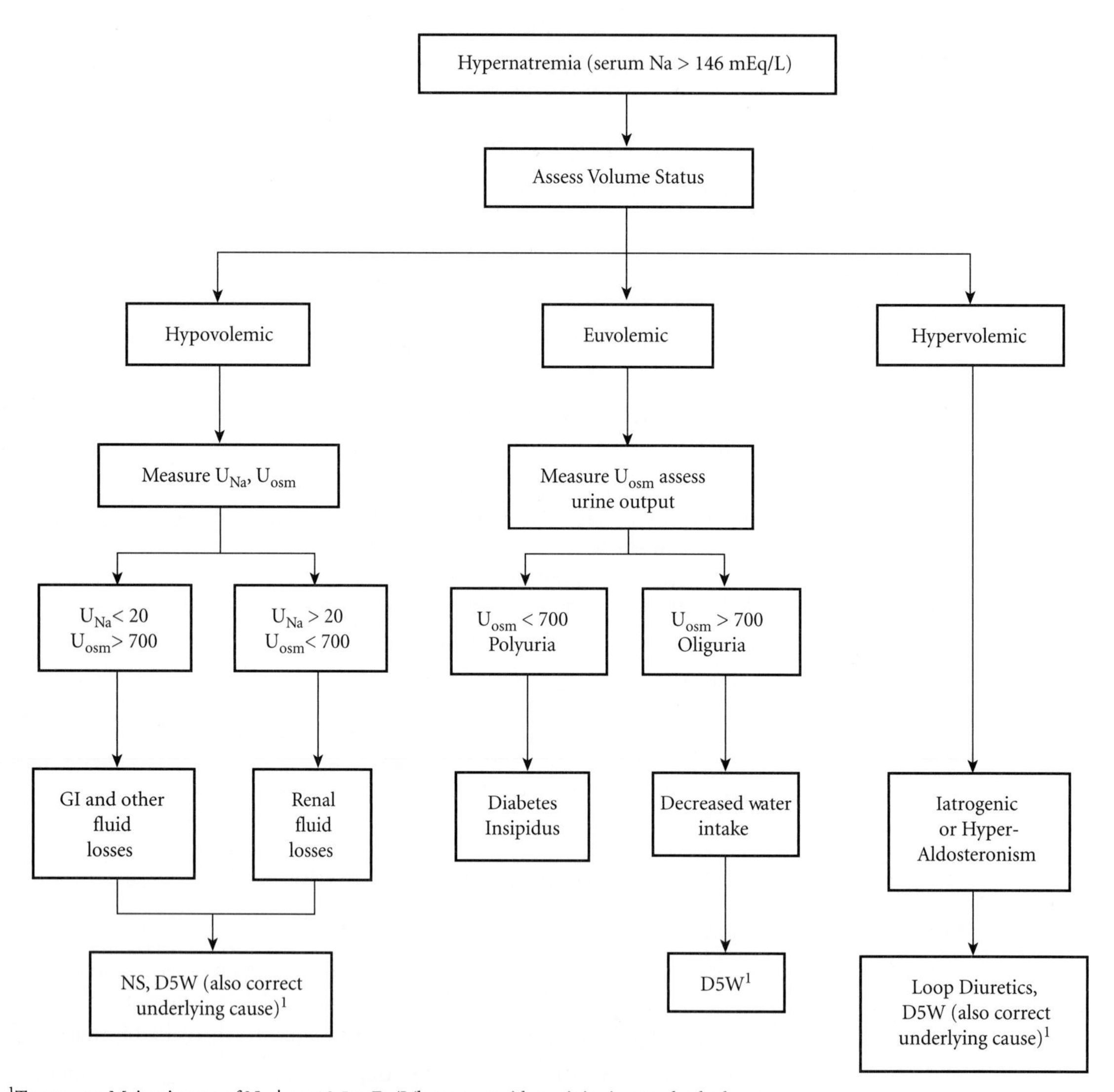

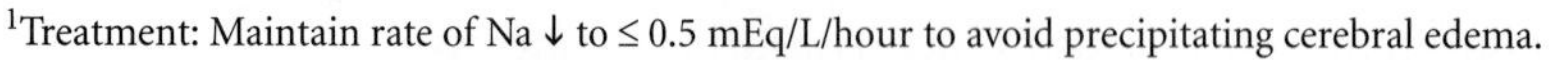
[1]Treatment: Maintain rate of Na ↓ to ≤ 0.5 mEq/L/hour to avoid precipitating cerebral edema.

FIGURE 7–5 Major etiologies, work-up, and treatment of hypernatremia.

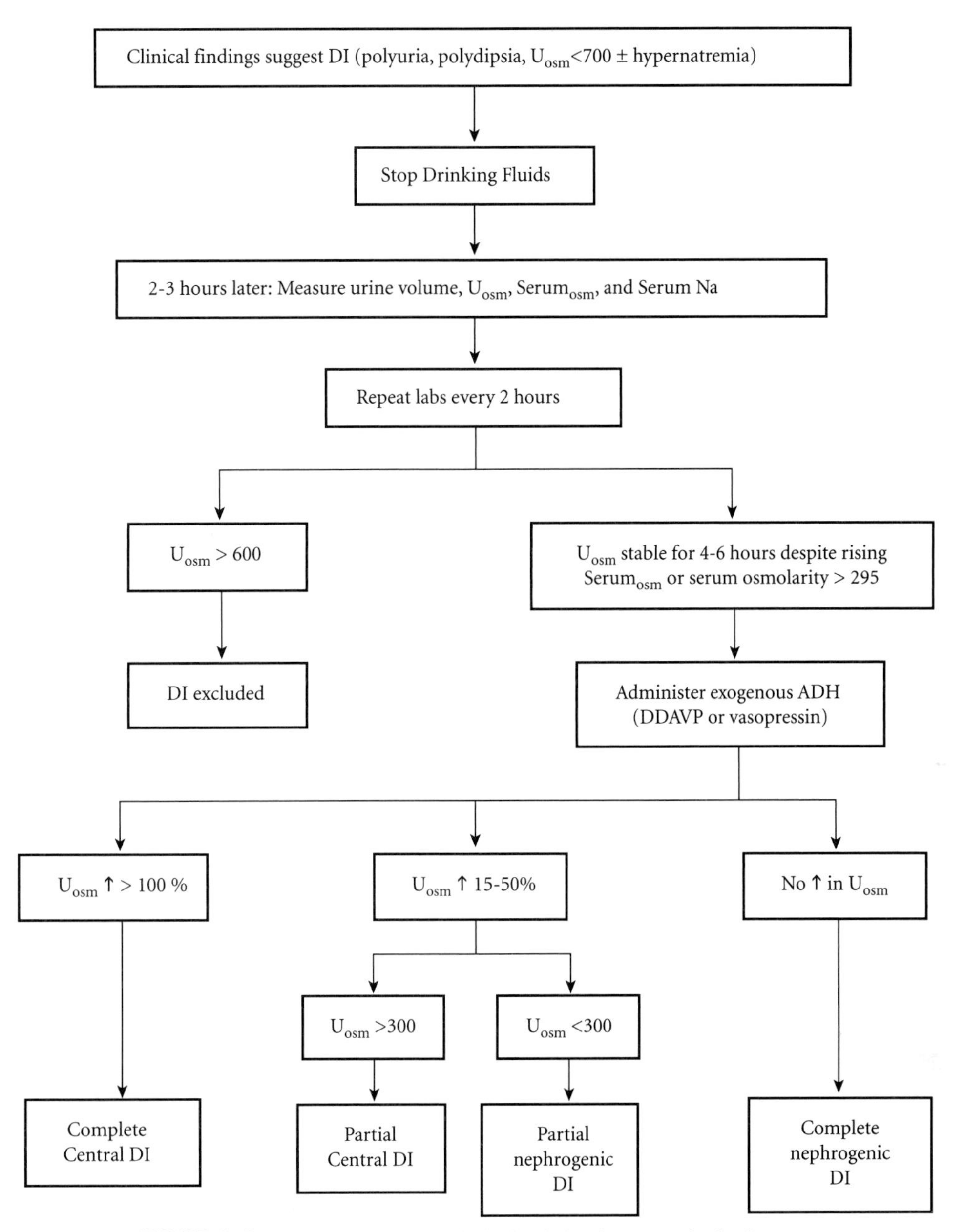

FIGURE 7–6 Diagnosis of diabetes insipidus (DI) using water deprivation test.

for decreased water reabsorption with increased water intake (increased thirst), so serum sodium is typically <150 mEq/L (high-normal or mildly elevated).

Alternative 7.6.1

A 55-year-old man with a history of cirrhosis caused by hepatitis C is hospitalized for hepatic encephalopathy. His mental status improves with lactulose. On hospital day 2, serum sodium is 158 mEq/L. On physical exam, oropharynx is dry and there is decreased skin turgor. Blood pressure is 108/95 supine and 90/80 sitting.

What is the most likely cause of hypernatremia?

Osmotic diarrhea as a result of lactulose is the most likely cause of hypernatremia in this clinically hypovolemic patient (see Fig. 7-5). Most clinicians would treat this patient without further work-up. If the diagnosis were less obvious, the next step would have been to obtain urine osmolarity and U_{Na}.

TABLE 7–4 Central Versus Nephrogenic Diabetes Insipidus

	Central DI	Nephrogenic DI
Pathophysiology	Hypothalamic lesion causes ↓ ADH production.	Kidneys cannot respond to ADH.
Causes	1. Strokes 2. Tumors 3. Neurosurgery 4. Infrequent causes[a]	1. Medications (lithium, amphotericin B) 2. Kidney disease (APKD) 3. Electrolyte imbalances (↓ K, ↑ Ca) 4. Hereditary
Clinical	Onset of polyuria and polydipsia is abrupt.	Onset of polyuria and polydipsia is gradual.
Treatment[b]	Treat with dDAVP (increase dose until polyuria resolves).	Step-wise therapy:[c] 1. Low-sodium, low-protein diet[d] 2. Thiazide diuretics 3. NSAIDs 4. dDAVP

Abbreviations: APKD, autosomal polycystic kidney disease; dDAVP, desmopressin; DI, diabetes insipidus; NSAID, nonsteroidal anti-inflammatory drug.

[a] Infrequent causes include hypothalamic infiltration due to sarcoidosis, hemochromatosis, tuberculosis, syphilis, and Langerhans histiocytosis.

[b] Correct hypernatremia in both types of DI with 5% dextrose in water (D5W).

[c] Add next medication to regimen only if polyuria does not resolve.

[d] Lithium-induced DI: Consider amiloride as part of initial therapy if you cannot discontinue lithium.

Dehydration: Loss of free water → increased serum sodium (hypernatremia).
Hypovolemia: Loss of sodium and water → decreased volume with hypo-, hyper-, or normonatremia.

How is hypovolemic hypernatremia treated?

First eliminate the offending agent (in this case, lactulose) and correct hypovolemia with normal saline or D5½NS (5% dextrose in half normal saline). Then correct hypernatremia with D5W.

Hypervolemic hypernatremia: First treat underlying cause and correct hypervolemia with loop diuretics. Then correct hypernatremia with D5W.

At what rate should you administer normal saline to a patient with mild-moderate hypovolemia (i.e., not in shock)?

Consider the following formula to estimate the rate of normal saline administration:

Rate = (Urine output/hour) + (30 to 50 mL/hour for insensible losses) + (50 to 100 mL).

Note that if the patient has fever, diaphoresis, or increased respiratory secretions, insensible losses are higher (80 to 150 mL).

The patient's diarrhea improves after withholding lactulose. His orthostatic hypotension and other signs of hypovolemia resolve with normal saline. He weighs 70 kg. His ideal body weight (IBW) is 60 kg.

How much replacement therapy with D5W will this patient require to correct hypernatremia and at what rate?

Step 1. Calculate total body water (TBW): TBW = 0.6 × IBW (×0.85 if female or elderly) = 0.6 × 60 = 36

Step 2. Calculate free water deficit (FWD): FWD = TBW × (serum Na – 140)/140 = 36 × (158 – 140)/140 = 36 × 18/140 = 4.6 L

Step 3. Calculate how much sodium needs to be lowered: In this case, we must lower sodium by $158 - 145 = 13$ mEq/L.

Step 4. Calculate over what period of time sodium should be lowered: To avoid cerebral edema, lower serum sodium by ≤ 0.5 mEq/L per hour. Therefore, lower this patient's sodium over 26 hours.

Step 5. Calculate rate of D5W administration: In this case, administer 4.6 L of D5W over 26 hours, or approximately 0.18 L/hour (180 mL/hour).

> **Replacement therapy:** correction of water and electrolyte deficits in patients with excessive fluid loss (e.g., diuresis, diarrhea, third spacing, burns, etc.).
> **Maintenance therapy:** replacement of water and electrolyte losses that occur normally as a result of urination, sweating, defecation, etc. Indicated for patients who are unable to eat (e.g., postoperative, anorexic, and mechanically ventilated patients).

After correcting hypovolemia and hypernatremia with the replacement therapy described earlier, the patient is unable to tolerate oral intake because of nausea and anorexia.

At what rate would you administer maintenance fluids?

Calculate the maintenance fluid rate using the 4/2/1 rule (4mL/kg for the first 10 kg, 2 mL/kg for the second 10 kg, and 1 mL/kg for every kg >20 kg). This 70-kg patient requires $(4 \times 10) + (2 \times 10) + (1 \times 50) = 40 + 20 + 50 = 110$ mL/hour. Also, monitor serum chemistries and replace as necessary.

When is artificial nutrition support indicated?

Consider enteral or parenteral nutrition if a patient has not eaten for 7 to 14 days. The other common indication for artificial nutrition is multiorgan dysfunction.

> **"If the gut works, use it":** Enteral feeding may prevent gut epithelium breakdown and thereby reduce bacterial translocation across the gut (i.e., reduce infection). As a result, the enteral route (via nasogastric or gastrostomy tube) is preferred if there are no contraindications (vomiting, GI tract obstruction/ischemia/ileus).

> **Parenteral nutrition:** Infuse feeding solution into a large blood vessel using a central venous catheter.

CASE 7–7 HYPOKALEMIA

A 65-year-old woman is admitted for treatment of COPD exacerbation. She also has type 2 diabetes mellitus. On admission, serum potassium is 4.0 mEq/L. She receives oxygen, albuterol/ipratropium, and oral steroids. She is started on a four-shot regimen of regular insulin with meals and NPH insulin at bedtime. On hospital day 2, serum potassium is 3.1 mEq/L.

What is the most likely cause of hypokalemia?

Based on the patient's history, the hypokalemia is most likely caused by albuterol and insulin (Table 7-5). These medications shift K^+ from the extracellular to the intracellular compartment. If the cause is not obvious, follow the diagnostic approach in (Fig. 7-7).

What are possible clinical manifestations of hypokalemia?

Patients with serum K^+ >3.0 mEq/L are usually asymptomatic (unless they are also taking digitalis). Most symptoms occur only after serum K^+ <2.5 mEq/L.

1. **Nausea and vomiting**
2. **Muscle weakness:** Symptoms begin in lower extremities and then spread to trunk and upper extremities. Weakness may progress to paralysis.

TABLE 7–5 Major Causes of Hypokalemia

↑ RENAL K^+ LOSSES

Hypertension and metabolic alkalosis

1. **Hyperaldosteronism**
2. **Cushing's syndrome**
3. **Renal artery stenosis**

In all three conditions, ↑ RAAS activity leads to ↑ Na and H_2O reabsorption (hypertension) plus ↑ K^+ and H^+ secretion (hypokalemia and metabolic alkalosis).

Hypo- or normotensive (*"If you don't correct hypokalemia, U R BAD M.D."*)

1. ***U*pper GI fluid loss (vomiting, nasogastric suction)**: Upper GI fluids are low in K^+, but patients have hypokalemia via two mechanisms: volume depletion activates RAAS, and ↓ gastric acid → metabolic alkalosis → ↑ HCO_3^- delivered to distal tubule (non-reabsorbable anion) → ↑ electrochemical gradient for K^+ secretion.
2. ***R*enal tubular acidosis (types 1 and 2)**
3. ***B*arter and Gitelman syndromes**: Mechanism similar to diuretics.
4. ***A*mphotericin B**: Increases renal membrane permeability for K^+ secretion.
5. ***D*iuretics (CAIs, loop and thiazide diuretics)**: Volume depletion activates RAAS.
6. ***M*agnesium depletion**: Mechanism unclear.
7. ***D*iabetic ketoacidosis**: Refer to Case 1.

↑ LOWER GI K^+ LOSSES

Diarrhea, laxatives, and villous adenoma of colon: K^+ content of lower intestinal secretions is high, so diarrhea leads to hypokalemia.

TRANSCELLULAR SHIFT (*"ALKALOSIS BRINGS POTASSIUM IN"*)

1. ***A*lkalosis**: H^+ leaves cells to raise serum pH; K^+ enters cells to maintain electrical neutrality.
2. **β-agonist drugs**: Activate β-2 receptors → ↑ Na/K/ATPase (drives K^+ into cells).
3. **Hypokalemic *P*eriodic paralysis**: Rare genetic (autosomal dominant) or acquired condition (in patients with thyrotoxicosis).
4. ***I*nsulin**: Activates Na/K/ATPase.

Abbreviations: CAI, carbonic anhydrase inhibitor; RAAS, renin-angiotensin-aldosterone system.

3. **EKG abnormalities**: The characteristic EKG triad in hypokalemia is ST depression, decreased T wave amplitude, and prominent U waves. Other nonspecific dysrhythmias can also occur.
4. **Rhabdomyolysis**: see Chapter 6: Nephrology.

> **U waves**: depolarizations that follow T waves with the same polarity but amplitude less than one third that of T waves. Suspect hypokalemia if increased U wave amplitude.

How is hypokalemia managed?

1. Obtain a baseline EKG.
2. Replace potassium and treat the underlying cause.
3. Monitor EKG, serum K^+, and other electrolytes.

> **Hypokalemia + metabolic acidosis**: Use potassium citrate or potassium bicarbonate.
> **Other patients with hypokalemia**: Use potassium chloride.

> **Transcellular shifts**: Close monitoring of serum K^+ is essential because potassium replacement and correcting underlying cause can lead to hyperkalemia.

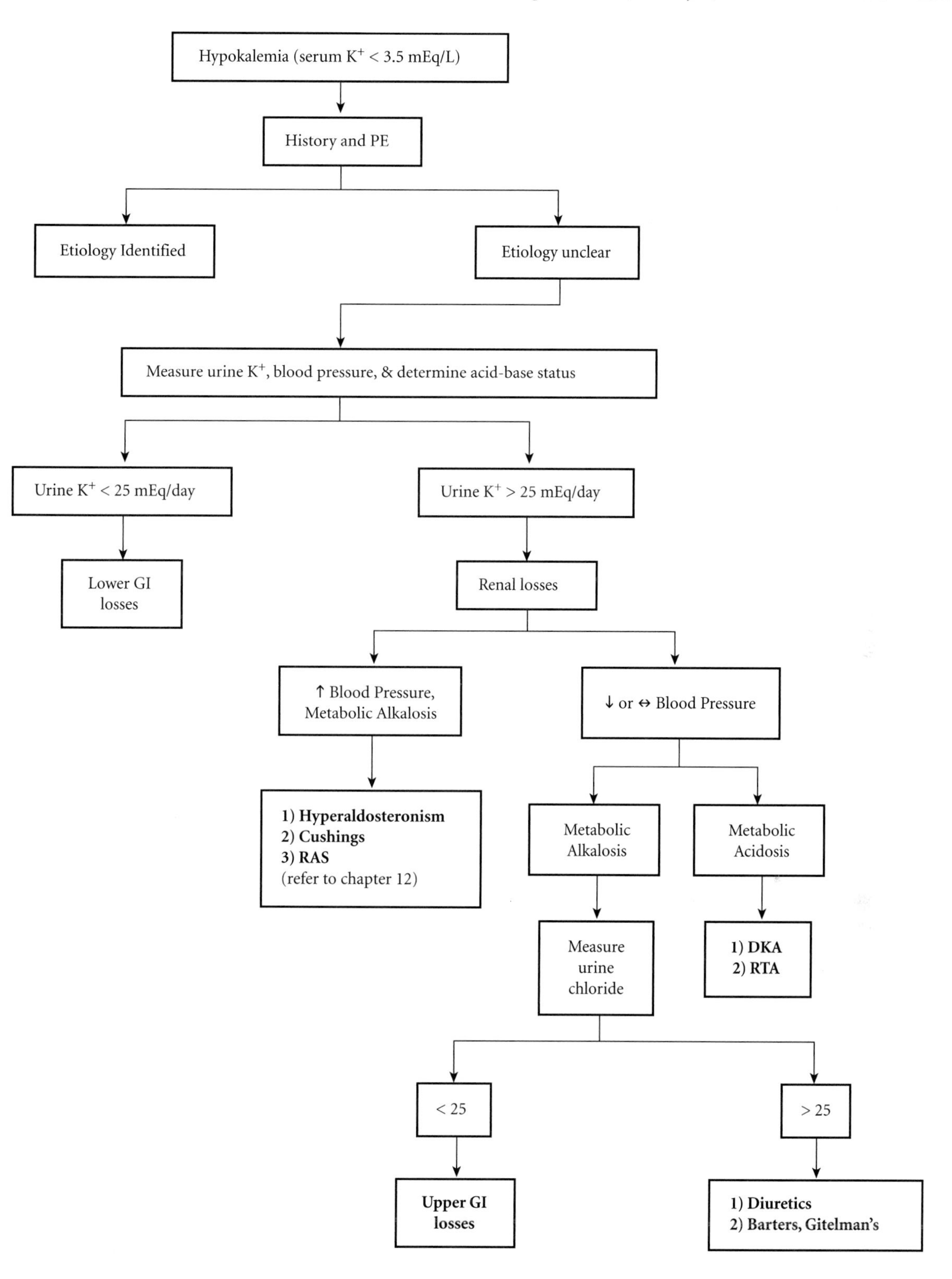

[1]= Identify etiologies that cause transcellular K+ shift based on history and assessment of acid-base status. Suspect hypokalemic periodic paralysis (rare) if patient has recurrent episodes of weakness/paralysis and hypokalemia but normal serum K+ between episodes.

FIGURE 7–7 Work-up and treatment of hypokalemia.

Hypomagnesemia: Can cause hypokalemia, hypocalcemia, and metabolic alkalosis. Decreased serum K^+ and Ca^{+2} are often refractory unless decreased serum Mg^{2+} is corrected first.

What are the indications for IV potassium administration?

The oral route is usually preferred. Use the IV route alone or as an adjunct to oral replacement if the patient has severe symptoms or cannot tolerate oral intake (vomiting, anorexia, etc.).

IV potassium tips:

1. **Infusion route**: Administer with saline-containing rather than dextrose-containing fluids (dextrose → increased insulin → shifts K^+ into cells).
2. **Infusion rate**: Do not infuse K^+ at a rate >10 to 20 mEq/hour. If infusing at a maximal rate, monitor EKG continuously.
3. **Infusion concentration**: Avoid K^+ concentration ≥60 mEq/L through a peripheral vein (painful).
4. **Infusion amount**: 10 mEq of K^+ (oral or IV) raises serum K^+ by 0.1 mEq.

Five years later, the patient presents to her primary care physician for a regularly scheduled visit. She was diagnosed with hypertension 2 years ago. Blood pressure has been well controlled with hydrochlorothiazide since then. Serum K^+ has ranged from 3.1 to 3.3 mEq/L for the last 3 months.

What the options for treatment of chronic hypokalemia?

1. **Oral potassium chloride or salt substitutes**: most common methods
2. **Dietary intake of potassium-rich foods (e.g., bananas)**: not as effective
3. **Potassium-sparing diuretics**: effective but poorly tolerated alternative.

Patients receiving chronic K^+ replacement should monitor serum K^+ every 3 to 4 months.

CASE 7–8 HYPERKALEMIA

A 57-year-old man is admitted to the hospital for treatment of severe community acquired pneumonia. On hospital day 2, serum potassium is 6.8 mEq/L. The laboratory report mentions "sample hemolyzed." Physical exam and vital signs are normal.

What are possible clinical manifestations of hyperkalemia?

Hyperkalemia is usually asymptomatic until serum K^+ >7 mEq/L (severe hyperkalemia). Clinical manifestations of severe hyperkalemia are:

1. **Muscle weakness**: Like severe hypokalemia, weakness begins in the lower extremities and progresses to the trunk and upper extremities. Weakness can progress to flaccid paralysis.
2. **EKG abnormalities**: The characteristic EKG triad in hyperkalemia is peaked T waves, prolonged PR interval, and wide QRS complex (Table 7-6). Untreated, patients progress to bundle branch block and finally to ventricular fibrillation and asystole.

Pathophysiology:

Initially: Increased extracellular K^+ → activated Na^+ channels → increased depolarization → increased action potentials (increased membrane excitability) → abnormal EKG.

Later: Persistent depolarization inactivates Na^+ channels → decreased membrane excitability → muscle weakness/paralysis.

TABLE 7-6 Characteristic EKG in Hyperkalemia Versus Hypokalemia

	Hypokalemia	Hyperkalemia
T-wave	↓ Amplitude	Tall and peaked
PR interval	Longer	Shorter
Other	U-wave	Wide QRS complex

What is the next step in management?

Suspect pseudohyperkalemia (Table 7-7) in the following situations:

1. Hemolyzed sample
2. Increased WBCs or platelets
3. Sample drawn from same site as IV fluids containing potassium.

The next step in this asymptomatic patient is to recheck serum K^+. If repeat serum K^+ is <5 mEq/L, the patient has pseudohyperkalemia and no further work-up is necessary. If repeat serum K^+ is >5, obtain an EKG and examine the patient for neuromuscular symptoms (see Fig. 7-7).

Repeat serum K^+ is 3.9. Two months later, serum K^+ is 6.1 on routine laboratory evaluation. There are no risk factors for pseudohyperkalemia. Physical exam and vital signs are normal. EKG is normal.

What is the next step in management?

The next step in an asymptomatic patient with serum K^+ between 5 and 7 mEq/L and normal EKG is to determine the underlying cause (see Table 7-7):

1. Take a detailed history (particularly medication history).
2. If history does not identify an obvious cause, order the following tests:
   - Serum chemistries (detects metabolic acidosis, renal failure, or hyperglycemia)
   - Serum osmolarity, spot urine osmolarity, and urine potassium (used to calculate transtubular K^+ gradient)

> **Transtubular K^+ gradient** = (urine K^+/serum K^+) × ($serum_{osm}/urine_{osm}$). If transtubular K^+ gradient is <7, suspect hypoaldosteronism. Differentiate the cause of hypoaldosteronism using plasma renin activity, serum aldosterone, and serum cortisol (see Chapter 8: Endocrinology).

What medications are available to treat hyperkalemia?

Remember drugs used to treat hyperkalemia using the mnemonic "***CIA Kills Fanatics***":

1. **C**alcium: $CaCl_2$ or calcium gluconate inhibit K^+-induced membrane excitability.
2. **I**nsulin and **A**lbuterol: Drives K^+ into cells. When using insulin, also give glucose to prevent insulin-induced hypoglycemia.
3. **K**ayexelate and loop diuretics (such as **F**urosemide): Kayexelate binds K^+ in the gut. Loop diuretics promote renal K^+ excretion. Monitor patients receiving kayexelate for abdominal tenderness (intestinal necrosis is a potential complication).

> Sodium bicarbonate also drives K^+ into cells. Not commonly used unless the patient has moderate to severe metabolic acidosis.

How should you treat this asymptomatic patient with serum K^+ of 6.1?

In addition to correcting the underlying cause, treat this patient with moderate hyperkalemia (serum K^+ 6 to 7) with kayexelate and loop diuretics (Fig. 7-8).

TABLE 7–7 Major Causes of Hyperkalemia

TRANSCELLULAR SHIFT

1. **Acidosis**
2. **β-Blockers**
3. **Hyperkalemic periodic paralysis**
4. **Deficiency of insulin**
5. **↑ Tissue breakdown:** Releases K^+ into plasma; causes include trauma and tumor lysis syndrome (refer to Chapter 14: Primary Care Gynecology and Urology)
6. **Pseudohyperkalemia:** Common causes are venipuncture with a tourniquet (predisposes to local hemolysis), venipuncture at IV fluid site (if IV fluids contain K^+), and ↑ WBCs or platelets (once blood clots, K^+ moves out of these cells).

Note: Notice that first four causes are exact opposite of transcellular hypokalemia.

↓ RENAL K^+ EXCRETION (*"U R AMA MEMBER"*)

1. ***U**reterojejunostomy*: Ureters inserted into jejunum, which absorbs urinary K^+ into the bloodstream.
2. ***R**enal failure*
3. **HypoAldosteronism**
4. ***M**edications*: Heparin, cyclosporine, pentamidine, and K^+ sparing diuretics cause hypoaldosteronism.[a]
5. **↓ Effective *A*rterial blood volume (heart failure, cirrhosis, nephrotic syndrome):** ↓ Fluid delivery to distal tubule inhibits RAAS.

Abbreviations: ACE, angiotensin-converting enzyme; IV, intravenous; WBC, white blood cells.
[a] Monitor serum K^+ closely when combining medications that cause hyperkalemia in a patient who is already predisposed to increased serum K^+. A common example is the combination of K^+-sparing diuretics and ACE inhibitors in a patient with heart failure.

How would management differ if serum K^+ were >7 (severe hyperkalemia)?

Hyperkalemia treatment may affect laboratory results, so the first step is to obtain blood and urine samples for diagnostic work-up. Initiate urgent treatment before laboratory results are available:

Step 1. Administer calcium ($CaCl_2$ or calcium gluconate). The American Heart Association recommends $CaCl_2$ over calcium gluconate, but many clinicians prefer calcium gluconate because peripherally administered $CaCl_2$ can cause tissue necrosis.

Step 2. Administer insulin with glucose and/or nebulized albuterol ± $NaHCO_3$.

Step 3. Recheck serum K^+. If the level is >6, re-administer insulin. When serum K^+ is <6, administer kayexelate. Consider dialysis if serum K^+ is >6 despite repeated doses of insulin.

Abnormal EKG or muscle weakness: Treat as severe hyperkalemia even if K^+ <7.

CASE 7–9 PHOSPHATE AND MAGNESIUM

An 18-year-old woman is hospitalized for inpatient management of severe anorexia nervosa. She has no other medical conditions. The patient receives thiamine and begins to ingest food under surveillance. On hospital day 7, she appears confused. She is oriented to person but not to place and time. Heart rate is 115 bpm and respiratory rate is 28/minute. Head CT is negative. Fingerstick glucose is 100 mg/dL. Serum chemistries are sodium 138, potassium 3.2, chloride 95, HCO_3 24, BUN 15, creatinine 0.8, calcium 9.0, magnesium 1.1, and phosphorus 1.0.

What is the most likely cause of this patient's symptoms?

Important causes of altered mental status after nourishment of malnourished patients are Wernicke's syndrome and re-feeding syndrome. Wernicke's syndrome is unlikely in this patient who received thiamine prior to alimentation. The most likely diagnosis is re-feeding syndrome.

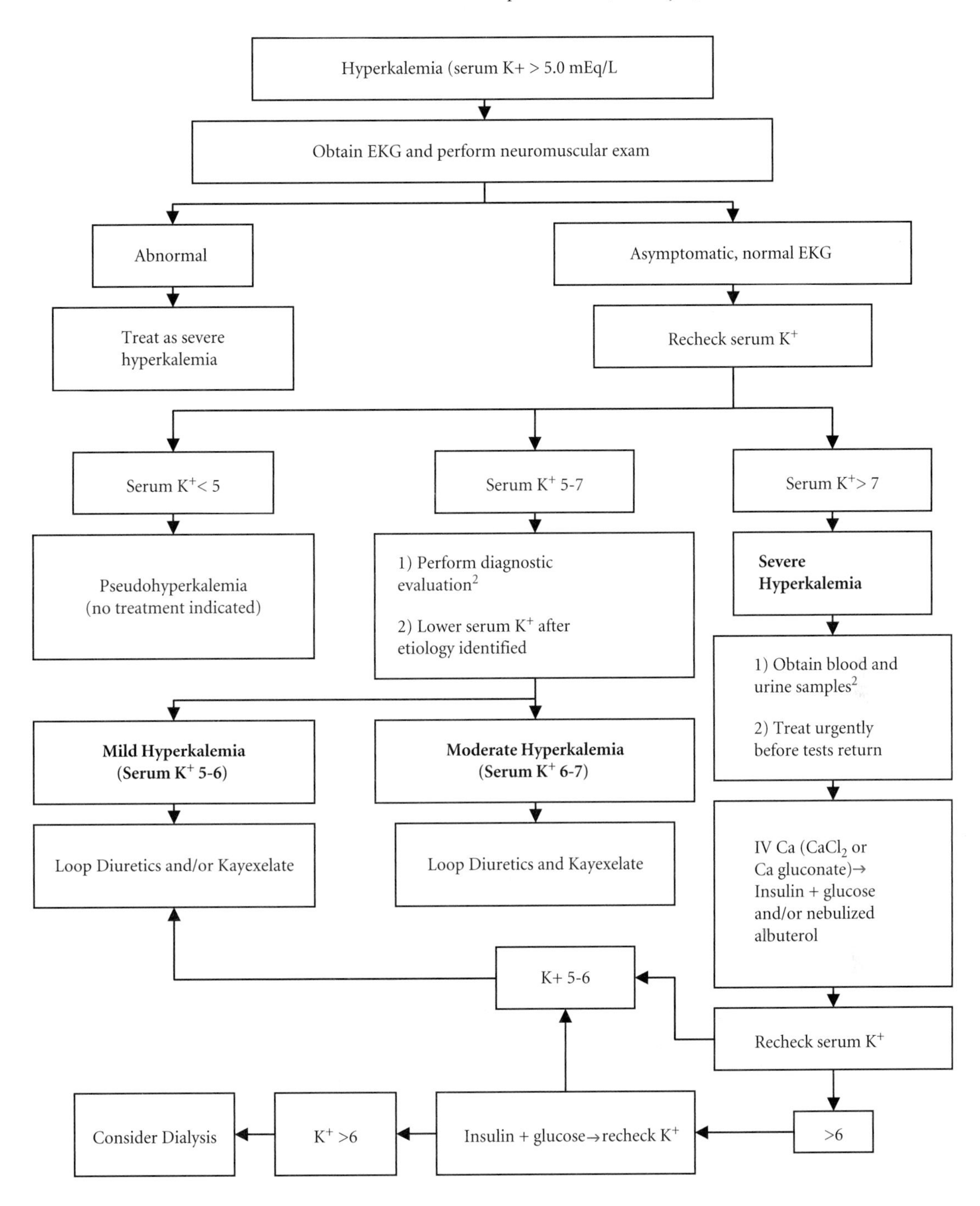

[1]= If neuromuscular exam is normal and you strongly suspect pseudohyperkalemia (hemolyzed sample, ↑↑WBCs or platelets, sample drawn from same site as IV fluids containing K+), consider repeat measurement before EKG.

[2]= Initial tests are serum chemistries, spot urine potassium and urine osmolarity.

[3]= 2005 AHA guidelines recommend calcium chloride as 1st line. However, many clinicians prefer calcium gluconate because peripherally administered $CaCl_2$ can cause tissue necrosis.

FIGURE 7–8 Management of hyperkalemia.

What causes the clinical manifestations of re-feeding syndrome? How is this condition treated?

Malnourished patients (alcoholics, anorexics, terminal cancer patients, etc.) have depleted intracellular phosphate, potassium, and magnesium stores despite normal serum values. Re-feeding → increased glucose load → increased insulin secretion → drives PO_4, Mg, and K into cells → hypophosphatemia (major abnormality), hypokalemia, and hypomagnesemia. Treatment is to correct these electrolyte abnormalities with IV PO_4, K, and Mg.

Prevention: Start feeds slowly. Monitor and aggressively supplement PO_4, K, and Mg.

What are the major causes of hypomagnesemia?

1. **Upper GI losses**: Upper GI fluids are rich in magnesium.
2. **Renal losses**: Mnemonic is "*Team kidneys **HAND** magnesium a loss*": **H**ypercalcemia, **A**lcohol, **N**ephrotoxins, and **D**iuretics (loop and thiazide).

What are important clinical manifestations of hypomagnesemia?

1. **Cardiac**: abnormal EKG findings and ventricular arrhythmias
2. **Serum electrolytes**: hypokalemia and hypocalcemia (see Chapter 8: Endocrinology)

How is hypomagnesemia treated?

1. Correct underlying cause.
2. Asymptomatic patients: Administer oral magnesium.
3. Abnormal EKG, hypocalcemia, or hypokalemia: Administer IV magnesium.

What are the major causes of hypophosphatemia?

1. **Transcellular shift**: Re-feeding syndrome and acute respiratory alkalosis (increased pH → increased phosphofructokinase → drives PO_4 into cells for glycolysis).
2. **Decreased GI absorption**: Antacids, malabsorptive diarrhea, decreased intake of PO_4 or vitamin D.
3. **Increased urine PO_4 excretion**: Hyperparathyroidism (see Chapter 8: Endocrinology), osmotic diuresis, carbonic anhydrase, inhibitors, and Fanconi syndrome.

What are important clinical consequences of hypophosphatemia?

Clinical manifestations are caused by decreased ATP production and decreased red blood cell diphosphoglycerate production (causes increased affinity of O_2 for hemoglobin → decreased O_2 delivery to tissues). Clinical manifestations usually occur only after serum PO_4 <2 mEq/L and include:

1. **CNS**: Tissue ischemia can cause paresthesia, confusion, seizures, and coma.
2. **Heart and lungs**: Decreased ATP → decreased heart and diaphragm contractility → dyspnea, tachypnea, and heart failure.
3. **Muscles**: Decreased ATP and tissue ischemia → myopathy and rhabdomyolysis (occurs when serum PO_4 <1).
4. **Bones**: Decreased PO_4 (chronic) → increased bone resorption → hypercalciuria, osteomalacia.
5. **Blood cells**: Rarely, decreased PO_4 causes hemolysis, decreased platelets, or decreased WBC function.

How is hypophosphatemia treated?

1. Correct underlying cause.
2. Asymptomatic and serum PO_4 >2: increase dietary PO_4 intake (e.g. milk).
3. Asymptomatic and serum PO_4 1 to 2: administer oral PO_4 (e.g., KPhos, NeutraPhos).
4. Symptomatic or serum PO_4 <1: administer IV PO_4; monitor closely for hyperphosphatemia.

The patient receives IV PO_4. Two days later, serum calcium is 7 mEq/L. Serum phosphate is 5.5 mEq/L. What is the next step in management?

IV phosphate administration carries a high risk of hyperphosphatemia, which leads to hypocalcemia ± calcium deposits in joints, subcutaneous tissues, and eyes. Treat this asymptomatic patient with acute hyperphosphatemia using normal saline and acetazolamide. Consider dialysis for symptomatic patients.

> Remember causes of acute hyperphosphatemia with the acronym "***TEAR***": **T**umor lysis syndrome, **E**xogenous PO_4 (IV PO_4 and laxatives like Fleets Phospho-Soda), **A**cidosis (ketoacidosis, lactic acidosis), **R**habdomyolysis.

How would treatment differ if the patient had renal failure and chronically increased serum PO_4?

1. First-line therapy is a low-phosphate diet and maintenance dialysis.
2. If serum PO_4 remains >5.5, add an oral Ca^{2+}-based PO_4 binder to the regimen (calcium acetate or calcium carbonate).
3. If the patient develops hypercalcemia due to the Ca^{2+}-based PO_4 binder, switch to sevelamer, a more expensive agent that binds PO_4 through ion exchange.

> Remember causes of chronic hyperphosphatemia with the acronym "***FRED***":
> **F**amilial tumoral calcinosis (rare, autosomal recessive condition)
> **R**enal failure (number one cause)
> **E**ndocrine: hypoparathyroidism and acromegaly (mild)
> **D**rug (bisphosphonate)

Alternative 7.9.1

A 19-year-old G_{0001} patient presents to her obstetrician with swelling of her hands and feet. She is in her twenty-eighth week of gestation. Her blood pressure is 150/100 on two separate occasions. Urine protein is 350 mg/day. Her obstetrician administers IV magnesium sulfate and IV corticosteroids.

What does G_{0001} mean?

The subscripts indicate the patient has had zero full-term pregnancies, zero pre-term pregnancies, zero abortions, and has one living child. The one living child is in her womb.

> "*Florida Power And Light*" = **F**ull-term, **P**re-term, **A**borted, **L**iving.

What condition does this patient have?

The patient has preeclampsia (hypertension + 300 mg/day proteinuria ± fluid overload). This condition usually manifests after the twentieth week of gestation (most commonly in the third trimester). The first pregnancy poses the highest risk for developing preeclampsia.

Why did she receive magnesium and IV steroids?

Treatment of preeclampsia is delivery. However, if the patient is not close to term (<34 weeks), the fetus' lungs are unlikely to have matured sufficiently. She received IV corticosteroids to promote fetal lung maturation. She received magnesium sulfate to prevent seizures (eclampsia).

> **Major complications of preeclampsia:** eclampsia (seizures) and HELLP syndrome (**H**emolytic anemia, **E**levated **L**iver enzymes, and **L**ow **P**latelets with schistocytes).

TABLE 7-8 Clinical Manifestations of Hypermagnesemia

Serum Mg Level	Cardiac	Serum Ca^{2+}	Neuromuscular	Other
4–6 mEq/L	None	⇆	1. ↓ DTRs 2. Headache 3. Lethargy	Nausea, vomiting, flushing
6–10 mEq/L	Hypotension and bradycardia	↓	1. ↓ DTRs 2. Somnolence	Nausea, vomiting, flushing
>10 mEq/L	Heart block and cardiac arrest	↓	1. ↓ DTRs 2. Muscle paralysis (includes respiratory muscles)	Nausea, vomiting, flushing

Abbreviation: DTR, deep tendon reflexes.

What are the possible complications of magnesium therapy?

Magnesium therapy (oral or IV) can lead to hypermagnesemia. Clinical manifestations of hypermagnesemia vary depending on the serum level (Table 7-8).

How is hypermagnesemia due to exogenous magnesium treated?

1. **Asymptomatic patients**: Discontinue magnesium.
2. **Symptomatic patients**: Discontinue magnesium and administer IV calcium (magnesium antagonist).

Renal failure also causes hypermagnesemia. Treat symptomatic patients with dialysis.

chapter 8

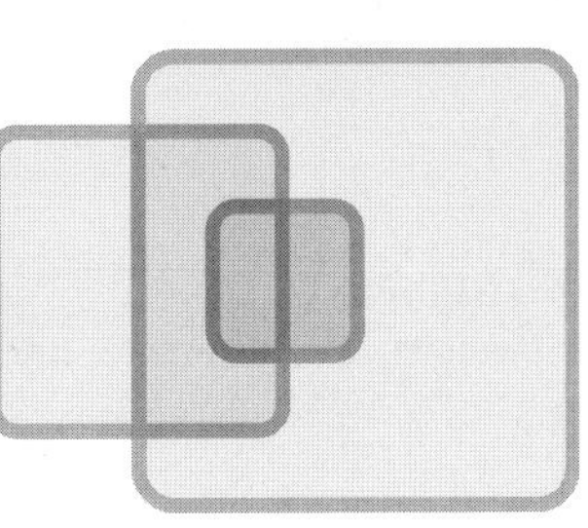

Endocrinology

CASE 8–1 INCREASED SERUM GLUCOSE

During routine screening of a 55-year-old patient, fasting blood glucose (FBG) is 110 mg/dL. He does not have any significant past medical history. His father had a myocardial infarction (MI) at age 50. He weighs 72 kg. Body mass index (BMI) is 30.

What does the serum glucose value indicate?

Interpret FBG as follows:

1. <100 mg/dL: normal
2. 100–125 mg/dL: impaired fasting glucose (IFG)
3. ≥126 mg/dL: diabetes mellitus (DM)

This patient has IFG. Although this condition does not cause microvascular complications of diabetes, it does increase the risk of macrovascular disease and diabetes.

Management of IFG:

1. Cardiovascular (CV) risk factor control (refer to Chapter 1: Health Maintenance and Statistics and Chapter 2: Cardiology).

2. Measure FBG annually to screen for DM.
3. Initiate lifestyle measures: weight loss, exercise, and diet (low intake of calories, and trans-fats and saturated fats <7% of total calories).

Two years later, random blood glucose is 220 mg/dL. The patient is asymptomatic.

What is the next diagnostic step?

There are three ways to diagnose DM. Each must be confirmed on a subsequent day:

1. FBG $\geq$ 126 mg/dL
2. Two-hour oral glucose tolerance test (OGTT) $\geq$ 200 mg/dL (most sensitive test)
3. Random serum glucose $\geq$200 mg/dL in a patient with classic symptoms (polyuria, polydipsia, fatigue, weight loss, and blurry vision)

The next step is to obtain FBG because random serum glucose >200 mg/dL is not diagnostic in asymptomatic patients.

OGTT: Have the patient fast for at least 8 hours. Measure serum glucose and then administer a glucose load. Measure blood glucose 2 hours later. Although OGTT is sensitive, it is cumbersome and expensive, so FBG is the preferred diagnostic test.

OGTT >140 mg/dL corresponds to IFG.

FBG is 150 mg/dL the next day and 147 mg/dL a week later.

What type of DM does this patient have?

This middle-aged, asymptomatic, overweight patient most likely has type 2 DM (Table 8-1). Suspect adult-onset type 1 DM if the patient's initial presentation is abrupt onset of polyuria, polydipsia, weight loss, or $\geq$2+ ketonuria.

Adult-onset type 1 DM: Also known as latent autoimmune disease of adults (LADA); accounts for 25% of all cases of type 1 DM.

What are the major long-term complications of type 1 and type 2 DM?

Macrovascular complications: DM greatly increases the risk of coronary artery disease (CAD), stroke, and peripheral vascular disease. DM is a considered CAD equivalent because it carries the same risk of MI as a prior MI.

TABLE 8–1 Type 1 versus Type 2 diabetes

	Type 1 diabetes	Type 2 diabetes
Pathophysiology	Autoimmune destruction of insulin-producing pancreatic beta-cells.	Obesity leads to insulin resistance (body's cells do not respond to insulin).
Age at diagnosis	Children & adolescents (75%) > adults (25%)[1]	Adults > children & adolescents
Frequency[2]	5–10% of diabetes	90% of diabetes
Genetics	Identical twins have 50% concordance	Identical twins have 90% concordance
Onset	Abrupt onset of symptoms	Prolonged asymptomatic phase with gradual onset of symptoms
DKA vs. HHNS	DKA much more common in type 1 diabetes	HHNS much more common in type 2 diabetes
Treatment	Insulin	Lifestyle measures, oral medications ± insulin

[1] Adult-onset type 1 DM is called LADA (Latent Autoimmune Diabetes of Adults).
[2] Gestational DM: DM that occurs during pregnancy and resolves with delivery (accounts for <5% of DM).

TABLE 8–2 Screening for microvascular complications of diabetes

	Nephropathy	Symmetric Neuropathy	Retinopathy
Screening Test	Measure urine albumin/creatinine in a spot urine sample. Level between 30 – 300 mg/day indicates microalbuminuria.	Foot exam[1] and pertinent history and physical exam	Ophthalmoscopy of dilated fundi[2]
When to start screening	Type 1 DM: 5 years after diagnosis. Type 2 DM: Soon after diagnosis.	Start screening soon after diagnosis (type 1 and 2 DM).	Type 1 DM: 3–5 years after diagnosis Type 2 DM: Soon after diagnosis
Screening interval	Annual	Annual	Annual
Follow-up of abnormal result	Diagnosis requires at least 2 abnormal results in a 6-month period, so repeat test at 3 and 6 months.	Refer to a foot specialist if patient has abnormal findings.	Eye specialist may recommend more frequent surveillance for patients with abnormal findings.
Treatment[3]	ACE inhibitor or ARB (regardless of whether patient has HTN)	Refer to Table 3	**Proliferative retinopathy (PR)**: first line therapy is laser retinal photocoagulation. If unsuccessful, perform vitrectomy. **PR with macular edema**: consider intravitreal steroids and subcutaneous VEGF inhibitors as adjuncts.

[1] Components of foot exam are "***RAM IT***": **R**eflexes (measure at Achilles tendon), **A**sk (about foot discomfort), **M**onofilament test (to assess pressure sensation), visual **I**nspection, and **T**uning fork (to assess temperature and vibration).
[2] Performed by eye specialist (ophthalmologist or optometrist)
[3] First line treatment to prevent and control all microvascular complications is tight glycemic control (HbA1c < 7%).

Microvascular complications (Table 8-2):

1. Nephropathy: Excess glucose can damage glomerular blood vessels, which causes them to "leak" protein into the kidneys. The earliest sign of diabetic kidney disease is microalbuminuria (occurs on average 15 years after DM onset). Approximately 25% to 45% of patients with microalbuminuria progress to diabetic nephropathy, which is the leading cause of end-stage renal disease in the United States (see Chapter 6: Nephrology).
2. Neuropathy: Exact mechanism is unclear. One theory is that nerves develop ischemic damage because they cannot utilize glucose-rich blood. The term "diabetic neuropathy" refers to symmetric polyneuropathy (Table 8-3).
3. Retinopathy: Excess glucose can damage blood vessels in the retina. Diabetic retinopathy is the leading cause of blindness in the United States. There are two stages:
   - Nonproliferative retinopathy: Initial asymptomatic stage; eye exam detects cotton wool spots ± superficial retinal bleeds.
   - Proliferative retinopathy: Severe nonproliferative retinopathy leads to retinal ischemia, which activates formation of friable new blood vessels (Fig. 8-1). Proliferative retinopathy is initially asymptomatic. If blood vessels grow in the anterior chamber, patients may develop glaucoma. If blood vessels rupture, patients may develop macular edema or retinal detachment.

Normal kidney albumin excretion: <20 mg/day
Microalbuminuria: 30 to 300 mg/day
Macroalbuminuria: >300 mg/day
Diabetic nephropathy: macroalbuminuria + azotemia (increased blood urea nitrogen (BUN) and serum creatinine)

TABLE 8–3 Diabetic neuropathies

Symmetric polyneuropathy (most common)

Clinical features: Affects both feet. Symptoms of burning, numbness, tingling, and aching progress to the mid-calf then appear in the hands ("stocking-glove pattern"). Signs include ↓ ankle reflexes and ↓ sensation (light touch, vibration, proprioception).

Foot complications: ***Cut If Pain Unbearable*** – **C**harcot arthropathy (arch of midfoot and bony prominences collapse), **I**nfection (erythema, warmth, tenderness, swelling, and pus), severe **P**ain (even to light touch), and **U**lcers.

Treatment: FDA-approved treatments for severe pain are pregabalin and duloxetine. Key management of ulcers is debridement. Amputation is often necessary in patients with refractory pain, infections unresponsive to antibiotics, or non-healing ulcers.

Pearl: a diabetic with an ulcer that can be probed all the way to bone likely has osteomyelitis.

Polyradiculopathies

Lumbar polyradiculopathy (amyotropy): Unilateral thigh pain and weakness for ~6 months followed by similar symptoms in contralateral leg months–years later.

Thoracic polyradiculopathy: Abdominal pain in a band-like distribution.

Mononeuropathies

Cranial mononeuropathies: CN 3 damage causes unilateral eye pain, diplopia, and ptosis. CN 4 and 6 damage cause unilateral eye pain and diplopia. CN 7 damage (Bell's palsy) is more common in diabetics than the general population.

Peripheral mononeuropathy: Most commonly affects median nerve, which leads to symptoms of carpal tunnel syndrome (refer to Chapter 12: Neurology).

Mononeuropathy multiplex (asymmetric polyneuropathy)

Multiple mononeuropathies in the same patient. Differential diagnosis is vasculitis.

Autonomic neuropathies (diagnoses of exclusion)

Sexual dysfunction: Erectile dysfunction is the most common autonomic neuropathy in DM (may respond to 5-PDE inhibitor like Viagra). Retograde ejaculation (another neuropathy) presents with cloudy post-coital urine (may respond to anti-histamine).

Gastroparesis: Presents with nausea, vomiting, postprandial fullness, and no evidence of obstruction. Treat with small, frequent meals ± metoclopramide or domperidone.

Enteropathy: Presents with chronic constipation or diarrhea of unknown etiology. Consider stool softeners for constipation and loperamide for diarrhea.

Neurogenic bladder: Present with urinary retention and incontinence. Confirm diagnosis with cystometrogram. Treat with scheduled urination + bethanechol.

Cardiovascular autonomic neuropathy: Causes exercise intolerance, orthostatic hypotension, and ↓ heart rate variability. Patients may not notice angina or MI. Treatment is to improve CV fitness and stand slowly in stages. Consider fludrocortisone + high salt diet for refractory orthostatic hypotension.

Autonomic foot dysfunction: Dry, scaly feet (because of ↓ sweat), edema (normal JVD distinguishes neuropathic from CV edema), and dilated veins with bounding pulses. Consider midodrine for neuropathic edema.

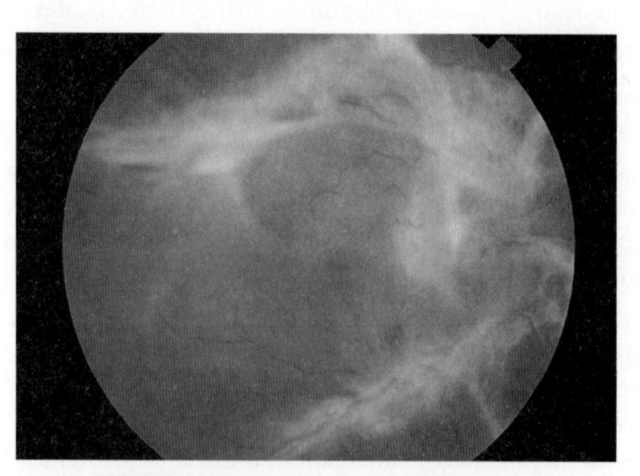

FIGURE 8–1 Eye: Proliferative retinopathy.

What initial therapeutic regimen is recommended for this asymptomatic patient with type 2 DM?

1. **Lifestyle measures**: Measures are similar to IFG management.
2. **CV risk factor control**: Measure blood pressure at every visit and fasting lipid profile annually. Prescribe aspirin if the patient has DM plus at least one other CV risk factor.
3. **Screen for microvascular complications** (Table 8-2).

> **Hypertension**: Target blood pressure is <130/80. First-line antihypertensive is a thiazide. If thiazide is not sufficient, add an angiotensin-converting enzyme (ACE) inhibitor or angiotensin receptor blocker.
> **Hyperlipidemia**: Add statins if low-density lipoprotein cholesterol ≥100 mg/dL.

How is glycemic control monitored in diabetic patients?

Glycemic control is monitored using HbA1c (glycated hemoglobin). This test gives a better estimate of glycemic control over the past 2 to 3 months than blood glucose values. Target HbA1c in diabetics is <7% (try to get as close to 6% as possible without causing significant hypoglycemia). HbA1c of 7.0% corresponds to mean blood glucose of 170 mg/dL. HbA1c of 6.0% corresponds to mean blood glucose of 135 mg/dL.

1. Initially, measure HbA1c every 3 months.
2. After HbA1c <7% on a stable regimen, measure HbA1c every 6 months.
3. If any changes are made to the treatment regimen or if glycemic control worsens, recheck HbA1c in 3 months.

> Tight glycemic control decreases risk of microvascular and macrovascular complications.

How would you monitor glycemic control if he were a 52-year-old with sickle cell disease?

Measurement of HbA1c is not as accurate in patients with hemolytic anemia or blood loss. Consider serum fructosamine (glycated albumin) instead. Serum fructosamine is also helpful for patients who require frequent changes (every few weeks) in their DM medication regimen, because it estimates blood sugar control over the last 2 to 3 weeks.

The 55-year-old patient initiates lifestyle measures. He begins to take aspirin. He undergoes initial screening for microvascular complications, which is negative. Three months later, HbA1c is 7.5%.

What is the next step in management?

Initiate metformin if the patient cannot reach target HbA1c within 3 months with lifestyle measures alone (see Table 8-4 and Fig. 8-2).

> **Chronic renal or liver disease**: Metformin is contraindicated. Consider a sulfonylurea instead.

How would the initial management have differed if the patient presented with fatigue, polyuria, polydipsia, weight loss, and blood glucose of 350 mg/dL?

Insulin is the preferred initial therapy in any patient with symptomatic DM (see Figs. 8-2 and 8-3). When symptoms and hyperglycemia resolve (FBG consistently 90 to 130 mg/dL), order c-peptide, islet cell antibodies, and anti–glutamic acid decarboxylase (anti-GAD) antibodies:

1. Low c-peptide and positive antibodies indicate LADA. Treat with lifelong intensive insulin therapy (oral hypoglycemics are not effective).
2. Near normal c-peptide and negative antibodies suggest type 2 DM. Discontinue insulin. Initiate metformin and lifestyle measures.

> **C-peptide**: component of endogenous but not exogenous insulin. Decreased in all patients with FBG >250 mg/dL. Suspect type 1 DM if c-peptide is low after correcting hyperglycemia.

TABLE 8–4 Oral hypoglycemic medications for type-2 DM

Drug class	Examples	Mechanism	Major side effects	Contraindications
Biguanides	Metformin	Exact mechanism unclear. One action is ↓ liver gluconeogenesis	Lactic acidosis and diarrhea	Liver or kidney disease. Discontinue 48 hours before surgery or use of radiocontrast dye.
Sulfonylureas	Glyburide Glipizide Glimeprimide ***Gle**eful Sulfonylureas (2nd generation sulfonylureas start with **Gly-** or **Gli-**)*	Block K-channels in pancreatic β cells, which activates opening of Ca-channels. Calcium influx stimulates insulin release	Weight gain and hypoglycemia	Use with caution in pregnant patients because sulfonylureas cross placental membrane.
TZDs[1] (Glitazones)	Rosiglitazone Pioglitazone	Bind to PPAR-receptors, which stimulates transcription of products that ↓ insulin resistance	Fluid retention and hepatitis	Heart failure and liver disease
Alpha-glucosidase inhibitors	Acarbose Miglitol ***Acarbose** the great is a **MIG**hty **Alpha** male.*	Inhibit alpha-glucosidase enzymes in small intestine brush border → ↓ carbohydrate digestion and absorption → ↓ postprandial hyperglycemia	GI symptoms (abdominal pain, diarrhea, flatulence)	
Meglitinides	Repaglinide Nateglinide *me**GLI**ti**NIDE** drugs end with **-glinide***	Mechanism similar to sulfonylureas	Weight gain and hypoglycemia (risk less than sulfonylureas)	

[1]: TZD = Thiazolidinediones

Islet cell and anti-GAD antibodies: Negative result does not rule out LADA.

Three months after starting metformin, HbA1c is 6.3%. The next few HbA1c measurements are <7%. Two years later, HbA1c is 7.6% despite maximal metformin dosage.

What is the next step in management?

Add a second drug (a sulfonylurea, thiazolidinediones, or insulin) if HbA1c is >7% despite maximal doses of metformin. Insulin is the most effective drug (it is the preferred agent if HbA1c >8.5%). Sulfonylureas are the least expensive agents. Thiazolidinediones have the lowest risk of hypoglycemia.

The patient adds glyburide to the regimen. Three months later, HbA1c is 7.3% despite metformin and the sulfonylurea. He is compliant with diet and lifestyle measures.

What are the next steps in management?

1. Add insulin augmentation to the regimen (Table 8-5). Common initial choices are:
   - Lantus (L) at bedtime or before breakfast (10 U).

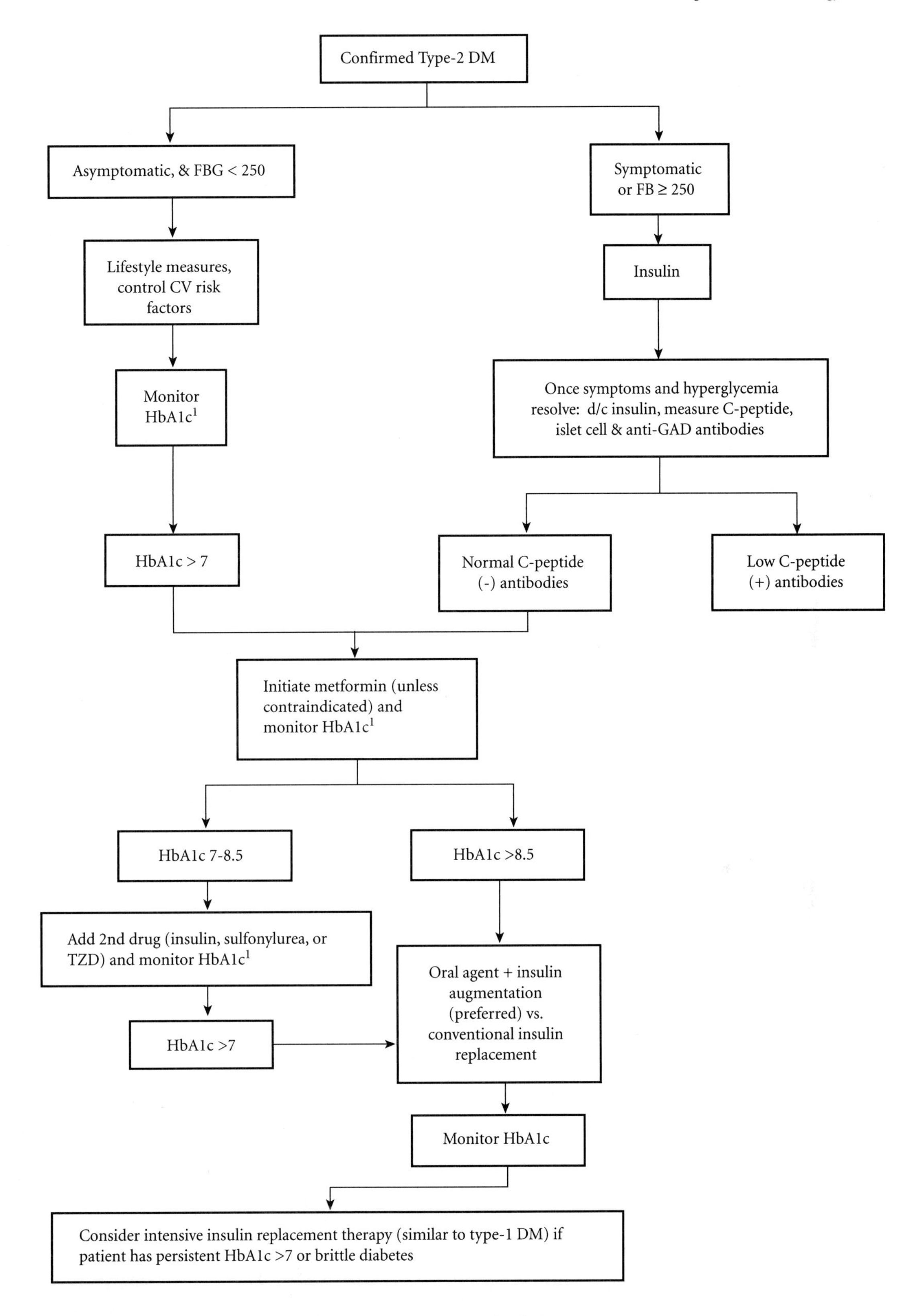

[1] = Monitor HbA1c every 3 months. Increase monitoring interval to 6 months if HbA1c < 7 for 6-9 months.

FIGURE 8–2 Algorithm for hypoglycemic therapy in type 2 diabetes mellitus.

- The most common insulin regimen is 2/3rd NPH and 1/3rd Regular.
- The total dose is 0.5 U/kg/day administered twice a day (2/3rd in the morning and 1/3rd at night).
- If this regimen does not correct hyperglycemia, increase insulin dose up to 1 U/kg/day.

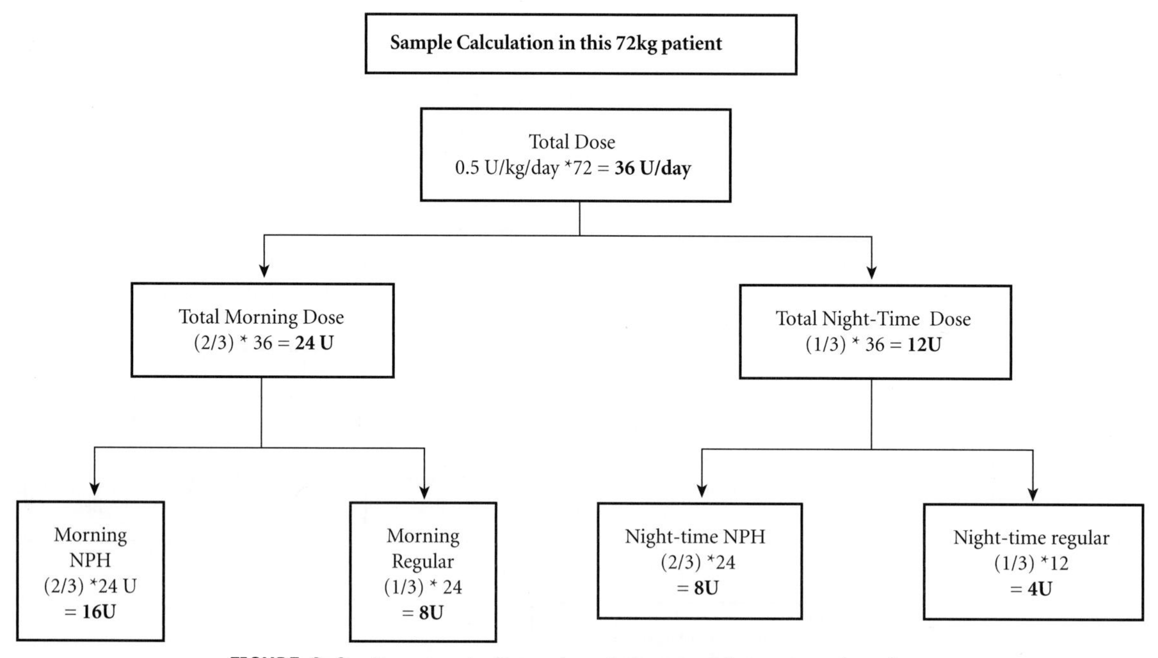

FIGURE 8–3 Management of hyperglycemia in an acutely symptomatic patient.

- Neutral protamine Hagedorn (NPH) or L at bedtime or before breakfast (10 U or 0.125 U/kg per day)
- Premixed 70/30 at bedtime or before breakfast.

2. Measure FBG every morning and postprandial blood glucose 2 hours after meals.
3. Increase insulin augmentation by 10% every week until typical FBG is 90 to 130 mg/dL.
4. Add short- or rapid-acting insulin before meals if FBG is well-controlled but postprandial blood glucose >180 mg/dL.

TABLE 8–5 Types of insulin

Type	Examples	Peak	Use	Mnemonics
Rapid acting	Humalog (Lispro) Novolog	30 minutes to 3 hours	Covers post-meal insulin requirements	**LOG** on **RAPID**ly
Short acting[1]	Regular (R)	2–5 hours	Covers post-meal insulin requirements	Con-men **SHORT**-change **REGULAR** people.
Intermediate acting[1]	NPH Lente (L)	3–12 hours	Covers basal insulin requirements	**INTER**ns are hospital's **N**ew **L**abor
Long acting	Lantus (glargine) Detemir Ultralente	Lantus and Detemir do not peak[2]. Ultralente peak is 10–20 hours.	Covers basal insulin requirements	At**LANTUS** was a **DETE**r**MI**ned civilization an **ULTRA LONG** time ago

[1] Premixed insulin = Contains set amounts of intermediate and short-acting insulin (70/30, 50/50, or 75/25). Not recommended for type 1 DM.
[2] Insulin delivered at a steady, physiologic level.

5. When the insulin regimen is stabilized, discontinue the sulfonylurea (mechanism of action is not useful in patients taking exogenous insulin). Continue metformin because it minimizes weight gain (side effect of insulin).

Triple oral therapy: Less effective than oral agent plus insulin.
Insulin monotherapy: Increased hypoglycemia and weight gain than insulin plus metformin.

Self-monitoring of blood glucose (SMBG): All diabetics should monitor blood glucose daily. Diabetics on insulin should monitor blood glucose before meals, at bedtime, and 1.5 to 2 hours after meals.

The patient is stabilized on the following insulin regimen: 28 U of NPH and 6 U of regular before breakfast; 16 U of NPH and 4 U of regular before dinner. HbA1c is 6.3%. He notices that blood glucose before breakfast is consistently in the 200s. Blood glucose ranges from 96 to 140 mg/dL before meals and at bedtime.

How can you determine the cause of the morning hyperglycemia?

Measure blood glucose levels throughout the night to distinguish between insufficient night-time basal insulin, dawn phenomenon, and Somogyi effect (Table 8-6). An alternative if night-long monitoring is too inconvenient is to measure 3 am blood glucose (increased blood glucose suggests insufficient insulin, stable blood glucose suggests dawn phenomenon, and decreased blood glucose suggests Somogyi effect).

Four months later, the patient is admitted to the hospital for elective cholecystectomy.

What changes should you make to his hypoglycemic regimen?

1. Discontinue oral hypoglycemics: In general, oral hypoglycemics are inappropriate in the inpatient setting. Most importantly, make sure to discontinue metformin 48 hours before surgery or contrast dye administration.
2. Insulin: Administer a continuous infusion of intravenous (IV) regular insulin (insulin drip) and dextrose-containing maintenance fluids such as 5% dextrose in half normal saline (D5½NS) while the patient is under nothing per oral (NPO) orders. As soon as the patient begins to eat, switch to a standing regimen of subcutaneous basal and meal-time insulin. Use sliding scale insulin regimens only as a supplement to standing insulin.

TABLE 8–6 Causes of early morning hyperglycemia in diabetics using insulin

Cause	Frequency	Mechanism	Diagnosis	Treatment
Insufficient insulin	Most common	Inadequate night-time basal insulin dose	Blood glucose rises continuously throughout the night	↑ Night-time intermediate or long-acting insulin dose
Dawn phenomenon	Common	Early morning physiologic surge in growth hormone and cortisol	Blood glucose stable all night, then sharp rise early in the morning	Eat a snack at bedtime
Somogyi effect	Least common	Excessive night-time basal insulin dose → hypoglycemia in the middle of the night → triggers release of counter-regulatory hormones	Hypoglycemia at 2 – 3 am[2]	↓ Night-time intermediate or long-acting insulin dose

[2] = Patients with long-standing DM may not have symptoms of hypoglycemia (discomfort, tremors, sweating, etc) because of autonomic diabetic neuropathy.

Steroids: Inhibit glucose uptake, which can cause hyperglycemia. Inpatients on steroids may need increased insulin. Inpatients taken off steroids may need decreased insulin dose.

Insulin can bind to IV apparatus. Avoid this problem by "priming" the apparatus: Allow the first 50 cc of insulin to run through the tubing; discard this fluid.

The patient begins eating 2 days after surgery and is ready for discharge. His blood sugars have been well controlled with a four-dose regimen of NPH at bedtime and regular insulin with meals. During evening rounds, he mentions that sometimes he finds it difficult to swallow. The attending decides to keep the patient in the hospital overnight and obtain an upper endoscopy the next morning. The patient is asked to remain NPO overnight.

How should you change his insulin regimen?

Decrease night-time NPH dose by 50% if a patient who is eating and is stabilized on an inpatient insulin regimen needs to fast. Obviously, he would not receive regular insulin either because this is only administered with meals.

Over the next 12 years, HbA1c slowly rises despite conventional insulin replacement. HbA1c is 10.5%. She reports frequent episodes of hypoglycemia.

How is an episode of hypoglycemia treated?

Treat hypoglycemia with 15 g of carbohydrate. Examples of foods that contain this much carbohydrate are 4 ounces of juice/soda or 1 slice of bread. If an outpatient with hypoglycemia cannot eat because of altered mental status, a caregiver can administer IM glucagon. Administer IV glucose (dextrose (D50)) if an inpatient with hypoglycemia cannot eat (e.g., NPO for a procedure or altered mental status).

Glucagon: Be sure to administer glucose after glucagon administration (oral if patient is able to eat, IV if patient cannot eat). Avoid glucagon in patients with chronic liver disease.

Hypoglycemia unawareness is common in patients with long-standing insulin-dependent DM because repeated lows impair the body's release of stress hormones.

What change should this patient with HbA1c of 10.5% institute to her regimen?

Patients with long-standing type 2 DM may develop progressive damage to pancreatic beta-cells, so conventional insulin replacement becomes insufficient. Such patients may require intensive insulin replacement similar to type 1 DM.

Brittle diabetes ("labile diabetes"): Frequent fluctuations of hypo- and hyperglycemia that cause significant functional distress. Occurs in <1% of DM.

Conventional insulin replacement: One to two doses of NPH and regular in the same syringe.
Intensive insulin replacement: One to two doses of long- or intermediate-acting insulin plus three or more doses of rapid- or short-acting insulin.

What newer agents are available for treatment of diabetes?

1. **Amylin and GLP-1 analogs**: Administer subcutaneously. These drugs slow gastric emptying and decreased postprandial insulin release, which improves response to insulin therapy in type 1 and 2 DM. Exenatide (GLP-1 analog) has added benefit of weight loss.
2. **Inhaled insulin**: Consider this rapid-acting agent for type 1 and type 2 diabetics who require insulin but refuse injections. Inhaled insulin is contraindicated in patients with lung diseases.

TABLE 8–7 DKA versus HHNS

	DKA	HHNS
Type of diabetes	More common in Type-1 DM[1]	More common in Type-2 DM
Symptoms	Polyuria, polydipsia, altered mental status, abdominal pain	Polyuria, polydipsia, and altered mental status but no abdominal pain
Serum glucose	250 - 800 mg/dL	> 800 mg/dL
Acid-base status	Anion gap metabolic acidosis	Normal acid-base status
Urine dipstick	4+ ketones	Negative for ketones
Other abnormal laboratory findings	↑ Serum osmolarity ↓ Serum Na (pseudohyponatremia) K and PO4 depletion[2] ↑ BUN/creatinine (dehydration) ↑ Amylase and lipase	Same as DKA
Treatment	Insulin, correct fluid and electrolyte deficits	Same as DKA

[1] = African-American and Hispanics often have a variant of type-2 DM that is prone to DKA (termed "ketosis-prone" type 2 DM or "Flatbush DM").
[2] Although there is total body potassium depletion, serum potassium may be low.

Insulin pump: An alternative to intensive insulin in type 1 DM, this device eliminates the need for frequent daily injections, but equipment is more expensive and obtrusive. There is an increased risk of DKA if patient discontinues pump use.

The patient begins an intensive insulin regimen. Six months later, he is brought to the emergency department for evaluation of altered mental status. Three days ago he was diagnosed with community-acquired pneumonia. He is oriented to person but not to place and time. Vital signs are temperature 37.4°C, pulse 112 bpm, respirations 29/min, and blood pressure 95/70. Serum chemistries are Na 130, potassium 4.0, chloride 102, HCO_3 24, BUN 25, Cr 2.0, and glucose 1200. Urine dipstick is negative for ketones.

What is the cause of his symptoms?

The two main causes of severe hyperglycemia and altered mental status in diabetics are diabetic ketoacidosis and hyperosmolar hyperglycemic nonketotic syndrome. Both conditions usually occur after a stressful precipitant such as infection, insulin noncompliance, or trauma. This patient with type 2 DM, altered mental status, serum glucose >1000, no ketonuria, and normal bicarbonate has hyperglycemic nonketotic syndrome (Table 8-7). Treatment is similar to diabetic ketoacidosis (refer to Chapter 7: Fluids and Electrolytes).

CASE 8–2 HYPERGLYCEMIA, DIARRHEA, AND WEIGHT LOSS

A 50-year-old man presents with a 2-month history of weight loss and watery diarrhea with steatorrhea. On physical examination, there are erythematous erosions and blisters on the face and buttocks. The patient reports that the rash is painful and pruritic. Abnormal laboratory findings are anemia and FBG of 145 mg/dL.

What is the most likely diagnosis?

This patient has the classic ***3 D's*** of glucagonoma: **D**M, **D**iarrhea, and **D**ermatological (necrolytic migratory erythema). Other findings commonly associated with this rare neuroendocrine α-islet cell tumor are weight loss, anemia, decreased albumin, and deep vein thrombosis.

What are the next diagnostic steps?

1. Confirm the diagnosis: Increased serum glucagon confirms the diagnosis.
2. Localize the tumor: First-line method is abdominal CT scan with contrast. If CT scan does not detect any lesion, perform endoscopic ultrasound (EUS).
3. Biopsy: If CT scan detects localized disease, perform EUS-guided biopsy. If CT scan detects liver metastases, perform CT-guided liver biopsy.

How is glucagonoma treated?

Although glucagonoma is a slow-growing tumor, most patients with symptoms have metastatic disease. Treatment of localized disease is surgery. Treatment of metastatic disease involves a combination of surgical resection and octreotide (somatostatin analog) ± debulking of liver metastases (resection, radiofrequency ablation, or chemoembolization).

Alternative 8.2.1

A 50-year-old woman presents with a 2-week history of right upper quadrant pain after heavy meals. She has also had watery diarrhea with steatorrhea and a 10-lb weight loss over the last 2 months. FBG is 145 mg/dL. Right upper quadrant ultrasound confirms the presence of gallstones.

What diagnosis should you support?

Diarrhea, DM, and gallstones are the classic triad of somatostatinoma, a rare neuroendocrine delta-islet cell or duodenal tumor. Most patients report abdominal pain and weight loss. Pancreatic somatostatinomas are more likely to present with the classic triad than duodenal somatostatinomas (typically presents with abdominal pain and obstructive jaundice).

Somatostatin inhibits cholecystokinin → decreased gallbladder contraction → gallstones, malabsorption.

What are the next steps in management?

1. Confirm the diagnosis: Fasting somatostatin >160 pg/mL confirms the diagnosis.
2. Localize the tumor: Options include CT scan, magnetic resonance imaging (MRI), or octreotide scan.
3. Biopsy: Perform EGD-guided biopsy for duodenal tumors, EUS-guided biopsy for localized pancreatic tumors, and CT-guided liver biopsy for people with liver metastases.
4. Treatment principles are similar to those for glucagonoma.

Alternative 8.2.2

A 32-year-old woman presents with a 2-month history of copious watery diarrhea and a 10-lb weight loss. Laboratory abnormalities include hypokalemia, hypochloridia, and hyperglycemia.

What diagnosis should you suspect?

Watery **D**iarrhea, **H**ypokalemia, **A**chloridia/hypochloridia (**WDHA** syndrome) are the characteristic findings of VIPoma (a rare neuroendocrine tumor). Other common clinical findings are weight loss, hyperglycemia, hypercalcemia, and flushing.

WDHA syndrome is also called Werner-Morrison syndrome or pancreatic cholera.

What are the next steps in management?

1. Confirm the diagnosis: Serum VIP >75 pg/mL confirms the diagnosis.
2. Localize the tumor: First-line test is CT scan. If CT scan is negative, perform EUS or octreotide scan.
3. Biopsy and treatment principles: Similar to glucagonoma and somatostatinoma.

Neuroendocrine pancreatic tumors: Gastrinoma, insulinoma, glucagonoma, somatostatinoma, and VIPoma. May occur in association with multiple endocrine neoplasia 1 (MEN 1).

MEN: Rare autosomal dominant mutations lead to endocrine tumors in multiple organ systems:

MEN 1: **P**arathyroid, **P**ancreas, **P**ituitary (*3 P's*).
MEN 2A: Pheochromocytoma, medullary thyroid carcinoma, parathyroid hyperplasia.
MEN 2B: Pheochromocytoma, medullary thyroid carcinoma, mucosal and gastrointestinal (GI) neuromas.

CASE 8–3 HYPERGLYCEMIA, HYPERTENSION, AND ABDOMINAL STRIAE

A 28-year-old woman presents to her physician with a 3-month history of weakness and fatigue. The weakness has increased to the point where she finds it difficult to climb stairs and to stand from a sitting position. She has only had one menstrual period in the last 3 months. She does not take any medications. She smokes a pack of cigarettes every day. Physical exam is significant for obesity most prominent around the abdomen and abdominal striae. Blood pressure is 160/100. Blood glucose is 294.

What cause should you suspect for this patient's symptoms?

Hypertension, hyperglycemia, weakness, and fatigue are nonspecific findings that require evaluation for a secondary cause given her young age. Increased serum cortisol is the most likely culprit in this patient with central obesity, abdominal striae, and oligomenorrhea (Table 8-8).

TABLE 8–8 Clinical manifestations of cortisol excess (Cushing's syndrome/disease)

General	**Weakness:** ↑ cortisol catabolizes skeletal muscle, which leads to proximal muscle wasting (difficult to stand from sitting position, difficult to climb stairs.
CV	**Hypertension:** ↑ cortisol activates mineralocorticoid receptors, which leads to HTN and hypokalemia (one mechanism). This mechanism is most common with *ectopic ACTH-producing tumors*.
Endocrine	**Hyperglycemia:** ↑ cortisol stimulates gluconeogenesis. **Central obesity:** ↑ abdominal fat but extremities wasted **Areas of fat accumulation:** face ("moon face"), neck ("buffalo hump") and behind orbits (exophthalmos). **Signs of androgen excess:** facial hirsutism, acne, oligomenorrhea, and ↑ sex drive. Usually due to *adrenal neoplasm*. Only occurs in women because source of androgens in males is testes not adrenals.
Bones	**Low back pain:** ↑ cortisol causes ↑ bone turnover, which predisposes to vertebral compression fractures and osteoporosis. **Aseptic necrosis of femoral head:** only in *chronic steroid users*.
Kidneys	**Calcium stones:** ↑ cortisol causes ↑ bone turnover.
Skin	**Bruises:** ↑ cortisol catabolizes subcutaneous connective tissue. **Striae:** ↑ cortisol causes skin atrophy, so veins in dermis visible as broad, red streaks. Abdomen is most common location. **Hyperpigmentation of sun-exposed areas:** only occurs if *↑ ACTH* (because ACTH stimulates melanocyte receptors).
Psych	Insomnia, emotional instability, depression, irritability

What are the causes of increased serum cortisol?

1. Iatrogenic: number one cause (due to chronic steroid use).
2. Pituitary adenoma or hyperplasia: number two cause (leads to bilateral adrenal hyperplasia).
3. Ectopic adrenocorticotropin-releasing hormone (ACTH)-producing tumors: most common are small cell lung carcinoma and bronchial or thymus carcinoid tumors.
4. Adrenal adenoma or carcinoma (Fig. 8-4).

> **Cushing's disease**: pituitary adenoma or hyperplasia.
> **Cushing's syndrome**: all other causes of increased serum cortisol.

What is the next diagnostic step?

The first step in this patient with no history of steroid use is to measure 24-hour urinary cortisol excretion (Fig. 8-5 and Table 8-8). Urinary cortisol more than three times the upper limit of normal indicates Cushing's syndrome/Cushing's disease.

> **Mildly increased urinary cortisol**: Equivocal finding; measure serum or salivary cortisol. If equivocal, recheck urine ± serum/salivary cortisol in a few weeks.

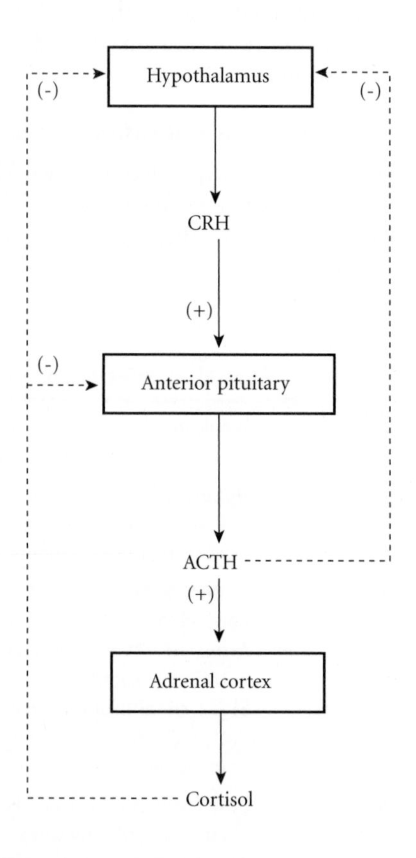

CAUSES OF CORTISOL EXCESS:

- Pituitary adenoma/hyperplasia → ↑ ACTH → ↑ Cortisol and ↑ CRH
- Ectopic ACTH → ↑ ACTH → ↑ Cortisol and ↓ CRH
- Adrenal neoplasia → ↑ Cortisol but ↓ CRH, ↓ ACTH
- Chronic glucocorticoid use → ↑ Cortisol but ↓ CRH, ↓ ACTH

CRH = Corticotropin releasing hormone
ACTH = Adrenocorticotropin releasing hormone

FIGURE 8–4 Control of cortisol secretion.

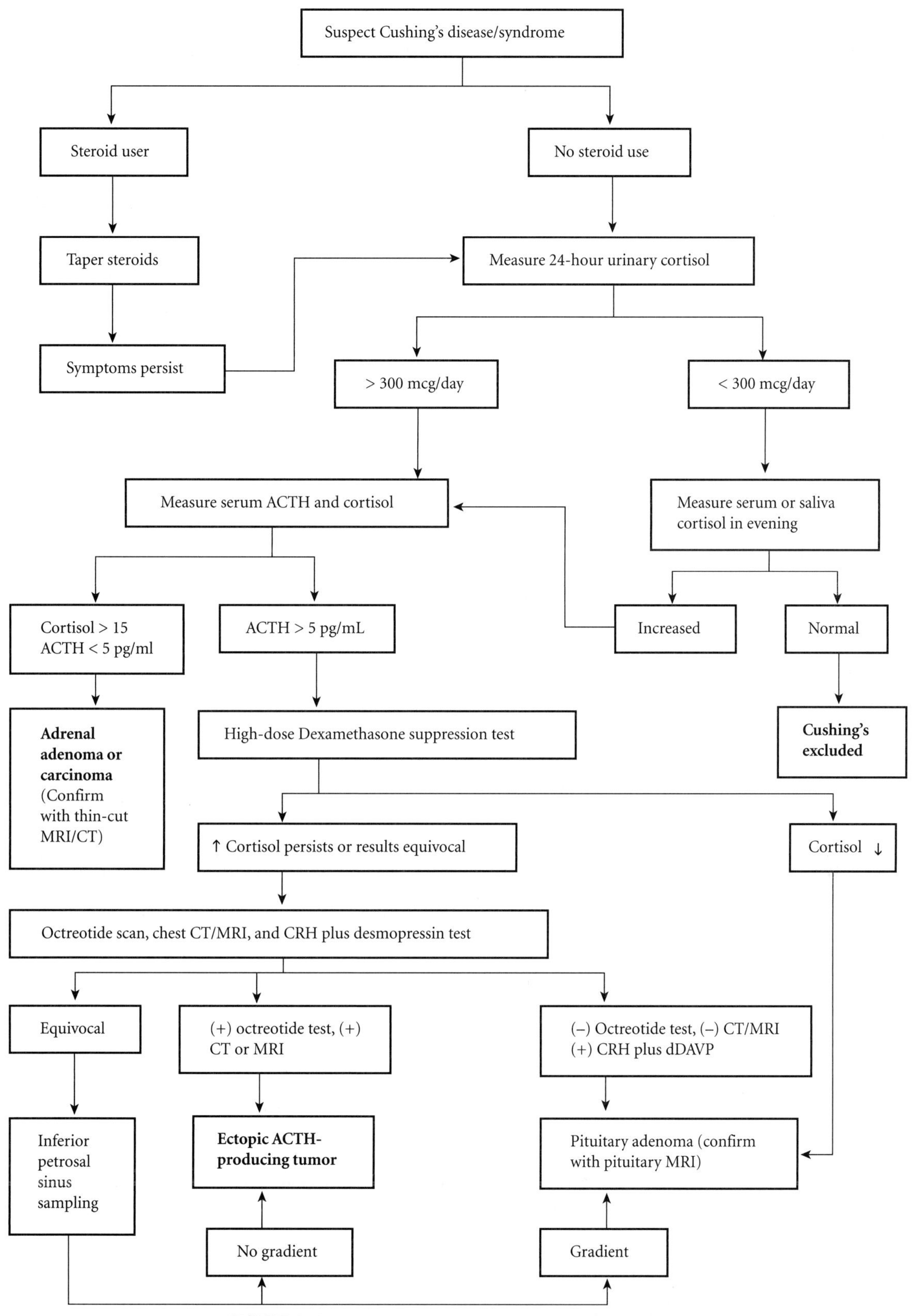

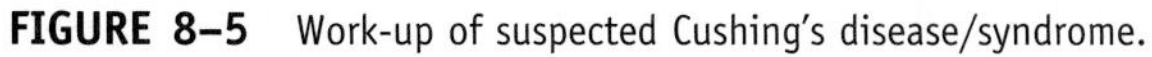
FIGURE 8–5 Work-up of suspected Cushing's disease/syndrome.

> **Causes of false-positive increased cortisol** (***IPOD***): **I**nfection, **P**COS, **O**besity, and **D**epression. Unlike true Cushing's syndrome/Cushing's disease, these causes do not have clinical features of cortisol excess.

Measurement of 24-hour urinary cortisol is 450 μg.

What is the next diagnostic step?

The next step is to measure plasma cortisol and ACTH. Low ACTH (<5 pg/mL) despite increased serum cortisol (>15 pg/mL) indicates an adrenal adenoma or carcinoma. ACTH >5 pg/mL indicates that she has Cushing's disease or an ectopic ACTH-producing tumor.

> Measure cortisol and ACTH between 11 pm and midnight, when serum levels are at their lowest.

Serum cortisol is 20 pg/mL and ACTH is 20 pg/mL.

What is the next diagnostic step?

Perform a 48-hour, high-dose, dexamethasone suppression test (DST). Pituitary tumors may respond partially, whereas ectopic ACTH-producing tumors do not respond at all.

> **48-Hour high-dose DST**: Administer 2 mg dexamethasone every 2 hours for 48 hours and measure serum cortisol every 2 hours. In normal patients, dexamethasone inhibits corticotropin-releasing hormone (CRH) and ACTH, which leads to decreased serum cortisol.

> **False-negative DST**: Pituitary tumors often do not respond to DST.

Serum cortisol levels do not decrease.

What is the next step in management?

Decreased serum cortisol would have ruled out an ectopic ACTH-producing tumor (with a few exceptions). However, this patient with no response to dexamethasone suppression may have Cushing's disease or an ACTH-producing tumor. The next step is to order the following tests:

1. Octreotide scan: Many ACTH-producing tumors demonstrate octreotide uptake (tumors appear as bright areas on the scan).
2. Chest CT or MRI: These imaging techniques detect mediastinal tumors that produce ectopic-ACTH.
3. CRH plus desmopressin test: ACTH and cortisol increase after administration of CRH and desmopressin in Cushing's disease but not ACTH-producing tumors.

> **Inferior petrosal sinus sampling**: Measure ACTH in petrosal sinus (drains pituitary) and peripheral veins. Administer CRH and repeat measurements. Petrosal ACTH: Peripheral ACTH >2 before CRH or >3 after CRH indicates Cushing's disease. Perform this test if all of the above tests are negative or equivocal.

How are the different causes of increased serum cortisol treated?

1. Iatrogenic Cushing syndrome: Taper steroid dose.
2. Pituitary tumor: Confirm diagnosis with pituitary MRI. Most tumors are amenable to surgery (trans-sphenoidal resection).
3. Adrenal tumor: Confirm diagnosis with thin-cut CT scan or MRI. Treat adenomas with surgery (adrenalectomy) and carcinomas with chemotherapy (mitotane).
4. Ectopic-ACTH producing tumor: Treat the underlying cancer.

CASE 8–4 EPISODES OF HYPOGLYCEMIA IN A NONDIABETIC PATIENT

A 43-year-old woman is brought to the emergency department for evaluation of altered mental status. There is no prior history of DM. Blood glucose is 45 mg/dL.

What are the symptoms of hypoglycemia?

There are no specific clinical manifestations of hypoglycemia. Patients with blood glucose <55 mg/dL often experience symptoms of sympathetic stimulation (e.g., sweating, anxiety, palpitations, and tremor). Patients with blood glucose <50 mg/dL may develop altered mental status.

> **Normal blood glucose during symptomatic period**: Hypoglycemia is excluded.
> **Asymptomatic + single low blood glucose value**: Repeat blood glucose measurement.
> **Asymptomatic + multiple low blood glucose values**: Perform hypoglycemia work-up.
> **Symptoms + one or more low blood glucose values**: Perform hypoglycemia work-up.

What is the next step in management?

First obtain a sample of blood for diagnostic workup. Then promptly administer thiamine followed by an IV bolus of 50% dextrose in water (D50).

> **Symptomatic hypoglycemia but normal mental status**: Give sugar-containing foods.

The patient receives thiamine and D50W. Blood glucose rises to 110 mg/dL. The patient recovers rapidly and is switched to D10W. She mentions that she has had several episodes of sweating, anxiety, palpitations, and tremors over the last 2 months.

How can you be sure her symptoms were caused by hypoglycemia?

Whipple's triad (symptoms, hypoglycemia during symptomatic period, and recovery when hypoglycemia corrected) establishes hypoglycemia as the cause of her symptoms.

The blood sample obtained in the emergency department was discarded because of an administrative error. During a follow-up appointment the next day, the patient is asymptomatic. Blood glucose is 115 mg/dL.

How can you determine the cause of hypoglycemia?

If lab work during a symptomatic episode is not available, induce hypoglycemia via a 24 to 72 hour fast. Obtain the following serum values at the end of the fast (see Table 8-9):

1. **Insulin**: Increased in insulin-mediated hypoglycemia, decreased in non–insulin-mediated causes.
2. **C-peptide**: Component of endogenous but not exogenous insulin. C-peptide is increased in patients with endogenous insulin-mediated hypoglycemia but decreased in factitious insulin use and non–insulin-mediated hypoglycemia.

TABLE 8–9 Etiologies of hypoglycemia and response to prolonged fast (≤ 72 hours)

Etiology	Insulin	C-peptide	Sulfonylurea	BHB	Post-glucagon glucose
Normal or non-insulin mediated	↓ (< 3)	↓ (< 200)	Negative	↑ (> 2.7)	↓ (< 25)
Insulinoma[1]	↑	↑	Negative	↓	↑
Factitious sulfonylurea use	↑	↓	**Positive**	↓	↑
Factitious insulin use	↑	↓	Negative	↓	↑

[1] = surgery is curative in 80-90% of patients.
BHB = β-hydroxybutyrate

3. **β-Hydroxybutyrate**: Helpful if insulin and c-peptide values are ambiguous. Insulin suppresses ketogenesis, so β-hydroxybutyrate decreases in insulin-mediated hypoglycemia, but increases in non–insulin-mediated hypoglycemia.
4. **Serum glucose immediately after glucagon administration**: Helpful if insulin and c-peptide values are ambiguous. Serum glucose increases in insulin-mediated hypoglycemia but remains normal in non–insulin-mediated causes (insulin prevents glycogenolysis, so patients have increased glycogen stores even after fasting) (Fig. 8-6).

Non–insulin-mediated hypoglycemia: Caused by decreased glucose production. Can occur in patients with severe underlying illnesses (renal or liver failure, sepsis, etc.).

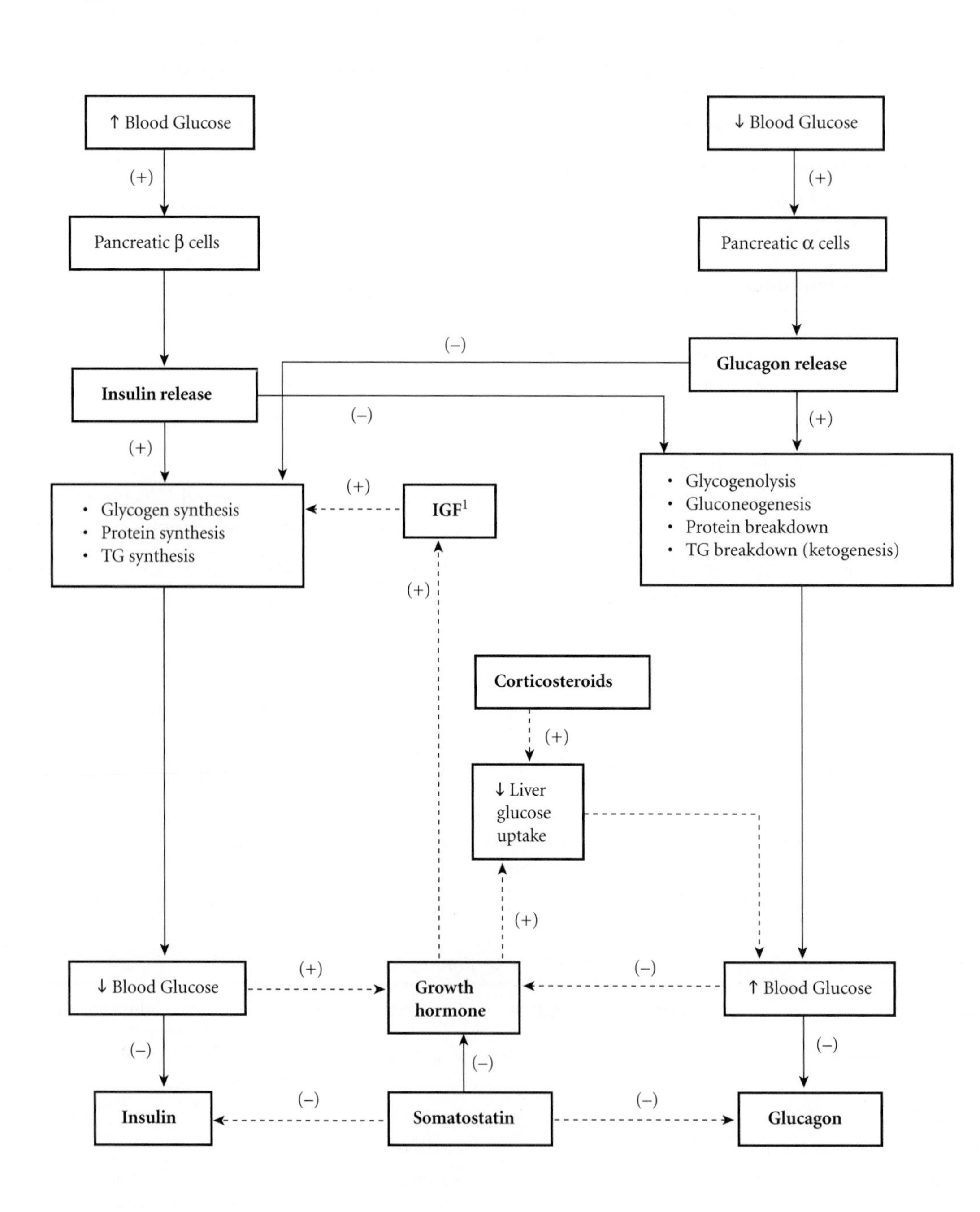

¹IGF = Insulin-like growth factor

FIGURE 8–6 Mechanism of insulin and glucagon release and action.

CASE 8–5 HEADACHES AND VISUAL FIELD DEFECTS

A 28-year-old woman presents with a 2-month history of progressively worsening headaches. The headaches are worse in the morning and increase on bending forward. On physical examination, there is bitemporal hemianopsia.

What is the next step in management?

Suspect an intracranial mass lesion in any patient with visual field defects ± increasingly severe headaches that are worse in the morning and on leaning forward (see Chapter 12: Neurology). The presence of bitemporal hemianopsia makes a sellar mass very likely (Fig. 8-7). The next step is to obtain brain MRI.

MRI shows a 10-mm sellar mass in the pituitary.

What is the differential diagnosis?

1. Non-neoplastic lesions: pituitary hyperplasia, cyst, or abscess.
2. Malignant lesions: metastases, lymphomas, germ cell tumors, and chordomas.
3. Benign neoplastic lesions:
   - Pituitary adenoma (number one cause): anterior pituitary neoplasm, classified as microadenoma (<10 mm) or macroadenoma (≥10 mm).
   - Craniopharyngioma (number two cause): embryological remnant of Rathke's pouch.
   - Meningioma.

> **MRI findings**: Sellar lesion outside pituitary rules out pituitary adenoma. Calcification suggests craniopharyngioma or meningioma.

In addition to headache and visual field defects, what are other possible clinical manifestations of sellar lesions?

Any sellar lesion can damage pituitary cells and cause one or more symptoms of hypopituitarism (Table 8-10). If the lesion is a pituitary adenoma, the patient may display symptoms of hormone excess that vary depending on the type of adenoma (Table 8-11).

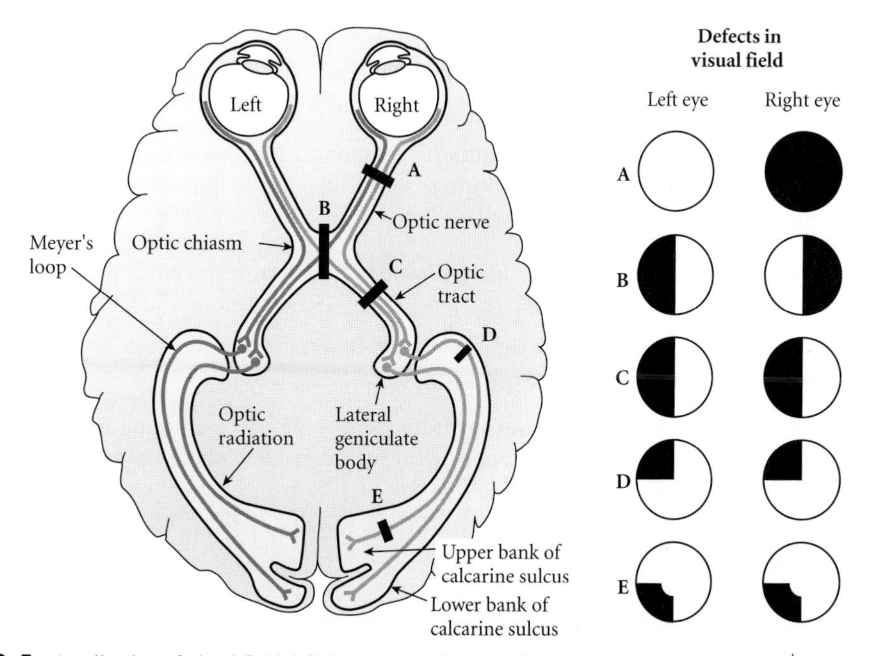

FIGURE 8–7 Localization of visual field deficits. From Ayala C, Spellberg B. *Boards and Wards*, 3rd ed. Lippincott Williams & Wilkins, 2007.

TABLE 8–10 Clinical manifestations of hypopituitarism

Damaged cell	Hormone deficiency	Clinical manifestations
Corticotrophs	ACTH	Secondary adrenal insufficiency (case 8-11)
Thyrotrophs	TSH	Hypothyroidism (case 8-6)
Somatotrophs	Growth hormone (IGF)	↓ Muscle mass, ↑ fat mass
Gonadotrophs	LH and FSH (women) Testosterone (men)	Men: ↓ energy and libido Women: oligo- or amenorrhea, hot flashes, and vaginal dryness
Lactotrophs	Prolactin	Inability to lactate after delivery

TABLE 8–11 Types of pituitary adenomas

Disorder	↑ Hormone	Clinical manifestations of hormone excess
Prolactinoma	Prolactin	Men: ↓ libido and impotence Premenopasual women: oligo- or amenorrhea, osteoporosis Men and premenopasual women: gynecomastia, galactorrhea Postmenopausal women: no symptoms of hormone excess
Somototroph adenoma (acromegaly)	Growth hormone[1]	↑ Bone thickness in jaw, fingers, and toes (leads to arthralgias) ↑ Skin thickness (leads to carpal tunnel syndrome) ↑ Tongue thickness (leads to sleep apnea) ↑ Heart thickness (leads to hypertrophic cardiomyopathy)
Corticotroph adenoma (Cushing's disease)	ACTH and cortisol	Refer to case 8-3
Gonadotroph adenoma	Testosterone, LH, FSH[2]	Men: ↓ Energy, ↓ libido, impotence Women: Menstrual irregularities, ovarian cysts[3]
Thyrotroph adenoma (2° hyperthyroidism)	↑/↔TSH and ↑T4, T3	Refer to case 8-7

[1] Measure serum IGF rather than growth hormone (inconsistent pulsatile release). If IGF values are equivocal, consider glucose tolerance test (serum growth hormone > 1 ng/mL 2 hours after receiving a 75g glucose load confirms the diagnosis).
[2] ↑ LH and FSH is diagnostic in men but not women. ↑ FSH, LH, or LH-β subunit in response to TRH administration is diagnostic in women.
[3] =Serum estradiol > 500 pg/mL in pituitary adenoma but < 500 in PCOS.

What is the next diagnostic step?

Measure levels of anterior pituitary hormones. Increase in any pituitary hormone establishes the diagnosis and type of pituitary adenoma. If no pituitary hormone is elevated, consider alternative diagnoses (Fig. 8-8).

How would the management have differed if the pituitary mass were detected incidentally in an asymptomatic individual?

Management depends on the size of the lesion:

1. >10 mm: Work-up is identical to symptomatic masses.
2. <10 mm: Measure serum prolactin level only (prolactinoma is the most common pituitary adenoma). If serum prolactin is normal, consider follow-up MRI only if the lesion is 5 to 9 mm (Fig. 8-9).

Serum prolactin is 1000 ng/mL. On further questioning, the patient mentions she has not had a menstrual period in 3 months.

What is the differential diagnosis of hyperprolactinemia (>20 mg/mL)?

Remember the causes of hyperprolactinemia with the mnemonic "*Prolactin **R**elease **S**timulates **D**airy **P**roduction*":

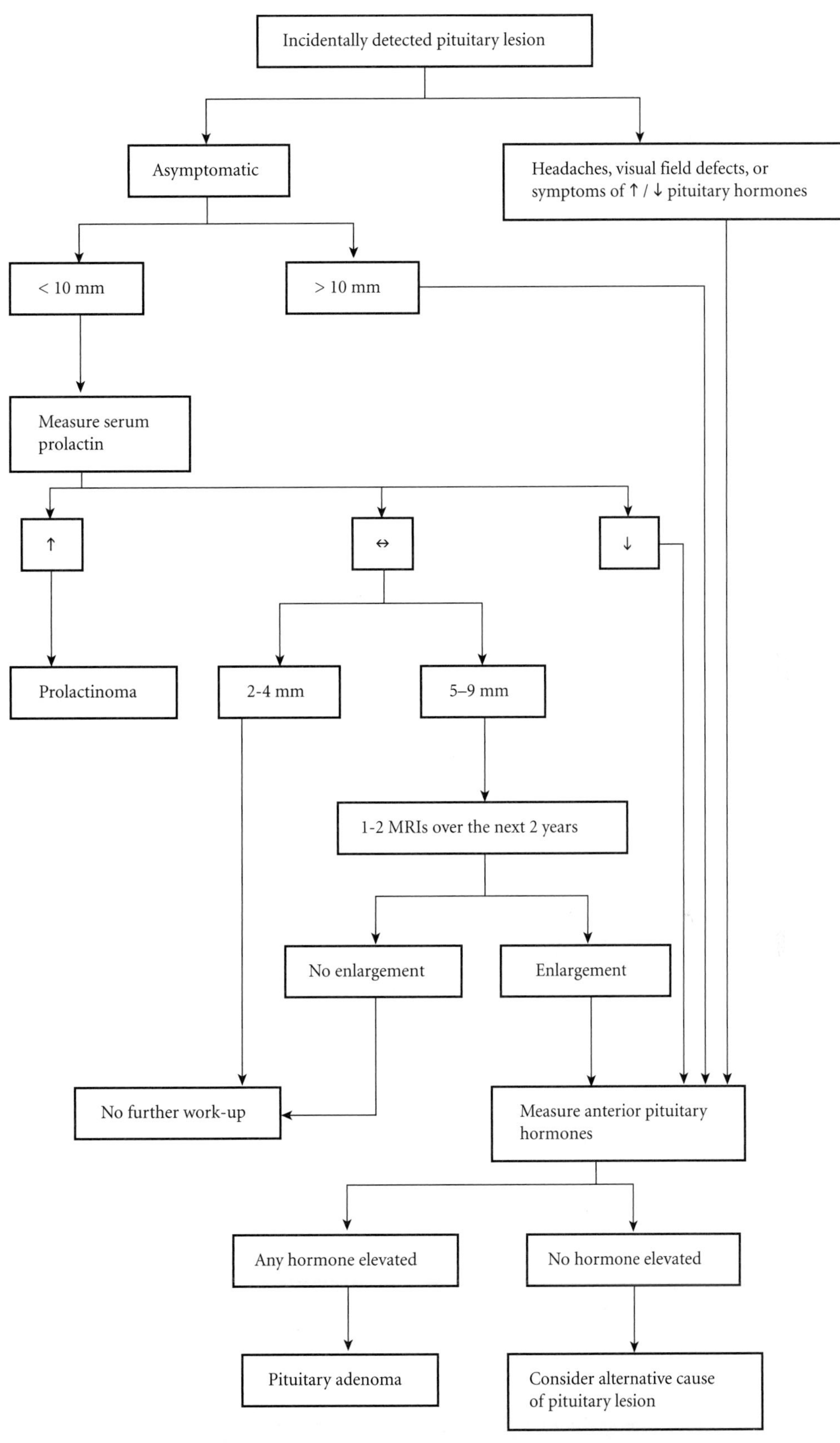

FIGURE 8–8 Work-up of incidentally detected pituitary lesions.

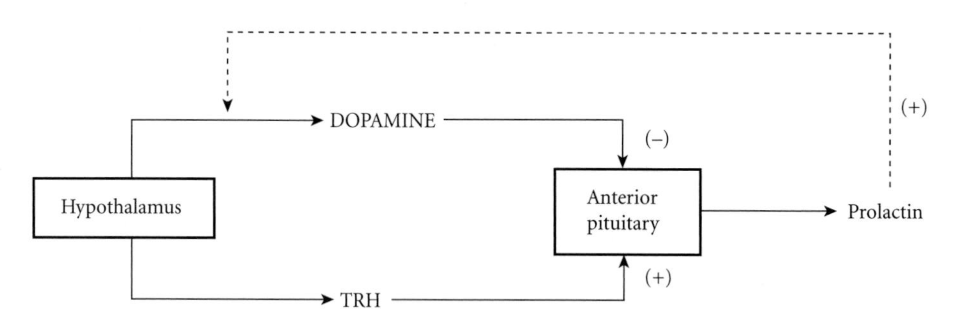

TRH=Thyroid releasing hormone

FIGURE 8–9 Regulation of prolactin secretion.

1. **P**ituitary adenoma: Prolactin ranges from mild increase to >10,000 ng/mL.
2. Chronic **R**enal failure: Variable increases.
3. **S**tress: Prolactin < 200 ng/mL.
4. **D**opamine antagonists: Prolactin < 200 ng/mL.
5. **P**regnancy (human chorionic gonadotropin (hCG) < 600 ng/mL).

The patient does not take any medications. β-hCG is negative. BUN and serum creatinine are normal.

How are prolactinomas treated?

1. Asymptomatic microadenoma: Obtain follow-up MRI scans and monitor symptoms. Treat if the lesion expands or if the patient develops symptoms.
2. Symptomatic or size ≥10 mm (this patient): First-line therapy is a dopamine agonist. Switch to another dopamine agonist if the patient has intolerable side effects. If increased prolactin or symptoms persist, consider trans-sphenoidal surgery. Consider estrogen as an alternative to surgery in patients with symptomatic microadenomas. Consider radiation therapy as an adjunct to surgery for large macroadenomas.

Dopamine agonists for prolactinoma: Cabergoline is the most effective agent and causes the fewest side effects. Bromocriptine is a less expensive alternative.

Patients who undergo pituitary surgery require lifelong anterior pituitary hormone replacement.

How would management differ if the prolactinoma were >3 cm (>30 mm) and the patient wanted to become pregnant soon?

Treat lesions <3 cm as described earlier. Treat lesions >3 cm with trans-sphenoidal surgery even if the patient responds to dopamine agonists because the lesion is likely to grow again during pregnancy.

How would management differ if the hyperprolactinemia were secondary to risperidone, which the patient needed to control schizophrenia?

Consider switching to quetiapine (an antipsychotic with less prolactin stimulating effects). Treat menstrual irregularities with estrogen and progesterone.

How would management differ if the patient had any other pituitary adenoma other than prolactinoma?

1. Asymptomatic microadenoma: Management is similar to prolactinoma.
2. Macroadenoma or symptomatic microadenoma: First-line treatment is trans-sphenoidal surgery ± radiation. Medical therapy is ineffective.

> Surgery ± radiation is also first-line therapy for symptomatic craniopharyngioma or meningioma.

Alternative 8.5.1

The patient is a 28-year-old G1P0001 woman. During the twenty-eighth week of her pregnancy, she develops sudden onset of excruciating headache and blurry vision. Physical exam is significant for bitemporal hemianopsia. T1- and T2-weighted MRI images demonstrate hypo-intensity in the pituitary gland.

What is the most likely diagnosis?

The clinical presentation along with pituitary hypo-intensity on T1- and T2-weighted MRI images (blood) is diagnostic of pituitary apoplexy (hemorrhage into the pituitary gland). The most likely cause of hemorrhage is pregnancy-induced growth of a previously latent prolactinoma.

What are the next steps in management?

1. Hemodynamic stabilization: Correct ***ABCs*** first (**A**irway, **B**reathing, **C**irculation; see Chapter 2: Cardiology).
2. High-dose steroids: This is the second step in management.
3. Labs: Obtain serum chemistries and anterior pituitary hormone levels.

If serum prolactin is elevated, administer dopamine agonists. Consider trans-sphenoidal surgery if symptoms do not improve in a few days.

> **Sheehan's syndrome**: Massive blood loss during childbirth can cause pituitary infarction (leads to pan-hypopituitarism). Severe infarction causes lethargy, anorexia, weight loss, and failure to lactate days to weeks after delivery. Diagnosis is often delayed in less severe cases because symptoms such as fatigue and oligomenorrhea are not specific. Treat with lifelong anterior pituitary hormones + estrogen + progesterone.

CASE 8–6 ELEVATED THYROID-STIMULATING HORMONE

A 51-year-old woman asks for a "thyroid blood test" because her sister was recently diagnosed with Hashimoto's thyroiditis. She is asymptomatic. She does not take any medications. Past medical history is negative. Physical exam and vital signs are normal.

What should you recommend to this patient?

Screening for thyroid disease in asymptomatic individuals is controversial. Some organizations (e.g., U.S. Preventive Task Force) recommend against screening, whereas others recommend screening older women (>50 to 60 years) for thyroid disease using serum thyroid-stimulating hormone (TSH).

Serum TSH is 6 mU/L (increased).

What is the next step in management?

Repeat TSH measurement in 2 weeks to 3 months. If TSH is normal, no further evaluation is necessary. If TSH is still increased, obtain free T4 (Figs. 8-10 and 8-11).

Repeat TSH is 6 mU/L (increased). Free T4 is 1.6 ng/dL (normal).

What is the diagnosis? How should you manage this condition?

The patient has subclinical hypothyroidism (Fig. 8-11). Patients may or may not have mild symptoms of hypothyroidism (Table 8-12). One management strategy is to measure fasting lipid profile and anti-thyroid peroxidase (TPO) antibody:

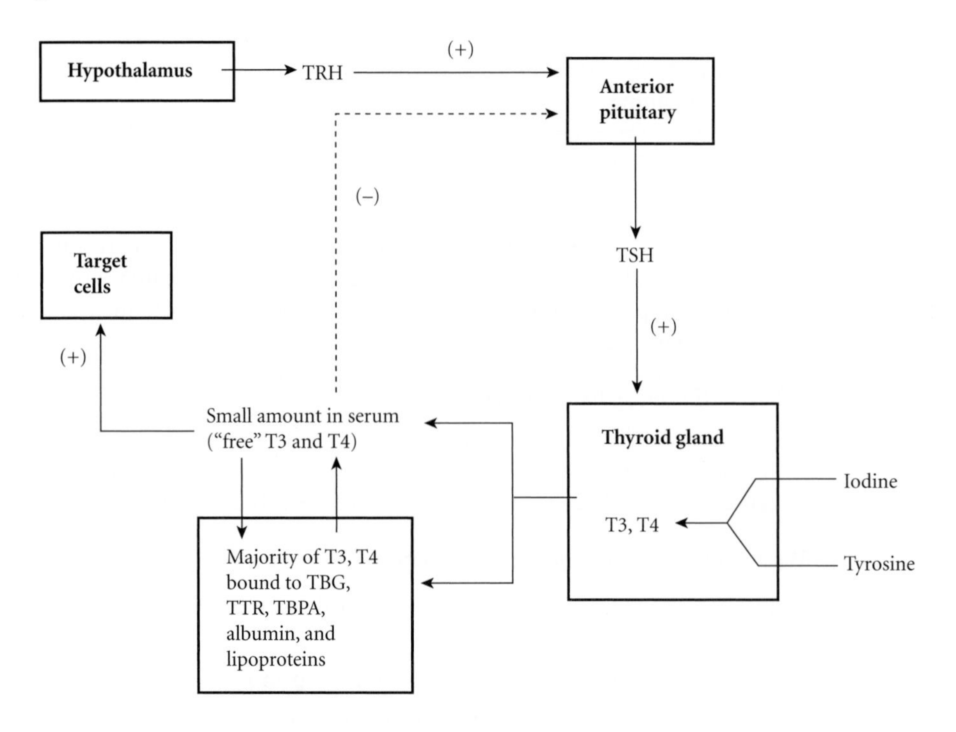

TRH = thyroid releasing hormone, TSH = thyroid stimulating hormone, TBG = thyroid binding globulin, TTR = transthyretin, TBPA = thyroxine binding prealbumin

FIGURE 8–10 Thyroid hormone regulation.

1. Asymptomatic, (−) TPO, and serum TSH <10: Monitor TSH every 6 to 12 months.
2. Symptoms, (+) TPO, or serum TSH >10: Treat with levothyroxine (T4).

> Subclinical hypothyroidism may increase risk of developing hypothyroidism, osteoporosis, atrial fibrillation, and cardiac dysfunction.

The patient does not return to measure serum lipids and anti-TPO. Two years later, the patient reports increased fatigue and constipation over 2 to 3 months. Serum TSH is 12 mU/L (increased), and free T4 is 0.6 ng/dL (decreased).

What is the diagnosis?

The patient has overt primary hypothyroidism. Clinical manifestations are often vague and nonspecific (e.g., fatigue and constipation).

> **Elderly patients**: Clinical findings are often misleading because many symptoms of hypothyroidism are also part of the normal aging process.

What are the causes of primary hypothyroidism?

Primary hypothyroidism makes up 95% of hypothyroidism cases. Remember causes of primary hypothyroidism by the ***5 I's***:

1. AutoImmune (Hashimoto's or chronic lymphocytic thyroiditis): Leading cause of hypothyroidism. (+) Anti-TPO is diagnostic. Patients may also have (+) anti-thyroglobulin.
2. Iatrogenic: Thyroidectomy, radioiodine ablation, neck irradiation, and drugs.
3. Iodine excess or deficiency: Increased iodine inhibits formation of T3 and T4; decreased iodine leads to hypothyroidism and enlarged thyroid gland (goiter).
4. Infiltration of thyroid (rare): Amyloidosis, sarcoidosis, leukemia, etc.
5. Inherited (rare): Autosomal recessive defect in T3 and T4 synthesis.

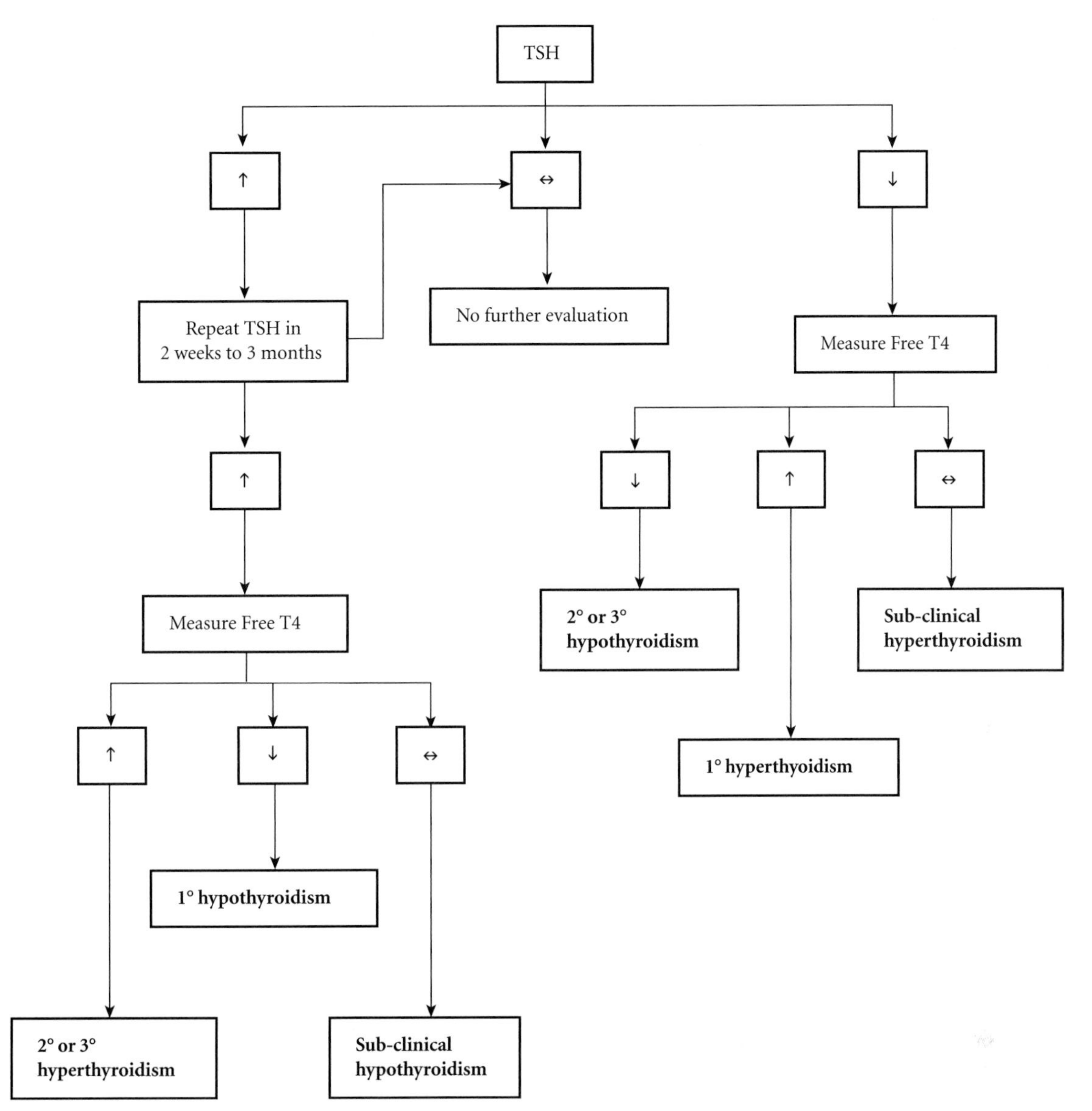

FIGURE 8–11 Approach to thyroid function tests.

What are causes of secondary and tertiary hypothyroidism?

Secondary and tertiary causes account for ≤5% of cases of hypothyroidism. Hypopituitarism can cause second-degree hypothyroidism. Hypothalamic lesions (rare) cause third-degree hypothyroidism. Laboratory tests do not distinguish second-degree from third-degree hypothyroidism, so obtain brain MRI if patient has decreased TSH and decreased free T4.

Drugs that cause hypothyroidism: **L**ithium, **A**miodarone, **M**ethimazole, **P**ropylthiouracil (***LAMP***).

Causes of subclinical hypothyroidism are the same as primary hypothyroidism.

What is the next step in management?

This patient with no history of iatrogenic damage or goiter on physical exam probably has Hashimoto's thyroiditis. Further diagnostic evaluation is not necessary. The next step is to initiate thyroid replacement (levothyroxine). Start at a low dose and check serum TSH every 6 to 8 weeks. Increase levothyroxine dose until serum TSH is normal. When the patient is stable on a particular dosage, monitor TSH annually.

TABLE 8–12 Possible manifestations of hypothyroidism and hyperthyroidism in adults

	Hypothyroidism	Hyperthyroidism
General	Fatigue and weakness Weight gain (not severe obesity)	Weight loss despite ↑ appetite
Temperature tolerance	Cold intolerance	Heat intolerance
Neuro	Slow DTR relaxation[1] ↑ Sleepiness	Brisk DTR relaxation[1] Insomnia Tremor
Eyes	Periorbital non-pitting edema[2] Loss of outer 1/3rd of eyebrows	Stare and lid lag Bilateral exophthalmos
Thyroid gland	Enlarged (goiter)	Enlarged (goiter)
CV	Bradycardia	Tachycardia (palpitations) Atrial fibrillation High-output heart failure (in severe disease)
Pulmonary	Dyspnea on exertion Hoarseness Sleep apnea (2° to macroglossia)	Dyspnea on exertion
GI	Constipation	Diarrhea
Reproductive system	Women: Menorrhagia or oligomenorrhea Men: ↓ Libido and erectile dysfunction	Women: Oligomenorrhea or amenorrhea Men: gynecomastia, ↓ libido and erectile dysfunction Both: Infertility, ↑ frequency
Skin	Coarse, dry, cool, and clammy ↓ Sweating Yellow discoloration	Smooth and warm ↑Sweating
Extremities	Non-pitting edema (myxedema)[2]	Pre-tibial myxedema[4]
Psych	Depression ↓ Concentration	Emotional instability ↓ Concentration
Hair	Coarse with hair loss	Thin hair
Nails	Brittle	Loose and soft
Rheumatologic system	Muscle cramps and weakness Carpal tunnel syndrome	Proximal muscle weakness Osteoporosis and fractures
Laboratory abnormalities	Hyperlipidemia Anemia of chronic disease Hyponatremia ↑ Creatinine kinase	↓ HDL and total cholesterol Anemia of chronic disease Hyperglycemia ↑ alkaline phosphatase
Speech	Slow and slurred	

[1] DTR = deep tendon reflexes
[2] Non-pitting edema (myxedema) is a sign of severe disease
[3] Hyperpigmented, violaceous, orange-peel textured papules on shins. Only occurs in Grave's disease (rare).

Over the next 4 years, the patient's levothyroxine requirement continues to increase. While on a trip to Disney World, she falls and hurts her back. The physician prescribes oxycodone. The next day, she presents to an emergency department with altered mental status. Her husband mentions that she forgot her thyroid pills at home. She is not oriented to person, place, or time. Her skin is cool and clammy. Deep tendon reflex relaxation is delayed. Vital signs are temperature 35°C, pulse 55 bpm, respirations 9/min, and blood pressure 100/80.

What condition should you suspect?

Suspect myxedema coma (severe hypothyroidism) in this patient with altered mental status plus hypothermia, bradycardia, decreased respiratory rate, and other signs of hypothyroidism.

This uncommon endocrine emergency can occur as a result of long-standing untreated hypothyroidism or after a stressful event (in this case, the combination of noncompliance plus opioids).

What are the next steps in management?

1. ABCs: The first step is to stabilize the patient. Correct hypothermia with a heated blanket (passive rewarming). Correct electrolyte deficits (hyponatremia is common).
2. Labs: In addition to serum TSH and free T4, order serum cortisol, serum chemistries, complete blood count (CBC), coagulation studies, and urine drug screen (to rule out other causes of altered mental status).
3. Medications: Initiate IV levothyroxine ± T3 urgently before laboratory results are available. Also administer IV hydrocortisone until adrenal insufficiency is ruled out with normal serum cortisol.

Alternative 8.6.1

A 39-year-old woman presents with a 6-month history of palpitations, tremor, heat intolerance, and insomnia. On physical exam, the thyroid gland is enlarged (goiter). Serum TSH is 10 mU/L (increased) and free T4 is 6 mU/L (increased).

What is differential diagnosis?

The patient has clinical manifestations of hyperthyroidism (Table 8-12). Increased TSH and T4 indicate secondary hyperthyroidism. The two important causes of secondary hyperthyroidism are:

1. Thyrotroph adenoma of the pituitary gland
2. Thyroid hormone receptor mutation (leads to thyroid hormone resistance).

What is the next step in management?

The next step is to obtain head MRI and T3. Patients with a thyrotroph adenoma will have a pituitary lesion on MRI and increased T3. Patients with thyroid hormone resistance have no pituitary lesion on MRI and decreased T3.

How does management of the two causes of secondary hyperthyroidism differ?

1. Thyrotroph adenoma: Treatment is somatostatin followed by trans-sphenoidal surgery ± radiation. If increased TSH persists, consider thyroidectomy or radioiodine.
2. Thyroid hormone resistance: Treatment is difficult; consider T3 replacement.

Euthyroid sick syndrome: 70% of inpatients with nonthyroid illness have nonspecific thyroid laboratory abnormalities (e.g., mild or decreased TSH and/or free T4). Laboratory values return to normal after illness resolves. No treatment is indicated.

CASE 8–7 LOW THYROID-STIMULATING HORMONE

A 68-year-old man is diagnosed with atrial fibrillation. He smokes a pack of cigarettes a day. On physical exam, thyroid gland is enlarged (goiter). TSH is 0.1 mU/L (decreased).

What is the next step in management?

The next step is to measure free T4. Increased free T4 indicates primary hyperthyroidism. Stable free T4 indicates subclinical hyperthyroidism (Fig. 8-11).

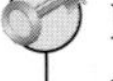

Elderly patients: Presentation of hyperthyroidism is often atypical (e.g., atrial fibrillation or weight loss with no other signs).

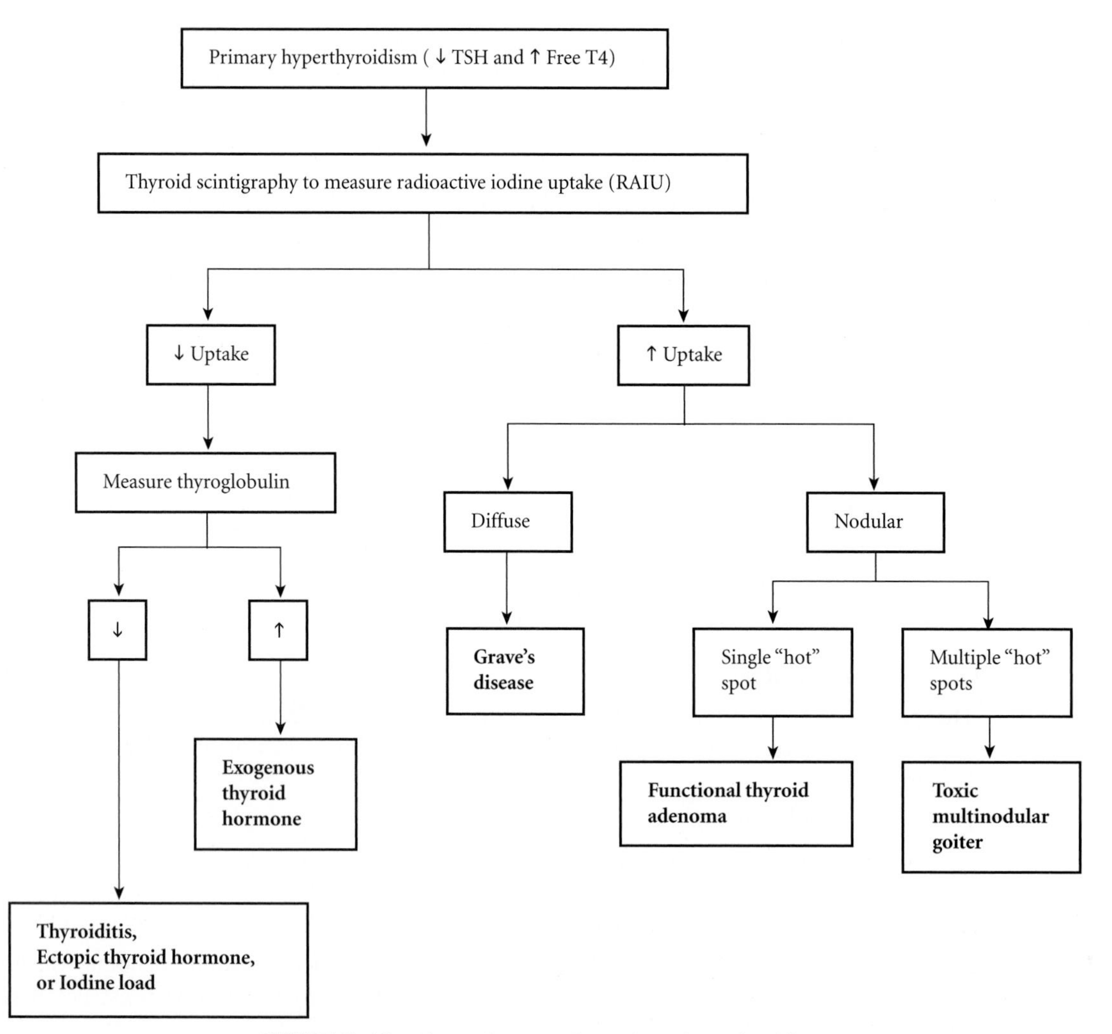

FIGURE 8–12 Diagnostic approach to primary hyperthyroidism.

> Screen all "*Grave Men And Women*" for hyperthyroidism with serum TSH: **G**ynecomastia, **M**enstrual disorders, **A**trial fibrillation, and unintentional **W**eight loss.

Free T4 is 7 mU/L (increased).

What is the next diagnostic step in management?

Perform radioactive iodine uptake test (RAIU) to determine the cause of primary hyperthyroidism (Fig. 8-12):

1. **Increased iodine uptake**: Indicates increased synthesis of thyroid hormone by the thyroid gland.
2. **Decreased iodine uptake**: Indicates either a nonthyroid source of hormone or thyroid gland inflammation (leads to thyroid hormone release into serum).

What are the causes of primary hyperthyroidism?

Causes associated with increased RAIU (mnemonic: "***I****odine* ***G****ets* ***T****hyroid* ***F****laming*"):

1. **I**odine load: Contrast agents or amiodarone (iodine-rich drug) can cause increased thyroid hormone production in patients with pre-existing iodine deficiency or toxic multinodular goiter (TMG).
2. **G**rave's disease: Leading cause of hyperthyroidism. Autoantibodies against the TSH receptor stimulate the thyroid gland to produce increased thyroid hormone.

3. **TMG or Plummer' disease**: Many autonomous nodules produce increased thyroid hormone. Frequency is higher in iodine-deficient areas.
4. **Functional adenoma**: Single autonomous thyroid nodule produces increased thyroid hormone. This is not related to iodine intake.

Causes associated with decreased RAIU:

1. Ectopic thyroid hormone: Struma ovarii (thyroid cells in an ovarian neoplasm).
2. Exogenous thyroid hormone: Factitious use or overdose of levothyroxine.
3. Thyroiditis (Table 8-13): The typical pattern in patients with thyroid inflammation is hyperthyroidism (acute phase) followed by hypothyroidism and finally resolution of abnormal thyroid tests. Patients often have goiter and increased erythrocyte sedimentation rate (ESR).

> **Goiter**: Enlarged thyroid caused by hypo- or hyperthyroidism. Goiter can be diffuse (e.g., Grave's disease) or nodular (e.g., toxic adenoma or TMG); <1% of nodular goiter is malignant. Leading cause of goiter worldwide is iodine deficiency.

There is increased diffuse RAIU. Serology is positive for thyroid-stimulating antibodies.

How is Graves' disease treated?

1. First, start the patient on a β-blocker and methimazole. The β-blocker controls symptoms secondary to increased adrenergic tone (tremor, palpitations, tachycardia, etc.). Methimazole (thionamide class of drugs) inhibits iodine organification.
2. When symptoms resolve and TSH normalizes, the options are radioiodine ablation (most popular), prolonged methimazole, or surgery (typically reserved for patients with large goiters that cause dyspnea, hoarseness, or dysphagia).

> **Toxic adenoma or TMG**: Treatment strategy similar to Grave's disease.

How would management have differed if the patient with Grave's disease was pregnant?

Avoid radioactive iodine and methimazole during pregnancy. Treatment is β-blockers for symptom control and propylthiouracil (another thionamide).

> Monitor CBC of patients on thionamides because a major complication is agranulocytosis.

How would management have differed if initial laboratory testing revealed decreased TSH but normal free T4?

Decreased TSH and normal free T4 suggest subclinical hyperthyroidism. The next step is to repeat TSH at a later date. If decreased TSH persists, perform RAIU and bone density scan. Consider use of thionamides or radioiodine ablation if the patient is a "***HoT SOB***": **H**ot nodule on RAIU, **T**SH < 0.1, **S**ymptomatic, **O**ld (elderly or postmenopausal female not taking estrogen), or decreased **B**one density.

The elderly patient decides to take prolonged methimazole. Two years later, he is admitted for treatment of community-acquired pneumonia. On his second day in the hospital, he appears confused and agitated. The nurse mentions that he keeps saying "Bobby, forgive me." Physical exam is significant for a thyroid bruit, hand tremor and brisk deep tendon reflexes. Vital signs are temperature 39°C, pulse 135 bpm, respirations 28/min, and blood pressure 170/100.

What is the most likely cause of his clinical deterioration?

Suspect thyroid storm (severe hyperthyroidism) in this patient with altered mental status, fever, tachycardia, and other manifestations of hyperthyroidism. This uncommon endocrine emergency can occur as a result of long-standing untreated hyperthyroidism or after a stressful event (in this case infection).

TABLE 8–13 Types of thyroiditis

Type	Cause	Tender thyroid	Classic symptoms	Management
Subacute thyroiditis (subacute granulomatous thyroiditis or de Quervain thyroiditis)	Viral infection	Yes	Flu-like prodrome followed by neck pain, thyroid tenderness and goiter. Self limited.	First line is NSAIDs. Consider prednisone if symptoms are severe or persistent.
Infectious thyroiditis	Bacterial infection (rare unless immune suppressed)	Yes	Fever, chills, unilateral thyroid pain, goiter ± fluctuance (indicates abscess).	Confirm diagnosis with FNA. Treat with drainage and antibiotics.
Radiation induced thyroiditis	Radio-iodine therapy for Grave's disease	Yes	Mild thyroid tenderness 5–10 days after giving radio-iodine. Self limited.	No further evaluation or treatment.
Iatrogenic	Surgery or biopsy of thyroid gland	Yes	Neck and thyroid tenderness after surgery or biopsy. Self limited.	No further evaluation or treatment.
Hashimoto's thyroiditis (chronic lymphocytic thyroiditis)	Anti-thyroid auto-antibodies	Yes	Rarely, initial manifestation is tender goiter, (+) anti-TSI, and ↑ thyroid hormone (similar to Grave's).	Initial management of hyperthyroidism similar to Grave's disease.
Silent thyroiditis (painless or subacute lymphocytic thryoiditis)	Variant of Hashimoto thyroiditis	No	Painless goiter. Self limited.	No treatment necessary
Post-partum thyroiditis	Variant of silent thyroiditis	No	Painless goiter ≤ 1 year after pregnancy. Self limited.	No treatment necessary
Drug-induced thyroiditis	Lithium, amiodarone, or interferon	No	Painless goiter	Discontinue or ↓ drug dose
Fibrous thyroiditis (Riedel thyroiditis)	Eosinophil infiltration leads to fibrosis	No	Hard, fixed goiter, ↓ neck mobility ± dysphagia.	Confirm with thyroid biopsy. Treat with prednisone ± surgery.

How is thyroid storm treated?

Initiate treatment before laboratory tests return (thyroid function tests, CBC, serum chemistries, cortisol, and coagulation studies). Treatment of thyroid storm is supportive care (ABCs), IV β-blockers (usually propranolol), and high-dose IV or oral thionamides (PTU or methimazole). Many physicians also administer iodine and corticosteroids.

Laboratory studies confirm the diagnosis of severe hyperthyroidism. Medical records reveal that the patient did not receive methimazole on his first day in the hospital. The patient recovers from the episode of thyroid storm and pneumonia. After discharge, he decides to take radioactive iodine.

How does this treatment work?

Radioactive iodine (^{131}I) is administered orally. ^{131}I enters many thyroid cells and destroys them. Iodine does not enter other cells, so no other tissue is affected. The major complication is hypothyroidism. Patients should avoid close contact with pregnant women and children for 24 to 72 hours because ^{131}I is excreted in feces, urine, and saliva.

Three months later, the patient complains of excessive tears and a feeling of discomfort in both eyes. On exam, the eyes bulge outward anteriorly (proptosis).

What is cause of his symptoms?

All causes of hyperthyroidism can cause stare and lid lag. However, this patient with proptosis, eye discomfort, and increased tears has bilateral exophthalmos (seen only in Grave's disease). Smoking and radioactive iodine increase the risk of this complication.

How is Grave's ophthalmopathy treated?

1. Mild symptoms (increased tears, discomfort): Supportive measures (e.g., artificial tears).
2. Proptosis or blurry vision: Consider oral steroids.
3. Loss of vision (medical emergency): Immediate oral steroids ± eye surgery.

> **Unique manifestations of Grave's disease:** Pre-tibial myxedema (treat with topical steroids), bilateral exophthalmos, and thyroid bruit.

> **Gender:** Hypo- and hyperthyroidism is much more common in women.

CASE 8–8 THYROID NODULE

During routine examination of a 28-year-old woman, a thyroid nodule is palpated. The patient is asymptomatic. There is no significant past medical history. She does not take any medications.

What is the differential diagnosis of thyroid nodules?

Nodules can be malignant (Table 8-14) or benign (much more common). Remember causes of benign nodules with the acronym "***CHICA***":

1. **C**olloid nodule: caused by normal tissue overgrowth (e.g., Hashimoto's).
2. **H**yperfunctional nodule: caused by Grave's disease, TMG, or functional adenoma.
3. **I**nflammatory nodule: caused by thyroiditis.
4. **C**ysts: Most cysts are benign; cysts rarely contain malignant cells.
5. **A**denomas (follicular and Hürthle cell).

What factors increase the likelihood that the nodule is malignant?

1. Family or personal history of thyroid or other endocrine malignancies.
2. Personal history of neck irradiation.
3. Age: <30 or >60 years.
4. Clinical findings: hard, fixed nodule, cervical adenopathy, or new-onset hoarseness (suggests recurrent laryngeal paralysis).

What is the next step in management?

First obtain serum TSH. Decreased TSH suggests one or more hyperfunctional ("hot") nodule, so the next step is RAIU. Normal TSH increases the likelihood of a hypofunctional ("cold") nodule, so the next step is fine-needle aspiration biopsy (FNA). Increased TSH increases the likelihood of Hashimoto's, so consider thyroid ultrasound as the next step (Fig. 8-13).

TABLE 8–14 Thyroid malignancies

Malignancy	Frequency	Treatment	Prognosis	Notes
Papillary carcinoma	70–75%	**< 1 cm**: lobectomy ± radioactive iodine. **> 1 cm**: thyroidectomy ± radioactive iodone. **Cervical LN spread:** also perform LN dissection. **Metastases:** also consider radiation or chemotherapy.	Very good	Cervical LN spread more common than recurrence or metastasis.
Follicular carcinoma	10–15%	Same as papillary carcinoma	Good	Recurrence or metastasis more common than LN spread.
Hurthle cell carcinoma	5%	Same as papillary carcinoma	Good	Aggressive variant of follicular cell carcinoma.
Medullary carcinoma	5–10%	Total thyroidectomy (radioactive iodine not helpful). **Cervical LN spread:** also perform LN dissection. **Metastases:** also consider radiation or chemotherapy.	Moderate	↑ Calcitonin. ~80% sporadic, 20% inherited (MEN IIA, IIB)
Anaplastic carcinoma	0.5–1.5%	Most patients are not candidates for surgery. Treatment is palliative (tracheostomy and neck radiation ± chemotherapy).	Very poor	Extremely rapid-growing.
Metastatic carcinomas	Rare	Total thyroidectomy, radiation, and chemotherapy	Very poor	Kidney is the most common tissue of origin

Hot nodule (increased uptake): Decreased risk of malignancy.
Cold nodule (decreased uptake): Increased risk of malignancy (20%).

Serum TSH is normal. FNA biopsy reveals follicular cells.

What is the next step in management?

Refer the patient for total thyroidectomy if FNA shows follicular or Hürthle cells (lobectomy acceptable if lesion <1 cm) because FNA cannot distinguish follicular or Hürthle cell adenoma (benign) from carcinoma (malignant).

Patients who undergo partial or total thyroid resection require lifelong levothyroxine.

The patient undergoes total thyroidectomy. Pathological examination reveals a 3-cm follicular carcinoma without any evidence of lymph node extension or distant metastases.

What surveillance strategy is recommended for the next 3 years?

Follow-up of papillary, follicular, and Hürthle cell carcinoma is as follows:

1. Every 6 months: serum TSH, free T4, and serum thyroglobulin.
2. Annually: CXR, thyroid ultrasound, and whole-body radioiodine imaging.

Medullary carcinoma: Surveillance also includes serum calcitonin every 6 months.

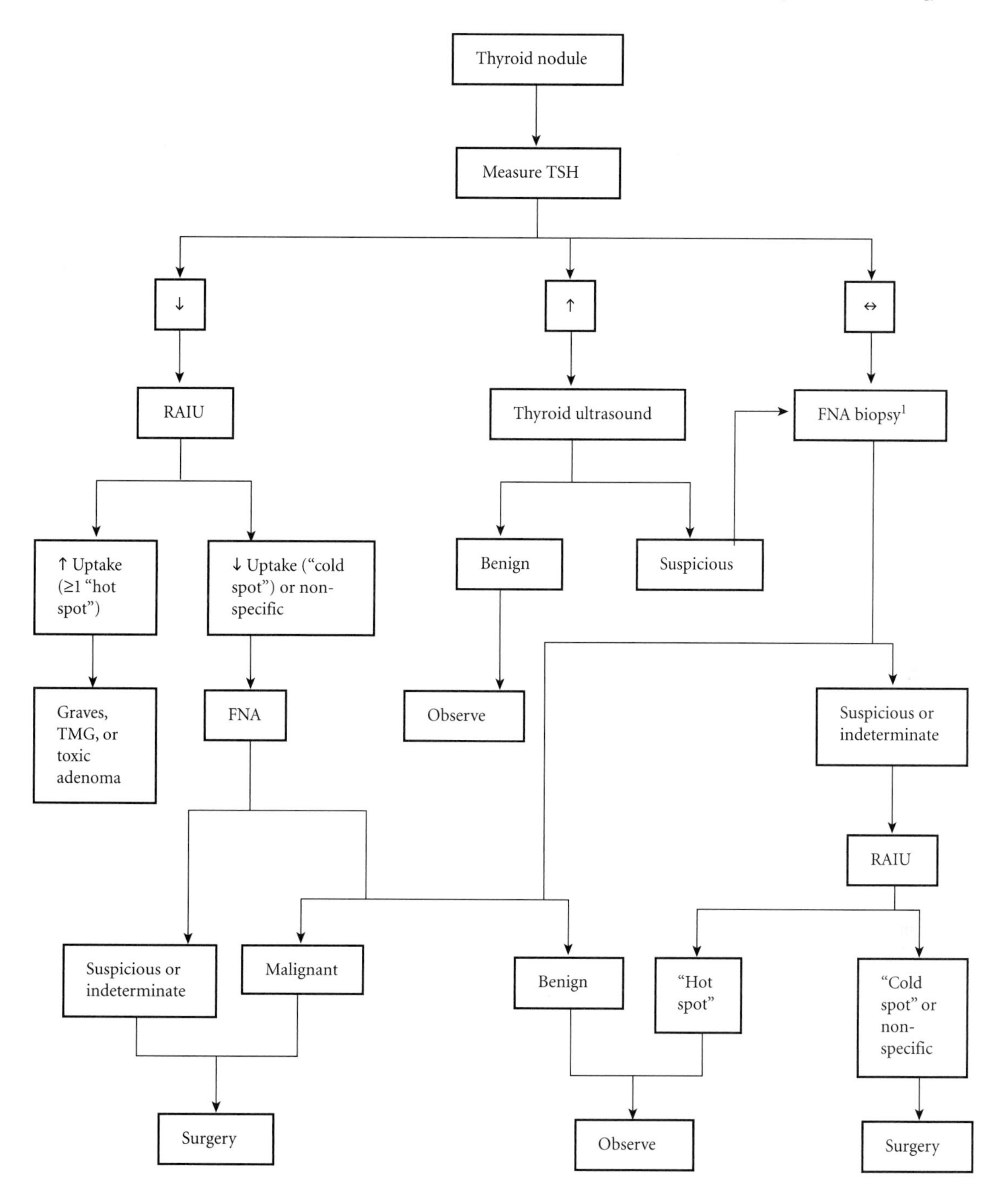

[1]If nodule is not palpable, perform under ultrasound guidance.

FIGURE 8–13 Work-up of thyroid nodule.

CASE 8–9 HYPERCALCEMIA

A 39-year-old woman presents with dysuria and colicky flank pain. She has been constipated for the last 4 weeks. She passes three calcium stones. Serum calcium is 11.7 mg/dL (increased). Other serum chemistries are normal.

What are the causes of hypercalcemia?

1. **Primary hyperparathyroidism**: Leading cause in outpatients (>90%); second most frequent cause among hospitalized patients. Causes include parathyroid adenoma (80% to 90%), hyperplasia (5% to 10%), or carcinoma (1% to 2%).
2. **Malignancy**: Leading cause among hospitalized patients; second most frequent cause in outpatients. The four major mechanisms of hypercalcemia in malignancy are:
   - Bone metastases cause increased bone resorption.
   - PTH-related peptide is released by many tumors (leads to increased bone resorption).
   - Lymphomas: cells release increased calcitriol (leads to increased intestinal Ca^{2+} absorption).
   - Multiple myeloma releases osteoclast-activating factor (increased bone resorption).
3. **Other causes of increased bone resorption**: Hyperthyroidism, Paget's disease, immobilization, excess vitamin A (e.g., oral isotretinoin), and tamoxifen.
4. **Granulomatous disease**: e.g., Sarcoidosis, TB. Exact mechanism is unknown. Granulomatous cells may increase conversion of calcidiol to calcitriol.
5. **Increased calcium intake (Milk-alkali syndrome)**: More common in the past when calcium carbonate (TUMS) and milk was the primary treatment available for ulcers.
6. **Increased vitamin D intake**: Leads to increased intestinal Ca^{2+} absorption (Fig. 8-14).
   Other medications: Thiazides (decreased urinary Ca^{2+} excretion) and lithium (increases set point for PTH suppression).
7. **Familial hypocalciuric hypercalcemia (FHH)**: Rare autosomal dominant mutation in calcium sensor in parathyroid gland and kidneys leads to mild hypercalcemia.

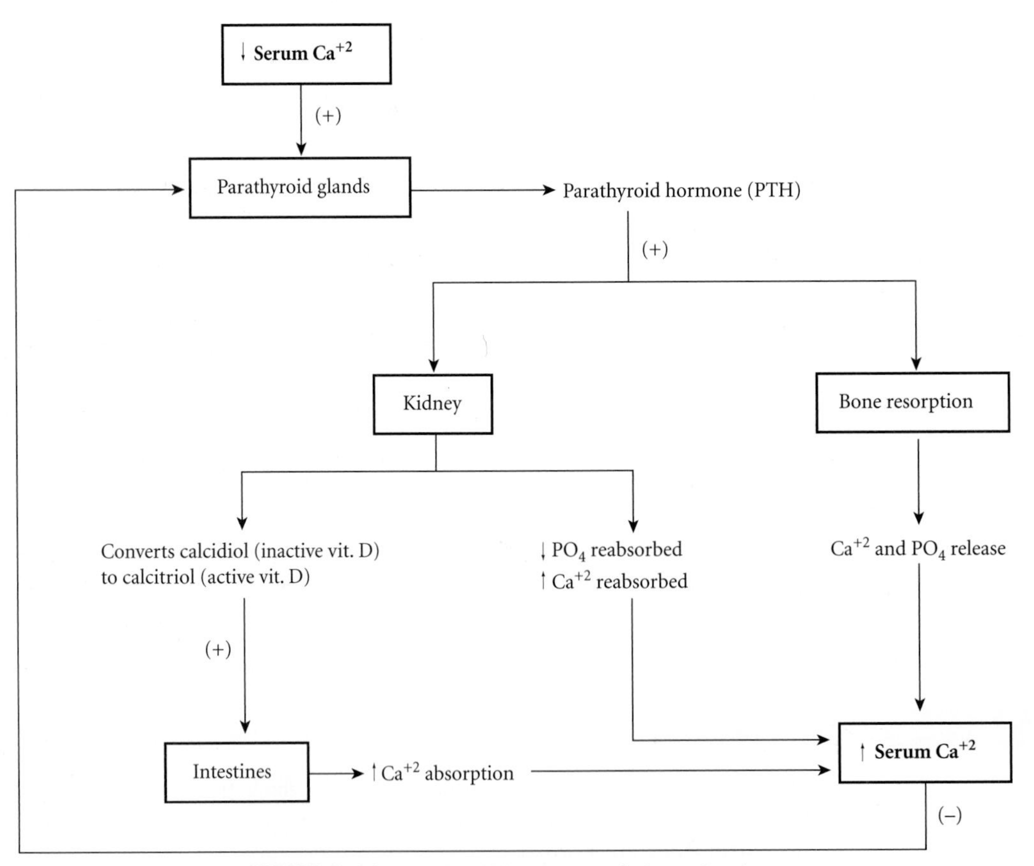

FIGURE 8–14 Parathyroid hormone regulation and actions.

What are possible clinical manifestations of hypercalcemia?

Patients with mild hypercalcemia (10 to 12 mg/dL) are often asymptomatic or have nonspecific symptoms (fatigue, constipation, depression, etc.). Moderate (12 to 14 mg/dL) or severe (>14 mg/dL) hypercalcemia causes multi-organ symptoms:

1. **"Stones" (renal symptoms)**: Nephrolithiasis (caused by increased urine Ca^{2+}) and nephrogenic diabetes insipidus occur with long-standing hypercalcemia (e.g., hyperparathyroidism or sarcoidosis).
2. **"Bones" (skeletal symptoms)**: Acute hypercalcemia can cause bone pain. Long-standing hypercalcemia can cause arthritis and osteoporosis.
3. **"Constipated groans" (GI symptoms)**: Constipation is the most common GI symptom. Patients occasionally develop acute pancreatitis.
4. **"Psychotic moans" (neuropsychiatric symptoms)**: Weakness, depression, and anxiety are common psychological symptoms. Severe hypercalcemia can cause cognitive dysfunction and psychosis.

> **Osteitis fibrosa cystica**: Severe primary hyperparathyroidism can cause replacement of bone by fibrous tissue, which leads to increased pain and fractures.

> **EKG**: Hypercalcemia can cause decreased QT interval. Hypocalcemia can cause increased QT interval.

What are the next steps in management of this patient with mild hypercalcemia?

First obtain serum albumin and calculate corrected calcium value. If corrected calcium is high, discontinue any medications associated with hypercalcemia and check serum Ca^{2+} and phosphorus. If corrected Ca^{2+} is still high, obtain serum PTH (Fig. 8-15).

> **Corrected calcium**: Majority of calcium is bound to albumin, so increased albumin can cause increased serum calcium and vice versa even if biologically active ("free" or "ionized") calcium is normal. Corrected calcium = (4 − serum albumin) × (0.8 + serum calcium).

Corrected calcium is high. The patient does not take any medications. She denies any fever, night sweats, weight loss, or anorexia. Serum PTH is 80 pg/ml (increased).

What is the next step in management?

The most likely diagnosis is primary hyperparathyroidism. The next step is to rule out FHH (the only other cause of hypercalcemia with increased/normal PTH). Obtain 24-hour urine calcium (decreased in FHH, increased or normal in primary hyperparathyroidism). Many clinicians also calculate Ca/Cr clearance (Ca/Cr >0.01 rules out FHH).

> **Ca/Cr clearance** = (urine Ca/creatinine)/(serum Ca/creatinine)

Measurement of 24-hour urine calcium is 500 mg (increased). BUN and serum creatinine are normal. Ca/Cr clearance is >0.01.

How is primary hyperparathyroidism treated?

Consider surgery for patients who meet any of the following criteria:

1. Age <50 years
2. Serum calcium >11.5 mg/dL
3. Urine calcium >400 mg/day
4. Symptomatic patient

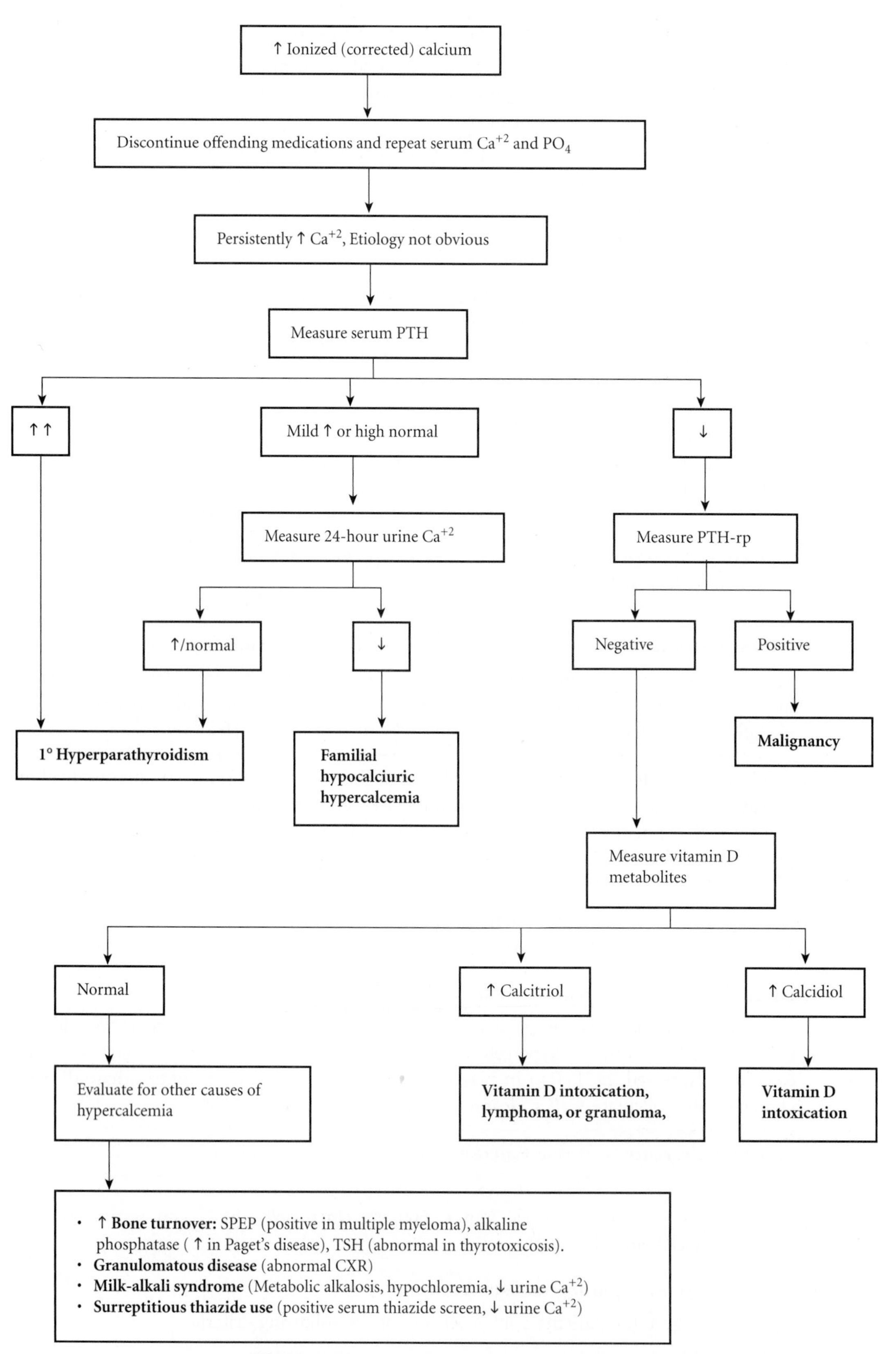

FIGURE 8–15 Diagnostic approach to hypercalcemia.

This young patient with serum Ca 11.9 mg/dL, urine Ca 500 mg/dL, and nephrolithiasis should undergo surgery (bilateral neck exploration + parathyroidectomy).

How would management have differed if the patient were an asymptomatic 60-year-old woman with serum Ca 11 mg/dL, PTH 80 pg/ml, and urine Ca 300 mg/day?

This older patient with primary hyperparathyroidism does not have any indications for surgery. Medical management of mild hypercalcemia is increased salt and fluid intake.

How would initial management have differed if the patient with nephrolithiasis had serum Ca 13.8 mg/dL?

Initial therapy for any patient with severe hypercalcemia or symptomatic moderate hypercalcemia is to increase calcium excretion with normal saline. If saline hydration causes fluid overload (e.g., peripheral or pulmonary edema), add loop diuretics to the regimen. Then, perform diagnostic evaluation to determine the underlying cause.

> **Serum Ca^{2+} > 18 mg/dL**: This is a rare finding; in addition to hydration and diuresis, consider hemodialysis.

How would you manage a patient with severe hypercalcemia due to increased bone resorption (hyperparathyroidism, solid tumors, etc.) that is refractory to fluids and diuretics?

In addition to continuing hydration, second-line therapy is calcitonin (peak effect in 1 to 2 days) and bisphosphonates (peak effect in 2 to 4 days). Both calcitonin and bisphosphonates decrease bone resorption by inhibiting osteoclasts. After correcting hypercalcemia, treat the underlying cause.

> **Calcitonin**: Decreases serum calcium by 1 to 2 mg/dL; not indicated for long-term treatment of hypercalcemia because tolerance develops after 48 hours.
> **Bisphosphonates**: Main drug class used for long-term control of hypercalcemia caused by an incurable malignancy (first-line agent is zoledronic acid, second-line agent is pamidronate).

> **Bisphosphonate side effects**: The most concerning side effects are esophagitis and jaw osteonecrosis (occurs mainly in cancer patients; presents with jaw pain, numbness, loose teeth, and exposed bone in oral cavity).

How would you manage a patient with severe hypercalcemia caused by increased vitamin D, granulomatous disease (e.g., sarcoidosis), or hematological malignancies (lymphoma, multiple myeloma) that is refractory to fluids and diuretics?

In addition to continued hydration, the major second-line therapy is glucocorticoids ± calcitonin and bisphosphonates. Also, discontinue any supplements containing vitamin D and minimize sun exposure. After correcting hypercalcemia, treat the underlying cause.

CASE 8–10 HYPOCALCEMIA

A 56-year-old man is found to have serum calcium of 7.6 mg/dL (decreased). Physical exam and vital signs are normal.

What are the causes of hypocalcemia in adults?

The major categories of hypocalcemia are the ***2 P's*** and the ***3 D's***: **P**TH abnormalities, acute increase in serum **P**O_4, **D**eposits (bone, pancreas, and intravascular), decreased vitamin **D**,

TABLE 8–15 Etiologies of hypocalcemia

PTH abnormalities	**Hypoparathyroidism**: Number one cause of hypocalcemia is surgical removal of parathyroid or thyroid gland (iatrogenic hypoparathyroidism). Less common causes are autoimmune parathyroid destruction or parathyroid infiltration by disorders like sarcoidosis, Wilson's disease, hemochromatosis, etc. **Pseudohypoparathyroidism**: Rare autosomal dominant mutation leads to PTH resistance, so patients have ↑ PTH but ↓ Ca^{+2}. Some patients are not diagnosed until adulthood. Two main types are: Type 1a (Albright's hereditary osteodystrophy): PTH-resistance in all tissues leads to hypocalcemia, short stature, short bones, and round face. Type 1b: PTH-resistance confined to the kidney causes isolated hypocalcemia. **Secondary hyperparathyroidism**: In chronic renal failure, kidneys do not respond to PTH so patients have ↑ PTH and PO_4 but ↓/normal serum calcium. ↓ **Serum magnesium**: ↓ Mg causes PTH resistance.
↑ **Serum phosphate**	↑ **PO_4 administration** **Acute renal failure**: Refer to Chapter 6: Nephrology **Tumor lysis syndrome**: Refer to Chapter 10
↓ **Vitamin D**	↓ **Vitamin D intake** ↓ **GI absorption of vitamin D**: Celiac disease, gastric bypass, etc. ↓ **Hydroxylation of calcidiol to calcitriol**: Chronic renal failure
↑ **Deposits**	↑ Bone deposits: **Osteoblastic metastases**: Metastatic breast or prostate cancer can cause calcium to deposit on bone. **Hungry bone syndrome**: Complication of iatrogenic hypoparathyroidism. ↓ PTH causes calcium to deposit on bone ↑ Pancreas deposits **Acute pancreatitis** Intravascular binding: Substances that bind to Ca^{+2} can cause ↓ ionized Ca^{+2} despite normal serum Ca^{+2}. **Massive blood transfusion**: Blood banks use citrate to prevent clotting of stored blood. Citrate binds to calcium. **Foscarnet**: Also binds to calcium and forms complexes. **Acute respiratory alkalosis**: ↑ binding of Ca^{+2} to albumin.
Drugs	Bisphosphonates, carbamazepine, cisplatin, calcimimetics, etc
Severe illness	E.g., sepsis

and **D**rugs (Table 8-15). In addition, patients with severe illness (e.g., sepsis) often have hypocalcemia.

Urine cAMP: increased in primary but not secondary hypoparathyroidism.

Pseudopseudohypoparathyroidism: Mutations similar to pseudohypoparathyroidism can cause symptoms of Albright's hereditary osteodystrophy but no hypocalcemia.

What are the clinical manifestations of hypocalcemia?

Many patients are asymptomatic. Chronic hypocalcemia can make a patient "***Fat, slow, blind, and stupid***" (**Fat**: puffy face, prolonged QT; **Slow**: Parkinsonian signs; **Blind**: cataracts; **Stupid**: cognitive impairment). Clinical manifestations of severe, acute hypocalcemia are mostly neurologic (tetany, papilledema, and seizures).

> Bone abnormalities (occur only in certain hypocalcemic disorders):
> 1. **Vitamin D deficiency** (osteomalacia)
> 2. **Type 1a pseudohypoparathyroidism** (Albright's hereditary dystrophy)

How does tetany typically manifest in a patient with hypocalcemia?

Patients usually do not develop tetany until serum calcium is <7.5 mg/dL. Initial symptoms are hand, foot, and mouth paresthesia (tingling). Later on, patients develop muscle spasms and cramps. Classic but insensitive signs are:

1. **Chvostek sign**: Tapping the facial nerve leads to twitching of facial muscles.
2. **Trousseau sign**: Carpal spasms when a blood pressure cuff is inflated to a pressure higher than systolic pressure for 3 minutes.

> Metabolic alkalosis, hypokalemia, and hypomagnesemia can exacerbate tetany.

> Trousseau sign ≠ Trousseau syndrome (migratory thrombophlebitis due to malignancy).

What is the next step in management?

First determine whether the patient is symptomatic (e.g., tetany, seizures, prolonged QT interval). If the patient is symptomatic and serum magnesium is normal, the first step is to treat with IV calcium gluconate. If serum magnesium is low or unknown, first administer IV magnesium sulfate, then calcium gluconate. After initiating therapy, proceed with the diagnostic evaluation (Fig. 8-16).

The patient is asymptomatic.

In addition to a thorough history and physical exam, what is the next diagnostic step?

Measure serum albumin to confirm whether the hypocalcemia truly represents decreased ionized calcium (Table 8-15). Ionized calcium = (4 − serum albumin) × (0.8 + serum calcium).

Ionized calcium is low. The patient does not have any history of parathyroidectomy. He does not take any medications. Serum phosphate is 4.7 mg/dL (increased), amylase is 36 (normal), magnesium is 2.2 mg/dL (normal), and creatinine is 2.3 mg/dL. Serum PTH and vitamin D metabolites (calcidiol and calcitriol) are pending.

What is the most likely cause of this patient's hypocalcemia?

This patient with increased serum phosphate and increased serum creatinine likely has chronic renal failure. PTH and vitamin D metabolite tests usually take 3 to 5 days to return. Increased PTH, increased/normal calcidiol, and decreased calcitriol would support the diagnosis (Fig. 8-16).

How is asymptomatic hypocalcemia treated?

1. **Serum calcium > 8 mg/dL**: Increase dietary calcium intake.
2. **Serum calcium < 8 mg/dL**: First-line therapy is to increase dietary intake as well as take oral calcium supplements. If hypocalcemia persists, add calcitriol ± thiazide diuretics to the regimen. Monitor urine calcium in patients receiving calcium supplements (major toxicity is hypercalciuria).

> Avoid calcium citrate in patients with renal failure (leads to increased aluminum).

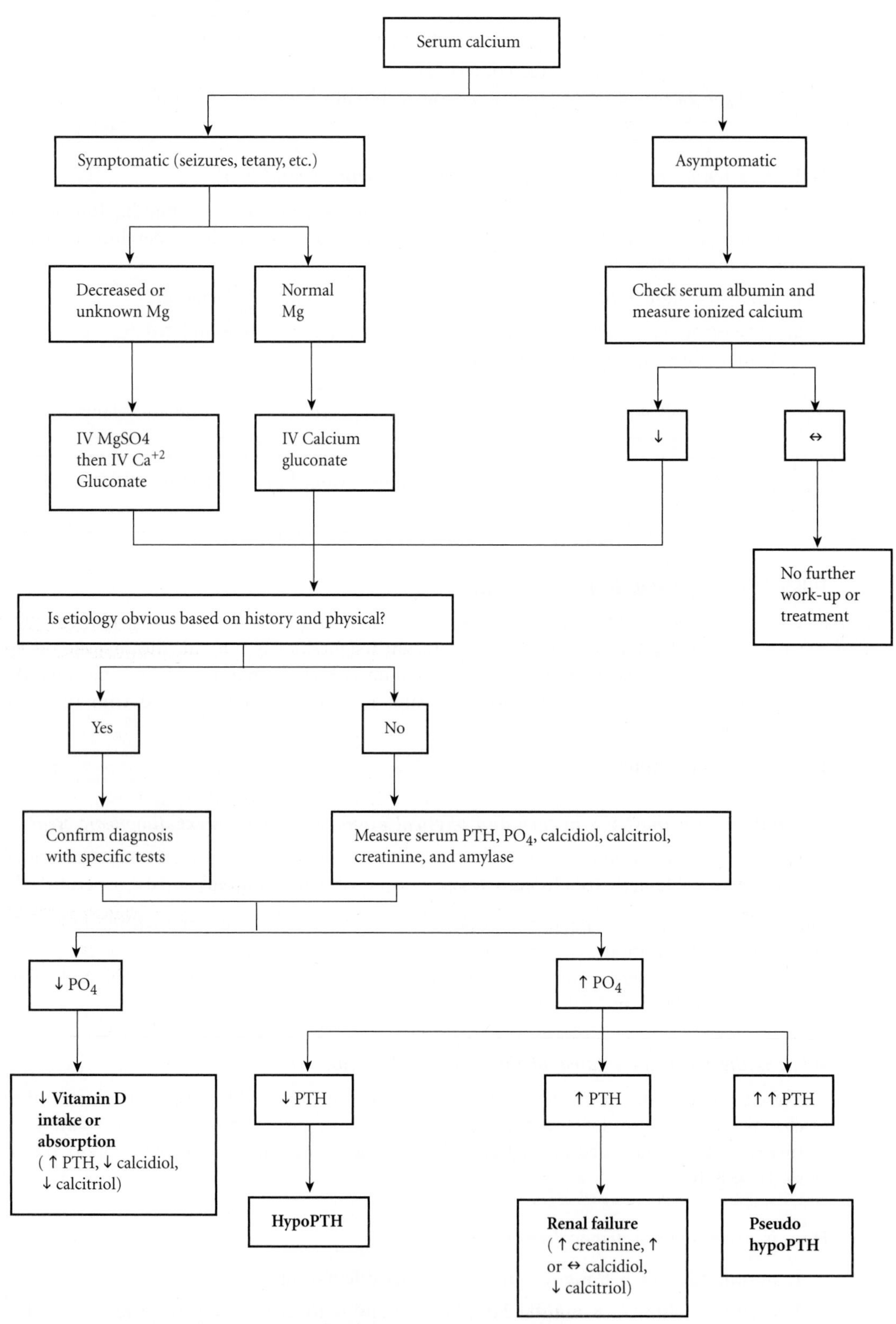

FIGURE 8–16 Evaluation of hypocalcemia.

CASE 8–11 ORTHOSTATIC HYPOTENSION AND HYPERKALEMIA

A 34-year-old man presents with a 2-month history of weakness and fatigue. Physical exam is significant for hyperpigmentation. Blood pressure is 100/80 in the supine position and falls to 90/65 upon standing. Temperature, pulse, and respiratory rate are normal. CBC, ESR, TSH, and creatinine kinase are normal. Abnormal serum chemistries are sodium 128 mEq/L, potassium 5.2 mEq/L, and chloride 114 mEq/L.

What is the most likely cause of the patient's symptoms?

Weakness and fatigue are nonspecific symptoms. However, orthostatic hypotension and hyponatremia should raise suspicion for hypoaldosteronism. Primary hypoaldosteronism (Addison's disease) is the most likely diagnosis in this patient with hyperkalemia and hyperpigmentation.

> Hypoaldosteronism = mineralocorticoid deficiency = adrenal insufficiency.

What is the next diagnostic step?

Obtain early morning serum cortisol and ACTH:

1. **Increased/normal cortisol**: Adrenal insufficiency is ruled out.
2. **Decreased cortisol, increased ACTH**: Primary adrenal insufficiency (Addison's disease).
3. **Decreased cortisol, decreased ACTH**: Secondary or tertiary adrenal insufficiency. Use MRI to distinguish pituitary from hypothalamic lesions. If MRI is nondiagnostic, consider CRH stimulation test (CRH administration leads to increased ACTH in tertiary but not secondary adrenal insufficiency).
4. **Decreased cortisol, inconclusive ACTH**: Perform ACTH stimulation test. Measure baseline ACTH and serum cortisol. Administer synthetic ACTH (cosyntropin) and measure serum cortisol 30 to 60 minutes later. Unchanged serum cortisol confirms Addison's disease.

Serum cortisol is 3 μg/dL (decreased) and serum ACTH is increased.

What causes Addison's disease?

Autoimmune adrenal gland destruction causes 70% to 90% of cases of Addison's disease. The remaining cases are caused by adrenal infiltration by infections (e.g., tuberculosis), hemorrhage (complication of anticoagulation), and malignancy (e.g., metastases).

What are the clinical manifestations of adrenal insufficiency?

1. **General**: fatigue, malaise, weight loss
2. **CV**: orthostatic hypotension
3. **GI**: nausea, vomiting, anorexia, and increased craving for salt and ice
4. **Women**: amenorrhea, decreased axillary and pubic hair
5. **Addison's**: hyperpigmentation and hyperkalemia
6. **Autoimmune Addison's**: increased autoimmune disorders (e.g., vitiligo)

What is the next diagnostic step in this patient with Addison's disease?

The next step is abdominal CT to visualize the adrenal glands. An adrenal mass or calcification indicates infiltration by an infection, hemorrhage, or malignancy. Absence of an adrenal mass suggests autoimmune Addison's disease.

> **Nonhemorrhagic adrenal mass**: Consider CT-guided FNA biopsy to establish the cause of the adrenal mass.

Abdominal CT does not detect any mass or calcification.

How is Addison's disease treated?

Treat chronic Addison's disease with oral glucocorticoids, increased salt intake, and oral mineralocorticoids (fludrocortisone).

> **Second- or third-degree adrenal insufficiency**: Patients generally produce sufficient aldosterone, so fludrocortisone is not necessary.

Two years later, the patient presents to the emergency department with abdominal pain, nausea, and vomiting. The symptoms started a few hours after he ate custard at a restaurant 2 days ago. On examination, he appears confused. Vital signs are blood pressure 88/60, pulse 120 bpm, respirations 28/min, and temperature 38.1°C. SaO_2 is 98% on room air.

What is the most likely cause of his symptoms?

This patient with altered mental status and hypotension is in shock (see Chapter 2: Cardiology). The most likely cause is acute adrenal insufficiency (Addisonian crisis). Addisonian crisis usually occurs after a stressful event such as infection in a patient with pre-existing adrenal insufficiency. In his case, the combination of infectious gastroenteritis and an abrupt decrease in glucocorticoids (due to vomiting) is the most likely precipitant.

What are the next steps in management?

1. Airway and breathing: Give this patient with tachypnea and O_2 saturation of 98% supplemental oxygen. Continue to monitor oxygenation using a pulse oximeter.
2. Circulation: Obtain IV access. Draw blood for electrolytes, serum cortisol, and ACTH. Administer 2 to 3 L of normal saline and IV dexamethasone before lab studies return. When the patient is stable and can tolerate oral intake, switch to oral steroids and oral fludrocortisone.

> **No history of adrenal insufficiency**: Suspect Addisonian crisis if the patient has signs of shock + hyperkalemia ± abdominal pain. Administer saline and IV steroids before serum cortisol and ACTH measurements are back.

> **Fludrocortisone**: Use of this agent is not indicated for initial stabilization because effects are not evident for days. Also, normal saline is more effective at rapidly replacing sodium.

> Instruct patients with adrenal insufficiency to increase steroid dose during infections and other stressful events.

CASE 8–12 HYPERTENSION AND HYPOKALEMIA

During a routine evaluation of a 23-year-old man, blood pressure is 160/100. Hypertension persists 1 week and 3 weeks later. He does not have any known medical conditions. There is no family history of CV disease. He does not take any medications. Physical exam is normal. BMI is 22. Serum potassium is 2.8 mEq/L. EKG, fasting lipid profile, and other serum electrolytes are normal.

What diagnoses should you suspect?

Suspect a secondary cause in any hypertensive patient <30 years old, particularly if they are not obese and have no family history of heart disease. The major causes of hypertension and hypokalemia are:

1. **Primary hyperaldosteronism (Conn's syndrome)** is caused by aldosterone-producing adrenal hyperplasia, adenoma, or carcinoma.

2. **Secondary hyperaldosteronism** is usually caused by renovascular disorders such as renal artery stenosis (kidneys sense decreased volume, which leads to increased renin secretion). A rare cause is renin-producing tumors.
3. **Non–aldosterone-mediated mineralocorticoid excess**: Cushing's disease and chronic licorice ingestion (less common causes).

> **Diuretics** comprise a major cause of hypokalemia in patients with pre-existing hypertension.

What are the next diagnostic steps?

The next step is to measure plasma renin activity (PRA) and plasma aldosterone concentration (PAC). Interpret the values as follows:

1. **Increased PRA and increased PAC**: Suspect secondary hyperaldosteronism.
2. **Decreased PRA and increased PAC**: Suspect primary hyperaldosteronism.
3. **Decreased PRA and decreased PAC**: Suspect non–aldosterone-mediated mineralocorticoid excess.

> Discontinue diuretics and angiotensin-converting enzyme inhibitors before measuring PRA and PAC.

PRA is decreased and PAC is increased.

What is the next step in management?

The findings suggest but do not confirm primary hyperaldosteronism. The next step is to measure aldosterone after a period of oral or IV sodium loading. Urine aldosterone >14 ng/dL after a 3-day oral load or serum aldosterone >14 ng/dL after a 4-hour IV load confirms primary hyperaldosteronism.

Sodium loading confirms primary hyperaldosteronism.

What is the next step in management?

The next step is to obtain abdominal CT or MRI. A unilateral abdominal mass indicates adenoma or carcinoma. Nonspecific bilateral adrenal abnormalities indicate adrenal hyperplasia.

What test is recommended if abdominal imaging does not detect any mass or bilateral abnormalities?

Consider adrenal vein sampling. The physician obtains blood samples for measurement of aldosterone from both adrenal veins. Unilaterally elevated aldosterone indicates an adrenal adenoma, whereas normal or symmetrically elevated aldosterone indicates bilateral adrenal hyperplasia.

How do treatment of adrenal adenoma, carcinoma, and hyperplasia differ?

1. **Adrenal adenoma or carcinoma**: First-line treatment is surgery (unilateral adrenalectomy). Patients who are not candidates for surgery should take aldosterone receptor antagonists. First-line aldosterone blocker is spironolactone; the second-line agent is eplerenone (because of higher cost). If neither drug is effective or well-tolerated, consider amiloride.
2. **Adrenal hyperplasia**: First-line treatment is aldosterone receptor antagonists (first-line agent is spironolactone; second-line agent is eplerenone, third-line agent is amiloride).

CASE 8–13 EPISODES OF HYPERTENSION, HEADACHES, AND PALPITATIONS

A 29-year-old man presents with episodes of headaches, palpitations, and diaphoresis. The episodes occur almost every day. The patient is currently asymptomatic. Physical exam is normal. Blood pressure is 150/90. Remaining vital signs are normal.

What diagnosis should you suspect?

Suspect secondary hypertension in this patient <30 years old. Episodes of headaches, palpitations, and sweating are the classic triad of pheochromocytoma (catecholamine-secreting tumor of the adrenal medulla). Pheochromocytoma usually causes sustained or paroxysmal hypertension.

> **Pheochromocytoma rule of 10s**: 10% malignant, 10% multiple, 10% familial, 10% bilateral (suspect MEN 2A or 2B), 10% extra-adrenal, 10% occur in children.

What is the next diagnostic step?

Obtain a 24-hour urine sample and measure fractionated metanephrine levels (catecholamine breakdown products). If urine metanephrine is elevated, obtain abdominal CT or MRI.

> **Personal or family history of MEN 2A or 2B tumors**: Initial testing includes urine fractionated metanephrine + fractionated catecholamines.

> **MIBG scan**: This test measures uptake of MIBG (metaiodobenzylguanidine, an adrenaline analog) and is indicated if CT or MRI is negative in a patient with increased urinary metanephrine or catecholamines.

How is pheochromocytoma treated?

Treatment is administration of an α-blocker such as phenoxybenzamine followed by a low-dose β-blocker followed by surgery (adrenalectomy).

> Hypertension is often the only abnormality in patients with renovascular disease, pheochromocytoma, or Conn's syndrome. Rule out these conditions in any hypertensive patient <30 years old who is not obese and has no family history of premature heart disease.

How would management have differed if an adrenal mass were discovered incidentally during abdominal imaging in an asymptomatic patient (adrenal incidentaloma)?

Rule out pheochromocytoma (with urine fractionated metanephrine and catecholamines) and Cushing's syndrome (with serum cortisol ± DST). If the patient has hypertension, obtain PRA and PAC to rule out hyperaldosteronism. If any of the laboratory tests are positive, treat the conditions as described earlier.

How is an adrenal incidentaloma managed if laboratory testing is not diagnostic?

Features that should cause suspicion of malignancy are size >4 cm, irregular borders, calcifications, or nonhomogenous appearance. Patients with any of these features should undergo adrenalectomy. Otherwise, obtain a follow-up CT scan or MRI at 3 to 6 months and then every 12 months.

CASE 8–14 MANAGEMENT OF OBESITY

A 24-year-old man presents for a routine evaluation. He is 5 feet 6 inches tall and weighs 200 lbs. His only exercise involves walking up the stairs to his apartment.

How can you determine if the patient is overweight or obese?

Clinically, BMI is used to determine whether a patient's weight is appropriate. BMI equals weight (kg)/height^2 (m^2). On the basis of BMI, patients are categorized as follows:

1. BMI <18.5 = underweight
2. BMI 18.5 to 25 = normal weight

3. BMI ≥25 but <30 = overweight
4. BMI ≥30 but <40 = obese
5. BMI ≥40 = severely obese

Asians: BMI ≥24 and <30 is considered overweight.

Adjustment for waist circumference (for patients with BMI 22 to 29):
Men: Add 2 to BMI if waist is 32 to 40 inches; add 4 to BMI if waist >40 inches.
Women: Add 2 to BMI if waist is 28 to 35 inches; add 4 to BMI if waist >35 inches.

BMI overestimates obesity in patients with a high amount of muscle mass and underestimates obesity in elderly patients with less lean mass and in short patients.

What is this patient's BMI?

Weight (kg) = weight (lbs)/2.2 = 200/2.2 = 91 kg

Height (cm) = height (in.) × 2.54 = 66 × 2.54 = 168 cm = 1.68 m

BMI = weight (kg)/height^2 (m^2) = 91/(1.68 × 1.68) = 32

This patient's BMI places him in the obese category. Correction for waist circumference is not necessary because BMI >29.

What evaluation is indicated for obese patients?

1. Focused history and physical to detect underlying causes of obesity (Table 8-16).
2. Evaluate for comorbidities that increase CV risk: Measure blood pressure, fasting lipid profile, FBG. Ask whether the patient smokes. Also, inquire about symptoms of sleep apnea.

How is overweight/obesity managed?

Treat comorbid conditions and counsel the following patients about diet, exercise, and weight loss:

1. Adjusted BMI >30
2. BMI >27 in the presence of comorbidities.

Consider drug therapy if the patient cannot achieve weight loss goals with diet and exercise alone. The first-line drug for patients without any comorbidity is sibutramine. The second-line drug for patients with one or more comorbidities is orlistat. Avoid combining the two drugs.

TABLE 8–16 Important causes of obesity in adults

Behavioral
↑ Dietary caloric intake
Sedentary lifestyle
Smoking cessation
Iatrogenic
1. Medications: Diabetes drugs (insulin and sulfonylureas), psychiatry drugs (e.g., neuroleptics), and steroids
2. Hypothalamus surgery
Endocrine
1. Cushing's syndrome/disease
2. Polycystic ovarian syndrome (see Chapter 14: Primary Care Gynecology and Urology)
3. Albright's hereditary osteodystrophy
Psychiatric
1. Depression (particularly seasonal affective disorder)

> In the absence of exercise, humans require 22 to 25 kCal/kg to maintain body weight.

> **Sibutramine**: sympathomimetic drug that causes early satiety.
> **Orlistat**: inhibits pancreatic lipase, which leads to decreased fat absorption.

When is surgery indicated for treatment of obesity?

Consider bariatric surgery for the following patients who have failed diet, exercise, and drug therapy:

1. BMI > 40
2. BMI > 35 with severe comorbidities

CASE 8–15 PATHOLOGICAL FRACTURES

A 75-year-old Caucasian woman presents with acute onset of severe low back pain after stepping out of her bathtub. The pain radiates to the anterior abdomen. The pain improves somewhat in the supine position. Walking and standing upright exacerbate the pain. She has smoked a pack of cigarettes every day for the last 55 years. There is tenderness over the L4–L5 area of the lower back. Straight leg test and neurological exam are normal. Vital signs are normal. BMI is 16.

What cause should you suspect is responsible for this patient's symptoms?

The patient has the characteristic features of a compression fracture of the spine: acute onset of back pain and tenderness ± radiation to the anterior abdomen. Only one third of compression fractures cause characteristic symptoms; two thirds of cases are not diagnosed because they are asymptomatic or cause mild, slowly progressive back pain.

What is the next diagnostic step?

Obtain plain frontal and lateral radiographs of the spine in any patient >50 years old with acute onset of severe back pain to rule out compression fracture.

> **Wedge fracture**: compression fracture limited to anterior part of vertebral body.
> **Burst fracture**: severe compression fracture that compresses entire vertebral body.

Plain radiographs confirm the presence of a compression fracture.

What causes compression fractures?

1. Major trauma in a patient with normal bone.
2. Minor trauma in a patient with abnormal bone (pathological fracture): An innocuous event such as stepping out of a bathtub, sneezing, or lifting a very light object can cause a compression fracture in patients with pre-existing bone disease. Osteoporosis causes 85% of all compression fractures. Malignancy and infection (osteomyelitis) are other important causes.

> Osteoporosis is usually asymptomatic until the patient has a compression fracture. Over time, multiple compression fractures can cause chronic back pain, decreased stature (due to kyphosis), and lordosis.

How is a compression fracture treated?

1. **Unstable fractures**: Immediate surgery is indicated for patients with neurological signs or bone fragments in the spinal canal on imaging.
2. **Stable fractures**: Initial management of this patient without neurological signs or bone fragments in the spinal canal is conservative. Administer analgesics such as nonsteroidal

anti-inflammatory drugs, muscle relaxants, and calcitonin nasal spray. Advise her to take a few days of bed rest (but avoid prolonged bed rest!). Consider surgery (kyphoplasty or vertebroplasty) only if symptoms persist after 6 to 12 weeks.

What tests are indicated to determine the etiology of compression fracture?

Osteoporosis is the leading cause of osteopenia and compression fractures. Perform a dual-energy x-ray (DXA) scan to confirm osteoporosis. Order the following laboratory tests to screen for other causes of compression fractures and decreased bone mineral density: serum chemistries, CBC, TSH, ESR, C-reactive protein, and alkaline phosphatase.

DXA scan: two x-ray beams of different energies measure BMD.
T-score: difference between patient's BMD and an average, sex-matched 30-year-old.
Osteopenia: T score 1 to 2 standard deviations (SDs) below average.
Osteoporosis: normal labs and T score $\leq$2.5 SDs below average.
Other causes of decreased BMD: osteomalacia, hyperthyroidism, and hyperparathyroidism.

The two chief causes of osteopenia are osteoporosis and osteomalacia.

The patient's T score is <2.5 SDs below the mean. Laboratory tests are normal.

How is osteoporosis treated?

First-line therapy is lifestyle measures and bisphosphonates. Lifestyle measures include smoking cessation, weight-bearing exercise, adequate caloric intake, and calcium and vitamin D supplements.

Treatment of osteoporosis lowers the risk of subsequent compression fracture.

How is response to therapy monitored?

Many clinicians repeat DXA scan after 1 to 2 years to assess response to therapy. Some also obtain baseline and follow-up markers of bone turnover (urine NTX and serum CTX). Lack of increase in bone density or decrease in bone turnover markers indicates poor response to therapy.

What second-line drugs are available for patients with a poor response to therapy or intolerable bisphosphonate side effects?

1. Raloxifene (selective estrogen receptor modulator): second-line drug for most patients.
2. Recombinant PTH: second-line drug for patients who continue to have fractures despite bisphosphonate therapy.
3. Estrogen $\pm$ progesterone: second-line treatment for subset of postmenopausal women with intolerable menopausal symptoms.

What other fractures commonly occur in patients with osteoporosis?

Compression fracture of the spine is the most common fracture. Others include:

1. Hip fracture: second most common fracture (major cause of death and disability)
2. Distal radius (Colle's) fracture: caused by a fall on an extended, outstretched hand
3. Long bone fractures (humerus, femur, etc.)

Alternative 8.15.1

A 38-year-old dark-skinned South Asian woman with a history of celiac disease presents with a 9-month history of progressively worsening back, hip, and thigh pain unresponsive to conservative therapy. On physical exam, she has a waddling (Trendelenburg) gait. There is point tenderness in the hips and knees. Vital signs are normal. X-ray of the hip and femur reveals osteopenia as well as partial fractures (Looser pseudofractures).

What is the most likely diagnosis?

Partial fractures (Looser pseudofractures) in the hip and pelvis are pathognomonic for osteomalacia. Patients with osteomalacia have soft and fragile bones because of defective bone mineralization. Initial symptoms are usually limited to nonspecific bone pain, so diagnosis is often delayed for years. As the disease progresses, patients develop a waddling gait and pseudofractures.

> The femur is one of the strongest bones in the body. Femoral fracture in the absence of major trauma indicates a pathological fracture.

What causes osteomalacia? What risk factors does this patient have for osteomalacia?

The major causes of defective bone mineralization in adults are:

1. **Inadequate mineral stores (calcium, phosphate, or vitamin D)**: primarily due to malabsorption or renal wasting (nephrotic syndrome, renal tubular acidosis, etc). Vitamin D deficiency can also result from decreased sunlight exposure or impaired hydroxylation (cirrhosis, chronic renal failure, or hypoparathyroidism). Other causes of calcium and phosphate deficiency were described earlier.
2. **Inhibition of bone mineralization**: Caused by increased fluoride, aluminum, or bisphosphonates.

Malabsorption as a result of celiac sprue, bariatric surgery, etc., is the major cause of osteomalacia in the United States. Worldwide, the most common cause of osteomalacia is dietary vitamin D deficiency. South Asians have a higher prevalence because their chief bread (chapatti) is low in vitamin D. Also, dark-skinned individuals cannot utilize sunlight to synthesize vitamin D as effectively.

> Prevalence of osteomalacia is higher among elderly patients in the United States because of decreased sunlight exposure and poor diet.

What is the next step in management?

Order the following laboratory tests to determine the cause of osteomalacia: serum chemistries, serum alkaline phosphatase, and calcidiol.

Abnormal laboratory values are serum phosphate 1.7 mg/dL (decreased), alkaline phosphatase 350 U/L (increased), and decreased calcidiol.

What is the next step in management?

The laboratory studies indicate secondary hyperparathyroidism caused by vitamin D deficiency. Treat this patient with high doses of vitamin D supplements. Also, maintain calcium intake $\geq$1000 g/day. This regimen should resolve symptoms and cause bone healing over weeks to months.

Alternative 8.15.2

A 68-year-old man presents with a 12-month history of bone pain in his hips and thighs. Vital signs are normal. Plain radiographs show fractures in the left femur and left hip. Serum chemistries and calcidiol are normal. Serum alkaline phosphatase is 450 U/L.

What condition should you suspect?

Normal serum chemistries and calcidiol make osteomalacia unlikely. Suspect Paget's disease in this older man with bone pain, pathological fractures, and elevated alkaline phosphatase. In this disorder, patients have accelerated resorption and formation (i.e., increased bone turnover), but the newly formed bone is more fragile than normal bone. Bone pain and deformity are the most common symptoms, and patients often develop pathological fractures. The disease is frequently asymptomatic, and patients are often diagnosed after laboratory studies incidentally detect elevated alkaline phosphatase.

> **Bone scan** is the most sensitive test to identify lesions in Paget's disease, which appear as areas of increased uptake ("hot spots"). Follow up positive bone scan with plain radiograph.
> **Urinary hydroxyproline** is often increased in Paget's disease. This test is not widely available.
> **Serum calcium** is usually normal, but some patients with immobilization or trauma have hypercalcemia.

> **Osteoporosis circumscripta**: Paget's disease often causes radiolucent areas in the skull followed years later by enlargement and "cotton wool" appearance. Skull enlargement can cause cranial nerve palsies.

What causes Paget's disease?

Although the precise cause is unclear, both genetic factors and viral infection likely play a causative role.

How is Paget's disease treated?

First-line therapy is oral pamidronate. Other bisphosphonates are equally effective but are associated with increased GI side effects. Measure alkaline phosphatase every 2 months to assess response to therapy (alkaline phosphatase should decrease).

How would management differ if Paget's disease were suspected in an asymptomatic patient with elevated alkaline phosphatase?

Obtain bone scans followed by plain radiographs to assess bone involvement. Initiate therapy only if the disorder affects the pelvis or weight-bearing long bones.

Symptoms resolve and alkaline phosphatase declines with pamidronate therapy. The patient is placed on a long-term pamidronate regimen. Ten years later, he presents with new-onset pain and swelling in the right femur.

What is the next step in management?

New-onset symptoms are unusual in patients successfully treated for Paget's disease. Maintain a high index of suspicion for malignancy because this disorder greatly increases the risk of bone tumors (particularly osteosarcoma). The next step is to obtain plain radiographs of the entire femur. If plain radiographs detect a tumor, obtain MRI to evaluate the extent of the primary tumor and perform bone scans to search for distant metastases.

> Summary of abnormal labs in patients with pathological fractures:
> **Osteoporosis**: no abnormal labs
> **Vitamin D deficiency osteomalacia**: normal or mildly decreased Ca, decreased PO4, increased alkaline phosphatase, decreased calcidiol
> **Paget's disease**: normal or increased Ca, increased alkaline phosphatase
> **Albright's hereditary osteodystrophy**: decreased Ca, increased PTH

chapter **9**

Rheumatology

CASE 9–1 CHRONIC AND SYMMETRIC POLYARTICULAR PAIN

A 35-year-old woman presents with a 9-month history of episodic joint pain (arthralgia). The symptoms began with mild pain in the left metacarpophalangeal (MCP) joint, but now she has pain in both MCPs, both proximal interphalangeal joints (PIPs), and both knees. Her joints feel "stiff" for about an hour every morning. The stiffness improves with activity. The MCP and PIP joints are tender, swollen, and boggy. Vital signs are normal.

What is the most likely diagnosis?

Chronic polyarticular pain with features of inflammatory arthritis is most commonly caused by an autoimmune arthritis or spondyloarthropathy. This patient with symmetric involvement of the MCPs and PIPs meets diagnostic criteria for rheumatoid arthritis (RA). Patients must meet four of seven criteria (mnemonic: ***Rheumatoid Hands Require Some PM&R***):

1. **R**heumatoid nodules: freely moving subcutaneous nodules on bony prominences
2. **H**and joint symptoms (wrist, MCP, PIP) for ≥6 weeks
3. **R**heumatoid factor (RF): IgM RF sensitive (positive in 70% to 80%) but not specific
4. **S**ymmetric joint involvement for ≥6 weeks
5. **P**ain in three or more joints for ≥6 weeks
6. **M**orning stiffness that lasts ≥60 minutes for ≥6 weeks
7. **R**adiographic findings: joint space narrowing; bone and cartilage erosions

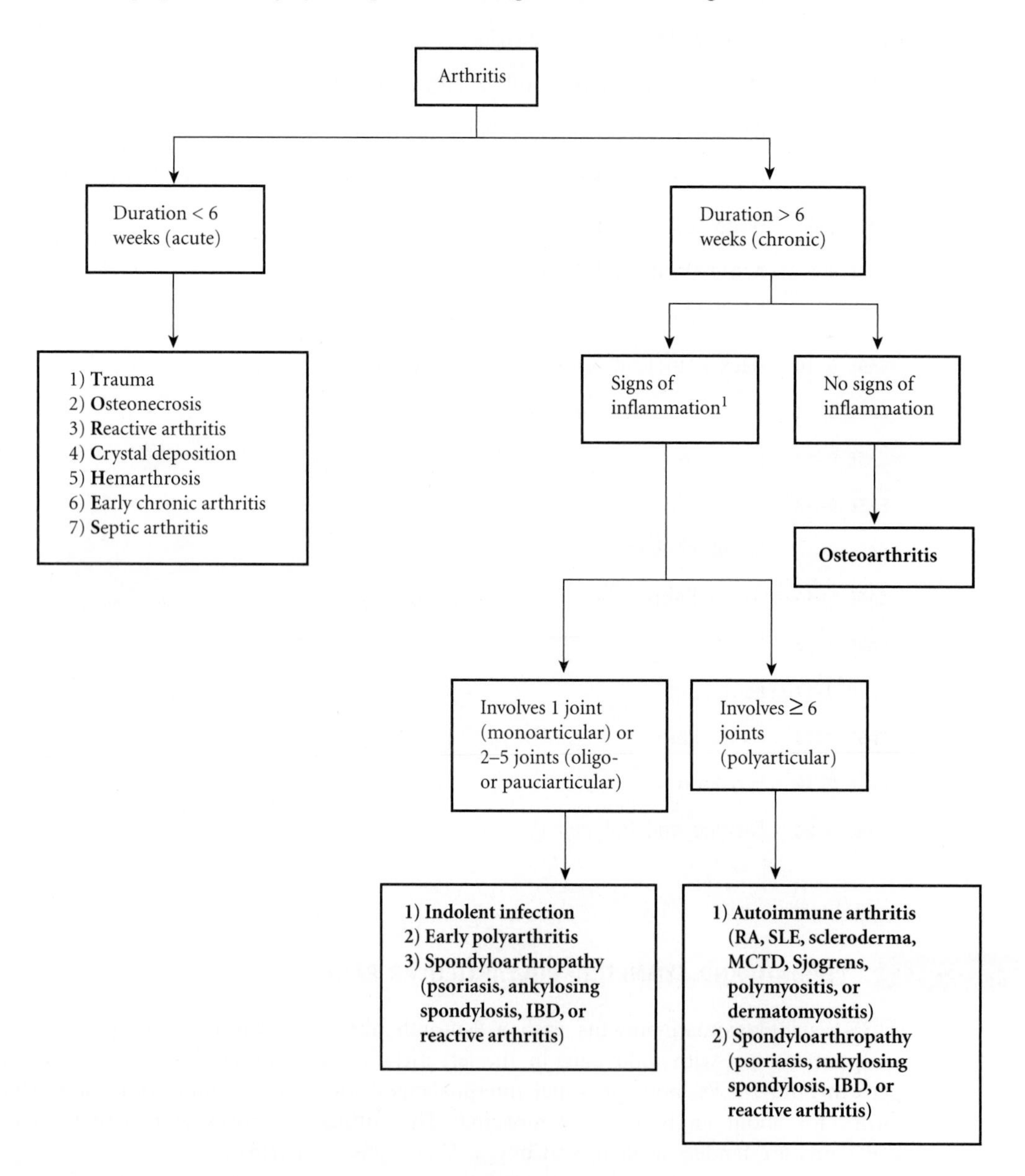

[1]Signs of inflammation include (a) morning stiffness > 30 minutes (b) ↓Pain with activity (c) tender, swollen, or boggy joint
Adapted from Sabatine M. Pocket medicine 2nd edition

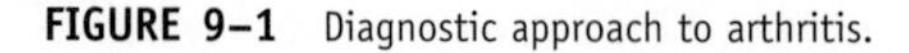

FIGURE 9–1 Diagnostic approach to arthritis.

TABLE 9–1 Classification of Rheumatoid Arthritis

	Mild	Moderate	Severe
No. of involved joints	<6	6–20	>20
Extra-articular	No	No	Yes
Functional disability[a]	Mild	Moderate	Severe
RF and anti-CCP	(+) or (−)	(+)	(+)
ESR, CRP	Negative	Occasionally positive	Often positive
X-ray	Normal	Periarticular swelling ± mild joint space narrowing and erosions	Substantial joint space narrowing and erosions ± joint malalignment

Abbreviations: CCP, anti-cyclic citrullinated peptide; CRP, C-reactive protein; ESR, erythrocyte sedimentation rate; RF, rheumatoid factor.

[a] Assessed using questionnaires such as Stanford Health Assessment Questionnaire.

This patient with symmetric involvement of the MCPs and PIPs meets diagnostic criteria for rheumatoid arthritis (RA) (Table 9-1). In this condition, an autoimmune lymphocytic infiltrate in the synovium forms a pannus. Pannus growth destroys joint cartilage and bone.

Rheumatoid arthritis (RA) diagnostic dilemmas:

1. There is no single clinical or laboratory feature that is diagnostic of RA.
2. Patients with early-stage RA may not meet diagnostic criteria.
3. Laboratory and imaging tests are often negative in early-stage RA.

Features of chronic inflammatory arthritis:

Symptoms: Morning stiffness >30 minutes, decreased joint pain with activity
Signs: Tender, boggy, swollen joint
Laboratory features: ↑ Erythrocyte sedimentation rate (ESR) and ↑ C-reactive protein (CRP)

What factors increase the risk of developing RA?

Both genetic and environmental factors are involved in RA pathogenesis. Known risk factors are HLA-DR1 and HLA-DR4, female sex, smoking, and positive family history. Typical age of onset is 20 to 40 years of age.

Autoimmune arthritides are also collectively referred to as connective tissue disorders. All connective tissue disorders are more common in women.

The patient asks about her long-term prognosis.

What should you tell her?

1. Approximately 80% of patients have episodes of exacerbations (active disease) and remissions.
2. Approximately 10% have a single episode followed by complete remission.
3. Approximately 10% have severe, progressive arthritis despite treatment.

Markers of poor prognosis: Erosions on x-ray, rheumatoid nodules, ↑ ESR or CRP, and high-titer RF (e.g., 1:160 is a higher titer than 1:64).

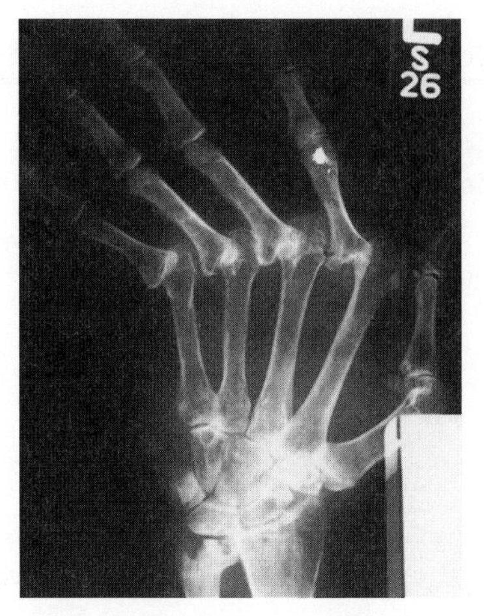

FIGURE 9–2 X-ray in rheumatoid arthritis showing periarticular swelling but no erosions. From Harris JH Jr., Harris WH, Novelline RA. *The Radiology of Emergency Medicine*, 3rd ed. Lippincott Williams & Wilkins, 1993.

What imaging and laboratory studies are indicated initially?

Obtain the following laboratory and imaging studies to increase diagnostic certainty, assess disease severity, and establish a baseline for comparison:

1. X-rays of involved joints
2. Auto-antibodies: Obtain RF ± anti-cyclic citrullinated peptide (anti-CCP). RF is more sensitive, but anti-CCP is more specific. Combination is more sensitive and specific than either test alone.
3. CBC: Patients may have anemia of chronic disease, increased platelets, and increased white blood cells (WBCs).
4. Liver function tests (LFTs) and serum chemistries: Establish baseline because RA drugs can affect liver and kidney function.
5. ESR and CRP: Nonspecific markers of inflammation that are used to monitor disease progression.

Figure 9-2 is the patient's x-ray. RF and anti-CCP are positive. Remaining tests are normal.

What stage disease does she have?

X-rays demonstrate periarticular swelling but no erosions. This patient with six involved joints, no extra-articular symptoms or joint malalignment, positive auto-antibodies, and normal complete blood count (CBC), ESR, and CRP has moderate-stage RA (Tables 9-1, 9-2, and 9-3).

Palindromic RA: Recurrent episodes of oligo-articular inflammatory arthritis that last for hours to weeks and then subside; ESR, CRP, RF, and anti-CCP are usually positive.

How is RA treated?

1. **Patient education and exercise**: Indicated for all patients. Patients with signs of joint deformity (severe RA) should undertake weight-bearing exercise cautiously.
2. **Pharmacotherapy**: There are four major drug categories used in RA treatment: nonsteroidal anti-inflammatory drugs (NSAIDs), corticosteroids, disease-modifying antirheumatic drugs (DMARDs), and biological agents. NSAIDs and steroids rapidly decrease inflammation but do not slow disease progression. DMARDs and anti-cytokine therapies take weeks to months to take effect but can slow disease progression. Therapeutic choices depend on disease severity and the individual patient's response (Fig. 9-3).

TABLE 9–2 Extra-articular Complications of Rheumatoid Arthritis

Constitutional
Fatigue, anorexia, and weight loss
Bones
Osteopenia/osteoporosis (additive increased in risk with steroid use)
Muscle
1. Inflammation and disuse atrophy 2. Polymyositis (rare)
Peripheral nerves
Carpal tunnel syndrome and other hand/foot paresthesias
Skin
1. Rheumatoid nodules 2. Neutrophil dermatoses (see Chapter 13: Dermatology)
Eyes
1. Scleritis and episcleritis (see Chapter 16: Ophthalmology) 2. Sjögren's syndrome
Lungs
1. Pleural effusions 2. Empyema (uncommon; due to rheumatoid nodules in the lungs) 3. Interstitial lung disease
Heart
1. Pericarditis 2. Myocarditis 3. ↑ Risk of heart failure and myocardial infarction 4. Heart block (uncommon; due to rheumatoid nodules in heart)
Blood vessels
Rheumatoid vasculitis
Hematological
Felty's syndrome

TABLE 9–3 Joint and Tendon Manifestations in Severe or Long-standing Rheumatoid Arthritis

Joint	Clinical Manifestations
Hand and wrists	Mnemonic: "***Fingers BUST***" 1. **F**usiform swelling and tenderness 2. **B**outonnière deformity: hyperflexed PIP and hyperextended DIP 3. **U**lnar deviation: fingers displaced towards the little finger 4. **S**wan-neck deformity: hyperextended PIP and hyperflexed DIP 5. **T**endon rupture: causes inability to bend or straighten fingers
Feet	1. Tenderness of the metatarsal joints 2. Cock-up deformity: toe phalanx articulates at 90° with metatarsal 3. Rupture of Achilles tendon: rare; presents with pop or snap followed by sharp pain in back of ankle and inability to walk
Elbows	Most common site of rheumatoid nodules
Shoulder	Shoulder stiffness due to adhesive capsulitis ("frozen shoulder")
Knees	Popliteal (Baker) cyst (see Chapter 2: Cardiology)
Vertebrae	1. Atlanto-axial subluxation 2. Subaxial subluxation

Abbreviation: DIP, distal interphalangeal; PIP, proximal interphalangeal.

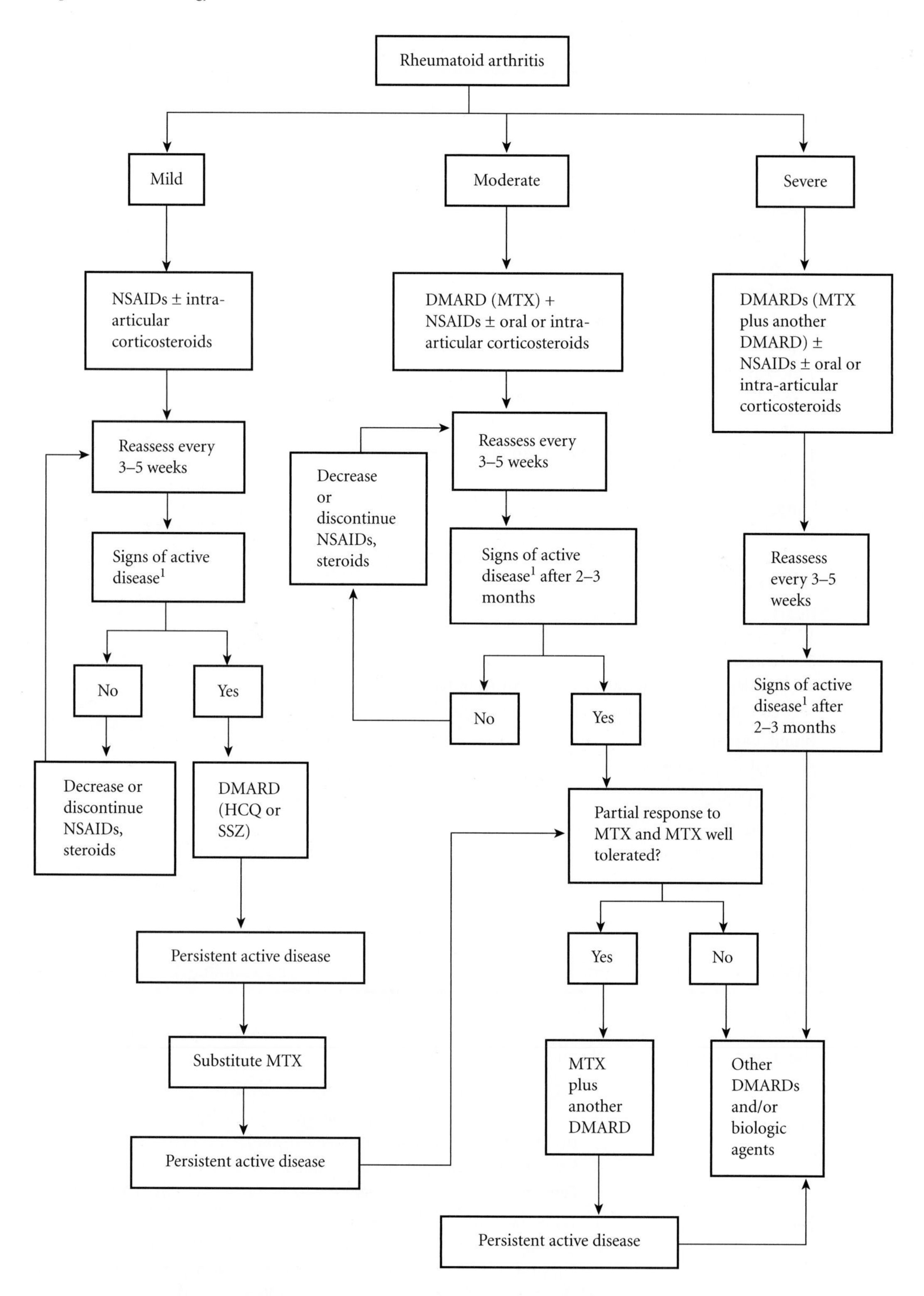

[1]Physical signs of inflammation, ↑ESR or CRP, progressive erosion on x-ray
HCQ = hydroxychloroquine, SSZ = sulfasalazine, MTX = methotrexate

FIGURE 9–3 Therapeutic approach to rheumatoid arthritis.

What are some examples of DMARDs?

1. **Hydroxychloroquine (HCQ) and sulfasalazine (SSZ)**: safest side effect profile
2. **Methotrexate (MTX)**: relatively rapid effect (4 to 6 weeks)
3. **Azothioprine, cyclosporine, gold, and leflunomide**: less popular because of side effects

What are some examples of biological agents?

1. **Anti–tumor necrosis factor-α drugs** (e.g., Etanercept and Infliximab)
2. **Anti-interleukin-1 drugs** (e.g., Anakinra)
3. **Anti-CD 20 drugs** (e.g., Rituximab)

> Combination therapy:
> 1. **MTX + azothioprine**: Avoid because increased risk of serious febrile reaction.
> 2. **MTX + leflunomide**: Monitor LFTs monthly.

Alternative 9.1.1

A 60-year-old woman presents with a 2-month history of symmetric joint pain in her neck, shoulders, and hips. She also reports 30 to 40 minutes of stiffness every morning. Hand joints are not affected. There are no rheumatoid nodules. Plain radiographs are normal. RF, CCP, and LFTs are normal. ESR is 60 mm/hour (↑) and CBC shows anemia of chronic disease.

What is the most likely diagnosis?

This patient with morning stiffness, symmetric joint pain, and elevated ESR but no evidence of arthritis on plain radiographs most likely has polymyalgia rheumatica (PMR). This idiopathic condition almost exclusively affects patients >50 years of age and typically affects the neck, shoulders, and hips.

> The term "polymyalgia" is misleading because PMR typically causes joint pain.

How is PMR treated?

First-line therapy for PMR is low-dose oral corticosteroids, which usually causes prompt symptom resolution. Laboratory abnormalities (increased ESR, increased CRP, and anemia of chronic disease) should also revert to normal with steroids.

The patient's symptoms and laboratory abnormalities improve with oral prednisone. Five years later, she presents with a 2-month history of headache, jaw pain, fatigue, and a 10-lb weight loss. Temperature is 38.1°C.

What complication should you suspect?

PMR greatly increases the risk of developing giant cell arteritis (GCA), also known as temporal arteritis. The major clinical manifestations of this large- and medium-vessel vasculitis are systemic symptoms (fever, fatigue, and weight loss), headache (often in the region of the temporal artery), visual loss, and jaw pain. Patients with GCA also have elevated ESR.

> Approximately 10% to 15% of patients with PMR develop GCA.
> Approximately 50% of patients with GCA have PMR.
> Both PMR and GCA are associated with HLA-DR4 (more common in Europeans).

What is the next step in management?

Confirm the suspected diagnosis with temporal artery biopsy. Like PMR, first-line therapy is systemic corticosteroids.

CASE 9–2 RHEUMATOID ARTHRITIS COMPLICATIONS

A 48-year-old woman with a 10-year history of RA presents with a 2-month history of difficulty climbing stairs and combing her hair. Her current medications include MTX, infliximab, and prednisone. Physical exam is significant for proximal muscle weakness. There is no sensory loss. There is mild ulnar deviation but no tenderness or bogginess. ESR and CRP are normal. Creatinine kinase is normal.

What is the most likely cause of her symptoms?

The most likely cause of her symptoms is steroid-induced myopathy, which presents with proximal muscle weakness (symptoms like difficulty climbing stairs and combing hair) but normal ESR. Treatment is to taper down and then discontinue steroids.

What are other important causes of weakness in patients with RA?

1. **Disuse atrophy**: Patients have signs of atrophy ± active inflammation.
2. **Neuropathy**: Patients also have paresthesia or sensory loss.
3. **Polymyositis (rare)**: Patients exhibit proximal muscle weakness and increased ESR (see Chapter 12: Neurology).

Alternative 9.2.1

A 51-year-old woman with a 25-year history of RA presents with a 2-day history of numbness and tingling in her left foot. She also reports increased fatigue and unintentional weight loss over the last 6 weeks. On physical exam, there is ulnar deviation, swan-neck deformity, and rheumatoid nodules. There are petechiae on her fingertips. There is an ulcer with a violaceous border on her right foot. Vital signs are normal. ESR and CRP are elevated. RF and anti-CCP are positive.

What is the most likely diagnosis?

Suspect rheumatoid vasculitis in any patient with long-standing RA who has new onset of fatigue, fever, or weight loss. Other signs of this small and medium vessel vasculitis are:

1. Nervous system: mononeuritis multiplex
2. Skin: digital petechiae/infarcts, lower extremity ulcers, and palpable purpura
3. Eyes: scleritis and keratitis

Long-standing severe RA: Physical signs of inflammation are often absent because erosive process "burns itself out." ESR and CRP are still elevated; RF and anti-CCP are usually positive.

How can you confirm the diagnosis?

Confirm the diagnosis with biopsy at the border of the affected skin. Rheumatoid vasculitis is histologically identical to polyarteritis nodosa (see Chapter 6: Nephrology). The clinical setting of RA distinguishes rheumatoid vasculitis from polyarteritis nodosa.

Scleritis or keratitis: Biopsy is not necessary.
No skin lesions: Consider nerve and/or muscle biopsy.

Pyoderma gangrenosum: This rare complication in RA presents with fever and foot ulcer with violaceous border. Biopsy distinguishes pyoderma gangrenosum from rheumatoid vasculitis.

How is rheumatoid vasculitis treated?

No additional treatment is necessary for isolated digital petechiae. This patient with systemic signs of rheumatoid vasculitis should receive glucocorticoids and cyclophosphamide (or azothioprine).

Alternative 9.2.2

A 60-year-old man with long-standing severe RA presents with a 7-day history of neck tenderness radiating to the occiput. There are no neurological deficits.

What diagnosis should you suspect?

Suspect cervical spine involvement in any patient with long-standing RA who presents with neck pain. The most common cervical deformity is atlanto-axial (C1–C2) subluxation. Some patients may have sub axial cervical subluxation. The next step is to obtain cervical spine radiographs.

Cervical spine radiographs show a 5-mm interval between the atlas (C1) and odontoid (C2).

What is the next step in management?

C1–C2 interval >3 mm indicates C1–C2 subluxation, which is treated as follows:

1. **Neurological deficits**: Treatment is emergent surgery.
2. **C1–C2 interval >8 mm but no neurological deficits**: Consider elective surgery.
3. **C1–C2 interval <8 mm and no neurological deficits**: Continue medical therapy with DMARDs and analgesics. Monitor with physical exam and x-rays ± magnetic resonance imaging (MRI).

Obtain cervical spine radiographs in all patients with RA before elective intubation.

Alternative 9.2.3

A 57-year-old woman with long-standing severe RA presents for a routine evaluation. She takes Anakinra. Physical exam is significant for rheumatoid nodules, boutonnière deformity, and splenomegaly. RF is positive (1:640 titer). Leukocyte count is 2000 U/L (↓) and absolute neutrophil count is 700 U/L (↓).

What is the most likely diagnosis?

Neutropenia and splenomegaly in a patient with long-standing RA are the characteristic manifestations of Felty's syndrome. Confirm the diagnosis with bone marrow biopsy (usually demonstrates myeloid hyperplasia).

Bone marrow biopsy confirms the diagnosis.

How is Felty's syndrome treated?

The pathogenesis of Felty's syndrome is similar to RA. First-line DMARD for Felty syndrome is MTX; second-line therapy is gold. Also, consider granulocyte colony-stimulating factor (G-CSF) to rapidly raise neutrophil count. Consider splenectomy for patients with multiple infections due to neutropenia that is unresponsive to DMARDs and G-CSF.

Alternative 9.2.4

A 69-year-old man with long-standing RA presents with a 6-month history of dry mouth and eye irritation. He describes the ocular symptoms as a "feeling of grit." The parotid gland is firm and enlarged but not tender.

What diagnosis should you suspect?

Dry mouth and dry eyes ("sicca syndrome") along with salivary gland enlargement are the characteristic manifestations of Sjögren's syndrome (SS). In this disorder, lymphocytes infiltrate multiple organs, particularly the lacrimal and salivary glands. SS can be primary or secondary to autoimmune arthritides such as RA, systemic lupus erythematosus (SLE), or scleroderma.

How can you confirm the diagnosis?

To fulfill the criteria for secondary SS, the patient must have either oral or ocular symptoms plus characteristic findings on one objective test (Table 9-4).

What are other important complications of SS besides dry eyes and dry mouth?

Lymphocytes can also infiltrate the following organ systems:

1. Skin: dry skin, pruritus, and nonpalpable purpura
2. Bones: arthralgia (independent of underlying cause)
3. Upper airway: dry cough

TABLE 9–4 Diagnostic Criteria for Sjögren's Syndrome

Indications

1. Ocular symptoms
2. Oral symptoms
3. Ocular signs: Schirmer's or Rose Bengal test[a]
4. Positive salivary gland biopsy
5. Salivary gland test: salivary flow or salivary scintigraphy or parotid sialography
6. Autoantibody: positive SSA/Ro and/or SSB/La

Primary SS (no underlying cause):

- 4 of 6 criteria are positive (as long as one of them is #4 or #6) ***OR***
- 3 of the last 4 criteria are positive.

Secondary SS (secondary to underlying disorder like RA):

- #1 or #2 is positive ***AND***
- #3, 4, or 5 is positive.

Abbreviation: RA, rheumatoid arthritis; SS, Sjögren's syndrome.

[a] **Schirmer test:** Place a strip of paper under the lower eyelid for 5 minutes, then measure the length of paper that is wet with tears. In SS, decreased length is wet compared to reference. **Rose Bengal test:** Apply Rose Bengal stain to conjunctiva. If conjunctiva is stained, the test is positive for dry eye, suggesting SS.

4. Bone marrow: non-Hodgkin's lymphoma (major cause of mortality)
5. Kidneys: glomerulonephritis

How is SS treated?

For most patients, treatment is symptomatic:

1. Dry mouth: First try sucking on sugarless candy and drinking sips of water. If symptoms persist, try artificial saliva gels. If these are unsuccessful, treat with muscarinic agonists (pilocarpine or cevimeline). Patients should also maintain good oral hygiene because they have an increased risk of dental caries.
2. Dry eyes: First-line treatment is artificial tears; second-line treatment for refractory symptoms is punctal occlusion.

CASE 9–3 OTHER AUTOIMMUNE ARTHRITIDES

A 26-year-old woman reports 6 months of fatigue, asymmetric migratory polyarthralgias, and morning stiffness for >30 minutes that improves with activity. She also mentions getting sunburned very easily. She does not take any medications. On physical exam, her joints are tender, boggy, and swollen. RF is negative.

What diagnosis should you suspect?

Although RA is the most common cause of chronic inflammatory polyarthritis, this diagnosis is less likely because RF is negative and the joints are affected in an asymmetric pattern. The additional complaint of photosensitivity should raise suspicion for systemic lupus erythematosus (Table 9-5). A patient must meet four of the 11 diagnostic criteria to receive a diagnosis of lupus (mnemonic: "***A RASH POINts MD to lupus***"):

1. **A**rthralgias
2. **R**enal disease: proteinuria or cellular casts (see Chapter 6: Nephrology)
3. **A**NA: positive anti-nuclear antibody
4. **S**erositis: pleuritic chest pain or pericardial friction rub
5. **H**ematologic abnormalities: ↓ RBCs, ↓ WBCs, or ↓ platelets
6. **P**hotosensitivity
7. **O**ral ulcers

TABLE 9–5 Important Clinical Manifestations of Systemic Lupus Erythematosus

Constitutional	Fever, fatigue, weight loss
Neuropsychiatric	Seizures, psychosis, depression, ↑ risk of thromboembolic stroke
Hair	Alopecia
Eyes	Dry eyes (SS)
Mouth	Nasopharyngeal ulcers
Skin	Malar rash, discoid rash, photosensitivity
Heart	Pericarditis, Libman-Sach's endocarditis, ↑ risk of CHD
Lungs	Pleuritis, interstitial lung disease
Kidneys	Nephrotic or nephritic syndrome (see Chapter 6: Nephrology)
Blood	↓ WBCs, ↓ RBCs, ↓ platelets, ↓ complement, ↑ ESR, ↑ CRP
Musculoskeletal	Migratory asymmetric polyarthritis, myalgias, Raynaud phenomenon

RBC, red blood cell; WBC, white blood cell.

8. **I**mmunological tests: anti-double stranded (ds) DNA, anti-Smith Abs, Leukocyte esterase (LE), Anti-phospholipid Abs (APLA), or false (+) RPR/VDRL
9. **N**europsychiatric symptoms: seizures or psychosis
10. **M**alar rash
11. **D**iscoid rash

Note: This mnemonic was adapted from Leonard R. A mnemonic for SLE diagnostic criteria. *Ann Rheum Dis* 2001; 60: 638.

> RF is not positive in up to 30% of RA patients, so negative RF does not necessarily rule out RA.

What is the next step in evaluating the possibility of SLE?

The next step is to order ANA. This test is very sensitive test for SLE (most patients have ANA titer ≥1:160).

ANA is 1:32.

What is the next step in management?

ANA is not specific for SLE (often positive in other autoimmune arthritides). Obtain the following tests to establish a baseline as well as to increase diagnostic probability: anti–double-stranded DNA (anti-dsDNA), anti-Smith antibodies, CBC, serum creatinine and urinalysis, LFTs, ESR, and CRP.

> **Anti-dsDNA and anti-Smith antibodies**: specific but not sensitive for SLE.

> **SLE with negative ANA**: <2% to 5% of SLE. Patients often have anti-Ro (anti-SSA) or anti-La (anti-SSB) antibodies.

> **Discoid lupus**: Subtype with discoid erythematous plaques but no other systemic signs of SLE. ANA often negative.

What other diagnostic test would have been indicated if the patient had a 10-year history of hydralazine use?

A number of drugs can cause drug-induced lupus erythematosus (DILE) with long-term use. The most common offenders are hydralazine, procainamide, and quinidine. DILE is associated with all the clinical manifestations of SLE except for neurological and kidney dysfunction. If you suspect DLE, obtain anti-histone antibodies (extremely sensitive and specific). Treatment is to discontinue the offending drug. Prognosis is good.

> ANA often positive but anti-dsDNA and anti-Smith antibodies are negative in DILE.

Anti-dsDNA is positive. Serum chemistry is normal.

What initial treatment is indicated?

Consider an NSAID and an anti-malarial (e.g., HCQ) as initial therapy for this patient. NSAIDs are the first-line drug for arthralgias. HCQ is the first-line drug for skin manifestations and second-line therapy for arthralgias.

When are corticosteroids and other immunosuppressive therapies indicated?

Consider corticosteroids and other immunosuppressive medications (cyclophosphamide, mycophenolate) for SLE that involves organ systems like the central nervous system, lungs, or kidneys.

> **SLE prognosis**: Variable course (exacerbations and remissions); can be life-threatening.

The patient' symptoms improve with NSAIDs and HCQ.

What tests should you routinely order to monitor patients with SLE?

Routinely obtain CBC, serum chemistries, urinalysis, LFTs, ESR, and CRP.

The patient wishes to become pregnant at some point in the near future.

What should you recommend?

SLE is not a contraindication to pregnancy, although patients should try to avoid becoming pregnant for at least 6 months after an exacerbation. First-line therapy for an exacerbation during pregnancy is corticosteroids.

Alternative 9.3.1

A 32-year-old woman presents with a 2-month history of fatigue and asymmetric polyarthralgia. She also mentions that over the last 5 months she has had episodes where her fingers become cold, numb, and white/blue when exposed to cold temperature. The episodes typically improve 15 to 20 minutes after placing her fingers in warm water (Raynaud's phenomenon). On physical exam, the joints are tender and swollen. There are patches of tight, thick skin on the trunk and arms (sclerosis).

What is the most likely diagnosis?

Suspect scleroderma in this patient with sclerotic skin lesions (*sclero* = tight, *derma* = skin). Systemic abnormalities such as polyarthralgia and Raynaud's phenomenon indicate systemic sclerosis (Ssc). The location of sclerotic lesions on the trunk and arms suggests diffuse Ssc (Fig. 9-4).

> Although both localized and systemic forms of scleroderma exist, the term "scleroderma" is typically used interchangeably with Ssc.

What causes scleroderma?

In scleroderma, an autoimmune insult stimulates excessive collagen deposition in the skin and other organs. The exact cause of this autoimmune insult is unknown.

What systemic manifestations commonly occur in systemic scleroderma?

Raynaud's phenomenon is the most common initial manifestation in both limited and diffuse systemic scleroderma. Other systemic manifestations occur years later in patients with limited scleroderma but only months later in patients with diffuse scleroderma.

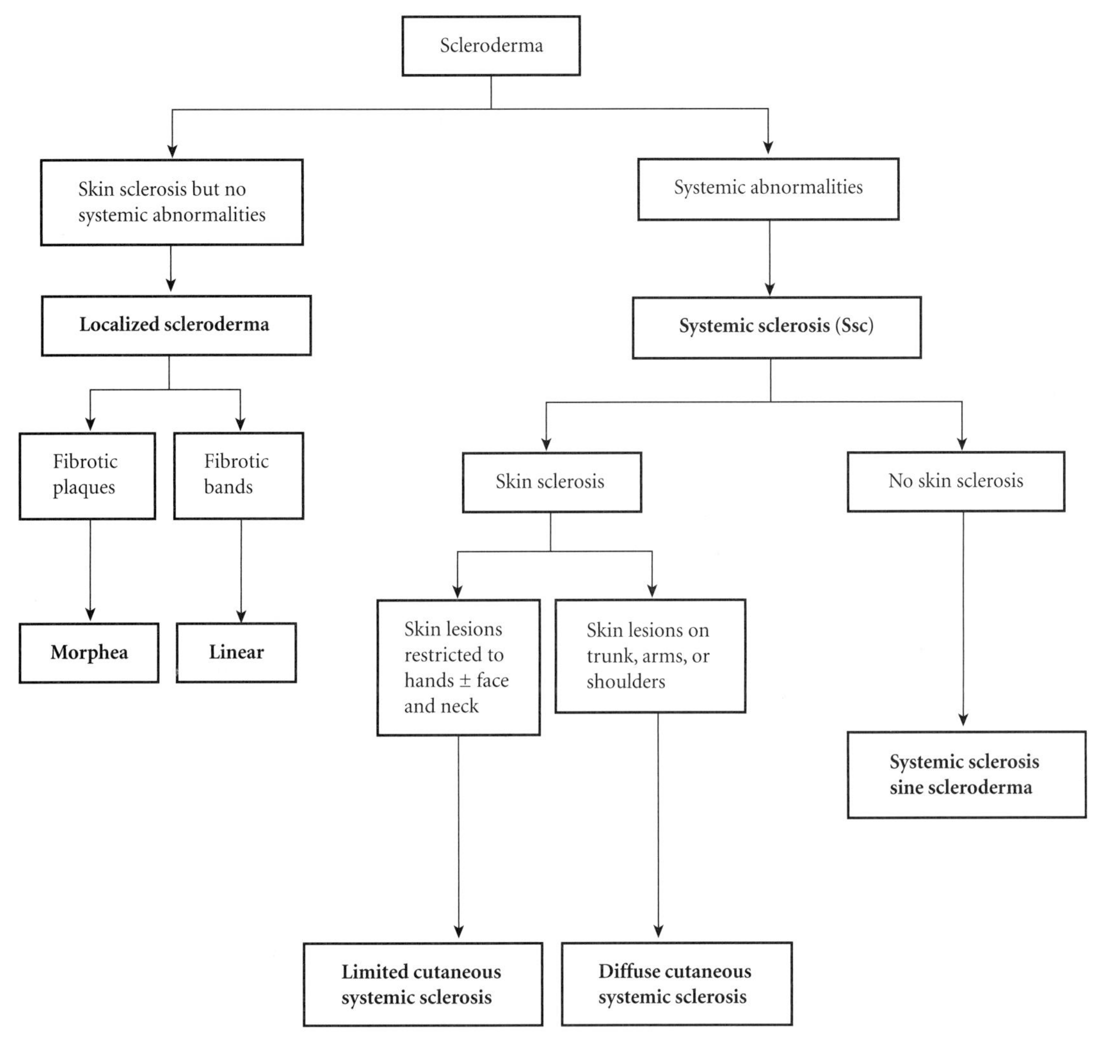

FIGURE 9–4 Classification of scleroderma.

1. **Limited cutaneous Ssc**: Systemic manifestations are usually limited to the CREST syndrome (other abnormalities do occur but less frequently):
   - **C**alcinosis: small, hard Ca^{2+}-containing masses on fingers and pressure points
   - **R**aynaud's phenomenon: often the earliest clinical manifestation
   - **E**sophageal dysmotility: leads to dysphagia and heartburn
   - **S**clerodactyly: thickening of hand and foot digits
   - **T**elangiectasias: can occur on face, trunk, hands, gastrointestinal (GI) tract and oral mucosa
2. **Diffuse scleroderma**: Systemic findings include CREST syndrome as well as:
   - Constitutional: fatigue
   - Heart: myocardial fibrosis, pericarditis, and arrhythmias
   - Lungs: interstitial lung disease and pulmonary hypertension are the leading causes of death.
   - GI: peri-oral fibrosis (leads to pursed-lips), constipation, and diarrhea.
   - Kidneys: scleroderma renal crisis (acute onset of hypertension and ARF)
   - Genitourinary: erectile dysfunction, decreased vaginal lubrication, increased miscarriages
   - Musculoskeletal: arthralgias (often out of proportion to inflammation)
   - Cancer: increased risk of lung (most significant), skin and blood cancers

Rayanaud's disease: Idiopathic hand and/or foot pain, numbness, and discoloration in response to stress or cold.
Raynaud's phenomenon: Symptoms are due to secondary causes. Mnemonic is "***CCold IS BAD***": **C**arpal tunnel syndrome, **C**hemical exposure to vinyl chloride, **I**njury to hands or feet, **S**moking, **B**lood vessel occlusion due to vasculitides such as Buerger's disease, **A**utoimmune arthritides, and **D**rugs (Bleomycin, controversial association with β-blockers and oral contraceptive pills).

Buerger's disease (thromboangiitis obliterans): Suspect this small- to medium-vessel vasculitis if the patient is a 20- to 40-year-old male cigarette smoker with severe Raynaud's and no other underlying cause. Confirm the diagnosis with angiography. Treatment is to stop smoking.

What antibodies are often positive in patients with systemic scleroderma?

1. **ANA**: often positive in both limited and diffuse forms of Ssc.
2. **Anti-centromere Ab**: specific but not sensitive for limited Ssc.
3. **Anti-scleroderma-70 Ab**: specific but not sensitive for diffuse Ssc.

Scleroderma is a clinical diagnosis. Negative antibody tests do not rule out the diagnosis.

Antiscleroderma-70 is positive.

How is scleroderma (Ssc) treated?

There is no effective therapy for scleroderma. Treatment targets correction or minimization of specific abnormalities. For example, treat arthralgias with NSAIDs and heartburn with PPIs or H2-blockers. Although not very effective, corticosteroids ± cyclophosphamide is sometimes considered for skin sclerosis.

The patient is particularly distressed with the Raynaud's symptoms.

How is this condition managed?

First-line treatment is lifestyle measures (often sufficient for primary Raynaud's). If lifestyle measures fail (most cases of secondary Raynaud's), treat with a long-acting calcium-channel blocker such as amlodipine or nifedipine. If a maximal dose of one calcium-channel blocker is ineffective, switch to another calcium-channel blocker. If symptoms persist, add topical nitroglycerin to the regimen (vasodilator). Surgery (sympathectomy) is a last resort for severe refractory symptoms.

Lifestyle measures: Remind the patient to avoid cold temperatures, smoking, caffeine, stress, and sympathomimetic drugs, and to wear warm clothes (thermals, mittens, etc.).

The major complications of secondary Raynaud's syndrome are digital ulcers and gangrene.

Mixed connective tissue disease: Autoimmune polyarthritis that combines features of RA, SLE, scleroderma, and polymyositis. Key laboratory feature is (+)-anti-U1-RNP antibody. ANA is often positive (Table 9-6).

CASE 9–4 CHRONIC SERONEGATIVE INFLAMMATORY ARTHRITIS

A 38-year-old man presents with a 7-month history of asymmetric oligoarthralgia, morning stiffness >30 minutes, and symptom improvement with activity. The symptoms occur in the back,

TABLE 9–6 Summary of Immunological Tests in Autoimmune Arthritides

Autoantibody	Main Indication	Comments
RF	RA	Neither sensitive nor specific
Anti-CCP	RA	Specific but not sensitive
ANA	SLE	97% sensitive for SLE but not specific
Anti-dsDNA	SLE	Specific for SLE but not sensitive
Anti-Smith	SLE	Specific for SLE but not sensitive
Anti-histone	DILE	Approximately 100% sensitive and specific for DLE
Anti-SSA (anti-Ro)	Sjogren's	Neither sensitive nor specific; often positive in ANA-negative SLE
Anti-SSB (anti-La)	Sjogren's	Neither sensitive nor specific; often positive in ANA-negative SLE
Anti-centromere	Limited Ssc	Specific for limited Ssc but not sensitive
Anti-Scl 70	Diffuse Ssc	Specific for diffuse Ssc but not sensitive
Anti-U1 RNP	MCTD	Fairly sensitive and specific for MCTD

Abbreviation: ANA, antineutrophilic antibody; MCTD, mixed connective tissue disease; SLE, systemic lupus erythematosus; Ssc, systemic sclerosis

right hip, left knee, and right heel. Physical exam is significant for diffuse swelling of the digits (dactylitis), nail pitting, and erythematous plaques on his elbows and behind his ears. The plaques are covered by a silvery scale. RF and ANA are negative.

What is the most likely diagnosis?

Consider spondyloarthropathy in patients with asymmetric oligoarthralgia and negative autoantibodies, particularly if the pain affects vertebrae (suggests spondylitis) and heel (suggests Achilles tendon enthesitis). Patients often have "sausage-like" digits (dactylitis). The characteristic skin lesions and nail pitting indicate that the patient has psoriatic arthritis (see Chapter 13: Dermatology).

> Remember important spondyloarthropathies with the mnemonic "***Kelly RIPA***": **R**eactive arthritis, **I**nflammatory bowel disease (IBD)-associated arthritis, **P**soriatic arthritis, and **A**nkylosing spondylitis.

What are spondyloarthropathies?

Spondyloarthropathies (seronegative arthritis) are a group of inflammatory arthritides that share the following common features (***AEIOU***):

1. **A**rthritis pattern: Classic pattern is asymmetric oligoarthritis (although some patients have a symmetric or polyarticular pattern), which often affects vertebrae (spondylitis) and buttock joints (sacroiliitis).
2. **E**nthesitis: In addition to synovial inflammation, spondyloarthropathies can cause joint inflammation at the attachment of bone to muscle or ligaments.
3. **I**nheritance: This is more common in patients with HLA-B27 antigen.
4. Ser**O**negative: Autoantibodies are usually negative (not always the case).
5. **U**veitis: This is a common extra-articular manifestation.

What patterns of arthritis can occur in patients with psoriasis?

There are five possible patterns of joint involvement in psoriatic arthritis:

1. Asymmetric or symmetric polyarthritis: most common pattern.

2. Oligoarthritis with spondyloarthropathy (spondylitis and sacroiliitis): common.
3. Arthritis mutilans: marked destruction of hand digits (uncommon pattern).
4. Isolated distal interphalangeal (DIP) involvement: characteristic but uncommon pattern; x-ray often shows "pencil-in-cup" appearance at the DIP.

How is psoriatic arthritis treated?

First-line treatment for arthralgias is NSAIDs. If symptoms persist, consider oral corticosteroids. Immunosuppressants are sometimes used for refractory cases.

Alternative 9.4.1

A 28-year-old man presents with a 2-year history of progressively worsening back pain, fatigue, and morning stiffness. He also reports pain in his left hip and right heel. The symptoms improve with activity. Past medical history is negative. Physical exam is significant for reduced spinal range of motion. ESR is elevated. RF and ANA are negative.

What is the most likely diagnosis?

This patient has many features of seronegative spondyloarthropathy. Ankylosing spondylitis is the most likely diagnosis in this patient with no history of IBD, genital symptoms, or psoriasis. This condition occurs most frequently in men between the ages of 20 and 30 years. The next step is to obtain plain radiographs of the spine. The characteristic findings on plain radiographs are fusion of lumbar vertebrae ("bamboo spine") and bilateral sacroiliitis (Fig. 9-5).

> Ulcerative colitis is a risk factor for ankylosing spondyloarthropathy. IBD-associated arthritis may be part of the spectrum of ankylosing spondyloarthropathy.

> **Schober test**: Have the patient stand erect. Mark L5 and the spot 10-cm above L5 with a pen. Ask the patient to bend. The patient has decreased range of motion if the distance between the two marks is <14 cm.

What would be the next step in management if plain films are nondiagnostic?

Obtain MRI and HLA-B27 if plain films are nondiagnostic but clinical suspicion is high.

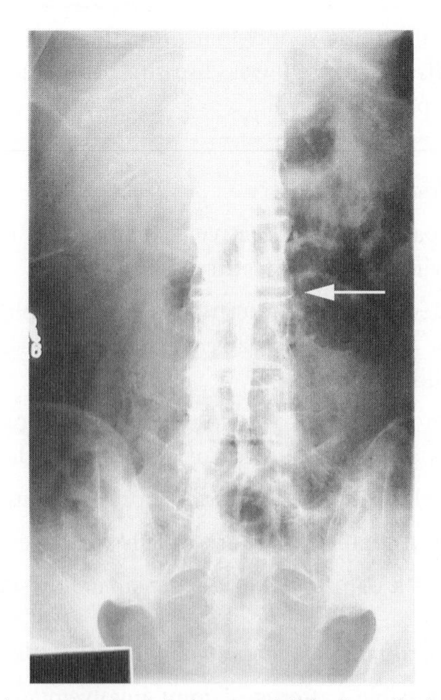

FIGURE 9–5 X-ray vertebrae: Bamboo spine of ankylosing spondylitis. From Ayala A, Spellberg B. *Boards and Wards*, 3rd ed. Lippincott Williams & Wilkins, 2007.

How is ankylosing spondylitis treated?

First-line therapy is NSAIDs, physical therapy, and smoking cessation (ankylosing spondyloarthropathy can cause decreased chest expansion). If the patient continues to have intolerable symptoms, consider SSZ for peripheral joint-predominant symptoms and anti–tumor necrosis factor drugs for axial-predominant symptoms. Consider surgical referral in patients with severe joint deformities.

CASE 9–5 CHRONIC NONINFLAMMATORY POLYARTHRITIS

A 66-year-old man presents with an 8-month history of polyarthralgias. He reports bilateral knee, hip, and finger pain. Physical activity makes the pain worse. He also has morning stiffness that resolves in 10 to 15 minutes. On physical exam, there is joint tenderness and effusions. Vitals signs are normal.

What is the most likely diagnosis?

Osteoarthritis (OA) is the most likely diagnosis in this patient with chronic, noninflammatory joint pain. The disorder can be mono-, oligo-, or polyarticular (usually symmetric). OA most frequently affects fingers and weight-bearing joints (knees, hips, and spine). Characteristic symptoms are morning stiffness lasting <30 minutes and increased joint pain with activity. Early signs are joint tenderness and effusions. Patients with advanced disease may have crepitus (grating sensation in the joints), osteophytes (hard, bony swelling in the joints), and limitation of joint movement.

Heberden nodes: hard, bony swelling around DIP.
Bouchard nodes: hard, bony swelling around PIP.

What causes OA?

Both genetic and environmental factors are responsible for articular cartilage degeneration. Risk factors include joint injury, joint overuse, and obesity. Unlike connective tissue disorders, onset typically occurs after age 60 years.

What are the characteristic x-ray findings of OA?

The diagnosis of OA is largely based on history and physical exam. Imaging and laboratory tests are not indicated in this patient with characteristic findings. On the other hand, plain radiographs can provide objective evidence of OA in atypical cases (x-ray findings are specific but not sensitive). The four key features of OA are osteophytes, joint space narrowing, subchondral sclerosis, and subchondral cysts (Fig. 9-6).

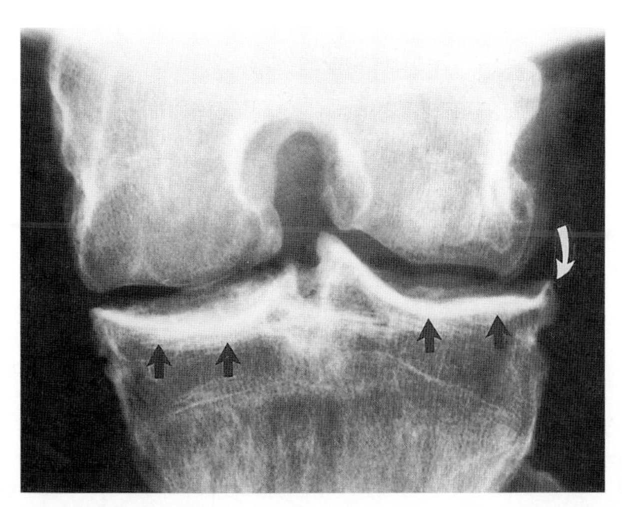

FIGURE 9–6 Knee x-ray showing all four features of osteoarthritis. From Daffner RH. *Clinical Radiology: The Essentials*, 3rd ed. Lippincott Williams & Wilkins, 2007.

What initial management is recommended?

Initial therapy of OA involves lifestyle measures:

1. Exercise: Exercise strengthens the muscles around joints. Recommend exercises that don't stress weight-bearing joints (e.g., aquatic aerobics).
2. Cane or crutch: Use if the patient has symptoms in weight-bearing joints. Hold the cane contralateral to the most symptomatic joint. The cane should contact ground at the same time as contralateral foot.
3. Weight loss.

If symptoms persist, first-line medication is acetaminophen (Fig. 9-7). NSAIDs are as effective as acetaminophen, but they are not first-line because of potential GI toxicity.

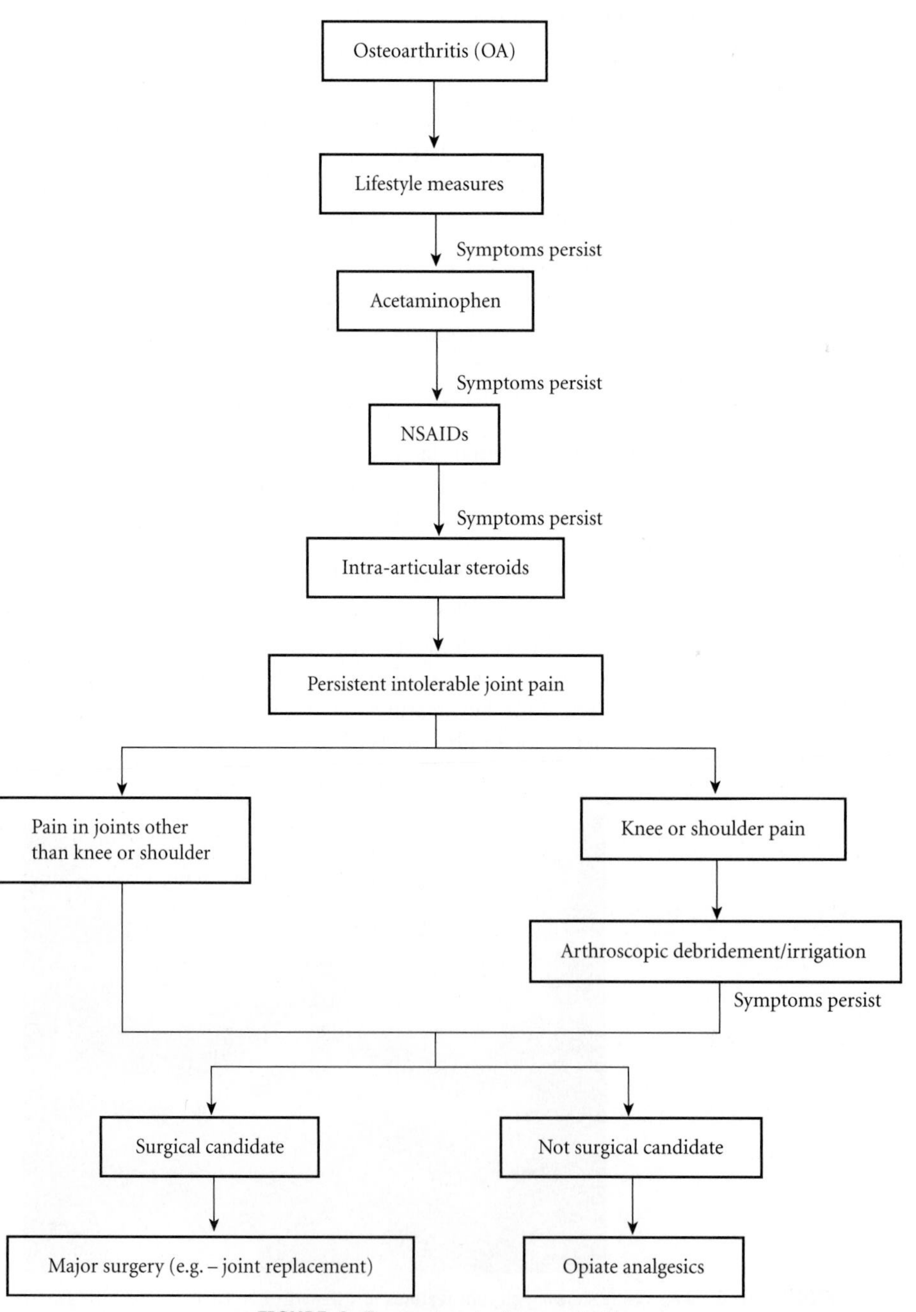

FIGURE 9–7 Treatment of osteoarthritis.

Glucosamine and chondroitin: Although safe and widely used to treat OA symptoms, their efficacy is actually unclear.

When should you suspect a secondary cause is responsible for OA?

Secondary causes of OA include joint instability (e.g., RA and gout), deposition disorders (e.g., hemochromatosis and calcium pyrophosphate dihydrate (CPPD)), and bleeding disorders (e.g., hemophilia). In addition to findings of the underlying disorder, suspect secondary OA if symptoms occur in atypical joints like the shoulder, elbow, or wrist.

Bleeding disorders can cause secondary OA due to intra-articular bleeding.

CASE 9–6 ACUTE ONSET OF MONOARTICULAR PAIN, SWELLING, WARMTH, AND ERYTHEMA

A 36-year-old IV drug user presents with a 2-day history of fever and knee pain. HIV test 3 weeks ago was negative. On physical exam, the right knee is swollen, tender, warm and erythematous. Temperature is 38.9°C.

What is the differential diagnosis of fever and joint pain?

In immunocompetent patients, joint pain with swelling, warmth, erythema, and tenderness ± fever is most commonly caused by nongonococcal bacterial infection (infectious arthritis) or crystal-induced arthritis (gout or pseudogout). Occasionally, atypical cases of gonococcal arthritis, Lyme disease, reactive arthritis, or RA can cause these symptoms.

Pseudogout: The knee is the most commonly affected joint.
Gout: The great toe is the most commonly affected joint followed by the knee; 20% of cases have an oligo- or polyarticular initial presentation.
Infectious arthritis: The knee is the most commonly affected joint; 20% of cases have an oligo- or polyarticular presentation. *Staphylococcus aureus* is the most common organism.

What is the next step in management?

The next step is joint aspiration (arthrocentesis) and synovial fluid analysis (Table 9-7).

TABLE 9–7 Synovial Fluid Analysis

	Normal	Noninflammatory Arthritis	Inflammatory Arthritis	Infectious Arthritis
Appearance[a]	Transparent	Transparent	Translucent or opaque	Opaque
WBC/mm^3	<200	200–2000	2000–10,000	>10,000
PMNs	≤25%	≤25%	50–75%	≥75%
Culture	(-)	(-)	(-)	Often (+)
Glucose	Approximately = serum	Approximately = serum	Less than serum but >25 mg/dL	<25 mg/dL
Polarized light microscopy	(-)	(-)	Gout: Needle-shaped, negatively birefringent crystals Pseudogout: Rhomboid-shaped, positively birefringent crystals	(-)

Abbreviation: PMN, polymorphonuclear leukocytes.
[a] Red color indicates traumatic tap or hemarthrosis.

Synovial fluid is opaque. Synovial fluid analysis shows WBC count of 15,000/mm^3 with 80% neutrophils, and glucose of 20 mg/dL. There are no crystals on joint microscopy. Gram stain and culture are pending.

What is the diagnosis?

The patient has infectious arthritis. Most cases are caused by hematogenous spread. In this case, IV drug use is the likely source of bacterial entry into the bloodstream.

Gram stain shows Gram-positive cocci in clusters.

How should you treat this patient?

Treat septic arthritis with antibiotics and joint drainage:

1. Antibiotics: Initial antibiotic choice in this patient with probable *S. aureus* infection is vancomycin to cover methicillin-resistant *S. aureus* (MRSA). Switch to a β-lactam if the susceptibility pattern shows that the bacteria are sensitive to methicillin.
2. Joint drainage: Initial approach is daily closed-needle aspiration. If this method is unsuccessful, perform arthroscopic drainage. Analyze the synovial fluid obtained daily to monitor effectiveness of the treatment.

Treatment duration: Typical duration is 14 days of IV antibiotics followed by 14 days of oral antibiotics. Tailor treatment duration on the basis of the patient's response.

What treatment would you initiate if gram stain had showed Gram-negative bacilli?

Treat septic arthritis due to Gram-negative bacilli with joint drainage (as described earlier) and a third-generation cephalosporin. IV drug users should also receive gentamycin because infection with *Pseudomonas aeruginosa* is a possibility.

How would management have differed if the Gram stain were negative?

Negative Gram stain does not rule out infectious arthritis. Perform joint drainage and initiate empiric therapy. In this case, treat with vancomycin (to cover MRSA) and gentamycin (to cover *P. aeruginosa*). Tailor antibiotics when culture and sensitivity results return. If culture is negative, continue empiric antibiotics because negative culture does not rule out the diagnosis either.

Alternative 9.6.1

A 48-year-old man presents with a 6-hour history of excruciating pain in his left big toe (first metatarsophalangeal joint). He does not have any other medical conditions. He does not take any medications. He drinks 5 to 6 cans of beer every day. On physical exam, the joint is warm, tender, swollen, and erythematous. Vital signs are temperature 38.1°C, pulse 110 bpm, respirations 20/min, and blood pressure 160/90. BMI is 32.

What is the most likely diagnosis?

Acute monoarticular pain in the first metatarsophalangeal joint (podagra) strongly suggests an acute attack of crystal-induced arthritis due to gout. Patients often have a low-grade fever during acute attacks. This patient also has the classic risk factors for gout: overweight, middle-aged man who frequently consumes alcohol.

What causes gout?

The underlying cause of gout is hyperuricemia, which leads to uric acid or monosodium urate crystal deposition in joints. Patients often have asymptomatic hyperuricemia for years before presenting with an acute attack. Common precipitants of an acute attack are alcohol, trauma or surgery, and drugs (e.g., thiazides, salicylates, and cyclosporine).

Asymptomatic hyperuricemia: Most patients do not develop gout. Treatment to lower uric acid is only indicated when:

1. Serum uric acid >13 mg/dL in men or >10 mg/dL in women
2. Uric acid excretion >1100 mg

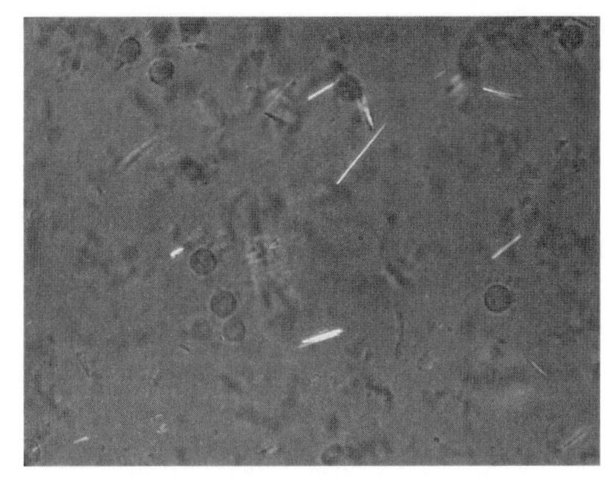

FIGURE 9–8 Gout: needle-shaped negatively birefringent crystals. From Ayala A, Spellberg B. *Boards and Wards*, 3rd ed. Lippincott Williams & Wilkins, 2007.

What is the next diagnostic step?

The next step is to obtain serum uric acid. In the acute setting, increased uric acid in a patient with podagra is reasonably accurate to diagnose a patient with gout. If symptoms affect a joint other than the great toe or if serum uric acid is normal, perform joint aspiration (arthrocentesis) and synovial fluid analysis to confirm the diagnosis (Fig. 9-8). Also, obtain CBC, LFTs, and serum chemistries in all patients to establish a baseline.

> One third of patients have normal serum uric acid even during an acute attack, so normal uric acid does not rule out gout.

Serum uric acid is elevated. CBC and serum chemistries are normal.

How are acute attacks of gout treated?

Without treatment, acute attacks usually resolve in a few days. The goal of therapy is symptom control:

- **NSAIDs**: First-line treatment; indomethacin (potent NSAID) is most commonly used.
- **Colchicine**: Second-line treatment; use if NSAIDs are ineffective or contraindicated. Many patients find the GI side effects intolerable.
- **Corticosteroids**: Third-line treatment; use if NSAIDs and colchicine are contraindicated, ineffective, or not tolerated. Use intra-articular steroids if symptoms are monoarticular. Consider oral or intramuscular steroids if multiple joints are affected.

> **Colchicine contraindications:** ↓ WBCs, ↓ platelets, severe liver or kidney failure.

The patient's symptoms resolve over the next few days.

What measures are recommended to prevent recurrent attacks?

The asymptomatic period after an acute attack has resolved is called intercritical gout. After the first attack, prevent future occurrences by controlling or eliminating risk factors (obesity, alcohol, hyperlipidemia, hypertension, and diuretics). Other important steps during the intercritical period are:

1. Perform synovial fluid analysis to confirm the diagnosis.
2. Obtain 24-hour urinary uric acid: Levels <800 mg/dL indicate that the defect is decreased uric acid excretion; levels >800 mg/dL indicate the main defect is uric acid overproduction.

> **Losartan**: Increases uric acid excretion. This drug is a commonly prescribed alternative to diuretics in hypertensive patients with hyperuricemia.

Over the next 12 months, the patient has two more attacks despite controlling risk factors. 24-hour urinary uric acid is consistently <800 mg/dL.

What is the next step to prevent recurrences?

Patients with three or more attacks per year should receive uric acid–lowering therapy to prevent recurrences. First-line therapy in underexcretors like this patient is probenecid (continued indefinitely). This drug reduces uric acid reabsorption, which leads to increased uric acid excretion. Probenecid is contraindicated in patients with renal failure (consider benzbromarone in these patients).

What uric acid–lowering therapy would you have recommended if 24-hour urine uric acid was >800 mg/day?

First-line therapy to prevent recurrences in overproducers is allopurinol (continue indefinitely). This drug reduces uric acid production by inhibiting the enzyme xanthine oxidase.

> Initially, allopurinol, probenecid, and benzbromarone can paradoxically increase risk of an acute attack. Therefore, continue colchicine or an NSAID after the acute attack and discontinue only after uric acid remains at target levels (5 to 6 mg/dL) for 6 months using uric acid–lowering therapy.

The patient is poorly compliant with probenecid. He resumes heavy alcohol intake. He typically presents for medical care only during acute attacks. During physical exam 15 years later, he has pain and stiffness in his knees and shoulders. There are painless, cream-colored nodules on his knees and behind his ears (Fig. 9-9).

What is this stage of disease called?

Poorly controlled gout can progress to chronic tophaceous gout 10 to 20 years after the initial attack. The name derives from the painless, cream-colored nodules (tophi) that develop on bones and behind the ears. These nodules contain chalky-white urate deposits and may have calcifications visible on x-ray. Polyarthritis symptoms result from bone erosion by tophi (x-ray appearance is sclerotic margins and overlying edges).

Alternative 9.6.2

A 45-year-old man presents with a 6-hour history of excruciating pain in the left knee. He does not have any other medical conditions. He does not drink alcohol or take any medications. On physical exam, the joint is swollen, tender, warm, and erythematous. Temperature is 38.3°C. Translucent fluid is aspirated from the joint. Synovial fluid analysis demonstrates 4000 WBCs/mm^3, 60% neutrophils, and glucose 60 mg/dL. Figure 9-10 is the specimen's appearance on polarized light microscopy. Gram stain is negative. Culture is pending.

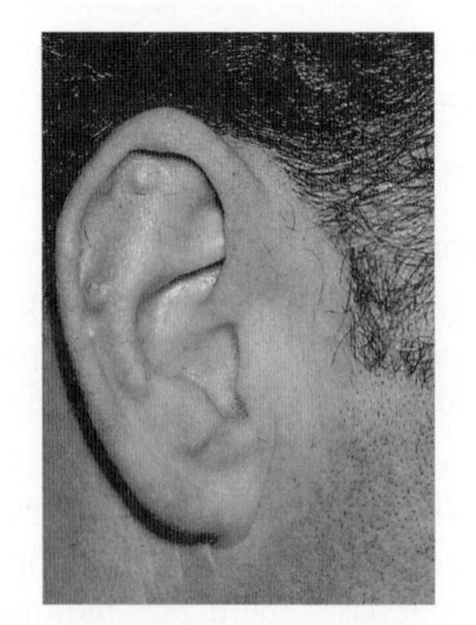

FIGURE 9–9 Gout: Tophi. From Ayala A, Spellberg B. *Boards and Wards*, 3rd ed. Lippincott Williams & Wilkins, 2007.

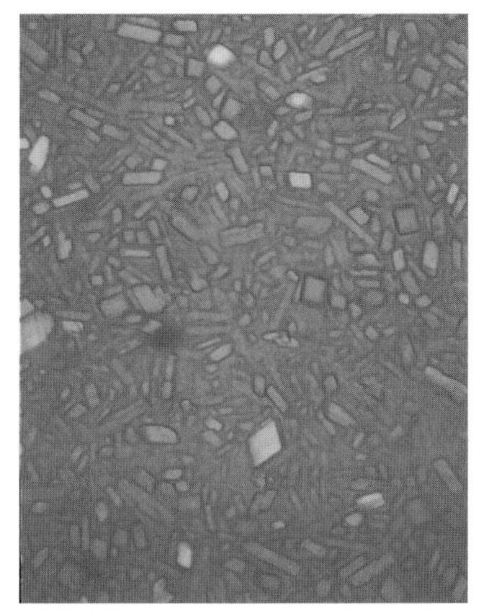

FIGURE 9–10 Pseudogout: Positive birefringent rhomboid crystals. From Ayala A, Spellberg B. *Boards and Wards,* 3rd ed. Lippincott Williams & Wilkins, 2007.

What is the diagnosis?

This patient with fever and monoarticular joint pain with positively birefringent rhomboid-shaped crystals on polarized microscopy has pseudogout due to CPPD crystal deposition.

Various manifestations of CPPD deposition: pseudo-OA (45%), asymptomatic (25%), pseudogout (25%), and pseudo-RA (<5%).

Polarized light microscopy: Unlike most materials, crystals are bright in one plane ("birefringent") but dark when the plane is turned 90°. When a red compensator plate is placed parallel to the long axis of the crystals, they appear blue if they are "positively birefringent" and yellow if they are "negatively birefringent."

What tests are routinely recommended in patients with CPPD deposition?

Obtain plain radiographs to evaluate the degree of chondrocalcinosis. Also, obtain the following labs to evaluate for predisposing factors: TSH (to detect hypothyroidism), iron studies (to detect hemochromatosis), and chemistries (to detect decreased PO_4, decreased Mg, and decreased PTH).

How is acute pseudogout due to CPPD crystal deposition treated?

1. Monoarticular: joint aspiration + intra-articular steroids.
2. Polyarticular: NSAIDs or colchicine.

Pseudogout prophylaxis: Consider colchicine if patient has three or more attacks per year.

Milwaukee shoulder-knee syndrome: This rare syndrome affects older women. Basic calcium phosphate crystals cause chronic shoulder and knee arthritis. Crystals are amorphous and nonbirefringent on polarized microscopy. X-rays show destructive arthritis and calcifications in knees and shoulders. Treatment is challenging.

CASE 9–7 OLIGO- OR POLYARTHRITIS AND GENITAL SYMPTOMS

A 27-year-old man presents with a 5-day history of dysuria and urethral discharge. Urethral swab demonstrates *Chlamydia trachomatis,* so he receives azithromycin and ceftriaxone. Three weeks later, he presents with joint pain. He reports pain in his back, left knee, right ankle, and left heel. The joints are swollen, tender, and erythematous. Arthrocentesis with synovial fluid analysis shows 8000 WBCs/mm^3 with 60% neutrophils and glucose of 50 mg/dL. There are shallow, painless ulcers on his penis. ESR and CRP are mildly elevated.

What is the diagnosis?

Suspect reactive arthritis in any patient with asymmetric inflammatory oligoarthritis that begins <6 weeks after a genitourinary or GI infection. Back and heel pain increase the likelihood that the joint pain is due to a spondyloarthropathy. Other common features of reactive arthritis are:

1. Mucosal lesions: Characteristic lesions include circinate balanitis (painless, shallow genital ulcers), keratoderma blennorrhagica (palm and sole vesicles that progress to macules, papules, and nodules), and painless oral ulcers.
2. Eyes: Most common disorder is transient conjunctivitis, followed by uveitis.

> **Reiter syndrome**: This older term is used to describe a subset of patients with the classic triad of reactive arthritis: Can't see (uveitis), can't pee (urethritis), can't climb a tree (arthritis).

What causes reactive arthritis?

Reactive arthritis occurs as an immune response to bacterial infection in genetically susceptible individuals (associated with HLA-B27). *C. trachomatis* is the most common bacteria. Others include Campylobacter, Salmonella, and Shigella.

> Not all patients with spondyloarthropathy are HLA-B27–positive. Diagnosis is based on history and clinical findings.

How is reactive arthritis treated?

Treat the infection with antibiotics and the acute arthralgias with NSAIDs. Symptoms resolve completely in about one third of patients, while others develop chronic arthritis with a waxing and waning course. First-line medications for persistent symptoms refractory to NSAIDs are SSZ and MTX.

Alternative 9.7.1

A 38-year-old Turkish woman presents with a 7-month history of fatigue and polyarthralgias. She also reports painful mouth sores over the last 3 months. Three days ago she developed burning vulvar pain. There is no history of antecedent infection. On physical exam, there are four large aphthous ulcers in the mouth. There are two painful vulvar ulcers. There is joint tenderness but no swelling in the elbows, knees, and shoulders.

What diagnosis should you suspect?

Suspect Behçet's disease in this young woman with polyarthralgia, painful genital ulcers, and painful aphthous ulcers. This vasculitis is most common in persons of Turkish or Iranian descent. HLA-B51 is a risk factor, although most people with this gene do not develop Behçet's.

> Oral and genital ulcers are painless in reactive arthritis but painful in Behçet's disease.

What other organs does Behçet's commonly affect?

Although Behçet's disease can affect virtually any organ system, frequently affected sites besides the ones mentioned earlier are:

1. Central nervous system: aseptic meningitis due to white matter demyelination
2. Eyes: uveitis

3. Lungs: hemoptysis due to ruptured pulmonary aneurysm
4. GI: symptoms and biopsy findings similar to IBD
5. Skin: folliculitis and erythema nodosum

What tests can aid in the diagnosis of Behçet's disease?

Although Behçet's disease is largely a clinical diagnosis, the following tests can aid in the diagnosis if positive:

1. **Biopsy**: Consider biopsy of genital or oral ulcer to confirm vasculitis.
2. **Pathergy test**: Prick forearm with a small needle. The test is positive if pustule formation occurs 1 to 2 days after the prick. The test is not sensitive, but it is relatively specific.

Biopsy of an aphthous ulcer demonstrates vasculitis. Pathergy test is positive.

How is Behçet's disease treated?

Topical steroids are sufficient for symptoms limited to the mouth or genitals. This patient with polyarthritis should receive systemic corticosteroids. Consider systemic corticosteroids plus immunosuppressive medications like cyclophosphamide for patients with eye or central nervous system involvement.

CASE 9–8 ACUTE ONSET OF MIGRATORY POLYARTHRALGIA

A 24-year-old woman presents with an 8-day history of joint pain. The symptoms started with pain and tenderness at the back of her hand with finger movement at the start of her menstrual period. She then had bilateral knee pain followed by left elbow pain and right wrist pain. She has had three sexual partners in the last 2 months. On physical exam, there are seven painless pustules on her trunk and arms. The joints are not swollen, warm, or erythematous. Vital signs are normal.

What is the most likely diagnosis?

This young, sexually active patient presents with the classic triad of disseminated gonococcal infection (DGI): tenosynovitis (typically the earliest symptom), dermatitis (most common lesion is painless pustules), and polyarthralgias (often migratory). Symptoms often begin at the start of menses. Interestingly, only a few patients with DGI actually have urethral symptoms of gonorrhea infection.

> The other common presentation of DGI is joint swelling, warmth, and tenderness with positive synovial fluid findings.

> **Tenosynovitis**: tenderness, swelling, and pain with movement of affected tendon sheath.

What laboratory testing is indicated in patients with known or suspected DGI?

1. Blood cultures: All patients should have at least two sets of blood cultures. Positive blood culture is diagnostic, but negative culture does not rule out DGI. Blood culture can also distinguish DGI from other infectious causes of arthritis such as *S. aureus* and *Neisseria meningitides.*
2. Urethral, rectal, skin, and synovial culture (grow on Thayer-Martin media).
3. Serology for syphilis (RPR/VDRL) and HIV antibodies.

> Synovial fluid analysis is usually negative in patients with tenosynovitis, dermatitis, and polyarthritis. However, blood culture is more likely to be positive than in patients with purulent arthritis.

The first set of blood cultures show Gram-negative diplococci. Remaining laboratory studies are pending.

What is the next step in management?

Gram-negative diplococci on blood culture are diagnostic of DGI. First-line therapy is a 7-day course of IV ceftriaxone or another third-generation cephalosporin PLUS oral doxycycline to cover possible concurrent Chlamydia infection. Also, treat sexual partners with a third-generation cephalosporin + doxycycline

> Treatment for patients with purulent arthritis should also include daily joint drainage.

The patient's symptoms resolve after 2 days of IV ceftriaxone.

What is the next step in management?

Consider switching to oral antibiotics if the patient's symptoms resolve within 1 to 2 days of IV therapy. First-line oral antibiotic is cefixime. Continue doxycycline.

Alternative 9.8.1

A 32-year-old woman presents to her physician in New Jersey with a 3-day history of arthralgias. She reports pain in the knees followed by the left elbow and the right wrist. About a week before her symptoms began, she experienced a flu-like illness and an erythematous rash on her right armpit. Vital signs are normal.

What diagnosis should you suspect?

The clinical picture should raise suspicion for Lyme disease, caused by transmission of *Borrelia burgdorferi* spirochetes by the deer tick (Table 9-8). Lyme disease is most prevalent in northeastern United States. Symptoms occur in three stages:

1. **Stage 1 (early localized disease)**: Nonspecific flu-like symptoms (fatigue, myalgia, and lymphadenopathy) typically occur 7 to 10 days after the tick bite. Approximately 90% of patients also report an erythematous rash (erythema migrans) at the site of the bite. The rash forms a central clearing ("bull's eye" appearance) in approximately 10% of patients.
2. **Stage 2 (early disseminated disease)**: Weeks to months after EM onset, patients develop one or more signs of disseminated disease:
   - Migratory mono-, oligo-, or polyarthritis occurs in approximately 60% of patients.
   - Neurological: Aseptic meningitis or cranial nerve palsy occurs in 10% of patients.
   - Cardiac: Arteriovenous block occurs in 5% of patients.
3. **Stage 3 (late chronic disease)**: Occurring months to years after the tick bite in untreated patients, clinical manifestations include chronic arthritis, neurological symptoms (neuroborreliosis), or dermatological features (rare).

TABLE 9–8 Important Tick-Borne Illnesses in the United States

Illness	Bacteria	Tick	First-line Therapy
Lyme disease	*Borrelia burgdorferi*	Ixodes (deer tick)	Doxycycline
Rocky Mountain spotted fever	*Rickettsia rickettsii*	*Dermacentor variabilis* (American dog tick)	Doxycycline
Babesiosis	*Babesia microti*	Ixodes	Atovaquone + azithromycin
Human granulocytic anaplasmosis	*Anaplasma phagocytophila*	Ixodes	Doxycycline
Human monocytic ehrlichiosis	*Ehrlichia chafeensis*	Lone star tick	Doxycycline

Patients can present with stage 2 or stage 3 disease with no signs of earlier stages.

What is the next step in management?

This patient from northeastern United States with erythema multiforme, objective signs, and constitutional symptoms has a high pretest probability for Lyme disease. The next step is to initiate antibiotics without further laboratory testing (Fig. 9-11). The choice of antibiotics is as follows:

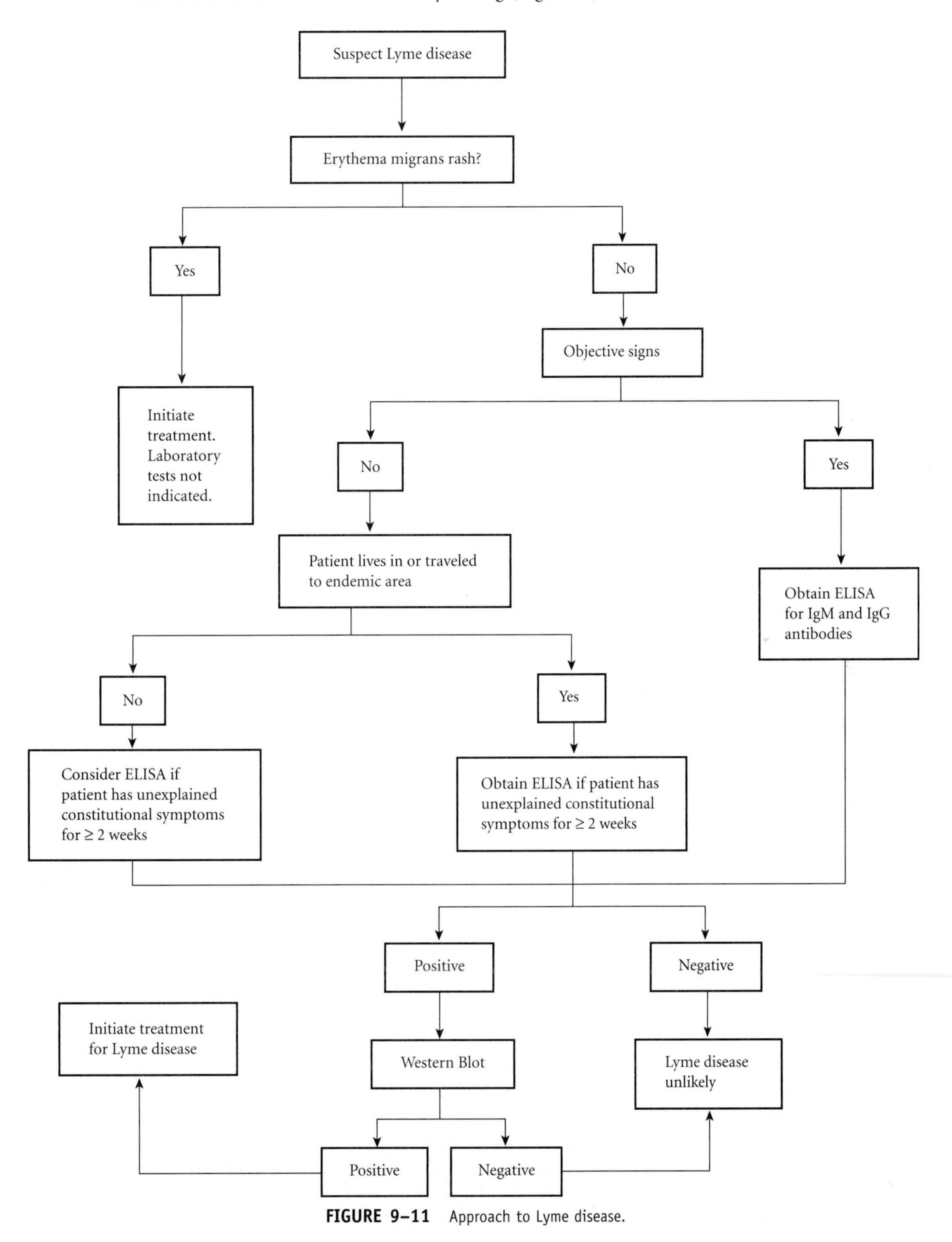

FIGURE 9–11 Approach to Lyme disease.

1. **Stage 1 disease**: Treat with a 10- to 14-day course of oral doxycycline, amoxicillin, or cefuroxime.
2. **Stage 2 disease**: Treat with a 14- to 28-day course of IV ceftriaxone or cefotaxime if patient has third-degree heart block or meningitis. Otherwise treat with a 10- to 14-day course of oral antibiotics similar to stage 1 disease (this patient).
3. **Stage 3 disease**: Treat with a 28-day course of IV ceftriaxone if the patient has encephalopathy (neuroborreliosis). Otherwise, treat with a 28-day course of oral doxycycline or amoxicillin.

Objective signs: arthralgia, heart block, aseptic meningitis, cranial nerve palsy
Constitutional symptoms: fever, fatigue, headache, myalgia, lymphadenopathy, etc.

Avoid doxycycline in pregnant patients (risk of fetal bone and teeth malformations).

How would management differ if the patient did not have erythema multiforme?

The next step would have been serology for IgM and IgG antibodies using ELISA. Positive ELISA requires confirmation with Western blot ("two-step approach").

False-positive ELISA: causes include syphilis, RA, infectious mononucleosis, and Lyme disease vaccine (withdrawn from market).
False-negative ELISA: usually occurs if patient is tested in the first 1 to 2 weeks of infection.

How would management differ if the patient presented after a tick bite while hiking in the Adirondacks (in New York) but was completely asymptomatic and had no signs of Lyme disease?

Do not test or treat asymptomatic individuals even if they have a history of recent tick bite. Advise the patient to return if she develops erythema multiforme, objective signs, or constitutional symptoms for $\geq$2 weeks.

What other illnesses are associated with Ixodes tick bites?

1. **Babesiosis**: Babesia infection can be asymptomatic, mild, or cause malaria-like symptoms (see Chapter 10: Hematology and Oncology). Diagnose with blood smear ("Maltese cross" inclusions in RBCs), serology, or polymerase chain reaction. Treat malaria-like symptoms with atovaquone plus azithromycin.
2. **Human granulocytic anaplasmosis (HGA)**: *Anaplasma phagocytophila* infection causes nonspecific constitutional symptoms. Preferred diagnostic test is immunofluorescence antibodies (IFA). Treat with doxycycline.

Alternative 9.8.2

A 28-year-old man presents to his physician in North Carolina in the month of May with migratory polyarthralgias. The arthralgias began after a 7-day period of fever, fatigue, headache, and nausea. On physical exam, there are petechiae on his palms and soles. CBC shows mild thrombocytopenia and serum chemistries show mild hyponatremia.

What is the most likely diagnosis?

Constitutional symptoms followed by arthralgias and a maculopapular rash during the spring or summer season in southern United States is the classic presentation of Rocky Mountain Spotted Fever (RMSF). Symptoms result from transmission of the Gram-negative bacterium *Rickettsia rickettsii* by *Dermacentor variabilis* (American dog tick). The tick is endemic throughout the United States, but most infections occur in the South. Patients with advanced disease may have hyponatremia, thrombocytopenia, and abnormal serum creatinine, or LFTs.

Classic triad of RMSF: Fever, rash, and history of tick bite. The characteristic petechial rash is usually not visible for approximately 1 week after symptom onset; 10% to 15% of patients do not have the characteristic rash. Many patients do not report any tick bite.

What is the next step in management?

Obtain IFA and then initiate empiric doxycycline immediately, before laboratory results return.

Give doxycycline to any patient in an endemic area who presents with fever and other constitutional symptoms for >3 days in the spring or summer months.

IFA IgM: Usually elevated after 5 to 7 days of symptom onset.
IFA IgG: Usually elevated after 7 to 10 days of symptom onset.

How would the choice of antibiotics differ if the patient were pregnant?

Avoid tetracyclines such as doxycycline during pregnancy; use chloramphenicol instead.

What other validated laboratory tests are available to aid in the diagnosis besides IFA?

1. **Polymerase chain reaction**: most rapid and specific test; not widely available.
2. **Skin biopsy immunostaining**: approximately 70% sensitive; often used in autopsies.

Human monocytic Ehrlichiosis (HME): Caused by *Ehrlichia chafeensis* infection transmitted by the lone star tick. Also known as "spotless" RMSF. The term "spotless" is misleading because 30% of HME presents with a rash. Preferred diagnostic test is IFA. Treat with doxycycline.

CASE 9–9 APPROACH TO LOW BACK PAIN

A 36-year-old man presents with a 7-day history of lower back pain. The symptoms began after a day of lifting heavy boxes. The pain radiates to the buttocks but not to the thighs or legs. He does not have any other medical conditions. He does not smoke or use illegal drugs. On physical exam, there is mild tenderness in his lower back. Lumbosacral neurological exam and vital signs are normal.

What is the most likely diagnosis?

This young patient does not have any alarm findings for fracture, infection, malignancy, or progressive neurological compromise (Table 9-9). Nonspecific soft-tissue strain (lumbago) is the most common cause in such patients. Back pain in lumbago may radiate to the buttocks but not to the thighs or legs.

What is the next step in management?

The next step is conservative therapy (see Fig. 9-12):

1. **Analgesics**: Take on a regular schedule rather than on demand. Options include NSAIDs, acetaminophen, or muscle relaxants such as cyclobenzaprine.
2. **Activity**: Continue regular activity as tolerated. Consider low-stress aerobic exercise (e.g., walking or swimming). Avoid lifting heavy objects and avoid prolonged bed rest.

Back pain is the fifth most common cause of physician visits. Most cases are benign and self-limiting (90% resolve in 4 weeks with conservative therapy).

Spinal manipulation: Chiropractic manipulation is as effective as conservative therapy.

TABLE 9–9 Alarm Findings in Low Back Pain

Alarm findings for infection

1. Systemic signs like fever, chills, or weight loss
2. Symptoms of urinary tract infection
3. IV drug use
4. Immunosuppression

Alarm findings for cancer (primary or metastasis)

1. Systemic signs like fever, chills, or weight loss
2. History of cancer
3. Age >50 years or <20 years
4. ↑ Pain at night or in the supine position

Alarm findings for cauda equina syndrome

1. Progressive or bilateral neurologic/motor deficits
2. Saddle anesthesia (numbness in groin and upper inner thighs)
3. Decreased anal sphincter tone
4. Bowel or bladder retention and/or incontinence

Alarm findings for vertebral fracture

1. Major trauma (e.g., motor vehicle accident, fall from height)
2. Minor trauma in a patient with risk factors for osteoporosis
3. Chronic corticosteroid use

Adapted from Bigos SJ. *Acute Low Back Problems in Adults*. Rockville, Md.: U.S. Department of Health and Human Services, Public Health Service, Agency for Health Care Policy and Research, 1994; AHCPR publication no. 95-0642.

The patient returns 4 weeks later. His symptoms have not resolved despite conservative therapy. Physical exam and vital signs are normal.

What is the next step in management?

If symptoms persist despite 4 weeks of conservative therapy, obtain ESR and x-rays of the spine (see Fig. 9-12).

ESR and plain radiographs are normal. The patient continues to have intermittent pain over the next 3 months.

How are such patients treated?

Consider the following measures to treat chronic back pain (duration >12 weeks):

1. **Analgesics**: first-line analgesics are NSAIDs or acetaminophen. Avoid opiates if possible because of the risk of side effects and dependence.
2. **Activity**: Adopt back protection strategies and begin an aerobic exercise program. Consider physical therapy if symptoms persist despite these measures.
3. **Monitor**: Monitor the patient for worsening pain, neurological compromise, or the development of other alarm findings.

Back protection strategies: Examples of the numerous strategies include (a) strengthen abdominal muscles, (b) avoid prolonged sitting or standing, (c) avoid bending when lifting a heavy object, (d) use a medium to firm mattress and sleep on one side.

CASE 9–10 BACK PAIN THAT RADIATES TO THE LOWER EXTREMITIES

A 48-year-old man presents with a 3-week history of back pain radiating to the back of his left thigh and calf. There is no history of trauma. He does not take any medications. On physical exam, straight leg raise (SLR) is positive. He has difficulty walking on his heels. Knee and ankle reflexes are normal. Vital signs are normal.

What is the differential diagnosis?

Back pain that radiates to the back of the thigh and/or calf is called sciatica (lumbar radiculopathy). Pain may increase with sneezing, cough, or valsalva. Symptoms usually occur in older patients with disk degeneration or trauma due to compression of lumbar or sacral nerve roots. The major causes of sciatica are:

1. Herniated disc
2. Spinal stenosis and spondylolisthesis
3. OA (degenerative disc disease in which osteophytes impinge on nerve roots).

> **SLR**: The patient lies supine. Raise symptomatic leg with knee kept straight. Pain in ipsilateral leg at 30° to 60° is sensitive but not specific for sciatica.
> **Contralateral SLR**: Perform SLR on asymptomatic leg. Pain in ipsilateral symptomatic leg is specific but not sensitive for lumbar disc herniation.

What is the next step in management?

Initial management of sciatica in the absence of alarm findings is conservative therapy. Consider MRI if symptoms do not resolve despite 4 weeks of conservative therapy (Fig. 9-12). MRI is also indicated if the patient develops bilateral or progressive neurological findings.

The patient's symptoms do not improve with conservative therapy. MRI is obtained (Fig. 9-13).

What is the diagnosis?

The patient has lumbar disc herniation at L4–L5 (Table 9-10). Herniation of the nucleus pulposus through a weakened annulus fibrosis typically causes pain that is worse with back flexion (bending or sitting) and improves with extension (standing or walking). L4–L5 is the most frequent site of herniation. MRI is the gold standard for diagnosis. Consider surgery (diskectomy) if the patient has severe disabling pain or develops signs of cauda equina syndrome. Otherwise, treat chronic back pain as described earlier.

> Disc herniation is a common incidental finding. Do not treat asymptomatic patients.

What condition would you diagnose if Figure 9-14 were the patient's MRI?

MRI shows the characteristic "trefoil" or "cloverleaf" pattern of spinal stenosis due to hypertrophy of the lamina and pedicles. In addition to back pain, patients often experience lower extremity burning or cramping with ambulation that resolves with rest (pseudoclaudication). Unlike lumbar disc herniation, symptoms increase with back extension and improve with flexion (mnemonic: "***STANding worsens STANosis***"). Consider surgery (laminectomy) if the patient has severe disabling pain or develops signs of cauda equina syndrome. Otherwise, treat chronic back pain as described earlier.

> **Ischemic claudication**: Symptoms don't change with flexion or extension.
> **Pseudoclaudication**: No decreased pedal pulse, impotence, cyanosis, pallor, or nail bed changes.

> **Type 3 spondylolisthesis**: Degenerative conditions like OA predispose to spinal instability, which can cause a vertebra to slip anteriorly and narrow the spinal canal. Symptoms and management are similar to spinal stenosis.

What condition should you suspect if a patient with sciatica has no abnormal findings on MRI, the pain is worse in a sitting position, and the patient reports increased sciatic notch and buttock pain on hip flexion, adduction, and internal rotation?

Consider the diagnosis of piriformis syndrome after other causes of sciatica have been ruled out. This condition occurs when the piriformis compresses the sciatic nerve as it traverses the muscle. Like disc herniation, symptoms are typically worse in the seated position. Electrophysiological testing or the FADIR maneuver may elicit positive findings (increased sciatic

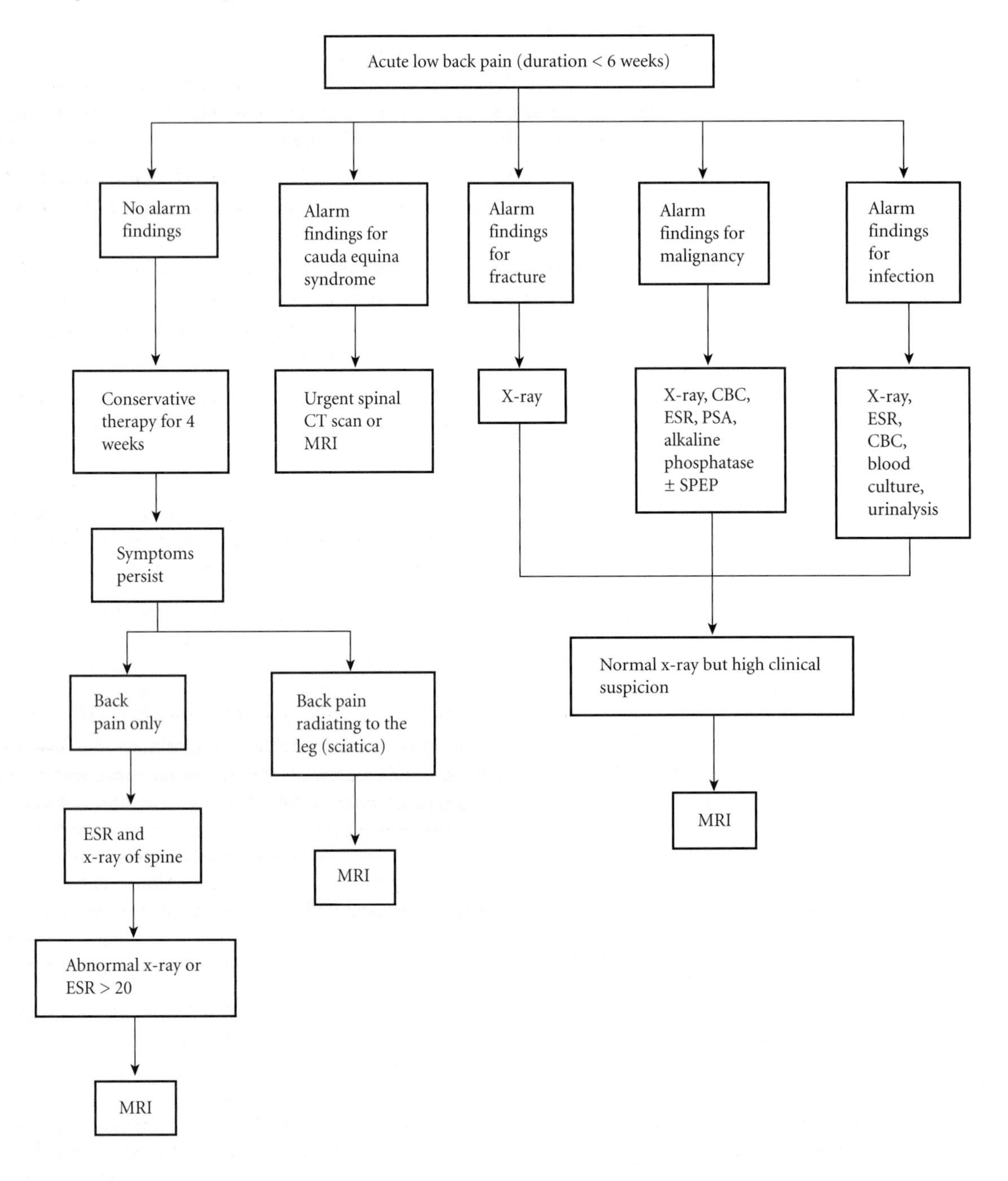

CT scan is a less accurate alternative to MRI in patients who are claustrophobic or have implanted metallic objects like pacemakers.

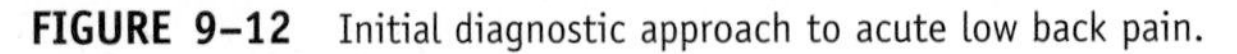

FIGURE 9–12 Initial diagnostic approach to acute low back pain.

notch and buttock pain on **F**lexion, **AD**duction, and **I**nternal **R**otation of the hip against resistance). Treatment is usually conservative (physical therapy). Consider corticosteroid injections into the piriformis muscle for refractory debilitating symptoms. Surgical resection of the piriformis muscle or tendon is a last resort measure.

Alternative 9.10.1

A 50-year-old man who was diagnosed with prostate cancer 6 months ago presents with a 2-week history of increasingly severe low back pain. Over the last 2 days the pain has begun to radiate to the back of the thighs and calves. Plantar flexion and ankle jerk reflex are diminished bilaterally. Physical exam is also significant for decreased anal sphincter tone.

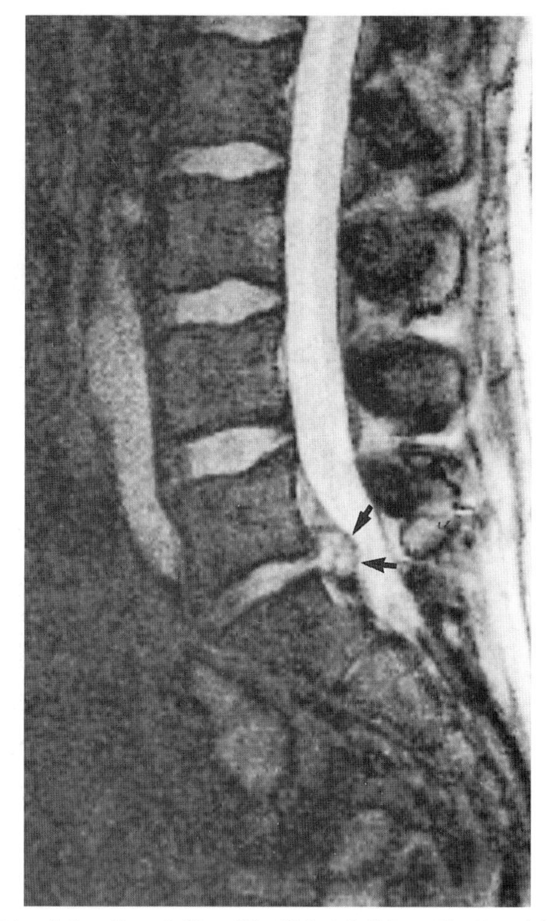

FIGURE 9–13 MRI: L4–L5 herniation. From Daffner RH. *Clinical Radiology: The Essentials*, 3rd ed. Lippincott Williams & Wilkins, 2007.

TABLE 9–10 Neurological Exam in Lower Back Pain

Nerve Root	Disc	Motor (weakness)	Sensory (numbness)	Reflexes
L3–L4	L4	Difficulty flexing knee (quadriceps flexion)	Numbness at quadriceps	↓ Knee jerk
L4–L5	L5	Difficulty walking on heels (ankle dorsiflexion) or positive Trendelenburg test[a]	Numbness over great toe	↓ Posterior tibial reflex
L5–S1	S1	Difficulty walking on toes (ankle plantarflexion)	Numbness at lateral malleolus	↓ Ankle jerk

[a] Tests hip abductors. Patient stands on one leg. Test is positive if opposite pelvis drops.

What is the differential diagnosis?

Bilateral neurological deficits and decreased anal sphincter tone are alarm findings for cauda equina syndrome. This syndrome results from compression of the thecal sac below the level of the spinal cord (L1–L2). Compression above L1 is called epidural spinal cord compression (ESCC). Because clinical manifestations and management of both conditions are similar, the terms are often used interchangeably. The major causes of cauda equina syndrome and ESCC are:

1. Malignancy (primary or metastasis): most likely cause in this patient
2. Musculoskeletal disorders

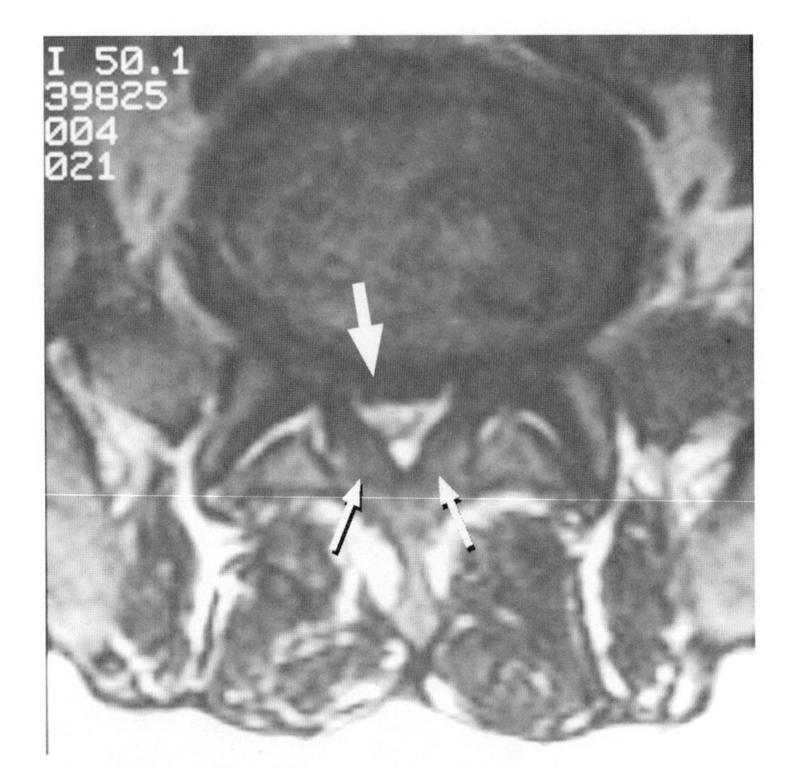

FIGURE 9–14 MRI: spinal stenosis. From Koval KJ, Zuckerman JD. *Atlas of Orthopedic Surgery: A Multimedia Reference*. Lippincott Williams & Wilkins, 2004.

3. Infection (spinal epidural abscess)
4. Traumatic injury to the spinal cord

> Prostate, breast, and lung cancer are the most common tumors to metastasize to vertebrae.

What is the next step in management?

Obtain emergent MRI in any patient with alarm findings for cauda equina syndrome or ESCC. This patient with a history of cancer should also receive IV corticosteroids prior to imaging (reduces swelling around the spinal cord).

MRI detects a metastatic lesion. What is the next step in management?

Refer the patient for emergent surgery to prevent further neurological deficits. If the patient is not a surgical candidate, treat with radiation therapy instead.

CASE 9–11 FEVER AND BACK PAIN

A 57-year-old woman presents with a 2-week history of fever and low back pain. She had a urinary tract infection 3 weeks ago. On physical exam, there is localized low back tenderness and reduced back mobility. Temperature is 38.2°C.

What is the next step in management?

Fever and history of urinary tract infection are alarm findings for infection. Localized back tenderness is the most frequently elicited sign in vertebral osteomyelitis. Many patients also have reduced back mobility. Hematogenous spread is the most common mode of infection. The next step is to obtain x-rays of the spine, CBC, ESR, and urinalysis (see Fig. 9-12).

> **Vertebral osteomyelitis epidemiology**: Most patients are >50 years old. Incidence is much greater in men for unknown reasons.

Laboratory studies demonstrate leukocytosis with a left shift and elevated ESR. Radiographs show destruction of L2 and L3 vertebral bodies and decreased disk space between L2 and L3. Blood cultures are negative.

What is the next step in management?

The radiographs findings are characteristic for vertebral osteomyelitis. The next step is CT-guided needle biopsy of the affected bone to determine the causative microbe.

> **Positive x-ray and blood cultures**: Consider foregoing needle biopsy and proceeding directly to treatment.

How is vertebral osteomyelitis treated?

When blood cultures or needle aspiration identify the causative microbe, treat with a 6- to 12-week course of IV antibiotics. Patients with a good response to IV antibiotics can switch to oral antibiotics after 2 weeks. Consider surgery if the patient develops signs of cauda equine syndrome or infection continues to progress despite appropriate antibiotics.

What additional test would have been indicated if the patient were an IV drug user or had a murmur on physical exam?

Perform echocardiography to rule out infective endocarditis as the source of osteomyelitis in the following patients:

1. History of heart disease or new murmur on physical exam
2. Recent IV drug use
3. *S. aureus* detected on blood cultures or CT-guided biopsy.

What would have been the next step if x-ray were normal?

Plain radiographs are often negative in the first 2 weeks. MRI would have been the next step in this patient with a high pretest probability of osteomyelitis. If MRI is positive, perform CT-guided needle biopsy of the affected bone.

What would have been the next step if CT-guided needle biopsy was negative?

Repeat CT-guided needle biopsy. If repeat biopsy is also negative, consider empiric IV antibiotics.

What would have been the initial diagnostic test if the patient presented with fever, back pain, altered mental status, and decreased knee jerk reflex?

Fever, back pain, and neurological deficits are the classic triad of spinal epidural abscess. MRI is the preferred initial diagnostic test. Confirm an MRI-detected abscess with needle aspiration. First-line therapy is surgical drainage and IV antibiotics.

CASE 9–12 HIP PAIN

A 61-year-old man presents with a 10-day history of anterior hip pain (groin pain). Past medical history is significant for chronic obstructive pulmonary disease requiring systemic steroids. He quit smoking 10 months ago but continues to drink a six-pack of beer every day. He has difficulty bearing weight and walking. Vital signs are normal.

What is the next step in management?

Groin pain suggests that the pain originates in the hip joint. Important causes of acute anterior hip pain are hip osteonecrosis (avascular necrosis), hip osteomyelitis, and hip fracture. The initial diagnostic study in any patient with acute onset of groin pain is AP (antero-posterior) and lateral (frog-leg) x-rays. If plain films are nondiagnostic, obtain MRI.

Plain films demonstrate sclerosis, cysts, and subchondral radiolucency ("crescent sign").

What is the diagnosis?

The findings are pathognomic for osteonecrosis. In this condition, bone marrow vasculature is compromised, which leads to bone marrow infarction. This patient has the two most common risk factors for osteonecrosis: chronic steroid and alcohol use. Other important risk factors include:

1. Inherited and acquired thrombophilias
2. Sickle cell disease
3. HIV and transplantation
4. Bisphosphonate or radiation therapies in patients with cancer

How is symptomatic osteonecrosis managed?

Refer any patient with symptomatic osteonecrosis for surgical management. Surgical options include decompression, osteotomy, or total hip replacement.

> **Asymptomatic osteonecrosis**: Management is controversial (conservative therapy with bed rest and partial weight bearing versus surgery).

Alternative 12.1

A 20-year-old varsity football player presents with a 3-week history of lateral hip pain. Direct pressure aggravates the pain. There are no neurological deficits. Plain films of the hips are normal.

What is the diagnosis?

The patient has trochanteric bursitis (Table 9-11). This overuse injury is common among athletes. Initial therapy is rest, ice, and NSAIDs.

TABLE 9–11 Common Causes of Hip Pain in Adults

Disorder	Clinical Presentation	Initial Diagnostic Steps
Trochanteric bursitis	Lateral hip pain that is worse with movement or direct palpation	Plain radiograph to rule out other conditions.
Meralgia paresthetica	Lateral hip pain, paresthesia and/or decreased sensation unaffected by movement or direct palpation	Plain radiograph to rule out other conditions.
Hip pointer	Iliac crest pain and tenderness	No diagnostic testing indicated.
Osteonecrosis	Acute onset of groin pain	Plain radiographs; if inconclusive, obtain MRI.
Osteomyelitis	Acute onset of groin pain	Plain radiographs; if inconclusive, obtain MRI.
Hip fracture	Acute onset of groin pain and inability to internally or externally rotate hip	Plain radiographs; if inconclusive, obtain MRI.
Inflammatory arthritides	Gradual onset of groin pain; pain in multiple joints; signs of inflammatory arthritis	Refer to Case 9-1 to Case 9-4.
Osteoarthritis	Gradual onset of groin pain; pain in multiple joints	Refer to Case 9-5.
Sciatica	Hip pain along with back or buttock pain; positive straight leg test; lower extremity neurologic deficits	Refer to Case 9-8 and Case 9-9.
Aortoiliac occlusion (Leriche's syndrome)	Hip and buttock cramps that worsen with ambulation; diminished popliteal and pedal pulses	See Chapter 2: Cardiology.

Abbreviation: MRI, magnetic resonance imaging.

What would the diagnosis have been if the patient had lateral hip pain unaffected by direct pressure or movement and reduced sensation over the lateral hips?

The diagnosis would have been meralgia paresthetica, caused by compression of the lateral femoral cutaneous nerve. Initial management is rest, ice, and NSAIDs.

How could you distinguish trochanteric bursitis from meralgia paresthetica if the diagnosis was uncertain?

Symptom relief with injection of local anesthetic into the trochanteric bursa indicates trochanteric bursitis, whereas symptom relief with injection of local anesthetic into the lateral femoral cutaneous nerve indicates meralgia paresthetica.

CASE 9–13 KNEE PAIN

A 23-year-old man complains of knee pain after a fall while playing basketball. He is walking with a limp. There is no warmth or erythema. The patient can tolerate passive knee flexion to 90°. There is no tenderness on palpation of the patella or fibular head. Tests of ligament and meniscus instability are negative.

What is the next step in management?

Recommend conservative therapy (rest, ice, and NSAIDs). Plain radiographs of the knee to rule out fracture are only indicated if patients have one or more Ottawa criteria:

1. Age >55 years
2. Tenderness at head of the fibula
3. Tenderness at patella
4. Inability to flex knees to 90°
5. Inability to bear weight

How would you diagnose and manage the patient if he had no Ottawa criteria but had a positive Lachman sign?

A positive Lachman sign indicates anterior cruciate ligament injury (Table 9-12). Plain radiographs are not indicated for suspected ligament injuries and meniscal tear unless patients have one or more Ottawa criteria. Treatment is conservative versus surgery depending on the desired functional status of the patient. Obtain MRI if surgery is being considered.

What diagnoses should you suspect if the patient presented with a 2-week history of patellar pain unrelated to trauma?

The differential diagnosis includes patellofemoral pain syndrome, prepatellar bursitis, and patellar tendonitis (Table 9-13). Radiographs are not indicated in the initial evaluation of nontraumatic knee pain unless you suspect arthritis or osteochondritis dissecans (a type of osteonecrosis). Initial therapy for most nontraumatic knee pain is conservative. Consider plain radiographs if nontraumatic knee pain persists despite 4 weeks of conservative therapy.

> **Osteonecrosis dissecans**: Radiographs may demonstrate sclerosis, cysts, subchondral radiolucency, or a loose body in the knee. Follow up such findings with MRI. Treatment is usually conservative, although arthroscopic surgery is sometimes necessary.

> **Patellofemoral pain syndrome**: This term is used to classify a number of syndromes. Important examples are chondromalacia patellae (degeneration of posterior patellar cartilage) and patellar subluxation (dislocation).

TABLE 9–12 Differential Diagnosis of Acute Knee Pain after Trauma

Disorder	Typical History	Characteristic Physical Findings
Anterior cruciate ligament injury	"Pop" in knee after an athlete suddenly changes position. Knee pain and swelling over the next 1 to 2 hours.	Anterior drawer sign: With patient seated, use one hand to stabilize the foot and the other to pull at tibia anteriorly. Test is positive if tibia moves excessively. Lachman sign: Similar to anterior drawer except knee is initially at 20° flexion instead of 90°. This is the most sensitive test.
Posterior cruciate ligament injury	"Pop" in knee immediately after force applied to bent knee. Knee pain and swelling over next 1 to 2 hours.	Posterior drawer sign: Similar to anterior drawer test except tibia is pushed posteriorly.
Medial collateral ligament injury	Blow to lateral knee. Knee pain and swelling over next 1 to 2 hours.	Valgus stress: Place knee in 30° flexion. Stabilize lateral thigh with one hand and abduct ankle with the other. Test is positive if knee moves excessively.
Lateral collateral ligament injury	Blow to medial knee. Knee pain and swelling over next 1 to 2 hours.	Varus stress: Place knee in 30° flexion. Stabilize medial thigh with one hand and adduct ankle with the other. This test is positive if knee moves excessively.
Meniscal tear	Similar to anterior cruciate ligament injury. Can also occur in older patients without any history of trauma.	McMurray sign: Rotate tibia with leg in flexion. "Click" on inward rotation indicates lateral meniscal tear; "click" on outward rotation indicates medial tear.
Fracture	History of trauma	≥1 Ottawa criteria

TABLE 9–13 Differential Diagnosis of Nontraumatic Knee Pain

Disorder	Age/Risk Factors	Typical History	Characteristic Physical Findings
Patellofemoral pain syndrome ("runner's knee")	Young active patients	Patellar pain and swelling ↑ with activity and prolonged sitting	Pain on palpation of the patella ± crepitus
Prepatellar bursitis ("housemaid's knee")	Repetitive kneeling in any age group; sometimes caused by trauma	Patellar pain and swelling with rest and activity; difficulty kneeling	Pain on palpation of the patella ± swelling, warmth, and erythema
Patellar tendonitis ("jumper's knee")	Young patients who play jumping sports like basketball.	Patellar pain and swelling ↓ with activity	Pain on palpation of inferior pole of the patella
Anserine (pes) bursitis	Underlying joint disease	Pain and swelling in medial knee	Pain on palpation of medial knee
Iliotibial band syndrome	Running or cycling	Lateral knee pain; pain ↑ with activity	Pain on palpation of lateral femoral condyle
Osteochondritis dissecans	Idiopathic condition more common in young women	Poorly localized knee pain in younger patients	Wilson's sign: Pain on extending and internally rotating flexed knee; loose body in knee
Baker cyst	Underlying joint disease	Posterior knee pain	Posterior knee swelling
Arthritides	Refer to Case 9-1 through Case 9-7.	Refer to Case 9-1 through Case 9-7.	Refer to Case 9-1 through Case 9-7

CASE 9–14 SHOULDER PAIN

A 30-year-old minor league baseball pitcher presents with a 3-week history of shoulder pain. The pain increases when the patient reaches for overhead objects. There is no history of trauma. There is no swelling, warmth, or erythema. Physical exam is significant for subacromial tenderness. Apley and Neer maneuvers increase shoulder pain. Range of motion is normal. Drop test is negative. Forearm flexion against resistance (Speed's test) does not increase pain.

What is the most likely diagnosis?

Rotator cuff tendonitis is the most likely diagnosis in this patient with increased pain on Apley and Neer tests (Table 9-14). Baseball pitching and overhead racquet sports are risk factors because they involve repetitive overhead motion. Patients often complain of increased pain on reaching for overhead objects and lying on the affected shoulder.

> **Rotator cuff muscles** ("*SITS*"): **S**upraspinatus (abduction past 20°), **I**nfraspinatus (external rotation), **T**eres minor, and **S**ubscapularis (internal rotation).

> **Neer and Hawkin's maneuvers**: These actions test for subacromial impingement. Because rotator cuff tendons pass under the acromion, tendon inflammation causes impingement.

What is the next step in management?

The next step in this patient with characteristic findings is conservative therapy (NSAIDs, decreased overhead arm activity, ice, and a weighted pendulum stretching exercise). After 2 to 3 weeks, begin internal and external shoulder rotation exercises to increased muscle strength.

TABLE 9–14 Physical Maneuvers to Test for Specific Shoulder Disorders

Disorder	Physical Findings
Rotator cuff tendon tear	• Apley scratch test: Reach behind head and scratch superior and inferior parts of opposite scapula. Positive test = ↓ range of motion. • Drop test: Fully abduct arm to 180° then slowly lower arm. Positive test = arm drops at 90° (specific but not sensitive).
Rotator cuff tendonitis (subacromial bursitis)	• Subacromial tenderness • Apley scratch test causes pain but normal range of motion • Neer's test: Fully pronate forearm then raise fully extended arm forward. Positive test = pain at 90° to 120°. • Hawkin's test: Flex elbow and raise arm forward to 90°, then pronate forearm. Positive test = pain on pronation.
Cervical nerve root impingement	• Spurling test: Extend neck and rotate it towards the side of pain while examiner applies axial pressure to the head. Positive test = ↑ shoulder pain.
Bicep tendonitis	• Yergason's test: Flex elbow 90°, then pronate forearm. Positive test = pain on pronation. • Speed's test: Flex elbow 30°, then flex forearm against resistance. Positive test = pain on resisted flexion.
Anterior glenohumeral instability	• Apprehension test: Examiner abducts shoulder 90° then externally rotates shoulder applying anterior pressure to head of humerus. Positive test = apprehension that shoulder is about to give way. • Relocation test: Performed immediately after positive apprehension test. Similar to apprehension test except examiner applies posterior pressure to head of humerus. Positive test = relief of apprehension.
Inferior glenohumeral instability	• Sulcus sign: Examiner pulls down on elbow or wrist. Positive test = depression lateral or inferior to acromion.

What would have been the next step in management if the patient had decreased range of motion due to excessive shoulder pain?

Inject lidocaine into the deltoid and subacromial bursa and then perform physical exam maneuvers. If the pain does not improve or if the patient continues to have decreased range of motion, order MRI of the shoulder to rule out rotator cuff tear.

What would have been the next step in management if the patient began experiencing shoulder pain after falling on his shoulder?

Plain radiographs are generally indicated in patients with traumatic shoulder pain.

What would be the next step in management if the patient were a 60-year-old diabetic with 2 hours of shoulder pain, normal shoulder exam, and no history of trauma?

Diabetes is a risk factor for "silent" myocardial infarct. Initiate evaluation for acute coronary syndromes in this patient with acute onset of shoulder pain in the absence of trauma or physical findings of a musculoskeletal problem (see Chapter 2: Cardiology).

The patient with rotator cuff tendonitis returns 2 months later with continued shoulder pain despite conservative therapy.

What is the next step in management?

If shoulder pain persists despite 4 to 6 weeks of conservative therapy, inject lidocaine into the deltoid and subacromial bursa and repeat physical exam maneuvers (see Table 9-14). If the patient has decreased range of motion or if the pain does not improve, obtain MRI to rule out rotator cuff tear. Otherwise, consider subacromial corticosteroid injection.

What measures are indicated if pain persists despite corticosteroid injection?

Consider repeat corticosteroid injection if the patient has <50% pain relief after 6 weeks. Consider imaging and referral to an orthopedic surgeon if pain persists after 3 months.

Suppose that instead of initiating conservative measures to treat rotator cuff tendonitis, the patient listened to a friend and wore a sling for the next 4 weeks. His pain improved considerably but he now complains of stiffness. He is unable to perform the Apley scratch test or drop test to due to shoulder stiffness. The shoulder will not passively abduct to 90°.

What complication should you suspect?

Suspect adhesive capsulitis ("frozen shoulder") in this patient with shoulder stiffness and decreased range of motion. Rotator cuff tendonitis is the most common cause of frozen shoulder, particularly in patients who keep the joint immobile. Although plain radiographs are not diagnostically helpful, they should be obtained to rule out glenohumeral OA. Symptoms usually resolve with conservative measures.

> **Glenohumeral OA**: This rare conditions presents in a manner similar to frozen shoulder. Also causes crepitus and subcoracoid tenderness. Consider this as a secondary cause if OA is present on shoulder films.

> **Rotator cuff tendonitis**: shoulder pain despite lidocaine test; normal range of motion.
> **Rotator cuff tear**: shoulder pain despite lidocaine test; decreased range of motion due to pain.
> **Frozen shoulder**: shoulder pain present or absent; decreased range of motion due to stiffness.

CASE 9–15 ELBOW PAIN

A 28-year-old man presents with a 2-week history of pain in the lateral elbow. He plays racquetball regularly. Physical exam is significant for tenderness at the lateral epicondyle. The pain increases with resisted wrist extension and gripping.

What is the diagnosis?

This patient has lateral epicondylitis ("tennis elbow"). This overuse injury presents with localized pain and tenderness over the lateral epicondyle. Pain is aggravated by wrist extension against resistance and strong gripping. Range of motion is normal.

> **Medial epicondylitis ("golfer's elbow")**: This overuse injury presents with localized pain and tenderness over medial epicondyle aggravated by resisted wrist flexion and strong gripping. Range of motion is normal. Management is similar to tennis elbow.

What is the next step in management?

No further diagnostic testing is indicated in patients with clinical features of lateral epicondylitis. Initial treatment is conservative (rest, ice, NSAIDs ± wrist orthotic device). Consider corticosteroid injection if symptoms persist despite 4 weeks of conservative therapy.

Alternative 9.15.1

A 34-year-old man presents with pain in the posterior elbow. There is erythema and swelling over the posterior elbow, but range of motion is normal.

What is the next step in management?

The patient has olecranon bursitis. Causes range from overuse to inflammatory arthritides. The next step in this patient with signs of inflammation is aspiration of the bursa to rule out infection or crystal-induced arthritis. If evaluation of the aspirated fluid is negative, treat with conservative measures.

> **Elbow joint disease**: Primary complaint is decreased range of motion.
> **Olecranon bursitis**: Primary complaint is swelling; range of motion is normal.
> **Epicondylitis**: Primary complaint is pain; range of motion is normal.

CASE 9–16 HAND PAIN

A 50-year-old construction worker presents with a 4-week history of right hand pain. The pain is most prominent in the thumb and first two fingers. He often wakes up at night because of tingling sensations in his thumb and first two fingers. Complete wrist-palmar flexion for 30 seconds reproduces tingling. There is no swelling or tenderness at the MCP, PIP, or DIP.

What is the diagnosis?

This patient with pain and paresthesia in the distribution of the median nerve and positive Phalen sign meets diagnostic criteria for carpal tunnel syndrome. Symptoms result from compression of the median nerve as it passes through the carpal tunnel.

> Diagnostic criteria for carpal tunnel syndrome:
> 1. **One or more symptoms**: pain, paresthesia, or numbness in the distribution of the median nerve (thumb and first two and a half fingers)
> 2. **One or more objective findings**: Phalen sign, Tinel sign, thenar atrophy, or decreased sensation in the distribution of the median nerve

> **Phalen sign**: Complete wrist palmar flexion for 30 to 60 seconds reproduces paresthesia.
> **Tinel sign**: Percussion of the median nerve reproduces paresthesia (less sensitive test).

What is the next step in management?

Initial management of carpal tunnel syndrome is nonsurgical. The first-line measure is to wear a splint at night. If symptoms persist despite 4 weeks of nocturnal splinting, consider corticosteroid injection. Oral steroids, yoga, and physical therapy are options for patients who decline corticosteroid injections or have persistent symptoms despite injection.

The patient continues to have severe pain despite 6 months of nonsurgical measures.

What is the next step in management?

If the patient has severe symptoms after 6 months of conservative therapy, confirm the diagnosis using nerve conduction velocity studies (electrodiagnostic tests). If electrodiagnostic testing is positive, consider surgical decompression.

Alternative 9.16.1

A 56-year-old diabetic man presents with a 2-week history of hand pain. The pain is most severe at the base of the third MCP. The pain worsens when the extended fingers are stretched. When he flexes and extends his fingers, the third finger gets "locked" in flexion. There is no swelling at the PIP or DIP joints.

What is the diagnosis?

The patient has flexor tenosynovitis ("trigger finger"). This overuse injury occurs due to inflammation of the flexor tendon sheath at the MCP joint. Incidence is higher in patients with diabetes mellitus. First-line therapy is ice and immobilization with a finger splint. If symptoms persist after ≥4 weeks of immobilization, consider corticosteroid injection (can repeat injection after 6 weeks if symptoms persist). Consider surgery for persistent symptoms despite two or more corticosteroid injections.

Alternative 9.16.2

A 42 –year old woman presents with a 10-day history of thumb pain. Gripping and grasping motions aggravate the pain. Physical exam is significant for tenderness at the radial styloid and increased pain while performing the Finkelstein maneuver. There is no swelling or tenderness at the PIP or DIP joints.

What is the diagnosis?

The patient has de Quervain's tenosynovitis. This overuse injury results from inflammation of the abductor pollicis longus and extensor pollicis longus and brevis tendons. Treatment is similar to flexor tenosynovitis.

> **Finkelstein maneuver**: Ask the patient to make a fist with the fingers over the thumb. Then bend the wrist in the direction of the little finger.

> Other common hand disorders:
>
> **Dupuytren contracture**: Painless thickening ± nodules in palmar fascia leads to flexion contracture and stiffness. Diagnosis is clinical. First-line treatment is to passively stretch the digits. Consider palmar fasciectomy for severe functional impairment.
>
> **Mallet finger ("baseball finger")**: Common avulsion injury that occurs when flexion force is applied to an extended DIP joint. Tip of finger droops down on physical exam. Confirm diagnosis and extent of injury with posteroanterior and lateral radiographs of the DIP joint. Treatment is usually conservative (ice, NSAIDs, splint) unless the injury is severe.

CASE 9–17 FOOT PAIN

A 20-year-old ballet dancer presents with a 4-week history of foot pain in the mid-sole. Physical exam is significant for point tenderness at the mid-sole, particularly when the foot is dorsiflexed. There is no swelling, warmth, or erythema.

What is the most likely diagnosis?

The history and physical exam are characteristic of plantar fascitis. Plantar fascitis is one of the most common causes of foot pain. Risk factors include flat feet and repetitive dancing. First-line therapy is conservative (rest, ice, NSAIDs, and silicone heel inserts). Consider x-rays if symptoms do not resolve after 4 weeks of conservative therapy.

What would be your diagnosis if a patient who frequently wears high heels complained of pain, numbness, and tingling in the third and fourth toes, and compression of the forefoot reproduced the symptoms?

The findings suggest Morton's neuroma, a benign growth of nerve tissue as a result of nerve entrapment. Wearing high heels is a risk factor. The region of the third and fourth toes is the most frequent site of Morton's neuroma. No laboratory or imaging tests are indicated. Initial management is conservative (metatarsal support devices, rest, ice, and NSAIDs). Corticosteroid injection is the second-line measure, and surgery is the last resort.

> **Tarsal tunnel syndrome**: Presents with pain and paresthesia in sole of foot with increased symptoms on dorsiflexion-eversion and tapping on posterior tibial nerve.

> **Hallux valgus (bunion)**: The big toe (hallux) deviates inward. First step is to change footwear.

CASE 9–18 ANKLE PAIN

A 23-year-old-man presents with ankle pain after a fall while playing basketball. The patient is able to bear weight but complains of lateral malleolar tenderness on physical exam. There is no tenderness at the medial malleolus, navicular, or base of the fifth metatarsal.

What is the next step in management?

The Ottawa ankle rules recommend plain radiographs to rule out fracture in the following patients after trauma:

1. Order ankle and foot x-rays if the patient cannot bear weight.
2. Order only ankle x-rays if the patient medial or lateral malleolar tenderness.
3. Order only foot x-rays if the patient has tenderness at the navicular or base of the fifth metatarsal.

The next step is to obtain plain films of the ankle in this patient with lateral malleolar tenderness.

> **Ankle tendonitis**: Suspect if a patient with no history of trauma has ankle tendon pain and tenderness but normal range of motion and no pain on joint palpation.

Plain films do not demonstrate a fracture.

What is the next step in management?

The Ottawa ankle rules are very sensitive but not specific. The patient likely has an ankle sprain. First line therapy is NSAIDs plus ***RICE*** (**R**est, **I**ce, **C**ompression, and **E**levation).

> **Anterior talofibular ligament**: This is the most commonly sprained ankle ligament, and it is located in anterolateral part of the ankle.

CASE 9–19 LEG PAIN

An 18-year-old varsity cross-country athlete presents with a 2-week history of gradually worsening leg pain. The pain is localized to the anterior compartment. She has no known risk factors for deep vein thrombosis. The anterior compartment is tender. There is no swelling or erythema. Neurological exam of the foot is normal. Vital signs are normal.

What is the most likely diagnosis?

The most likely diagnosis is shin splint syndrome, an overuse injury common among runners. The next step is conservative therapy with NSAIDs + RICE.

What diagnosis would you suspect if leg pain were accompanied by lower extremity weakness or numbness and/or a compartment of the leg felt tight on physical exam?

Suspect chronic compartment syndrome in patients with leg pain isolated to a specific compartment and positive neurological findings or compartment tightness. Confirm the diagnosis by documenting elevated compartment pressure in the leg. Treatment is elective surgical fasciotomy.

The patient with shin splints returns 4 weeks later with persistent pain. Recently obtained medical records mention that she has a history of anorexia nervosa.

What is the next step in management?

The clinical presentation of stress fracture is very similar to shin splints syndrome. Obtain plain radiographs to rule out stress fracture if a patient with symptoms of shin splints syndrome fails to improve despite 2-3 weeks of conservative therapy. Eating disorders and oligomenorrhea increase the risk of developing stress fractures.

CASE 9–20 FATIGUE AND POLYMYALGIA

A 37-year-old woman presents with a 2-year history of fatigue, stiffness, and body aches in multiple areas. Immunological tests for autoimmune arthritis have all been negative. Physical exam is significant for 13 areas of soft tissue tenderness. Vital signs are normal.

What tests are indicated in the initial evaluation of patients who present with chronic polymyalgia and multiple tender areas on physical exam?

Initial laboratory testing in patients with polymyalgia are CBC, serum chemistries, ESR, thyroid function tests, and muscle enzymes (creatinine kinase and lactate dehydrogenase).

Laboratory tests are all negative.

What is the most likely diagnosis?

The most likely diagnosis is fibromyalgia. This idiopathic condition is much more common women. Patients present with fatigue and polymyalgia. Physical exam should demonstrate tenderness to palpation in at least 11 of 18 specified symmetric areas. All laboratory evaluations are negative in these patients. Most fibromyalgia patients also meet criteria for chronic fatigue syndrome (see Chapter 12: Neurology).

What is the next step in management?

Explain the chronic nature of her symptoms and reassure her that she does not have an underlying life-threatening disorder. Treatment of fibromyalgia is challenging. Some treatment options of questionable efficacy include low-dose antidepressants, acupuncture, psychotherapy, chiropractic care, massage and physical therapy.

Myofascial pain disorder: a fibromyalgia variant (pain localized to one soft tissue area).

chapter 10

Hematology and Oncology

CASE 10–1 MICROCYTIC ANEMIA

A 48-year-old man presents with a 3-week history of fatigue. On physical exam, the oral and conjunctival mucosa appears pale. Vital signs are normal. Complete blood count (CBC) reveals hemoglobin (Hb) 11 g/dL, hematocrit (HCT) 30%, normal platelets, and normal white blood cell (WBC) count.

What do the abnormal values indicate?

Hb is the major oxygen-carrying pigment. Its concentration is typically expressed as grams per deciliter of whole blood. HCT is the percentage of whole blood that contains red blood cells (RBCs). Decreased Hb, HCT, or RBC counts are surrogate measures of anemia. The components of whole blood are as follow:

- **RBCs** account for 40% of whole blood. Contain Hb, which carries O_2 from lungs to tissues and CO_2 from tissues to lungs. Hb gives blood its red color. A decreased number of circulating RBCs is called anemia; an increased number of circulating RBCs is called polycythemia.
- **Platelets (thrombocytes)**: Whole blood typically contains one platelet for every 200 RBCs. Platelets are required for blood clotting. A decreased number of platelets is called thrombocytopenia; an increased number of platelets is called thrombocytosis.
- **WBC**: Whole blood typically contains one WBC for every 600 to 700 RBCs. WBCs defend the body against infection/foreign bodies. An increased number of circulating WBCs is

called leukocytosis; a decreased number of circulating WBCs is called leukopenia. The five types of WBCs are:

- Neutrophils or polymorphonuclear leukocytes (PMNs) are the most numerous type of WBC. They defend against bacterial and fungal infections.
- T-lymphocytes and natural killer cells kill viruses and some cancer cells; B-lymphocytes produce antibodies.
- Monocytes ingest dead or damaged cells.
- Eosinophils kill parasites and participate in allergic responses.
- Basophils participate in allergic responses.

- **Plasma**: This yellow-colored liquid component, which accounts for 55% of whole blood, consists of water, electrolytes, and soluble proteins (albumin, carbonic anhydrase, clotting factors, and immunoglobulins). Solid components of blood (RBCs, WBCs, and platelets) are suspended in plasma.

Note: Serum is the yellowish liquid that remains after plasma clots. It does not contain clotting factors.

Anemia in men: typically Hb <13.5 g/dL (men) or HCT <41%
Anemia in women: typically Hb <12 g/dL or HCT <36%

What are common symptoms of anemia?

Patients most frequently report vague, nonspecific symptoms such as fatigue, malaise, and decreased concentration. Patients with severe or long-standing anemia may experience palpitations, dyspnea on exertion, or syncope on exertion. Mild anemia is frequently asymptomatic.

What are common physical exam findings in anemia?

Pallor (of the skin, palms, nail bed, or oral or conjunctival mucosa) is an important physical finding, but it is not always apparent. Hypotension and tachycardia can occur in severe or long-standing anemia.

Additional findings in iron-deficiency anemia (neither sensitive nor specific):
Pica: Increased appetite for non-nutritive substances or atypical foods (e.g., chalk, ice etc.)
Koilonychia ("spoon nails"): Flat or concave shaped nails.
Cheilosis: Cracks or splits at the corner of the mouth (may bleed, crust, or ulcerate).

The patient does not have any family history of anemia.

What is the next diagnostic step?

The next step in this hemodynamically stable patient is to measure reticulocyte index (Fig. 10-1). Also, try to obtain prior RBC measurements if available.

Reticulocyte count: Normal reticulocyte count is 25,000 to 75,000/mL (0.5% to 1.5%).
Reticulocyte index (RI): Reticulocyte count × (patient's HCT/normal HCT)/Maturation factor
Maturation factor: HCT 36% to 45%, 1; 26% to 35%, 1.5; 20% to 25%, 2; ≤20%, 2.5.

Prior CBC measurements are not available. RI is 1.5%. Mean corpuscular volume (MCV) is 58 dL.

What is the next diagnostic step?

The patient has a microcytic anemia (see Fig. 10-1). Remember causes of microcytic anemia with the mnemonic "***TAILS***" (**T**halassemias, **A**nemia of chronic disease (ACD), **I**ron-

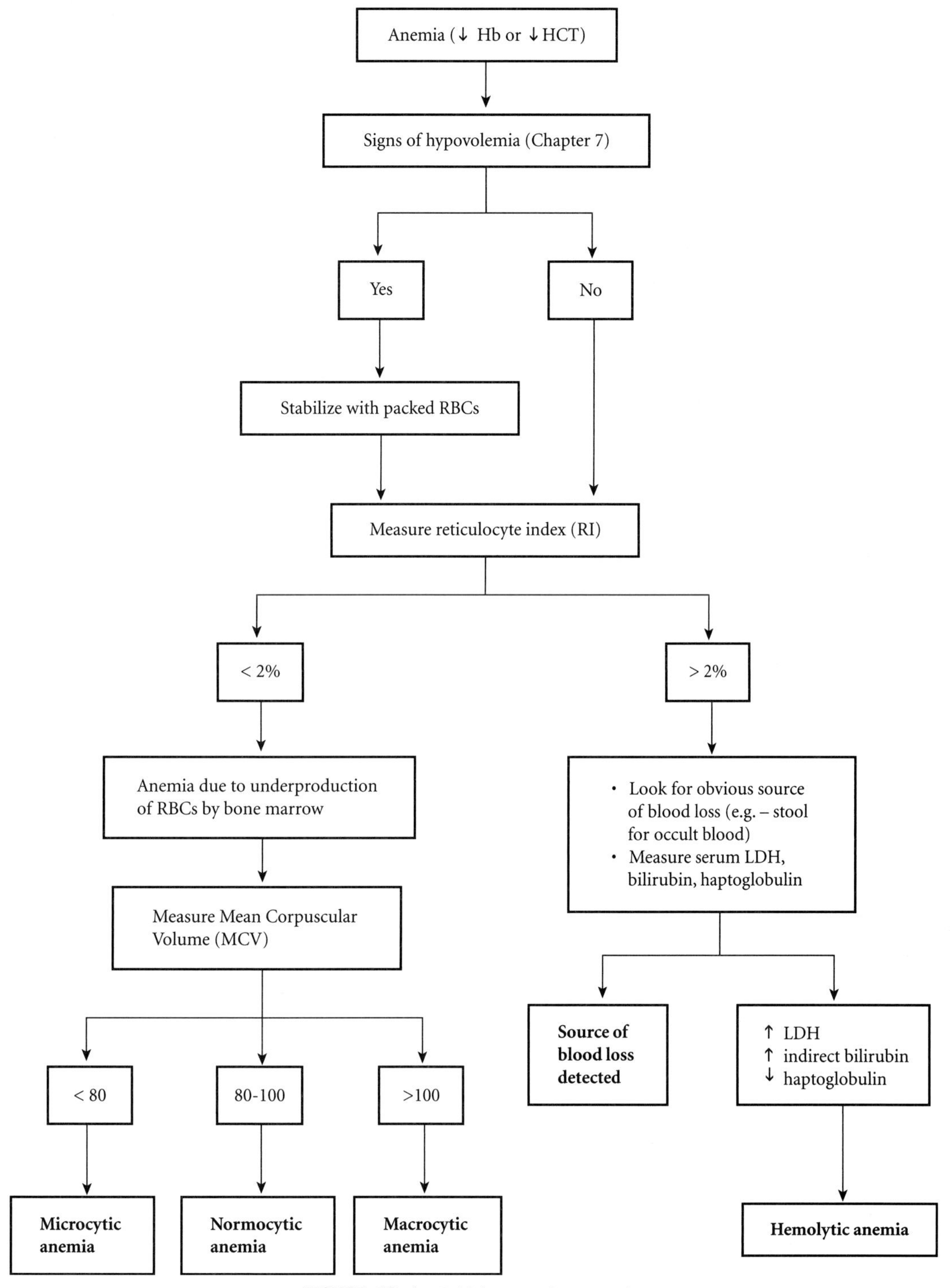

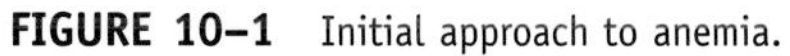

FIGURE 10–1 Initial approach to anemia.

deficiency anemia, **L**ead poisoning, and **S**ideroblastic anemia). Iron-deficiency anemia (IDA) is the most common cause of microcytic anemia, so the next step is to obtain iron studies (Fig. 10-2 and Table 10-1).

> **Hypochromia**: Increased central pallor in RBCs; occurs in most cases of microcytic anemia.

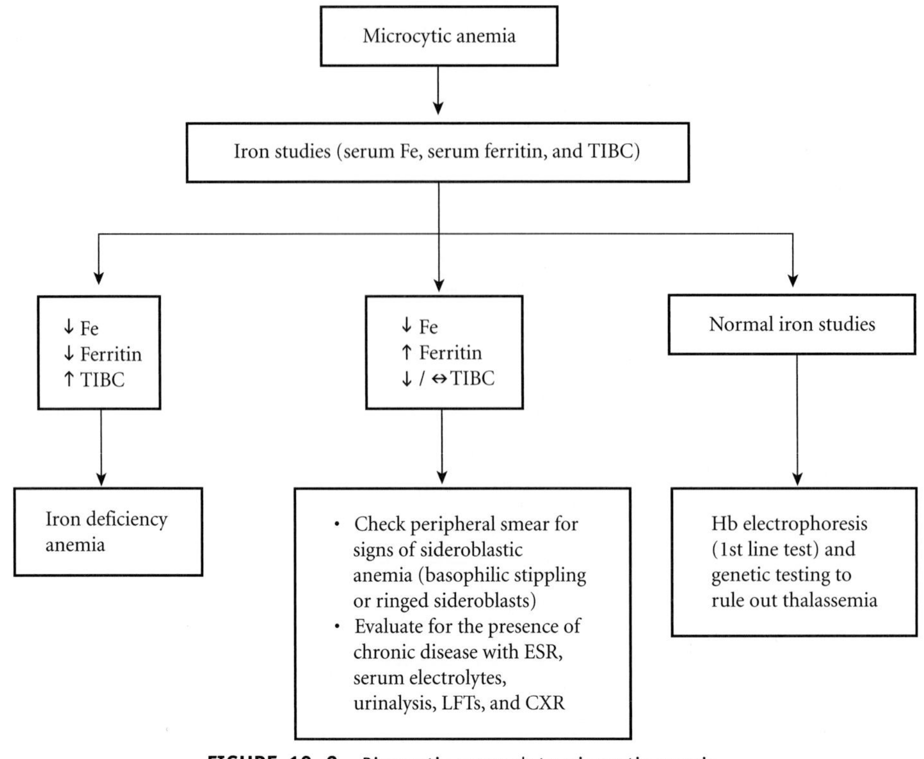

FIGURE 10–2 Diagnostic approach to microcytic anemia.

> **MCV**: measure of average RBC size. MCV = HCT/RBC count.

Serum iron is 30 µg/dL (decreased), serum ferritin is 5 ng/mL (decreased), and total iron binding capacity (TIBC) is 65% (increased).

What are the causes of this pattern of iron studies?

The patient has IDA, which causes anemia because it impairs synthesis of heme, a component of Hb. Important causes are blood loss, dietary deficiency, and malabsorption. Blood loss (gastrointestinal (GI) bleeding, menorrhagia, etc.) is the most common cause of iron deficiency among adults in the United States.

How is IDA treated?

The initial goal is to identify and treat the underlying cause. If it is not possible to definitively correct the cause of iron deficiency (e.g., hereditary hemorrhagic telangiectasia, gastric bypass, etc.), treat with iron replacement. Iron is available in both oral and intravenous (IV) forms.

> **Oral iron noncompliance**: 10% to 20% of patients discontinue oral iron replacement because of GI side effects. One strategy to minimize side effects is to take iron with meals.

What would have been the most likely cause of microcytic anemia if serum iron were 30 µg/dL (decreased), serum ferritin were 280 ng/mL (↔), and TIBC was low?

This pattern of iron studies usually indicates ACD. Although any chronic disease can cause ACD, most cases occur in patients with chronic infection, inflammation, or malignancy. Sideroblastic anemia can also cause a similar pattern but is far less frequent. The next step is to analyze the blood smear and obtain erythrocyte sedimentation rate, serum electrolytes, urinalysis, chest x-ray (CXR), and liver function tests (LFTs).

TABLE 10–1 Iron Studies

Study	Causes of Increased Levels	Causes of Decreased Levels	Notes
Serum Fe	• Iron overload[1]	• Iron deficiency • Chronic disease	Poor test because value varies daily and diurnally.
TIBC	• Iron deficiency	• Chronic disease • Iron overload	Pregnancy and oral contraceptives can ↑ TIBC.
Transferrin saturation	• Iron overload	• Iron deficiency • Chronic disease	Ratio of Fe/TIBC. Main use is to detect early iron overload.
Ferritin	• Chronic disease • Lead poisoning • Sideroblastic anemia	• Iron deficiency	Acute phase reactant, so concurrent infection, inflammation, or malignancy can increase ferritin to normal levels even if patient has iron deficiency.

Abbreviations: TIBC, total iron binding capacity; ↑, increased.
[1] Important causes of iron overload are hemochromatosis and hemosiderosis

Normocytic anemia is more common than microcytic anemia in ACD.

How is ACD treated?

First-line treatment is to correct or control the underlying disorder. If anemia persists, consider erythropoietin (EPO) or darbepoetin.

Alternative 10.1.1

Routine screening of an asymptomatic 30-year-old South Asian woman detects Hb of 11 g/dL and HCT of 30%. RI is 1.3%, and MCV is 60 dL. She has a history of heavy menstrual periods (menorrhagia) but is otherwise asymptomatic. The physician decides to start the patient on oral contraceptive pills and oral iron replacement. Three months later, her menstrual flow has lessened considerably. HG is 11.2, HCT is 33%, RI is 1.3%, and MCV is 60 dL.

What is the next step in management?

This patient with presumed IDA has failed to improve despite iron replacement. The next step is to obtain iron studies to check whether the patient truly has IDA.

Iron studies are normal.

What is the next step in management?

The next step is Hb electrophoresis to evaluate the patient for thalassemia.

What is thalassemia?

Hb contains one heme molecule surrounded by four globin chains (two α-globin and two non–α-globin chains). The predominant type of Hb in adults (HbA) contains two α-globin and two β-globin chains. α-Globins are encoded by four α-globin genes, and β-globins are encoded by two β-globin genes. Thalassemias are a heterogenous group of genetic mutations in α- or β-globin genes. They are inherited in an autosomal recessive pattern (Table 10-2).

Infants: Predominant Hb is HbF (has two α-globin and two γ-globin chains).
Adults: 97% HbA, 3% HbA2 (has two α-globin and two δ-globin chains), <1% HbF.

Hb electrophoresis is normal.

TABLE 10–2 Thalassemias

Disorder	Mutated Gene(s)	Hb Electrophoresis	Degree of Anemia	Symptoms of Anemia
α-Thalassemia silent trait	1 of 4 α-globin genes	Normal	None	Asymptomatic
α-Thalassemia minor (trait)	2 of 4 α-globin genes	Normal	Mild microcytic anemia	Asymptomatic
α-Thalassemia intermedia	3 of 4 α-globin genes	↑ HbH (group of 4 β chains)	Severe microcytic anemia	Severe
α-Thalassemia major	4 of 4 α-globin genes	Not applicable in adults	Not applicable in adults	Incompatible with life
β-Thalassemia minor (trait)	1 of 2 β-globin genes	↓ HbA, ↑ HbA2, ↑ HbF (mild abnormalities)	Mild microcytic anemia	Asymptomatic
β-Thalassemia major	Both β-globin genes	↓ HbA, ↑ HbA2, ↑ HbF	Severe microcytic anemia	Severe
β-Thalassemia intermedia	Less severe mutations in both β-globin genes	↓ HbA, ↑ HbA2, ↑ HbF (moderate abnormalities)	Moderate to severe microcytic anemia	Moderate[a]

Abbreviations: Hb, hemoglobin; ↓, decreased; ↑, increased.
[a] Patients often do not require packed red blood cell (PRBC) transfusions except during pregnancy and illness

What is the next step in management?

Patients with α-thalassemia do not usually have any abnormalities on Hb electrophoresis. The next step in the diagnostic evaluation is genetic testing.

Genetic testing reveals a mutation in two of the four α-globin genes.

What is the next step in management?

The patient has α-thalassemia minor. This condition is more common in South East Asian, South Asian, and Middle Eastern patients. No treatment is necessary for patients with α- or β-thalassemia minor.

How does management differ in α-thalassemia intermedia or β-thalassemia major?

Patients with these mutations become symptomatic at birth (α-thalassemia intermedia) or a few months after birth (β-thalassemia major). Untreated, patients often develop splenomegaly and skeletal abnormalities such as "hair on end" appearance on skull radiograph and "chipmunk facies" (maxillary overbite). Treatment is four-fold (mnemonic: "***PISS***"):

1. **P**acked red blood cell (PRBC) transfusions: Maintain Hb between 9 and 10 g/dL.
2. **I**ron chelation therapy: Chronic PRBC transfusions lead to iron overload (hemosiderosis), which can result in cardiac complications. First-line chelating agent in thalassemia major is deferoxamine. New oral agents are being investigated.
3. **S**plenectomy: Perform if transfusion requirements have increased by >50% over 12 months.
4. **S**tem cell transplantation: This is emerging as a viable option in carefully selected adults.

Alternative 10.1.2

Skin tuberculin testing of a recent Haitian immigrant who applies for a position as a respiratory technician reveals 12 mm of induration. CXR does not show any signs of active disease. He begins isoniazid (INH) to treat latent tuberculosis infection. Baseline labs are normal. During routine monitoring 2 months later, Hb is 10.7 and HCT is 30%. Figure 10-3 is the patient's blood smear.

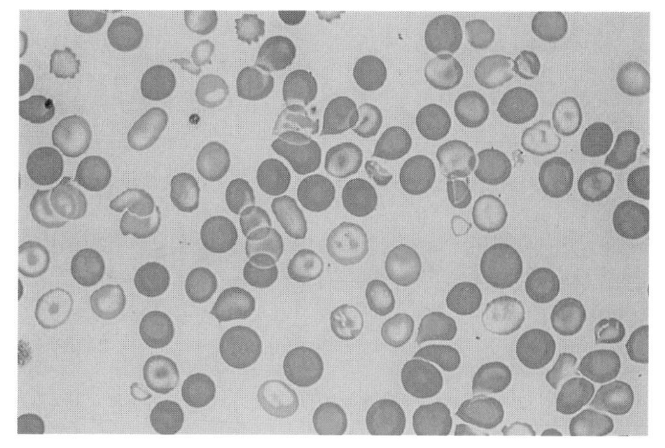

FIGURE 10–3 Blood smear containing siderocytes (sideroblastic anemia due to isoniazid). From McClatchey KD. *Clinical Laboratory Medicine, 2nd ed.* Lippincott Williams & Wilkins, 2002.

What is the abnormality?

The smear demonstrates microcytic, hypochromic RBCs. The RBCs contain bluish-green granules (siderocytes). This finding suggests sideroblastic anemia.

> **Sideroblastic**: inability to use iron to synthesize heme despite sufficient stores.

What are the causes of sideroblastic anemia?

1. Reversible causes: Alcoholism, drugs (INH and chloramphenicol), and mineral deficiency (decreased zinc or copper).
2. Acquired idiopathic sideroblastic anemia: Also called refractory anemia with ringed sideroblasts (RARS). RARS is one of the myelodysplastic syndromes (MDS). Incidence is highest in middle-aged men.
3. Hereditary causes: Most commonly cross-linked recessive (i.e., occurs in females).

> **Chloramphenicol**: This antibiotic is infrequently used in the west because it can cause aplastic anemia, pure red cell aplasia, and sideroblastic anemia.

What is the next step in management of this patient with sideroblastic anemia?

INH is the most likely cause in this young male. There are two options:

1. Switch from INH to rifampin monotherapy: Rifampin is not the first-line drug for latent tuberculosis, but discontinuing INH should correct the anemia.
2. Continue INH course and administer large doses of pyridoxine (vitamin B6).

How would management have differed if the patient with sideroblastic anemia were a young woman who ate a well-balanced diet and did not take alcohol or any medications?

Obtain bone marrow biopsy and free erythrocyte porphyrin (FEP) to distinguish between hereditary and acquired sideroblastic anemia. Hereditary sideroblastic anemia is associated with decreased FEP, whereas acquired sideroblastic anemia is associated with increased FEP.

How is hereditary sideroblastic anemia treated?

Treatment is pyridoxine, iron chelation (phlebotomy or deferoxamine), and supportive care. Consider PRBC transfusions for symptomatic anemia unresponsive to pyridoxine. Splenectomy is contraindicated (increased risk of postoperative thromboembolism).

> **RARS**: Pyridoxine is ineffective. Treat with iron chelation. Consider PRBC transfusion and EPO if the patient is symptomatic. Splenectomy is contraindicated.

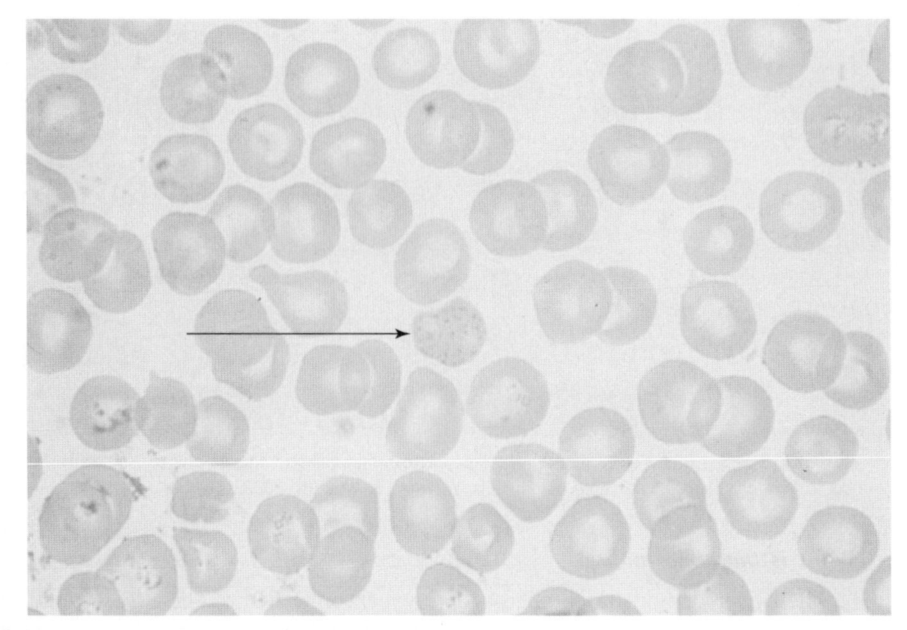

FIGURE 10–4 Blood smear with basophilic stippling (due to lead poisoning). From Anderson S. *Anderson's Atlas of Hematology*, Lippincott Williams & Wilkins, 2003.

Alternative 10.1.3

A 60-year-old man presents with episodes of colicky abdominal pain and arthralgias. He also reports fatigue and difficulty concentrating. He has a history of frequently drinking "moonshine" (illegally distilled alcohol). Oral and conjunctival mucosa is pale. There is a blue line at the gum–tooth border. Abdominal obstructive series is negative. Hb is 9.5 mg/dL and HCT is 29%. Figure 10-4 is the patient's peripheral blood smear.

What disorders can cause this pattern?

The blood smear of this anemic patient demonstrates microcytic hypochromic RBCs with basophilic stippling (dark-blue granular inclusions in RBCs). This pattern can result from lead poisoning, thalassemia, and sideroblastic anemia.

What is the most likely diagnosis in this patient?

The patient most likely has lead poisoning. Common causes in the United States are occupational exposure (to paint, wires, car radiators, etc.) and moonshine consumption. Remember the clinical manifestations of severe lead poisoning (serum level >80 μg/dL) with the mnemonic "***LEAD***":

1. **L**ead lines: bluish colored line at the gum–tooth border (specific but not sensitive)
2. **E**ncephalopathy: decreased short-term memory and concentration
3. **A**bdominal pain (colicky), arthralgias, and anemia (with basophilic stippling)
4. **D**rops: Wrist or foot drop

Serum lead = 30 to 70 μg/dL: nonspecific symptoms (fatigue, irritability, etc.)

What is the next step in management?

Obtain a serum lead level to confirm the diagnosis. The first-line measure in any patient with increased serum lead content is to remove the offending agent (in this case, moonshine). Lead chelation with calcium EDTA or succimer is indicated in the following situations:

1. **Serum lead ≥ 80 μg/dL**: Use lead chelation in any patient.

2. **Serum lead 60 to 80 μg/dL:** Use lead chelation in any symptomatic patient.
3. **Serum lead 40 to 60 μg/dL:** Consider lead chelation if symptoms persist for >2 weeks despite removing the offending agent.

CASE 10–2 NORMOCYTIC ANEMIA

A 43-year-old man presents with a 2-month history of fatigue, malaise, and dyspnea on exertion. He does not take any medications. CBC from 2 years ago was normal. On physical exam, there is conjunctival pallor. Hb is 5 g/dL, and HCT is 15%. Reticulocyte count is 20/mL, and RI is 0.1%. WBC and platelet counts are normal. There are very few normocytic RBCs on peripheral smear. CXR is normal except for an anterior mediastinal mass. EKG is normal.

What type of anemia does this patient have?

Profound normocytic anemia in a patient with normal WBC and platelet production suggests pure red cell aplasia (PRCA). This rare condition can be acute and self-limiting or chronic. The diagnosis can be confirmed with bone marrow biopsy (patients with PRCA have few RBC precursors but normal WBC and platelet precursors).

- Acute, self-limiting causes:
  1. Viral infection (parvovirus B19, viral hepatitis): PRCA is more likely if the patient has underlying thalassemia or hemolytic anemia (e.g., sickle cell anemia (SCA))
  2. Drugs:
     - **i.** Immune medicated injury (EPO)
     - **ii.** Direct toxic effects (anti-epileptic drugs, INH, procainamide)

- Chronic causes (mnemonic: "***Diamond TAIL***")
  1. **D**iamond-Blackfan syndrome: lifelong PRCA that presents in the neonatal period; autosomal dominant inheritance.
  2. **T**hymoma
  3. **A**utoimmune disorders (particularly SLE)
  4. **I**diopathic
  5. **L**ymphoproliferative disorders (leukemia, lymphoma, MDS)

Bone marrow biopsy confirms the diagnosis.

What is the most likely cause of PRCA?

The presence of an anterior mediastinal mass suggests the patient has a thymoma (rare neoplasm of the thymus). Confirm the diagnosis with CT-guided needle biopsy.

> **Thymoma presentation:**
> One third of patients are asymptomatic (detected incidentally).
> One third of patients are present with symptoms of local compression (cough, dyspnea, hoarseness, etc.).
> One third of patients are present as an autoimmune disorder (myasthenia gravis, PRCA).

What would have been the most likely cause of PRCA if CXR were normal but the patient had a history of chronic renal failure (CRF) on hemodialysis and took lisinopril, atorvastatin,, insulin, and EPO?

Patients with CRF often require EPO to treat CRF-induced anemia (normocytic anemia with Burr cells on peripheral smear). Ironically, EPO can sometimes induce PRCA. Confirm the diagnosis by measuring anti-EPO antibodies. Treatment is to administer PRBC transfusions and discontinue EPO.

> **Burr cells:** RBCs with regular, even projections (Fig. 10-5).

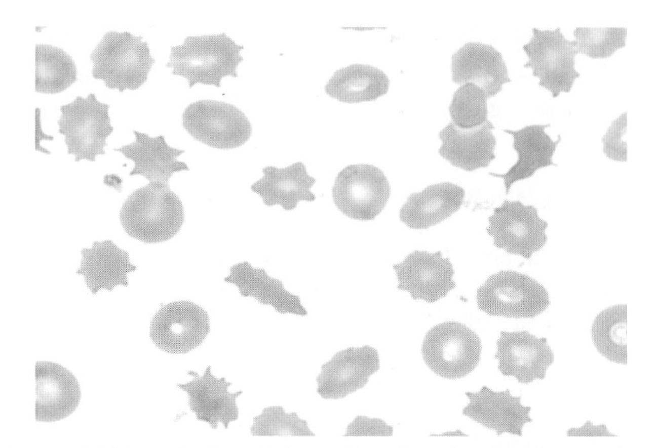

FIGURE 10–5 Blood smear with Burr cells. From Anderson S. *Anderson's Atlas of Hematology*, Lippincott Williams & Wilkins, 2003.

How would management differ if PRCA were caused by an autoimmune disorder?

First-line treatment of PRCA caused by autoimmune disorders is prednisone. Second-line treatment is cyclophosphamide.

Alternative 10.2.1

A 27-year-old G1P0001 woman in her 18th week of gestation has Hb of 11.5 g/dL. She is asymptomatic. There is no pallor or tachycardia. Reticulocyte count is 150,000, and RI is 1%. Iron studies are normal. Peripheral blood smear demonstrates normocytic RBCs.

What is the next step in management?

By the second trimester of pregnancy, RBC volume increases by approximately 30%. However, patients have mild anemia (mean Hb 11.5 g/dL) because plasma volume increases by approximately 50%. Dilutional anemia of pregnancy is a normal physiological condition that does not require any treatment. Consider treatment only if the patient develops symptoms of anemia or laboratory findings of a pathological anemia (e.g., iron deficiency).

Remember to supplement iron and folic acid during pregnancy.

Alternative 10.2.2

A 65-year-old man presents with a 3-month history of back pain, fatigue, and an unintentional 10-lb weight loss. The pain increases with movement. On physical exam, there is pallor and vertebral tenderness. Abnormal findings on CBC are Hb 9.7 mg/dL, HCT 29%, RI 0.5%, and MCV 90 dL. Figure 10-6 is the patient's peripheral smear.

What is the most likely diagnosis?

The patient with back pain has risk factors for malignancy (age >50 years and weight loss). The peripheral smear demonstrates rouleaux (RBCs stacked like coins), which occurs when a patient has increased serum protein. The most likely diagnosis is multiple myeloma (MM). MM is the neoplastic proliferation of a single plasma cell line to produce large amounts of monoclonal antibodies (M proteins), usually IgA or IgM. The disease is most common among elderly patients.

What are the clinical manifestations of MM?

Remember common clinical manifestations of MM with the mnemonic "***I, CRAB***":

1. **I**nfections: Increased production of defective antibodies (immunoglobulins) and decreased production of normal immunoglobulins leads to decreased humoral immunity.

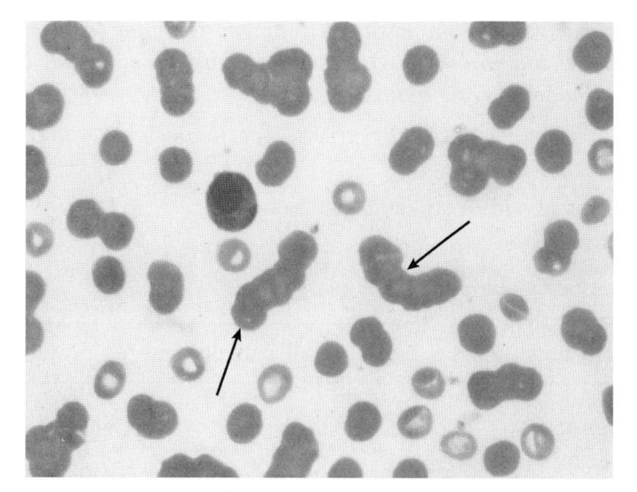

FIGURE 10–6 Blood smear showing rouleaux. From Rubin E, Farber JL. *Rubin's Pathology, 4th ed.* Lippincott Williams & Wilkins, 2004.

2. **C**alcium: Malignant plasma cells release osteoclast-activating factor, which breaks down bone and leads to hypercalcemia.
3. **R**enal failure: MM can cause chronic or acute renal failure. Most common causes are hypercalcemia and excretion of immunoglobulin light chains in the urine. In some patients, renal failure is caused by amyloidosis.
4. **A**nemia: MM can cause replacement of bone marrow by malignant plasma cells, which leads to normocytic anemia. MM also causes normocytic ACD. Rouleaux is the characteristic finding on peripheral smear.
5. **B**ones: Osteoclast-activating factor breaks down bone, which leads to bone pain (particularly in the chest and vertebrae) and pathological fractures. Classic x-ray finding is "punched out" lytic bony lesions.

> **Hyperviscosity syndrome**: Increased serum protein causes increased serum viscosity, which leads to easy bleeding, blurry vision, fatigue, hypoxia, and nonspecific neurological symptoms. Most common causes are Waldenström's macroglobulinemia and MM.

What are the next diagnostic steps?

Initial tests in the diagnostic workup besides CBC are serum chemistry, skeletal survey, serum protein electrophoresis (SPEP), and urine protein electrophoresis (UPEP). If diagnostic tests are suggestive, perform bone marrow biopsy to confirm the diagnosis. The Myeloma Working Group suggests three simplified criteria:

1. End-organ damage attributable to MM (I, CRAB)
2. SPEP or UPEP: increased M proteins (e.g., Bence Jones protein on UPEP)
3. Bone marrow biopsy: >10% clonal plasma cells

> **Skeletal survey**: X-rays of the skull, axial skeleton, and proximal long bones are more sensitive than a bone scan.

> **Erythrocyte sedimentation rate, lactic acid dehydrogenase (LDH), C-reactive protein, and β2-microglobulin levels** are not helpful diagnostically (nonspecific); however, they help assess prognosis when the diagnosis is established.

How is MM treated?

MM is associated with a poor prognosis. Treatment is either chemotherapy or autologous stem cell transplant.

What would have been the most likely diagnosis if the patient had 2.7 g/dL of M proteins on SPEP or UPEP but was otherwise asymptomatic with normal CBC, serum chemistry, skeletal survey, and bone marrow biopsy?

The patient meets diagnostic criteria for monoclonal gammopathy of uncertain significance (MGUS):

1. No signs of end-organ damage due to MM
2. SPEP/UPEP: M-protein spike <3 g/dL
3. Bone marrow biopsy: <10% plasma cells

> Obtain bone marrow biopsy in all patients with M-proteins >1.5 g/dL.

How is MGUS managed?

Repeat SPEP and UPEP after 6 months. If the level of M-proteins remains stable (↔), then monitor SPEP and UPEP annually because patients with MGUS have increased risk of MM.

> **Waldenström's macroglobulinemia:** This rare, low-grade (indolent), non-Hodgkin's lymphoma (NHL), which causes an IgM M-protein spike, presents with lymphadenopathy, easy bleeding, hepatomegaly, splenomegaly, and hyperviscosity.

> Causes of nonhemolytic normocytic anemia are ACD, PRCA, MM, chronic liver or kidney disease, dilutional anemia, endocrine disorders, and hemoglobinopathies.

CASE 10–3 MACROCYTIC ANEMIA

A 76-year-old woman presents with fatigue and short-term memory loss. She does not drink alcohol or smoke cigarettes. On physical exam, her tongue is shiny (atrophic glossitis). She walks with a broad-based clumsy gait (ataxia). There is decreased vibration and position sensation in both feet. Hb is 9 mg/dL, and HCT is 28%. Reticulocyte count is 40,000/mL, and RI is 0.4%. MCV is 114 dL. Figure 10-7 is her peripheral smear.

What is the most likely diagnosis?

In addition to macrocytes, the peripheral smear contains ovalocytes and hypersegmented neutrophils, which indicates that she has a megaloblastic anemia (Fig. 10-8). Atrophic glossitis and

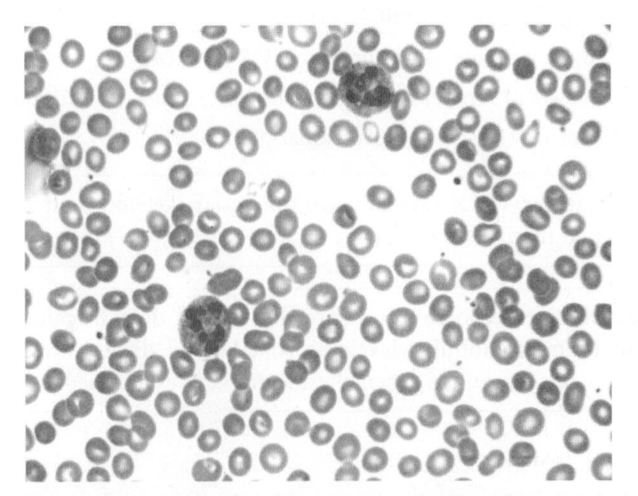

FIGURE 10–7 Blood smear showing macrocytosis and hypersegmented polymorphonuclear leukocytes due to vitamin B12 deficiency. From Rubin E, Farber JL. *Rubin's Pathology, 4th ed.* Lippincott Williams & Wilkins, 2004.

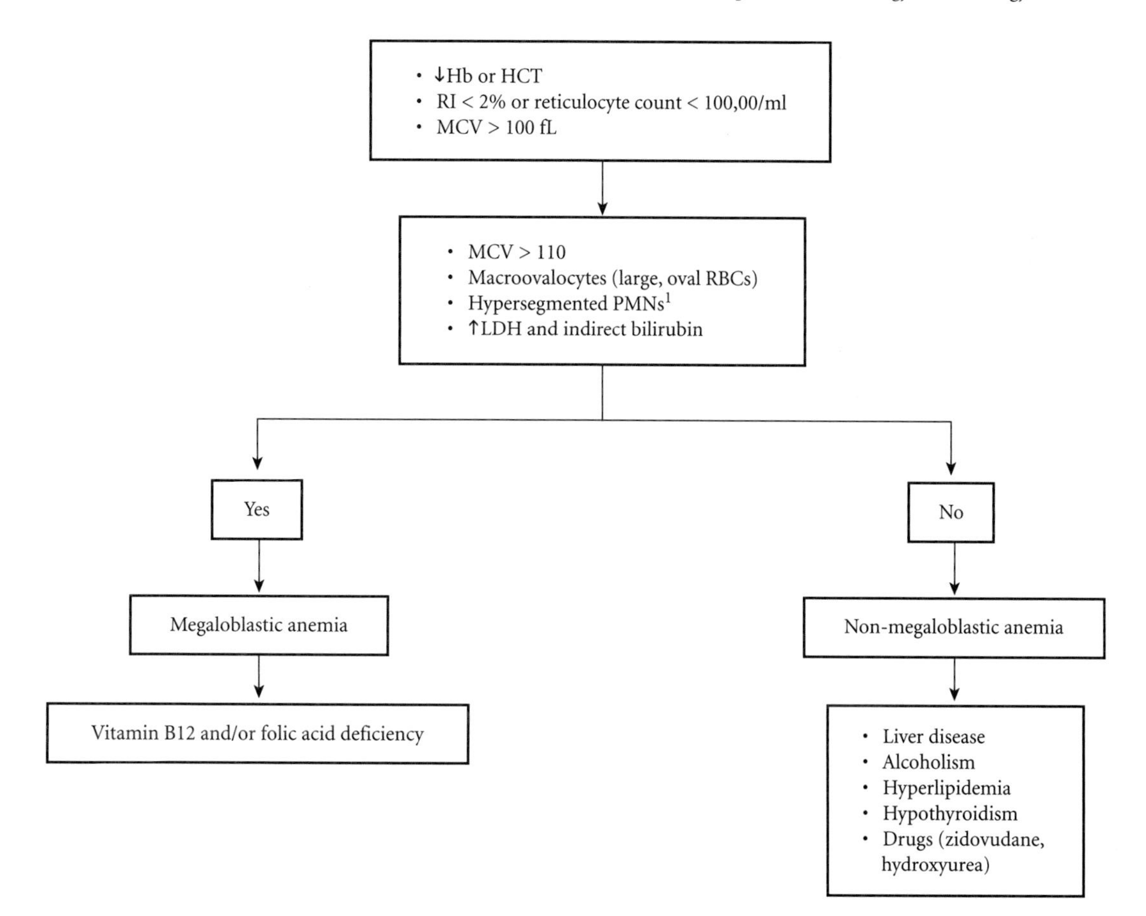

[1]≥ 5 % of PMNs with 5 lobes or ≥ 1 PMN with 6 lobes

FIGURE 10–8 Approach to macrocytic anemia due to underproduction of red blood cells.

neurological signs indicate that the patient has vitamin B12 deficiency. Concurrent folate deficiency is also possible, so the next step is to measure serum levels of folic acid and vitamin B12.

> **Peripheral smear**: Macrocytic cells are larger than a lymphocyte's nucleus.

What are common neurological signs of vitamin B12 deficiency?

1. **Autonomic dysfunction**: impotence and urinary or fecal incontinence
2. **Myelopathy**: ataxia, spasticity, and loss of deep tendon reflexes
3. **Peripheral neuropathy**: paresthesia, weakness, decreased vibration and position sense due to dorsal column degeneration
4. **Psychiatric**: dementia, depression, psychosis, and short-term memory loss

> Check for vitamin B12 deficiency in any patient with unexplained dementia.

Serum cobalamin is 120 pg/mL and folate is 4.5 mg/dL.

How should you interpret these values?

Serum vitamin B12 <200 pg/mL is diagnostic of vitamin B12 deficiency. Serum folate levels >4 mg/dL rule out folic acid deficiency.

> **Serum vitamin B12 >300 pg/mL**: no vitamin B12 deficiency.
> **Serum vitamin B12 200 to 300 pg/mL**: normal or subclinical deficiency.

How is vitamin B12 absorbed into the bloodstream?

Gastric acid cleaves vitamin B12 from other dietary proteins. Gastric parietal cells release intrinsic factor (IF), which binds to vitamin B12 in the stomach and duodenum. The IF-B12 complex facilitates absorption at the terminal ileum. This mechanism is responsible for 99% of vitamin B12 absorption.

The patient tells you she takes care to eat a balanced diet that contains meat, eggs, dairy products, and vegetables. She denies diarrhea, steatorrhea, or other symptoms of malabsorption. She has never had any surgeries. Her only medications are hydrochlorothiazide and lisinopril.

What are the next steps in management?

First, administer oral or intramuscular vitamin B12 to prevent further neurological degeneration. Then, search for an underlying cause for vitamin B12 deficiency (mnemonic: "***VITAMINS***"):

Vegan diet: Dietary sources of vitamin B12 are meat, eggs, and dairy products, so vegans who do not take vitamin B12 supplements develop deficiency.

Intestinal malabsorption: chronic pancreatitis, Crohn's disease, bowel resection, etc.

Tea and toast diet: Consumption of a nutritionally poor diet is common among alcoholics and the elderly.

Autoimmune gastritis (pernicious anemia): autoantibodies against parietal cells.

Medications (chronic use); remember the medications with the mnemonic "***PAM***":

1. **P**PIs: Decreased gastric acid leads to decreased cobalamin release from food.
2. **A**ntibiotics: Non-gut flora overgrowth causes malabsorption.
3. **M**etformin.

INtestinal tapeworm: *Diphyllobothrium latum* (fish tapeworm) was a notable cause in the past, but is less common today.

Surgery: Gastrectomy leads to decreased gastric acid production. Also, any abdominal surgery can cause strictures or blind loops that result in bacterial overgrowth.

This patient with no obvious cause should have serum levels of anti-parietal cell and anti-IF antibodies measured. Positive antibodies are diagnostic of pernicious anemia (common in the elderly and patients with other autoimmune disorders). Treatment of pernicious anemia is lifelong vitamin B12 replacement (oral or intramuscular).

Schilling test: an older, uncommonly used test used to diagnose pernicious anemia.

Large oral doses are as effective as intramuscular doses of vitamin B12 in pernicious anemia because 1% of vitamin B12 is absorbed by an alternative mechanism.

Alternative 10.3.1

A 60-year-old alcoholic man presents with fatigue and difficulty concentrating. His daughter mentions that he has not been eating well. On physical exam, the conjunctiva and nail beds are pale. Neurological exam is normal. Laboratory studies demonstrate macrocytic megaloblastic anemia.

What risk factors does this patient have for macrocytic anemia?

Chronic alcohol intake can cause nonmegaloblastic macrocytic anemia. Alcoholism also causes liver disease, which is associated with nonmegaloblastic anemia. Finally, malnutrition is common among alcoholic patients, which can lead to megaloblastic anemia because of folate and/or vitamin B12 (cobalamin) deficiency.

What is the most likely cause of macrocytic anemia in this patient?

Absence of neurological signs suggests that this patient's anemia is caused by folate rather than vitamin B12 deficiency. However, concurrent subclinical vitamin B12 deficiency is also possible.

Folate: Stores are small, so deficiency develops in a few weeks to months.
Vitamin B12: Stores are large, so deficiency requires years to develop.

What is the next step in management?

Obtain both vitamin B12 and folic acid levels. It is important to rule out concurrent vitamin B12 deficiency because treatment of folic acid deficiency will correct the anemia even if the patient has vitamin B12 deficiency, but it will not stop progression of neurological signs and symptoms.

Serum vitamin B12 is 250 pg/mL, and serum folate is 2 ng/mL.

What is the next step in management?

The laboratory tests confirm folic acid deficiency. However, this patient with serum cobalamin between 200 and 300 pg/mL may or may not have subclinical vitamin B12 deficiency. The next step is to obtain homocysteine and methylmalonic acid (MMA). If further testing confirms isolated folic acid deficiency, treat with oral folic acid.

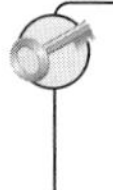

$\leftrightarrow$ **Homocysteine and** $\leftrightarrow$ **MMA**: Both vitamin B12 and folate deficiency are ruled out.
$\uparrow$ **Homocysteine and** $\uparrow$ **MMA**: Indicates $\downarrow$ vitamin B12 $\pm$ $\downarrow$ folate.
$\uparrow$ **Homocysteine and** $\leftrightarrow$ **MMA**: Indicates $\downarrow$ folate but not $\downarrow$ vitamin B12.

What are other important causes of folic acid deficiency?

In addition to malnutrition and malabsorption, folic acid deficiency can also result from pregnancy, hemolytic anemia, and drugs (trimethoprim-sulfamethoxazole, methotrexate, and phenytoin).

Alternative 10.3.2

A 57-year-old alcoholic man presents with fatigue and difficulty walking. He has an ataxic gait and mild hand tremor. There is no spasticity. Deep tendon reflexes are normal. Proprioception and vibration are intact. Laboratory studies reveal macrocytic anemia with MCV of 105 dL and no hypersegmented PMNs.

What is the most likely diagnosis?

Ataxia and tremor are signs of cerebellar degeneration as a result of chronic alcohol abuse. Chronic alcohol ingestion can cause macrocytic anemia with a mean MCV of 105 dL. Unlike vitamin B12 deficiency, alcoholic cerebellar degeneration does not cause myelopathy, peripheral neuropathy, or megaloblastic anemia.

Target cells: RBCs with a "bulls-eye" (due to liver disease, thalassemia, or splenectomy).
Spur cells: RBCs with irregular projections (due to liver disease). Spur cells have much fewer projections compared to Burr cells (due to kidney disease).

What are the next steps in management?

The next step is to measure serum vitamin B12 and folic acid levels to rule out concurrent deficiencies. Treatment of alcohol-induced macrocytic anemia is abstinence.

What would have been the most likely diagnosis if the patient with macrocytic nonmegaloblastic anemia had no history of alcohol use and presented with fatigue, difficulty concentrating, slow relaxation phase of deep tendon reflexes, and normal vitamin B12 and folic acid levels?

Fatigue, difficulty concentrating, and slow relaxation of deep tendon reflexes are features of hypothyroidism. The next step in this case is to obtain serum thyroid-stimulating hormone (see Chapter 8: Endocrinology).

Sideroblastic anemia, cold agglutinin disease, MDS, and aplastic anemia occasionally cause macrocytic nonmegaloblastic anemia. Rarely, when there are a large number of reticulocytes, the red cells may be measured as macrocytic.

CASE 10–4 HEMOLYTIC ANEMIA

A 50-year-old African-American man presents to the clinic with a 2-day history of fever, cough, and pleuritic chest pain. CXR shows a left upper lobe infiltrate. He is diagnosed with community-acquired pneumonia and is given azithromycin. One day later, he returns with abdominal pain and dark urine. Both sclera are icteric. LFTs detect increased indirect bilirubin. Hb is 10.2 mg/dL, HCT is 31%, reticulocyte count is 6%, RI is 3%, and serum haptoglobin is 25 mg/dL. Figure 10-9 is the patient's blood smear.

What are the causes of hemolytic anemia?

There are several ways to categorize hemolytic anemia. One way is to categorize them on the basis of whether the defect is intrinsic or extrinsic (Tables 10-3 and 10-4):

1. **Intrinsic**: Intracorpuscular defect (i.e., defective enzyme, membrane protein, or Hb) leads to formation of RBCs that are easily prone to intravascular destruction. With the exception of paroxysmal nocturnal hemoglobinuria (PNH), intrinsic hemolytic anemias are all hereditary.
2. **Extrinsic**: Acquired causes such as autoantibodies, trauma, infections, or splenic entrapment cause intravascular and extravascular RBC destruction.

Reticulocyte count is typically >4% to 5% in hemolytic anemia.

Other ways to categorize hemolytic anemia are:

1. Inherited versus acquired
2. Intravascular versus extravascular

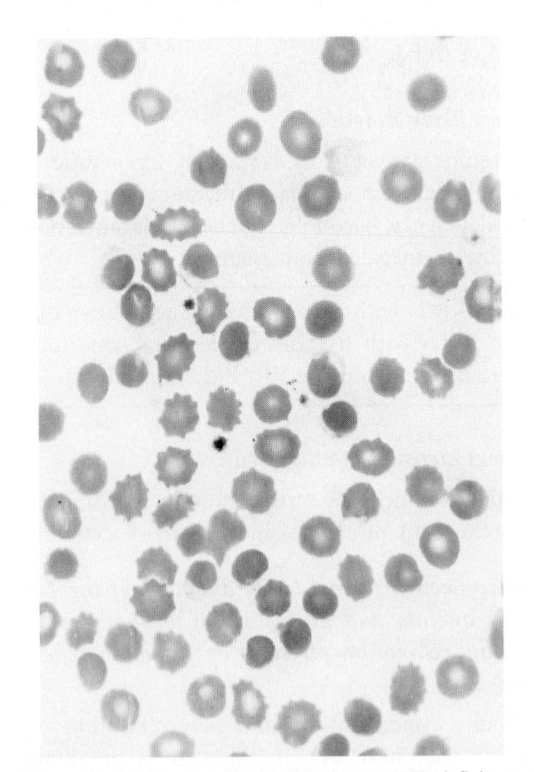

FIGURE 10–9 Blood smear showing bite cells and Heinz bodies due to G6PD deficiency. From McClatchey KD. *Clinical Laboratory Medicine, 2nd ed.* Lippincott Williams & Wilkins, 2002.

TABLE 10-3 Important Intrinsic Causes of Hemolytic Anemia

Disorder	Mechanism	Blood Smear	Characteristic Labs
SCA	Normal glutamic acid replaced by valine in β-globin gene; autosomal recessive inheritance.	Sickle cells	Hg electrophoresis detects HbS
G6PD deficiency	↓ Levels of enzyme necessary for pentose phosphate shunt (supplies energy to RBCs); cross-linked recessive inheritance.	Heinz bodies Bite cells	↓ NADPH formation on G6PD assay
Hereditary spherocytosis	Defect in RBC membrane proteins ankyrin or spectrin; autosomal recessive inheritance.	Spherocytes	Positive osmotic fragility test; ↑ MCHC
PNH	Acquired defect in GPI-linked RBC membrane proteins.	No specific findings	Flow cytometry (↓ GPI proteins)

Abbreviations: MCHC, mean corpuscular Hb concentration; PNH, paroxysmal nocturnal hemoglobinuria; RBCs, red blood cells; SCA, sickle cell anemia.

TABLE 10-4 Important Extrinsic Causes of Hemolytic Anemia

Disorder	Mechanism	Blood Smear	Characteristic Labs
Warm autoimmune hemolytic anemia	IgG antibodies bind to RBCs at room temperature and cause hemolysis.	Spherocytes	↑ MCHC; positive direct Coomb's test for IgG at room temperature
Cold autoimmune hemolytic anemia (cold agglutin disease)	IgM antibodies or complement (C3) binds to RBCs at cooler temperatures and causes hemolysis.	No specific findings	↑ MCHC, positive direct Coomb's test for anti-C3 at cooler temperatures
Microangiopathic hemolytic anemia	Physical injury to RBCs.	Schistocytes and helmet cells	↓ platelets
Malaria	Plasmodium parasites destroy RBCs.	Parasites inside RBCs	Antigen tests available but not first-line

Intravascular hemolysis: Hemolysis in the bloodstream can cause urinary hemosiderin (pink) and schistocytes on peripheral smear.

Extravascular hemolysis: The spleen or liver "pluck" out the RBCs. Splenomegaly and spherocytes are commonly seen.

All types of hemolysis can cause jaundice, increased indirect bilirubin, increased LDH, ↓ haptoglobin.

What is the most likely cause of hemolytic anemia in this patient?

Glucose 6 phosphate dehydrogenase (G6PD) deficiency is the most likely diagnosis in this patient with bite cells and Heinz bodies on peripheral smear (see Table 10-3). This X-linked disorder occurs in 10% of African-American men. G6PD deficiency is typically asymptomatic unless the patient undergoes oxidative stress (infection, diabetic ketoacidosis, and certain sulfa drugs like trimethoprim-sulfamethoxazole).

> **Favism:** Fava bean ingestion can cause severe hemolysis in this subtype of G6PD deficiency, which occurs mainly in Mediterranean men.

What is the next step in management?

The acute hemolytic anemia is usually self-limited and resolves with supportive care. In the long term, the key recommendation is to avoid precipitants.

How can you confirm the diagnosis?

G6PD assays that demonstrate reduced NADPH formation can confirm the diagnosis. The test is often falsely negative during acute hemolysis because the defective RBCs have been lysed. Consider testing this patient 2 to 3 months after the acute episode.

Alternative 10.4.1

An 18-year-old man presents with chronic fatigue. Vital signs are normal. Laboratory studies indicate the patient has a hemolytic anemia. In addition, mean corpuscular Hb concentration (MCHC) is increased. The patient's peripheral blood smear shows sphere-shaped RBCs with no central pallor.

What is the next step in management?

The peripheral smear contains numerous spherocytes. Both hereditary spherocytosis (HS) and warm autoimmune hemolytic anemia (AIHA) can cause increased MCHC and spherocytosis. Obtain osmotic fragility and Coomb's test to distinguish between these two disorders.

> **Positive Coomb's test:** RBCs agglutinate when antibodies or complement is added to blood sample.
> **Positive osmotic fragility test:** RBCs rupture easily when exposed to dilute saline.

Osmotic fragility test is positive, and Coomb's test is negative.

What is the diagnosis?

The patient has HS. In this autosomal dominant condition, abnormalities in RBC membrane proteins lead to decreased RBC surface area but not RBC volume. As a result, RBCs assume a spherical shape. Spherical RBCs become trapped in the spleen and are destroyed by splenic macrophages. The preferred treatment for anemic patients with HS is splenectomy.

> **Gallstones:** This common complication of HS due to chronic hyperbilirubinemia can be prevented by splenectomy.

Alternative 10.4.2

A 34-year-old woman with a history of systemic lupus erythematosus (SLE) presents with fatigue. On physical exam, she appears jaundiced. Laboratory studies reveal hemolytic anemia with spherocytosis on the peripheral smear. Osmotic fragility test is negative. Direct Coomb's test demonstrates RBC agglutination at room temperature (37°C) in response to IgG antibodies.

What is the diagnosis?

The patient has warm AIHA. Important causes of warm AIHA can be remembered with the mnemonic "***DIAL***": **D**rugs, (e.g., penicillin), **I**diopathic, **A**utoimmune disorders (particularly SLE), and **L**ymphoproliferative disorders (particularly chronic lymphocytic leukemia).

What is the next step in management?

First-line therapy for warm AIHA is PRBCs (if the patient is unstable) and urgent systemic corticosteroids. Also treat the underlying cause. If hemolytic anemia persists, consider splenectomy.

Alternative 10.4.3

A 22-year-old man complains of fever, sore throat, and fatigue over the last 3 days. Physical exam is significant for splenomegaly, cervical adenopathy, and jaundice. The fingertips and toes are dark purple. Pertinent laboratory findings are positive monospot test and hemolytic anemia.

What diagnosis should you suspect?

Hemolytic anemia and dark purple discoloration of the distal extremities in a patient with infectious mononucleosis should raise suspicion for cold AIHA (cold agglutinin disease). Other important causes of cold AIHA are mycoplasma pneumonia infection and lymphoproliferative disorders. Many cases are idiopathic.

> **Acrocyanosis:** In cold AIHA, distal extremities can turn dark purple in response to cold.

> **WARM** AIHA, Ig**G**: **WARM** weather is **G**reat (37°C).
> **COLD** agglutinins, **COMPLE**ment, Ig**M**: Cold weather is **COMPLE**tely **M**iserable (32°C).

Direct Coomb's test is positive for IgM binding to RBC membranes at 32°C.

How is cold AIHA treated?

First-line therapy for cold AIHA is to avoid cold temperatures. If the patient has severe symptoms refractory to cold avoidance, consider rituximab or cyclophosphamide. Also, treat the underlying cause.

> **Plasmapheresis:** Consider if a patient with severe cold AIHA requires surgery.

Alternative 10.4.4

A 32-year-old man presents with episodes of dark urine when he wakes up in the morning. The urine gets clearer over the day. He also reports erectile dysfunction and brief episodes of epigastric pain and dysphagia. On physical exam, there is jaundice and pallor. Laboratory studies indicate that he has a hemolytic anemia. On urinalysis, the sediment is clear and the supernatant is red. Urine dipstick is heme-positive with clear plasma. There are no characteristic findings on peripheral blood smear. Coomb's test is negative.

What diagnosis should you suspect?

Episodes of dark urine on waking along with hemolytic anemia should raise suspicion for PNH. Urinalysis demonstrates hemoglobinuria, which increases the likelihood of this rare condition. Confirm the diagnosis using flow cytometry to detect deficiency of GPI-linked proteins.

> **Ham's test, sucrose lysis test:** older tests for PNH (before flow cytometry was available).

Flow cytometry confirms the diagnosis.

What are possible complications of PNH?

Remember complications of PNH with the acronym "***TERM***":

1. **T**hrombosis: PNH increases risk of venous thrombosis in almost every organ (e.g., cerebral veins, hepatic vein, etc.).
2. **E**sophageal spasm and **E**rectile dysfunction: One possible mechanism is that free plasma Hb soaks up nitric oxide (smooth muscle relaxant).

3. **R**enal failure: PNH can cause acute renal failure as a result of massive hemoglobinuria or CRF from iron overload as a result of chronic hemolytic anemia.
4. **M**DS and leukemia: GPI-linked protein deficiency arises in hematopoietic stem cells, so patients have increased risk of MDS and leukemia.

How is anemia of PNH treated?

First-line therapy is supportive care (iron and folic acid supplements, PRBCs when necessary). Options for patients with severe anemia include systemic corticosteroids, EPO, danazol (androgenic hormone), eculizumab (anti-complement antibody), and stem cell transplantation.

Alternative 10.4.5

A 24-year-old man presents with a 3-day history of persistent fever, chills, fatigue, and myalgias. He recently returned from a monsoon wedding in India. Physical exam is significant for pallor, jaundice, and splenomegaly. Temperature is 102°F. Laboratory studies reveal the patient has a hemolytic anemia. Figure 10-10 is the patient's Giemsa-stained peripheral smear.

What is the diagnosis?

Suspect plasmodium infection (malaria) when a patient with a history of travel to an endemic area presents with fever and hemolytic anemia. This infection is transmitted by the Anopheles mosquito. Giemsa-stained thin and thick smears showing the parasites inside RBCs confirm the diagnosis.

What species of plasmodium is most likely to have infected this patient?

Noncyclical fever and symptomatic hemolytic anemia is most likely caused by *Plasmodium falciparum* infection. *P. vivax*, *P. ovale*, and *P. malariae* tend to cause cyclical fever (temperature spikes every 49 to 72 hours) and less severe hemolytic anemia.

How is P. falciparum infection treated?

Most cases of *P. falciparum* malaria are resistant to chloroquine. The most commonly prescribed regimen is quinine sulfate plus doxycycline or clindamycin. Alternative options are atovaquone-proguanil and mefloquine.

> **Primaquine**: G6PD deficiency was first discovered when this older antimalarial drug caused hemolytic anemia in African-American soldiers during World War II.

> **Babesiosis**: This uncommon parasite infection is transmitted by the deer tick. Clinical manifestations are similar to malaria. Classic finding on Giemsa-stained peripheral smear is a tetrad of organisms inside RBCs. Treat with quinine + clindamycin or atovaquone + azithromycin.

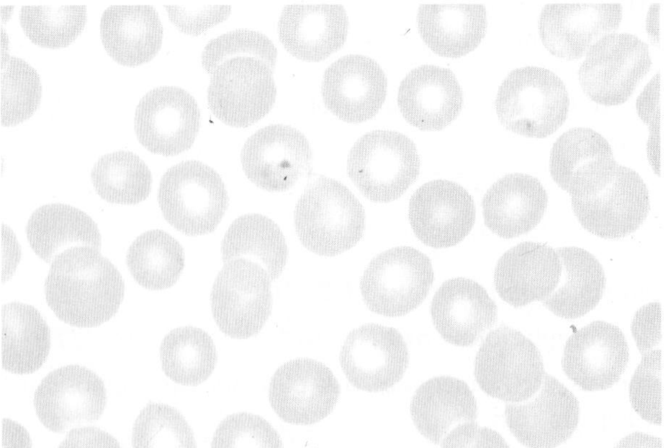

FIGURE 10–10 Giemsa-stained blood smear showing malaria. From Anderson S. *Anderson's Atlas of Hematology*, Lippincott Williams & Wilkins, 2003.

CASE 10–5 COMPLICATIONS OF SICKLE CELL ANEMIA

An 18-year-old African-American man with homozygous SCA presents for an initial evaluation. He recently moved from California to Boston. He is currently asymptomatic. His medical records mention that he had a splenectomy at age 3 years.

What was the most likely indication for splenectomy?

Splenic sequestration crisis is often the earliest sign of SCA, and it is the most common indication for splenectomy in these patients. This condition occurs because deformed RBCs become trapped in the splenic vasculature (Table 10-5). RBC entrapment leads to decreased RBCs in peripheral blood, which activates increased RBC production. Presenting signs are an enlarging spleen and hemolytic anemia. Splenectomy is indicated because splenic sequestration can cause life-threatening circulatory collapse.

TABLE 10–5 Complications of Sickle Cell Anemia

Anemia
• **Chronic hemolytic anemia:** ↑ Destruction of sickle-shaped RBCs.
• **Splenic sequestration crisis:** Caused by occlusion of sickle-shaped RBCs in splenic vessels (leads to ↓ RBCs in peripheral blood).
• **Aplastic crisis:** Parvovirus B12 (transient PRCA) is the most common cause in children and adolescents. Extensive bone marrow infarction by sickle-shaped RBCs (pancytopenia) is an important cause in adults.
Central Nervous System
• **Stroke:** Caused by occlusion of sickle-shaped RBCs in cerebral vessels.
Heart
• **High-output heart failure:** Caused by anemia or iron overload from chronic PRBC transfusions.
Lungs
• **Acute chest syndrome:** Major cause is occlusion of pulmonary vessels by sickle-shaped RBCs. Other causes are pulmonary thromboembolism, fat embolism (from bone marrow infarct) or infection.
• **Pneumonia:** Asplenic SCA patients have ↑ risk of infection with encapsulated organisms (e.g., *Streptococcus pneumoniae, Haemophilus influenza, Staphylococcus aureus* and *Klebsiella pneumonia*)
Gastrointestinal
• **Pigment gallstones:** Chronic hemolysis leads to ↑ bilirubin turnover.
• **Hepatic sequestration crisis:** Caused by occlusion of hepatic vessels by sickle-shaped RBCs.
• **Bowel infarct:** Caused by occlusion of gut vessels by sickle-shaped RBCs.
Kidneys
• **Painless hematuria:** Caused by mild papillary blood vessel occlusion. Suspect renal papillary necrosis if the patient has gross hematuria.
• **Acute and chronic renal failure:** Multiple causes.
Genitals
• **Priapism:** Prolonged erection caused by occlusion of penile vasculature by sickle-shaped RBCs.
Bones
• **Dactylitis:** Hand and foot swelling caused by occlusion of blood vessels supplying metacarpals and metatarsals. Most common initial symptom of SCA (occurs in infancy).
• **Painful crises:** Pain in multiple bones caused by occlusion of blood vessels supplying bones. Visceral blood vessels (abdomen, chest, etc.) can also be occluded during a pain crisis.
• **Avascular necrosis:** Caused by occlusion of blood vessels supplying bone.
• **Osteomyelitis:** Caused by infection by encapsulated organisms. Most common pathogen is salmonella followed by *S. aureus*.
Eyes
• **Retinal infarcts:** Caused by occlusion of blood vessels supplying the eyes.
• **Proliferative retinopathy**
Skin
• **Leg ulcers:** Caused by occlusion of skin vasculature by sickle-shaped cells.

Abbreviations: PRCA, pure red cell aplasia

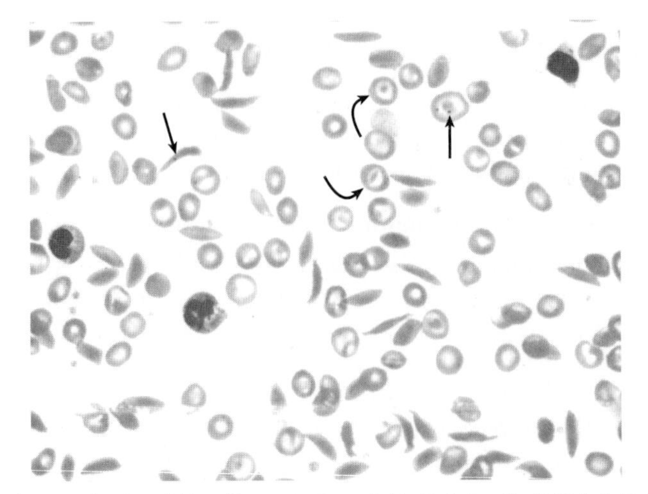

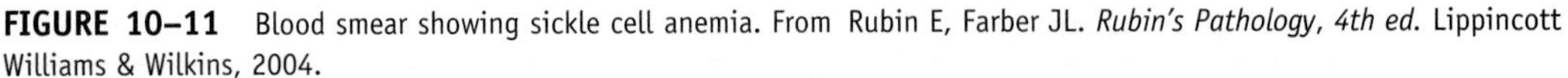

FIGURE 10–11 Blood smear showing sickle cell anemia. From Rubin E, Farber JL. *Rubin's Pathology, 4th ed.* Lippincott Williams & Wilkins, 2004.

> Splenic entrapment causes fibrosis and shrinking of the spleen by age 5 years, so SCA patients with no splenic sequestration crisis/splenectomy are functionally asplenic.

> **Howell-Jolly bodies:** Individual, round, red-purple inclusions in the periphery of RBCs. Seen in patients with functional or anatomic asplenia.

What testing and management is recommended for this asymptomatic patient?

1. CBC and peripheral smear: Monitor at every visit (Fig. 10-11).
2. Retinal examination: Refer to an ophthalmologist or optometrist annually.
3. Folic acid supplements.

> Granulocyte colony-stimulating factor (G-CSF) is absolutely contraindicated in patients with SCA.

Two months later, the patient presents to the emergency department with pain in his abdomen, chest, elbow, back, and knees. He has experienced similar episodes before. Vital signs are temperature 38.1°C, pulse 120 bpm, respirations 25/min, and blood pressure 120/80. Oxygen saturation is 99% on room air. CBC and peripheral smear are similar to baseline values.

What is the most likely complication?

Suspect acute pain crisis when a patient with SCA presents with pain in multiple sites. Acute pain crisis is the most common cause of hospitalization in SCA. Pain results from widespread vascular occlusion by sickle-shaped RBCs. Cold temperature and infection are common precipitants. The bones are the most common sites of pain. Other common sites are the abdomen and chest. Fever, tachycardia, and tachypnea are common physical findings.

> No precipitating cause is identified in >50% of acute pain crises.

How are acute painful episodes managed?

Obtain CXR, CBC, urinalysis, urine culture, and blood culture to rule out infection. If laboratory studies are negative, assess severity of pain using a visual or numeric scale:

1. Moderate to severe pain: Treat with IV fluids and opioids (first-line drug is morphine).
2. Mild pain: Treat with oral fluids and nonopioid analgesics (NSAIDs or acetaminophen).

Oxygen: Commonly administered during acute painful episodes; however, there is no evidence that supplemental oxygen is beneficial in the absence of hypoxemia.

If pain pattern is different from prior episodes or lasts >7 days, conduct a more detailed investigation to rule out other causes of chest pain, back pain, etc.

The patient's symptoms resolve with IV fluids and morphine, and he is discharged home. One week later, he presents with dyspnea and pleuritic chest pain. Physical exam is significant for bilateral crackles in the lower lobes. Vital signs are temperature 37.5°C, pulse 120 bpm, respirations 27/min, and blood pressure 125/85. CXR demonstrates patchy lower lobe infiltrates. Hb is 2 mg/dL below baseline.

What complication should you suspect?

This SCA patient with sudden onset of dyspnea, tachycardia, pleuritic chest pain, and pulmonary infiltrates meets diagnostic criteria for acute coronary syndrome (ACS). Approximately half of ACS cases are precipitated by an acute pain crisis. ACS is a broad description. The underlying cause of ACS is typically one or more of the following:

1. Occlusion of pulmonary vasculature by sickle-shaped cells (most common cause)
2. Atelectasis
3. Pneumonia
4. Pulmonary thromboembolism or fat embolism (from bone marrow infarct)

Obtain CXR, blood, and sputum cultures in all SCA patients with fever, chest pain, or respiratory symptoms (dyspnea, hypoxia, abnormal lung exam, etc.).

Diagnostic criteria for ACS: New infiltrate on CXR plus ≥1 of the following: pleuritic chest pain, increased work of breathing (tachypnea, retractions, etc.), temperature >38.5°C, or hypoxemia compared to baseline.

ACS is the second most common cause of hospitalization and the most common cause of death in adolescents and adults with SCA.

How is ACS managed?

Remember the treatment for ACS with the mnemonic: "***FAT ASS***":

1. **F**luids: Correct dehydration and then administer maintenance fluids.
2. **A**nalgesia: First-line is ketorolac. Consider morphine for severe pain.
3. **T**ransfusion: Administer PRBCs to maintain Hb >11 g/dL and HCT >30%.
4. **A**ntibiotics: Treat empirically with a third-generation cephalosporin (like ceftriaxone) and a macrolide (like azithromycin).
5. **S**upplemental oxygen: Maintain oxygen saturation >92%.
6. **S**pirometry: Patients receiving supplemental oxygen should perform incentive spirometry to prevent atelectasis.

Hydroxyurea: May decrease SCA complications by inducing increased HbF. Major indications are one or more episodes of ACS or multiple episodes of acute pain crisis.

Exchange transfusion: Remove the patient's RBCs and platelets, then transfuse donor RBCs and platelets; this method is indicated in ACS if vital signs or oxygen saturation deteriorate despite supportive therapy.

Two years later, the patient presents with a painful erection that has not returned to the flaccid state for the last 4 hours.

How would you treat this patient?

An erection that lasts >30 minutes is called priapism. Priapism that lasts >3 hours is a urological emergency. First-line therapy for priapism lasting <6 hours is oral terbutaline or pseudoephedrine. If the erection does not resolve within 30 minutes, perform aspiration of the corpus cavernosa (to remove clogged blood) and administer intracavernous α-agonists.

> **Chronic PRBC transfusion:** Consider if a SCA patient has one or more episodes of priapism or stroke. Most SCA patients do not require chronic PRBC transfusions.

What are other common causes of priapism?

1. Pharmacological injection therapy: Injection of greater-than-recommended doses of penile drugs for erectile dysfunction is the most common cause of priapism.
2. Psychiatric medications: Trazodone is the most frequently implicated drug.

Six months later, the patient presents with a 7-day history of fatigue and dyspnea on exertion. Physical exam is significant for pallor and tachycardia. He is afebrile. CXR is unchanged from baseline. Hb is 3 mg/dL, and HCT is 14%. Reticulocyte count is 0. Platelet and WBC counts are normal.

What complication should you suspect?

PRCA in a SCA patient is most commonly caused by a Parvovirus B19 infection. The next diagnostic step is to obtain serum IgM and IgG antibodies against Parvovirus B19. Positive IgM usually indicates acute infection. Treatment is PRBC transfusions until the patient's immune system clears the infection. After viral clearance, patients are immune from further infection (negative IgM and positive IgG).

Five years later, he presents with ulcers on his medial malleolus and anterior tibia.

How are these ulcers treated?

Leg ulcers are a common complication of SCA. They occur most frequently at the anterior tibia, medial malleolus, and lateral malleolus. Initial therapy is debridement of nonviable tissue. Use wet to dry dressings or hydrocolloid dressings to facilitate debridement. Once debridement is complete, wrap the patient's leg in an Unna boot (contains nitric oxide) to facilitate healing.

What complications commonly occur in patients with sickle cell trait?

Like homozygous SCA, sickle cell trait is predominantly found in African Americans. Patients with sickle cell trait have one abnormal gene (HbS) and one normal gene. They are usually asymptomatic and do not have anemia. They do, however, have a higher incidence of urinary tract infections than the general population. Also, African-American men with sickle cell trait have increased risk of renal medullary carcinoma.

> **HbSC disease, sickle α-thalassemia, and sickle β-thalassemia:** Patients are symptomatic but complications are less severe than homozygous SCA.

CASE 10–6 ISOLATED THROMBOCYTOPENIA

During routine screening of an asymptomatic 27-year-old white woman, platelet count is found to be 40,000/μL. RBC and WBC counts are normal. Physical exam is normal. Figure 10-12 is the patient's peripheral smear.

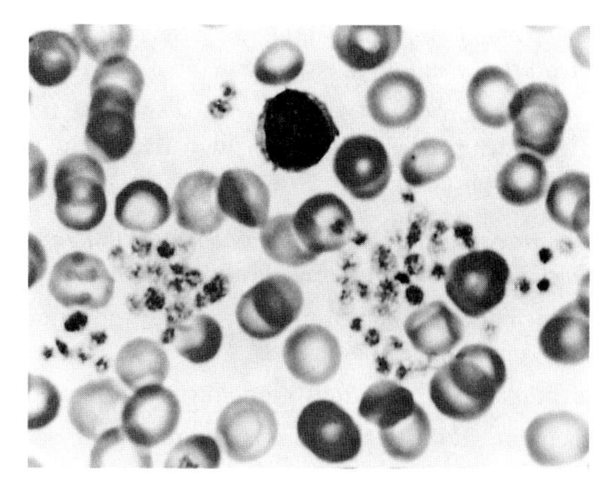

FIGURE 10–12 Blood smear showing pseudothrombocytopenia (clumped platelets). From McClatchey KD. *Clinical Laboratory Medicine, 2nd ed.* Lippincott Williams & Wilkins, 2002.

What are the clinical manifestations of thrombocytopenia?

Thrombocytopenia is often asymptomatic unless platelet levels fall to <20,000/μL (Table 10-6). Clinical manifestations in these patients are caused by increased bleeding risk:

1. Mucosal bleeding: Heavy menstrual periods, frequent nosebleeds, and gingival bleeding are common findings; GI bleeding is less frequent.
2. Cutaneous bleeding: Bleeding into skin manifests as petechiae or ecchymoses (larger purple patches that resemble a bruise).
3. Intracranial bleeding: This is a rare but serious complication of thrombocytopenia.

↓ **Platelets and IDA** can occur with increased mucocutaneous bleeding.
↓ **Platelets and megaloblastic anemia** can occur in vitamin B12 or folate deficiency.

Petechiae versus telangiectasias: Both appear as painless red-purple dots. Unlike telangiectasias, petechiae do not blanch when a glass slide is applied to the lesion.

What is the most likely diagnosis in this patient?

The initial step in the evaluation of any patient with thrombocytopenia is to examine the peripheral smear. This patient's smear contains a number of clumped platelets. The most likely diagnosis is pseudothrombocytopenia. This laboratory artifact commonly occurs when EDTA is used to anticoagulate the blood specimen. The next step is to repeat platelet measurement with citrate instead of EDTA anticoagulation. If platelet count is normal, no further workup is necessary.

TABLE 10–6 Thrombocytopenia and Risk of Mucocutaneous Bleeding

Platelets/μL	Bleeding Risk
>100,000	No ↑ risk
50,000–100,000	↑ Risk with major trauma; may proceed with general surgery
20,000–50,000	↑ Risk with minor trauma or general surgery
<20,000	↑ Risk of spontaneous bleeding
<10,000	↑ Risk of spontaneous, life-threatening bleeding

Adapted from Sabatine M. *Pocket Medicine*, 2nd ed.

What cause of thrombocytopenia would you suspect if the patient received 16 units of PRBCs a few hours ago after a motorcycle accident?

PRBCs do not contain any platelets, so massive PRBC transfusion causes dilutional thrombocytopenia. Consider platelet transfusion in patients who receive >20 units of PRBCs to prevent bleeding complications.

What are common causes of isolated thrombocytopenia in a patient with no evidence for pseudothrombocytopenia or dilutional thrombocytopenia?

Thrombocytopenia can result from decreased production, increased destruction, or splenic sequestration. Important causes are:

1. **Viral infections**: HIV, infectious mononucleosis, hepatitis C virus, and herpes simplex virus.
2. **Drugs**: heparin, GPIIb/IIIA inhibitors, quinine, gold, and sulfa drugs.
3. **Autoimmune disorders**: SLE, rheumatoid arthritis, etc.

> The most common cause of thrombocytopenia in intensive care unit (ICU) patients is septic shock.

What disorder would you suspect if the patient with isolated thrombocytopenia has no evidence for pseudothrombocytopenia, dilutional thrombocytopenia, viral infections, autoimmune disorders, or use of drugs associated with thrombocytopenia?

Idiopathic thrombocytopenia purpura (ITP) is a diagnosis of exclusion in patients with otherwise unexplained isolated thrombocytopenia. ITP is most likely caused by autoantibodies against platelets. The majority of affected patients are women.

> **Anti-platelet antibodies** are not seen in all patients with ITP, so this test is not used for diagnosis.

How is ITP treated?

No treatment is necessary for asymptomatic patients with platelet counts >20,000/μL. First-line therapy for symptomatic patients or those with platelet counts <20,000/μL is corticosteroids. If platelet count remains <20,000/μL despite corticosteroids, consider rituximab or cyclophosphamide. Treatment options for ITP refractory to first- and second-line drugs are IV immunoglobulin (IVIG) and splenectomy.

Alternative 10.6.1

Thirty hours after initiating heparin in a patient diagnosed with deep vein thrombosis (DVT), the platelet levels fall to 110,000/μL. Baseline platelets were 200,000/μL.

What is the next step in management?

Type 1 heparin-induced thrombocytopenia (HIT) causes a small drop in the platelet count within 2 days of heparin administration. This condition is not clinically significant and platelet levels tend to remain >100,000/μL. The optimal management for this patient who needs anticoagulation is to continue heparin. Platelet levels should return to baseline with continued treatment.

Alternative 10.6.2

Four days after initiating heparin and warfarin in a patient diagnosed with DVT, the platelet levels fall to 35,000/μL.

What complication should you suspect?

Suspect type 2 HIT in patients with a drop in platelet counts 4 days to 2 weeks after initiation of heparin. Because type 2 HIT is an immune-mediated disorder associated with platelet activation, the major clinical problem is thrombosis. Bleeding is not a significant problem with type 2 HIT because platelet counts rarely fall to <20,000/μL.

What is the next step in management?

Discontinue all exposure to heparin, including heparin flushes and heparin-bonded catheters. Also, discontinue warfarin until the thrombocytopenia resolves. This patient has a very recently diagnosed pulmonary embolism and requires some ongoing anticoagulation. Consider a direct thrombin inhibitor such as lepirudin or argatroban. Reinitiate warfarin when platelet levels are >100,000/μL, but do not use warfarin in the absence of other anticoagulants.

> **Serotonin release assay**: This is the gold standard to diagnose HIT type 2, but it has a slow turnaround time. Do not delay discontinuing heparin while waiting for the assay results.

Alternative 10.6.3

A 32-year-old woman is diagnosed with DVT. Past history is significant for three spontaneous abortions (miscarriages). There is no family history of thrombosis. Platelet count is 30,000/μL. Hb, HCT, and WBC counts are normal.

What diagnosis should you suspect?

Suspect anti-phospholipid antibody syndrome (APLA) in patients with the triad of thrombosis, thrombocytopenia, and recurrent fetal loss. This acquired disorder can be idiopathic (50% of cases) or secondary to syphilis, SLE, or another autoimmune condition. Although inherited thrombophilias can also cause thrombosis and recurrent fetal loss, thrombocytopenia and negative family history make them less likely (see Chapter 2: Cardiology).

How is APLA diagnosed?

One or more of the following must be positive on at least two occasions 6 weeks apart:

1. Anti-cardiolipin antibodies (IgA or IgM)
2. Anti-β2 glycoprotein 1 (IgA or IgM)
3. Lupus anticoagulant

What tests would you order if the patient with recurrent fetal loss had no thrombosis, thrombocytopenia, and no specific findings on history and physical examination?

Initial laboratory tests for recurrent unexplained fetal loss are:

1. Tests for inherited thrombophilia (see Chapter 2: Cardiology)
2. Tests for APLA
3. Thyroid-stimulating hormone and thyroid peroxidase test (to rule out Grave's disease)
4. Follicle-stimulating hormone and estradiol (to rule out decreased ovarian reserve)
5. Ultrasound of the uterus (to rule out structural abnormalities of the uterus)

CASE 10–7 THROMBOCYTOPENIA AND HEMOLYTIC ANEMIA

A 37-year-old, previously healthy African-American woman is brought to the emergency department for evaluation of acutely altered mental status. During the evaluation, she appears confused. She is not oriented to place or time. Vital signs are temperature 38.8°C, pulse 90 bpm, respirations 12/min, and blood pressure 120/80. CBC is significant for anemia and thrombocytopenia. Reticulocyte count is 7%. LDH and indirect bilirubin are increased. Figure 10-13 is the patient's peripheral smear. Serum creatinine is 3 mg/dL.

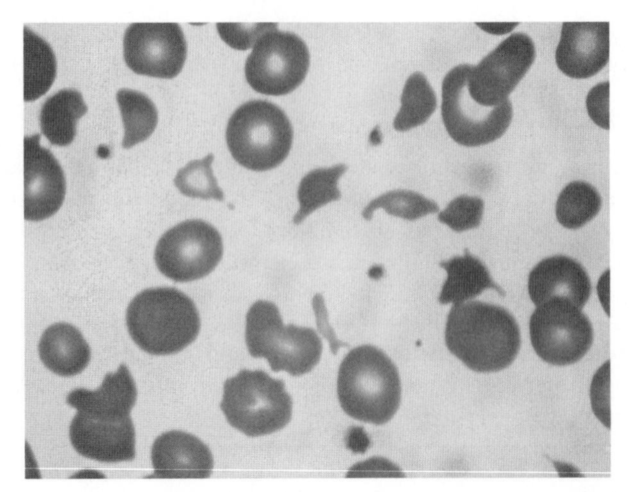

FIGURE 10–13 Blood smear showing schistocytes and thrombocytopenia purpura. From Rubin E, Farber JL. *Rubin's Pathology, 4th ed.* Lippincott Williams & Wilkins, 2004.

What significant findings are present on the peripheral smear?

The peripheral smear demonstrates numerous helmet cells and schistocytes (fragmented RBCs). These findings are indicative of microangiopathic hemolytic anemia (MAHA). There is also a paucity of platelets (thrombocytopenia).

> **March hemoglobinemia**: Prolonged marching or jogging can cause mechanical trauma to RBCs in blood vessels of lower extremities, leading to schistocyte formation. CBC abnormalities do not usually occur.

What is the most likely diagnosis?

This patient has the classic pentad of TTP/HUS (mnemonic: "***FART'N***"): **F**ever, microangiopathic hemolytic **A**nemia, acute **R**enal failure, **T**hrombocytopenia, and **N**eurological symptoms. In this disorder, increased formation of platelet thrombi leads to thrombocytopenia. Platelet thrombi occlude blood vessels, so RBCs are mechanically damaged as they pass through occluded blood vessels (MAHA).

> **Thrombocytopenia purpura (TTP)**: Neurological symptoms but minimal renal failure.
> **Hemolytic uremic syndrome (HUS)**: Acute renal failure but minimal neurologic signs.
> **TTP/HUS**: Distinction is not possible in most patients (both ARF and neurological signs).

What causes TTP/HUS?

Most cases of TTP/HUS are idiopathic. Occasionally, patients have a known risk factor like enterohemorrhagic *Escherichia coli* infection or recent stem cell transplantation.

> **Enterohemorrhagic *E. coli***: This bacteria causes HUS (one of the few instances where distinction between TTP and HUS is possible). Suspect if a patient has a history of bloody diarrhea and/or consumption of undercooked meat.

What is the next step in management?

Order coagulation studies to rule out disseminated intravascular coagulation (DIC). DIC is the other major disorder associated with MAHA and thrombocytopenia. DIC typically causes increased prothrombin time (PT), increased partial thromboplastin time (PTT), and decreased fibrinogen (Table 10-7). These values are normal in TTP/HUS.

> Dyad of MAHA and thrombocytopenia are sufficient to initiate treatment for TTP/HUS.

Coagulation studies are normal.

TABLE 10–7 Coagulation Tests Findings in Bleeding Disorders/Coagulopathies

	Platelets	PT	PTT	BT	FDPs (such as D-dimer)
Thrombocytopenia	↓	↔	↔	↑	↔
Thrombocytosis	↑	↔	↑/↔	↑/↔	↔
Abnormal platelet function	↔	↔	↔	↑	↔
vWD	↔	↔	↑/↔	↑	↔
Hemophilia A or B, heparin	↔	↔	↑	↔	↔
DIC	↓	↑	↑	↑	↑
Early liver disease	↔	↑	↔	↔	↔
Advanced liver disease	↓	↑	↑	↑	↔
Vitamin K deficiency	↔	↑	↑/↔	↔	↔
Warfarin	↔	↑	↑/↔	↔	↔
Heparin	↔	↔	↑	↔	↔
Thrombolytics	↔	↔	↑/↔	↔	↑

Abbreviations: DIC, disseminated intravascular coagulation; FDP, fibrin degradation products; PT, prothrombin time; PTT, partial thromboplastin time; vWD, von Willebrand disease; ↔, normal; BT, Bleeding Time.

How is TTP/HUS treated?

First-line therapy is plasma exchange. Also initiate corticosteroids unless a specific cause is apparent. Continue daily plasma exchange until platelet count >100,000/μL and LDH is normal (indicates cessation of hemolysis). Prognosis is good with prompt initiation of therapy. Without treatment, TTP/HUS is rapidly fatal in approximately 90% of patients.

Plasma exchange (plasmapheresis): Remove blood from the patient's body. Remove plasma from the blood cells. Add donor plasma to blood cells. Return the mixture to the body.

Platelets are contraindicated in TTP/HUS.

Alternative 10.7.1

A 27-year-old G1P0001 woman in her 32nd week of pregnancy presents with right upper quadrant pain, nausea, and malaise. On physical exam, there is right upper quadrant tenderness, jaundice, and pallor. Blood pressure is 160/100. Abnormal laboratory studies include decreased Hb, decreased HCT, decreased platelets, increased RI, increased indirect bilirubin, increased LDH, and increased transaminases. WBC count, coagulation studies, and fibrinogen are normal.

What is the most likely diagnosis?

The patient has HELLP syndrome (**H**emolytic anemia, **E**levated **L**iver enzymes, **L**ow **P**latelets). This condition is most common during the third trimester of pregnancy and may represent a severe form of preeclampsia. Treatment is immediate delivery.

The patient does not wish to deliver the baby at this time and leaves the hospital against medical advice. She presents to the emergency department 36 hours later with worsening abdominal pain and nausea. Physical exam is significant for petechiae and ecchymoses. Laboratory abnormalities include hemolytic anemia with schistocytes on peripheral smear, decreased platelets, increased PT, increased PTT, increased fibrinogen, increased transaminases, and increased creatinine.

What is the diagnosis?

Obstetric complications like HELLP syndrome are an important cause of acute DIC. In this disorder, there is widespread activation of the coagulation cascade. Clinical and laboratory findings in DIC include:

1. MAHA: Widespread clotting leads to occlusion of blood vessels.
2. Thrombocytopenia and mucocutaneous bleeding: Widespread activation of the coagulation cascade leads to platelet consumption.
3. Increased PT, increased PTT, and decreased fibrinogen: Widespread activation of the clotting cascade leads to consumption of clotting factors and fibrinogen.
4. Increased D-dimer and fibrin degradation products: End product of the coagulation cascade is fibrin.
5. Acute renal failure, acute liver failure, and stroke: Occlusion damages blood vessels supplying end organs.

What are the major causes of DIC?

Remember causes of DIC with the acronym "***STORM***": **S**epsis, **T**rauma (including surgery and burns), **O**bstetric complications, **R**BC transfusion reaction, and **M**alignancy.

How is acute DIC treated?

Acute DIC is associated with a very high mortality rate (40% to 80%). The most important component of management is to treat the underlying cause (in this case deliver the baby). Additional therapies are indicated in the following situations:

1. Platelets: Indications are platelet count $<20{,}000/\mu L$ or mucocutaneous bleeding.
2. Fresh frozen plasma (FFP): FFP, which contains all clotting factors, is indicated in actively bleeding patients with increased International Normalized Ratio (INR).
3. Cryoprecipitate: Contains fibrinogen, von Willebrand factor (vWF), and factors 8 and 13. Cryoprecipitate is indicated if fibrinogen <50 mg/dL (target ≥ 100 mg/dL).

> **Evan's syndrome**: Antibodies against RBCs and platelets cause AIHA and thrombocytopenia. Rare disorder. First-line therapy is steroids.

CASE 10–8 EASY BLEEDING WITH LITTLE OR NO THROMBOCYTOPENIA

A 22-year-old woman presents with a history of heavy menstrual periods. She has had frequent nosebleeds since childhood. She does not take any medications. She is an adopted child. There are no known medical conditions. On physical exam, there are petechiae and ecchymoses. There are no telangiectasias.

What is the next diagnostic step?

The initial screening tests in a patient with easy bleeding of unknown origin are platelet count, PT, and PTT.

PT, PTT, and platelet count are normal. The only abnormality on peripheral smear is microcytic anemia.

What is the differential diagnosis?

1. **Inherited platelet function abnormalities** (mnemonic: "***BAG***"): **B**enard-Soulier disease (decreased platelet adhesion due to decreased GPIb), **A**fibrinogenemia (decreased platelet aggregation due to decreased fibrinogen), **G**lanzmann's thrombasthenia (decreased platelet aggregation due to decreased GPIIb/IIIa).
2. **Acquired platelet function abnormalities**: Chronic kidney or liver disease, myeloproliferative or myelodysplastic disorders.

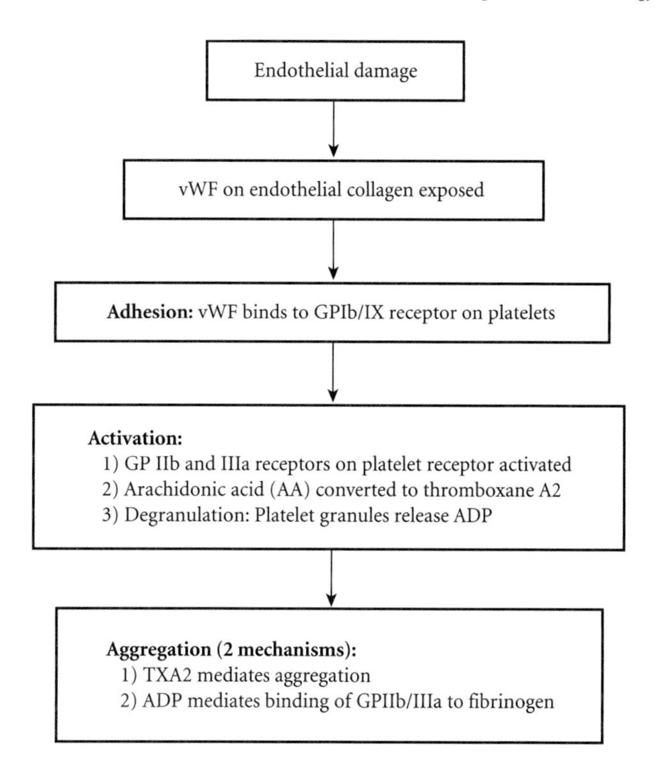

Anti-platelet drug class	Mechanism	Examples
Thienopyridines	Inhibit ADP	Clopidogrel and ticlopidine
NSAIDs	COX inhibitors prevention conversion of AA to TXA2	Aspirin, Naproxen, Ibuprofen
GPIIb/IIIa inhibitors	Inhibit GPIIb and IIIa receptors	Abciximab, Eptifibitide, Tirofiban

vWF: von Willebrand factor

FIGURE 10–14 Formation of platelet plugs and antiplatelet drugs.

3. **Drugs** (Fig. 10-14).
4. **Von Willebrand disease (vWD)**: Usually causes increased PTT, but sometimes PTT is normal.

> **PT**: ↑ if patient has ↓ clotting factors 2, 7, 5, or 10.
> **PTT**: ↑ if patient has ↓ in any clotting factor (except factor 7).

What is the next diagnostic step?

History, physical exam, and peripheral smear rule out drugs and MDS or myeloproliferative disorders. The next step is to assess platelet function using platelet function analyzer test (PFA-100). Also obtain serum chemistries and LFTs (to evaluate for liver or kidney disease).

> **Bleeding time**: A less sensitive alternative if PFA-100 test is not available.

Serum creatinine and LFTs are normal. PFA-100 is abnormal.

What is the next diagnostic step?

The next step is to order platelet aggregation studies (to detect an inherited platelet function abnormality) and tests to rule out vWD.

What tests help diagnose vWD?

Suspect vWF if any of the following tests are positive:

1. vWF antigen: positive in vWD
2. Ristocetin co-factor activity: measures vWF activity; decreased in vWD.
3. Ristocetin induced platelet aggregation (RIPA): decreased in vWD.
4. Factor 8: A second function of vWF is to carry factor VIII in the bloodstream, so factor VIII is often decreased in vWD (which is why PTT is often increased in vWD).

What are the different subtypes of vWD?

There are three major subtypes of this autosomal dominant condition:

Type 1: Mild decrease in vWF may cause increased bleeding during surgery or trauma but is otherwise asymptomatic. Type 1 is the most common and least severe subtype.

Type 2: Intermediate decrease in vWF (intermediate severity and frequency).

Type 3: Least common subtype (absent vWF leads to severe disease)

How is vWD treated?

First-line therapy for type 1 and type 2 vWD is desmopressin (DDAVP). If a trial of DDAVP increases vWF levels, use this drug whenever the patient is bleeding or prior to surgery. If the patient does not respond to DDAVP, consider Humate P (intermediate purity factor 8, which also contains vWF).

> **Type 3 vWD**: DDAVP is ineffective. First-line therapy is Humate P.

Alternative 10.8.1

A 22-year-old man requires extraction of his wisdom teeth. He recently emigrated from Sudan. He was separated from his family at the age of 5. During the procedure, he bleeds excessively and is referred for medical evaluation. On physical exam, there are two large ecchymoses. Review of systems is positive for joint pain. CBC is normal, PT is normal, but PTT is elevated.

What is the next step in diagnosis?

The next step in a patient with unexplained increase in PT or PTT is to perform a mixing study (mix patient's plasma 1:1 with normal plasma). If coagulation studies normalize, the patient has an inherited clotting factor deficiency (vWD or hemophilia). Otherwise, suspect an acquired clotting factor inhibitor such as heparin.

> **Thrombocytopenia and functional platelet disorders**: mucocutaneous bleeding.
> ↓ **Clotting factors**: deep tissue bleeding (large ecchymoses, hemarthroses, hematomas).
> ↓ **vWF**: leads to mucocutaneous bleeding; ↓ Factor VIII causes deep tissue bleeding.

Mixing study shows correction when normal plasma is mixed with the patient's plasma, so he is suspected to have an inherited coagulopathy (clotting factor deficiency).

What is the next diagnostic step?

Obtain vWF assays (positive only in vWD) and factor VIII levels (factor VIII coagulant, factor VIII antigen, and factor VIII vWF). In hemophilia A, factor VIII coagulant level is low, but other factor VIII levels are normal. In vWF all three levels are low. If all three factor VIII levels are normal, obtain factor IX coagulant level (decreased in hemophilia B).

vWF assay is negative. Factor VIII level is reduced.

How is hemophilia treated?

Both hemophilia A and B are inherited in an X-linked recessive pattern (hemophilia A is much more common). Most cases are detected in childhood, but milder cases may not be diagnosed until early adulthood. Management of hemophilia A is as follows:

1. Bleeding: DDAVP is the first line therapy in mild disease (>5% factor VIII). Factor VIII concentrates are first-line therapy in moderate to severe disease. Also, treat pain from hematomas or hemarthroses with non-NSAID analgesics.
2. Head trauma: Obtain CT scan to rule out intracranial bleed, even in minor trauma.
3. Pre-operative treatment: administer factor VIII until level is at least 30% to 50%.

> Hemophilia can also cause ↑ PTT that does not normalize after a mixing study. The mechanism is development of factor VIII antibodies after a blood transfusion.

> **Hemophilia B (Christmas disease)**: Treat with factor IX instead of factor VIII.

Alternative 10.8.2

A 70-year-old man is admitted to the ICU for severe pneumonia. He is placed on broad-spectrum antibiotics and mechanical ventilation. On his second day in the ICU, the nurse notices blood oozing from his catheter sites. Platelets and PTT are normal, but PT is prolonged.

What disorders commonly cause increased PT?

1. Early liver disease: The liver produces almost all clotting factors. Factor 7 is the first clotting factor to be reduced, so early liver disease causes prolonged PT. As liver disease advances, both PT and PTT are prolonged.
2. Vitamin K: Because vitamin K is necessary for synthesis of factors 2, 7, 9, and 10, as well as protein C and protein S, decreased vitamin K causes prolonged PT. Eventually, patients may also develop prolonged PTT (see Table 10-7). Another cause of isolated increase in PT is excess warfarin (which inhibits vitamin K).

> **Advanced liver disease**: Also causes anemia (with spur cells on peripheral smear) and thrombocytopenia (one mechanism is decreased thrombopoietin production by liver).

LFTs are normal.

What is the most likely diagnosis?

The major sources of vitamin K are dietary intake and synthesis by gut flora. This patient is nothing per oral (due to mechanical ventilation) and likely has gut flora suppression due to broad-spectrum antibiotics. Treatment is vitamin K replacement. Also consider FFP if the patient with vitamin K deficiency is bleeding.

CASE 10–9 TRANSFUSION REACTIONS

A 36-year-old woman has IDA caused by hereditary hemorrhagic telangiectasia. Hb is 6.8 mg/dL despite iron replacement. Her physician decides to transfuse two units of PRBCs. Thirty minutes into the transfusion, she complains of itching. Vital signs are normal.

What are the next steps in management?

Hb <7 mg/dL is an indication for PRBC transfusion (Table 10-8). The most common cause of itching and/or urticaria during a blood transfusion is a mild allergic reaction. However, pruritus can also be caused by a severe anaphylactic reaction. The next steps in management are as follows:

TABLE 10–8 Transfusion Therapy

Blood Product	Indications
PRBCs	• Any patient with Hb <7 mg/dL • Active bleeding with estimated blood loss ≥40% • Consider in patients with cardiopulmonary comorbidities and Hb <10 mg/dL
Platelets	• Any patient with platelets <10,000/μL • Bleeding disorder and platelets <20,000/μL • Preoperative patient with platelets <50,000/μL • Contraindicated in TTP/HUS, HIT, and HELLP
FFP	• Preoperative patient with PT >17 seconds • Multiple clotting factor deficiency (e.g., TTP/HUS, DIC, and advanced liver disease)
Irradiated blood products	• Immunosuppressed patient (risk of GVHD)
Leuko-reduced blood products	• History of anti-leukocyte antibody induced transfusion reaction (ANHFR, TRALI)
CMV-negative blood products	• Pregnant CMV-negative patients • HIV-positive patients • Pre- and posttransplant patients

Abbreviations: CMV, cytomegalovirus; FFP, fresh frozen plasma; GVHD, graft versus host disease; HELLP, obstetric complication (hemolytic anemia, elevated liver enzymes, and low platelet count); HIT, heparin-induced thrombocytopenia; HUS, hemolytic uremic syndrome; TRALI, transfusion-related acute lung injury; TTP, thrombocytopenia purpura;

Adapted from Sabatine M. *Pocket Medicine, 2nd ed.* Lippincott Williams and Wilkins, 2001.

1. Stop the transfusion.
2. Administer diphenhydramine (Benadryl).
3. Monitor for signs of anaphylaxis (Chapter 2: Cardiology).
4. If no signs of anaphylaxis develop, resume the transfusion.

PRBC transfusion pearls:

1. One unit of PRBCs raises Hb by approximately 1 g/dL and HCT by approximately 3% to 4%.
2. Do not infuse anything in the same line as PRBCs except normal saline.
3. Typical dose is two units over 1.5 to 2 hours.

The patient does not develop any signs of anaphylaxis, so the transfusion is resumed. Approximately 15 minutes before the transfusion is complete, she develops rigors (chills). Temperature is 38.7°C, pulse is 110 bpm, respirations are 15/min, blood pressure is 139/80, and oxygen saturation is 99% on room air.

What is the differential diagnosis?

The main causes of fever within 2 to 4 hours of starting the transfusion are:

1. **Acute nonhemolytic transfusion reaction** (**ANHTR**): Caused by preformed anti-leukocyte antibodies in the recipient's blood. In addition to fever, patients may experience tachycardia, tachypnea, dyspnea, or rigors. This self-limiting condition is the most common cause of fever soon after transfusion.
2. **Acute hemolytic transfusion reaction** (**AHTR**): Transfusion of ABO-incompatible RBCs as a result of clerical error leads to cytokine release and in vivo intravascular hemolysis. The classic triad of AHTR is fever, flank pain, and hemoglobinuria. Also, cytokines can cause

vasodilation (risk of hypotension and shock) and bronchoconstriction (risk of bronchoconstriction and respiratory collapse).

> **Transfusion-related acute lung injury (TRALI):** Although TRALI can cause fever within 2 to 4 hours of starting the transfusion, the predominant symptom is dyspnea.

What are the next steps in management?

Rule out AHTR in any patient with fever during or immediately after a transfusion even if ANHTR is more likely. Perform the following steps (mnemonic: "***Saturday Night Live***"):

1. **S**top the transfusion.
2. **N**ormal saline: Infuse normal saline to keep the IV line open, avoid hypotension, and maintain diuresis. Increase the rate of administration to 100 to 200 ml/hour if the patient has any sign of AHTR (hypotension, flank pain, pink urine, etc.).
3. **L**abs: Obtain CBC, type and crossmatch, and Coomb's test. Do not draw labs from the same IV line used for transfusion.

There is no hemolytic anemia. Coomb's test is negative. Type and crossmatch reveals no mismatch. She does not have any dyspnea.

What is the next step in management?

Treat ANHTR with NSAIDs or acetaminophen (for fever) ± meperidine (for chills). Consider leukocyte-reduced blood components for future transfusions.

> **AHTR:** Associated with hemolytic anemia, positive Coomb's test, and mismatched type and crossmatch. Treatment is aggressive fluid replacement to prevent shock.

During a follow-up examination 6 days after the transfusion, temperature is 38.4°C. On physical exam, there is mild scleral icterus and conjunctival pallor.

What is the next step in management?

The most likely cause of the patient's symptoms is delayed hemolytic transfusion reaction. This reaction typically occurs 5 to 7 days after the transfusion and presents with fever and mild hemolytic anemia. The cause is recipient antibodies against a mild RBC antigen encountered during a previous transfusion. Although no specific treatment is required, obtain CBC and perform Coomb's test to confirm the diagnosis. Also, identify the culprit antibody to avoid during future transfusions.

Four months later, the patient is involved in a motor vehicle accident and loses a large amount of blood. Blood pressure is 80/60. She receives 12 L of normal saline and 10 units of PRBCs. Blood pressure increases to 130/80. However, oxygen saturation begins to decrease, and she requires intubation. There are bilateral rales. There is 13 mm of jugular vein distension (JVD). CXR reveals bilateral infiltrates.

What is the next step in management?

Hypoxemia along with new pulmonary infiltrates and elevated JVD after large amounts of fluid and blood transfusions suggests that the patient has transfusion-associated circulatory overload (TRACO). Treat this hemodynamically stable patient with diuretics to relieve cardiogenic pulmonary edema.

> Do not withhold transfusion based on normal Hb and HCT immediately after blood loss. These values take 36 to 48 hours to accurately reflect patient's volume status.

The patient recovers from the accident and returns home. Two years later, she is admitted for transfusion of two units of PRBCs to treat IDA. During the transfusion, she begins to feel short of breath. Oxygen saturation falls to 92%. There are bilateral rales. JVD is not elevated.

Temperature is 38.3°C. The transfusion is stopped, and the patient begins to receive oxygen and normal saline. There is no evidence of hemolytic anemia or ABO mismatch. Coomb's test is negative. CXR demonstrates bilateral infiltrates.

What complication should you suspect?

Dyspnea, hypoxemia, bilateral chest infiltrates, and fever in the absence of massive transfusion or elevated JVD are most likely caused by TRALI. This condition results from donor blood anti-leukocyte antibodies attacking recipient WBCs. TRALI is a spectrum that ranges from mild cough and fever to symptoms like acute respiratory distress syndrome. Most patients recover in 3 to 4 days with supportive care (supplemental oxygen or mechanical ventilation). Use leuko-reduced blood components for future transfusions.

CASE 10–10 LEUKOCYTOSIS

A 65-year-old man presents with a 2-month history of fatigue and dyspnea on exertion. He also reports frequent nosebleeds in the last 2 months. On physical exam, there is conjuctival pallor and petechiae. WBC count is 20,000/μL, Hb is 8 mg/dL, and platelets are 40,000/μL.

What is the differential diagnosis?

Although a number of conditions can cause leukocytosis (Table 10-9), concurrent anemia and thrombocytopenia should raise suspicion for neoplastic WBC proliferation (Table 10-10). The differential diagnosis for a neoplastic process includes:

1. Lymphoma: A neoplastic WBC clone originates and proliferates in lymphoid organs (lymph nodes, spleen, and thymus). Lymphoma is broadly classified as Hodgkin's disease (HD) and NHL.
2. Leukemia: Neoplastic WBCs originate in bone marrow and proliferate in peripheral blood. Classified as acute myelogenous leukemia (AML), acute lymphocytic leukemia (ALL), chronic myelogenous leukemia (CML), and chronic lymphocytic leukemia (CLL).
3. MDS: As in leukemia, bone marrow produces abnormal clones of one or more blood cells, but the percentage of abnormal bone marrow cells is less than in leukemia. Approximately 30% of MDS progresses to AML (former term for MDS was "pre-leukemia.")

TABLE 10–9 Causes of Leukocytosis in Adults (*"VINDIcATE"*)

Vascular	• Myocardial infarct: can cause neutrophilia. • Cholesterol emboli syndrome: can cause eosinophilia.
Infections	• Bacterial infections: cause neutrophilia. • Viral infections: cause lymphocytosis. • Tuberculosis and fungi: cause monocytosis. • Parasites: causes eosinophilia.
Neoplasms	• Myeloproliferative disorders: variable; can cause pancytopenia. • MDS: variable; may cause pancytopenia. • Leukemia: variable; can cause pancytopenia. • Lymphoma: variable; can cause pancytopenia. • Paraneoplastic syndromes: variable. • Hodgkin's disease: can cause eosinophilia.
Drugs	• Steroids, β-agonists, and G-CSF: can cause neutrophilia.
Allergic	• Asthma, eczema, ABPA, CSS, etc.: can cause eosinophilia.
Immune	• Autoimmune disorders: can cause lymphocytosis ± eosinophilia.
Trauma	• Surgery, burns, and other trauma: can cause neutrophilia.
Endocrine	• Adrenal insufficiency: can cause eosinophilia.

Abbreviations: ABPA, allergic bronchopulmonary aspergillosis; CSS, Churg-Strauss syndrome; G-CSF, granulocyte colony-stimulating factor; MDS, myelodysplastic syndromes.

TABLE 10–10 Diagnostic Studies in White Blood Cell Disorders

Disorder	WBCs	RBCs	Platelets	Smear	Biopsy	Other
CLL	↑	Varies	Varies	Smudge cells	↑ B lymphocytes	↑/↓ gamma globulins
CML	↑	Varies	Varies	WBCs in various stages of maturation	↑ Myelocytes (granulocytes)	↓ LAP, t(9:22) or Bcr-Abl
ALL	Varies	↓	↓	Blast cells	↑ Lymphoblasts	95% tDT positive
AML	Varies	↓	↓	Blast cells ± Auer rods	↑ Myeloblasts (contain granules)	Positive MPO or NSE in many subtypes
Hodgkin's disease	Varies	Varies	Varies	No specific findings	Reed Sternberg cells (B-cells with bilobed nucleus)	
NHL	Varies	Varies	Varies	No specific findings	Varies depending on sub-type of NHL	
MDS	Varies	Varies	Varies	Blast cells ± RS	Blast cells (<20% to 30%) ± RS	
AMM	Varies	Varies	Varies	Teardrop cells	Severe fibrosis	Bone marrow aspirate often yields "dry tap"
MM	Varies	Varies	Varies	Rouleaux	↑ Plasma cells	↑ M-proteins on SPEP or UPEP

Abbreviations: ALL, acute lymphocytic leukemia; AML, acute myelogenous leukemia; AMM, agnogenic myeloid metaplasia (idiopathic myelofibrosis); TdT, terminal deoxynucleotidyl transferase; CLL, chronic lymphocytic leukemia; CML, chronic myelogenous leukemia; MM, multiple myeloma; MPO, myeloperoxidase; NSE, Non-specific esterase; NHL, non-Hodgkin's lymphoma; RS, ringed sideroblasts; SPEP, serum protein electrophoresis; UPEP, urine protein electrophoresis.

4. Idiopathic myelofibrosis/agnogenic myeloid metaplasia (MF/AMM): One of the myeloproliferative disorders in which bone marrow produces excessive amounts of a blood cell type. Initiating event in MF/AMM is clonal proliferation of abnormal myeloid cells in the bone marrow. Clonal cells release growth factors that activate bone marrow fibrosis.

Myeloid cells differentiate into PMNs, eosinophils, and basophils.

Pancytopenia: All cell lines are down (decreased WBCs, RBCs, and platelets). Lymphoma, acute leukemia, MDS, and myelofibrosis can present with pancytopenia rather than leukocytosis. Other causes include advanced MM and aplastic anemia.

Chronic leukemia almost always causes leukocytosis and not leukopenia.

Figure 10-15 is the patient's peripheral smear.

What is the most likely diagnosis?

The peripheral smear contains a number of blast cells, which suggests the patient has an acute leukemia (see Table 10-10). Some of the blast cells contain needle-like inclusions (Auer rods), which are specific (but not sensitive) for AML. AML is most common in older persons (mean age is approximately 65 years).

Blast cells: primitive WBCs. Cells are large with big nuclei that contain nucleoli.

What is the next step in management?

The next step is to perform bone marrow biopsy. Bone marrow morphology showing >20% to 30% infiltration by myeloid blast cells (granulocytes) confirms the diagnosis.

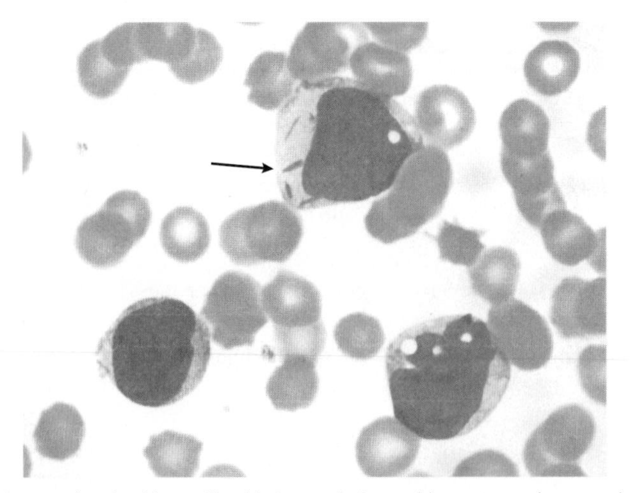

FIGURE 10–15 Blood smear showing blast cells with Auer rods (caused by acute myelogenous leukemia). From Rubin E, Farber JL. *Rubin's Pathology, 4th ed.* Lippincott Williams & Wilkins, 2004.

MDS: Based on the French-American-British system, <30% blasts is considered MDS. According to the World Health Organization classification system, <20% blasts is considered MDS. MDS patients also often have ringed sideroblasts on peripheral smear.

How is AML treated?

Treatment depends on the specific subtype (M0 to M7) as determined by morphology, cytochemistry, and cytogenetics. The presence of cardiopulmonary and other comorbidities also plays a role in assessing whether the patient can tolerate aggressive chemotherapy. In general, treatment involves the following (Tables 10-11 and 10-12):

1. Induction chemotherapy: Goal is to induce complete remission (i.e., no evidence of leukemia on bone marrow biopsy).
2. Consolidation therapy: Goal is to eliminate any residual disease.

TABLE 10–11 AML versus ALL

	AML	ALL
Age	Most common leukemia in adults (uncommon in children)	Most common leukemia in children (less common in adults)
Peripheral smear	Blasts ± Auer rods	Blasts (no Auer rods)
Bone marrow	Morphology: granulocytes	Morphology: no granules Cytochemistry: 95% is tDT-positive
Induction therapy	Cytarabine plus daunorubicin	***CHOP***: **C**yclophosphamide **H**ydroxydaunomycin (doxorubicin) **O**ncovin (vincristine) **P**rednisone
Consolidation therapy	Cytarabine plus daunorubicin versus stem cell transplant	Multiple regimens are being used and studied. Stem cell transplant is also an option
Maintenance	Not effective	Debatable benefit
CNS leukemia	Less common	More common

Abbreviation: CNS, central nervous system.

TABLE 10–12 Types of Hematopoietic Stem Cell Transplants (bone marrow transplant)

Type	Description	Advantages	Disadvantages
Autologous	Patient's stem cells are harvested and frozen. After chemotherapy/radiation to ablate the bone marrow, stem cells are returned to marrow.	No risk of GVHD	Risk of harvesting cancer cells along with normal cells
Allogeneic	HLA-matched donor's stem cells are harvested and injected into patient's ablated bone marrow.	No risk of harvesting cancer cells; donor's cells destroy cancer cells	Risk of GVHD
Syngeneic	Identical twin's stem cells are harvested and injected into patient's ablated bone marrow.	No risk of GVHD and no risk of harvesting cancer cells.	Donor cells do not attack cancer cells.

Reference: American Cancer Society, www.cancer.org.

AML M3 (acute promyelocytic leukemia): Initial choice for induction chemotherapy is all-trans retinoic acid (ATRA) plus an anthracyclin. Monitor for chronic DIC (due to release of procoagulants from the granules of the cells). Prognosis is better than other AML subtypes.

Alternative 10.10.1

During routine testing of a 55-year-old man, WBC count is found to be 80,000/μL. Hb is 12.2 mg/dL and platelets are 300,000/μL. Figure 10-16 is the patient's peripheral smear.

What is the most likely diagnosis?

Suspect CML in this patient with WBCs of the granulocyte series at different stages of maturation on peripheral smear (see Table 10-10). This condition most frequently occurs in middle-aged persons. Almost half of patients are asymptomatic at diagnosis. Other common presentations are one or more of the following:

1. Fatigue and other constitutional complaints (due to anemia)
2. Easy bleeding (due to thrombocytopenia)
3. Splenomegaly, hepatomegaly, and recurrent infections (due to abnormal WBCs)

CML is classified as leukemia and as a myeloproliferative disorder.

What diagnostic studies can help confirm the diagnosis?

First obtain serum leukocyte alkaline phosphatase (LAP). LAP is decreased in CML but increased in leukemoid reaction. If serum LAP is low or absent, obtain cytogenetics and molecular studies from bone marrow cells. The diagnosis is confirmed if one or more of the following are present:

1. Cytogenetics: Philadelphia chromosome (chromosome 9;22 translocation)
2. Molecular studies: Fluorescence in situ hybridization or polymerase chain reaction demonstrates Bcr-Abl protein or mRNA.

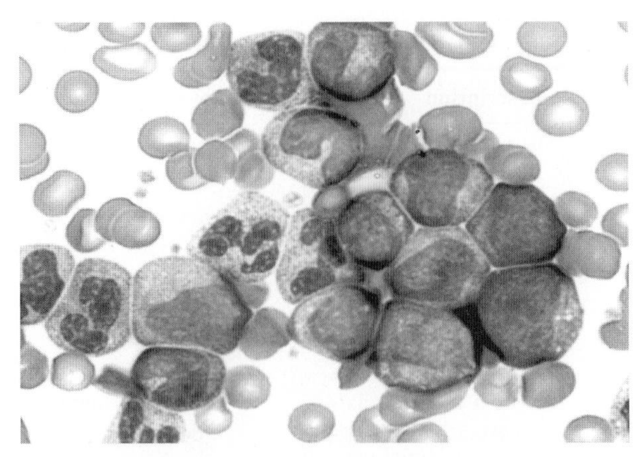

FIGURE 10–16 Blood smear in chronic myelogenous leukemia (granulocytes in different stages of maturation). From Anderson S. *Anderson's Atlas of Hematology*, Lippincott Williams & Wilkins, 2003.

> **Leukemoid reaction**: Although myeloproliferation caused by infection, drugs, etc., can cause leukocytosis with increased PMNs and peripheral smear similar to CML, LAP is high or normal. Cytogenetics is normal. This condition is benign and transient.

> **Bone marrow biopsy in CML**: many granulocytes (nonspecific finding).

How is CML treated?

In general, first-line therapy for older patients is imatinib (Bcr-Abl tyrosine kinase inhibitor). First-line therapy for younger patients is stem cell transplant.

> **Blast crisis**: The natural history of CML is to stay indolent for years then enter an accelerated phase that resembles AML and is called "blast crisis."

What diagnosis would have been more likely if Figure 10-17 were the patient's peripheral smear?

The peripheral smear demonstrates the characteristic "smudge cell" of chronic lymphocytic leukemia (CLL). CLL is the most common leukemia in patients older than 60 years. CLL has 3 stages:

1. Stage 1: bone marrow and blood lymphocytosis
2. Stage 2: lymphadenopathy or hepatosplenomegaly
3. Stage 3: anemia and/or thrombocytopenia

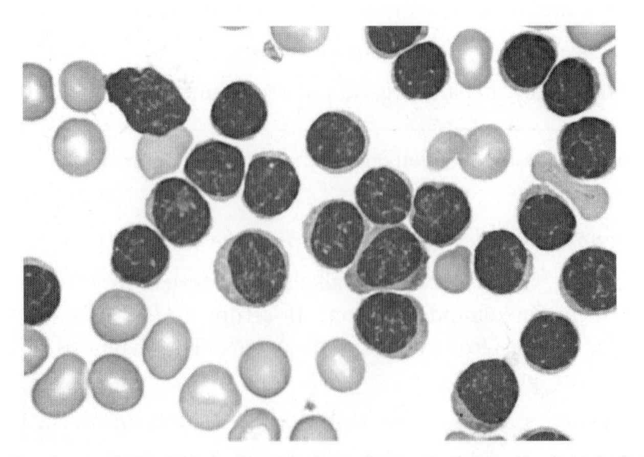

FIGURE 10–17 Reed-Sternberg cell (Hodgkin's disease). From Rubin E, Farber JL. *Rubin's Pathology, 4th ed.* Lippincott Williams & Wilkins, 2004.

> **CLL treatment:** In general, CLL is the most indolent leukemia. Chemotherapy does not alter survival, but it is indicated for palliation in stage 3 disease.

CASE 10–11 LYMPHADENOPATHY

A 24-year-old medical student presents with a 2-month history of enlarged lymph nodes in her neck. She is otherwise asymptomatic. Physical exam reveals 2 to 3 mm of rubbery, nontender, cervical lymph nodes. Vital signs are normal.

What disorders can cause lymphadenopathy?

Lymphadenopathy (enlarged lymph nodes) is a common finding in the adult population. Remember causes of lymphadenopathy with the acronym "***MIAMI***": **M**alignancy, **I**nfections, **A**utoimmune disorders, **M**iscellaneous disorders (e.g., sarcoidosis), and **I**atrogenic (e.g., serum sickness, reaction to phenytoin, etc.).

> Malignancy accounts for <2% of lymphadenopathy in primary care. Malignancy is unlikely if lymphadenopathy resolves within 2 weeks or remains stable for >1 year.

What is the next step in management?

No specific cause of lymphadenopathy is obvious in this asymptomatic person. Consider excisional lymph node (LN) biopsy to rule out malignancy if any of the following are present:

1. Age >40 years
2. Duration >1 month
3. Size >1.5 to 2 cm
4. Supraclavicular location
5. Hard, rubbery, and nontender consistency

> **Shotty lymphadenopathy:** Matted lymph nodes with tiny bumps (feels like a bird shot) or larger bumps (that feel like a buck shot). Requires monitoring for growth.

The patient undergoes LN biopsy (see Fig. 10-17).

What is the diagnosis?

The figure shows a Reed-Sternberg cell (clonal B cell with "owl's eye" appearance), which is pathognomic for HD. HD occurs predominantly in two age groups: young adults (20 to 30 years old) and older patients (>50 years old). Painless lymphadenopathy is the sole finding at presentation in two thirds of patients with HD. One third of patients present with lymphadenopathy plus "B symptoms" (fever, night sweats, and weight loss), which are associated with a worse prognosis.

> **Pruritis:** This common symptom in HD may begin even before lymphadenopathy occurs. It is not included as a B symptom because its presence does not change the prognosis.

> **Pel-Ebstein fever:** High-grade fever (39°C to 40°C) that keeps rising and falling every 7 to 10 days is highly suggestive of HD (relatively specific but not sensitive finding).

How is HD classified?

1. Histology: HD is classified into four major sub-types (Table 10-13).

TABLE 10-13 Histological Classification of Hodgkin's Disease

Subtype	Frequency	Prognosis	Age and Gender
Nodular sclerosing	60% to 80%	Excellent	Young women
Mixed cellularity	15% to 30%	Intermediate	Older men
Lymphocyte predominant	5%	Excellent	Young men
Lymphocyte depleted	<1%	Poor	Older men

Adapted from Sabatine M. *Pocket Medicine, 2nd ed.*

2. Numerical stage: Each subtype is assigned a stage from I to IV. Stage I disease affects only a single LN region. Stage II disease affects more than one contiguous LN regions on the same side of the diaphragm. Stage III disease affects contiguous LN regions on both sides of the diaphragm. Stage IV disease involves multiple organ systems (disseminated disease).
3. Alphabetical stage: Each numerical stage is assigned alphabetical modifiers as follows: A (no symptoms), B (B symptoms), X (at least one LN >5 to 10 cm indicates bulky disease), E (at least one contiguous extranodal site involved).

How is HD treated?

The most commonly used initial regimen is ABVD chemotherapy followed by radiation directed at the affected lymph node regions.

ABVD: **A**driamycin (doxorubicin), **B**leomycin, **V**inblastine, and **D**acarbazine.

The patient is diagnosed with stage IIA nodular sclerosing HD. She undergoes ABVD chemotherapy followed by radiation therapy of the involved LNs.

What is the most concerning long-term complication of radiation therapy?

Radiation therapy increases the risk of another neoplasm at the radiated site decades later. For example, this patient who receives neck and mediastinal radiation has an increased risk of thyroid cancer, breast cancer, and NHL. Also, monitor for hypothyroidism.

NHL: More common than HD.
NHL subtypes: More than 30 subtypes, which are grouped on the basis of histological grade and whether they arise from B or T cells.
NHL staging: Similar to HD, NHL presents with B symptoms more frequently than HD.
NHL grade: NHL is divided into high and low grade. Grade is a more reliable indicator of prognosis than stage.

Burkitt's lymphoma: High-grade (aggressive) B cell NHL with "starry sky" pattern on histology. Three subtypes are epidemic (due to EBV infection; common in African children and presents with jaw swelling); sporadic (uncommon; presents with abdominal swelling); and HIV-associated Burkitt's lymphoma.

CASE 10-12 Complications of Cancer Therapy

A 63-year-old man is diagnosed with AML. He undergoes induction chemotherapy with cytarabine and daunorubicin. Ten days later, he presents with abdominal pain, nausea, vomiting, and diarrhea. There is abdominal distension and right lower quadrant pain. Temperature is 38.9°C. Blood pressure is 110/80. Obstructive series is negative. WBC count is 2000/μL. Absolute neutrophil count is 200/μL.

What is the next step in management?

Neutropenia (absolute neutrophil count <500/μL) is a common complication of induction chemotherapy. Infections account for 75% of chemotherapy related mortality, so fever and neutropenia is a medical emergency. Important diagnoses to consider besides appendicitis in a neutropenic patient with right lower quadrant pain are typhlitis and pseudomembranous colitis. The next step in this hemodynamically stable patient is CT scan. Also order blood and stool assays of *C. difficile* toxin. Avoid colonoscopy or barium enema in patients with neutropenic fever (increased risk of cecal rupture).

CT scan of this hemodynamically stable patient with abdominal pain shows cecal thickening and inflammation. *C. difficile* toxin is pending.

What are the next steps?

CT scan is diagnostic for typhlitis (necrotizing colitis localized to the cecum). This uncommon condition is also called necrotizing enterocolitis. The next steps are:

1. Initiate supportive care: nothing per oral, IV fluids, NG suction, and frequent reassessment for signs of peritonitis.
2. Obtain blood and stool cultures.
3. Initiate empiric, broad-spectrum antibiotics against Gram-negative organisms. Cefepime is a frequently used initial antibiotic.

How would management differ if the patient's blood pressure were 80/60?

If a patient with neutropenic fever and abdominal pain is unstable, forego CT scan and refer the patient for emergent laparotomy. Emergent surgery is also indicated if a patient with known typhilitis develops signs of peritonitis on repeat assessment.

What laboratory tests would you order if the patient with fever and neutropenia did not have any abdominal pain or other GI symptoms?

Standard initial tests for neutropenic fever of unknown origin are CXR, CBC, serum chemistries, LFTs, and PAN cultures (blood, sputum, urine, and catheter sites). After cultures are drawn, begin broad-spectrum antibiotics and supportive care.

How would you tailor therapy if a patient with fever and neutropenia of unknown origin were found to have mucosal inflammation or pus at a catheter site?

Mucositis or signs of catheter-site infection increase the likelihood of a Gram-positive infection. Add vancomycin to the empiric antibiotic regimen. Also, remove the infected catheter.

> Vancomycin is also indicated if neutropenic fever persists in any patient despite 2 days of cefepime.

The patient with typhlitis is started on cefepime. Two days later, fever persists so vancomycin is added. Five days later, temperature is still 38.4°C, and the patient continues to experience abdominal pain. Vitals signs are normal. *C. difficile* toxin is negative. Blood and stool cultures are negative. Absolute neutrophil count is 210/μL.

What is the next step in management?

Add empiric antifungal therapy to the regimen if fever persists for >5 to 7 days in a neutropenic patient. Options include amphotericin B, caspofungin, or voriconazole.

> Cultures are positive in less than 30% of patients with neutropenic fever.

> **G-CSF**: Consider if a patient is neutropenic prior to potentially curative consolidation chemotherapy to increase neutrophil count. G-CSF is not recommended prior to palliative chemotherapy.

After discharge, the patient undergoes allogeneic bone marrow transplant (consolidation therapy). One week after the transplant, he presents with a burning maculopapular rash on his neck, shoulders, and palms. He also reports abdominal pain and 10 loose watery stools a day.

What is the most likely cause of his symptoms?

The patient has acute graft versus host disease (GVHD), which can occur in the first 100 days after allogenic stem cell transplant. The most common manifestations are one or more of the following: burning maculopapular rash, abdominal pain, diarrhea (watery or bloody), and cholestatic LFTs (increased alkaline phosphatase and direct bilirubin). This patient with classic findings does not require further diagnostic testing. If the diagnosis is less obvious, perform biopsy of the affected site.

How is acute GVHD treated?

First-line therapy for acute GVHD is low-dose methylprednisolone. If symptoms fail to resolve within 5 days, switch to high-dose methylprednisolone.

Acute GVHD prophylaxis: Most common regimen is methotrexate plus cyclosporine. Other drugs used to prevent acute GVHD include tacrolimus, sirolimus, and mycophenolate.

The patient recovers from acute GVHD. He remains in clinical remission for the next 2 years. During a follow-up evaluation, he presents with shiny, flat, violaceous, polygonal papules and white, lacelike striae on his nails and mouth. Laboratory testing reveals a cholestatic pattern of LFTs.

What is the most likely diagnosis?

The most likely diagnosis is chronic GVHD, which can occur after 100 days posttransplant. The most common manifestations are one or more of the following: a rash resembling lichen planus (this patient), a rash resembling scleroderma or Sjögren's syndrome, and a cholestatic pattern of LFTs. Some patients may also have oral ulcers and bronchiolitis obliterans. The next step is to confirm the diagnosis with a punch biopsy of the affected skin. If biopsy is positive, treat with prednisone ± cyclosporine or tacrolimus.

Limited chronic GVHD: Limited skin manifestations are the only abnormality. No specific therapy beside symptomatic treatment is indicated.

Alternative 10.12.1

An 18-year-old man with ALL is admitted for induction chemotherapy with "***CHOP***" (**C**yclophosphamide, **H**ydroxydaunomycin (doxorubicin), **O**ncovin (vincristine), **P**rednisone). You notice the attending also ordered allopurinol.

Why was this drug ordered?

Increased cell turnover after chemotherapy can lead to a host of metabolic abnormalities including hyperkalemia, hyperphosphatemia, hyperuricemia, and hypocalcemia. These metabolic abnormalities are collectively termed tumor lysis syndrome (TLS). Acute leukemias (particularly ALL) and high-grade lymphomas (e.g., Burkitt's lymphoma) carry the highest risk of TLS, so allopurinol is usually prescribed prior to chemotherapy to prevent hyperuricemia-induced ARF (uric acid nephropathy).

Shortly after completing the course of induction chemotherapy, his serum creatinine is 3.0 mg/dL.

What electrolyte is most likely responsible for ARF?

With the routine use of prophylactic allopurinol, uric acid nephropathy is uncommon after chemotherapy. The most common likely cause of acute renal failure is hyperphosphatemia. First-line therapy is hemodialysis.

Pre-chemotherapy TLS: Acute renal failure can occur prior to chemotherapy in acute leukemias and high-grade lymphomas. The most common cause is increased serum uric acid. First-line therapy is rasburicase. If hyperuricemia persists, consider hemodialysis.

CASE 10–13 POLYCYTHEMIA AND THROMBOCYTOSIS

A 50-year-old man presents with a 4-week history of fatigue, headache, blurry vision, and pruritus. He also reports episodes of burning and erythema in his hands and feet (erythromelalgia). He does not take any medications. He does not smoke cigarettes or drink alcohol. There is splenomegaly on physical exam. Vital signs and oxygen saturation are normal. Body mass index is 23. LFTs and serum chemistries are normal. Abnormal findings on CBC are Hb 20 g/dL, HCT 60%, and platelets 500,000/μL.

What are the most common causes of polycythemia?

Polycythemia is defined as increased Hb (>16.5 mg/dL in women and >18.5 mg/dL in men), increased HCT (>48% in women or >52% in men), or increased RBC count (less commonly used). The differential diagnosis includes:

1. First-degree polycythemia: The most important first-degree cause of polycythemia is polycythemia vera (PV).
2. Second-degree polycythemia: The most important second-degree causes are EPO-secreting tumors and hypoxemia-induced increased EPO secretion.
3. Pseudopolycythemia: caused by fluid depletion (polycythemia resolves with fluids), chronic smoking, living at a high altitude, or spurious elevation (Gaisboch's syndrome).

Tumors secreting EPO (mnemonic: "***PUR H2O***"): **P**heochromocytoma, **U**terine myomata, **R**enal cell carcinoma, **H**epatocellular carcinoma, and **H**emangioblastoma.

Hypoxemia caused by pulmonary disease (COPD, obesity hypoventilation syndrome, etc.) is the leading cause of polycythemia.

What diagnosis do the history and physical exam findings suggest?

The most likely diagnosis is PV. In this rare, idiopathic, myeloproliferative disorder there is excessive production of RBCs independent of EPO. Many PV patients also have increased platelet and WBC production. Increased RBCs makes the blood thicker than normal (increased viscosity), which causes most clinical manifestations of PV. Remember symptoms of PV using the mnemonic "***Carolina Tar Heels Play Excellent BasketBall***":

1. **C**onstitutional symptoms (e.g., headache, fatigue, decreased concentration, etc.)
2. **T**hrombosis
3. **H**ypertension
4. **P**ruritus (unknown mechanism)
5. **E**rythromelalgia
6. **B**lurry vision
7. **B**leeding (because increased thrombosis consumes vWF and leads to vWF deficiency)

Remember signs of PV with the acronym "***GAPS***":

1. **G**outy **A**rthritis (due to breakdown of large numbers of RBCs)
2. **P**lethora (face appears red because of hyperviscosity)
3. **S**plenomegaly ± hepatomegaly (increased RBCs ± platelets get stuck in splenic and hepatic vasculature)

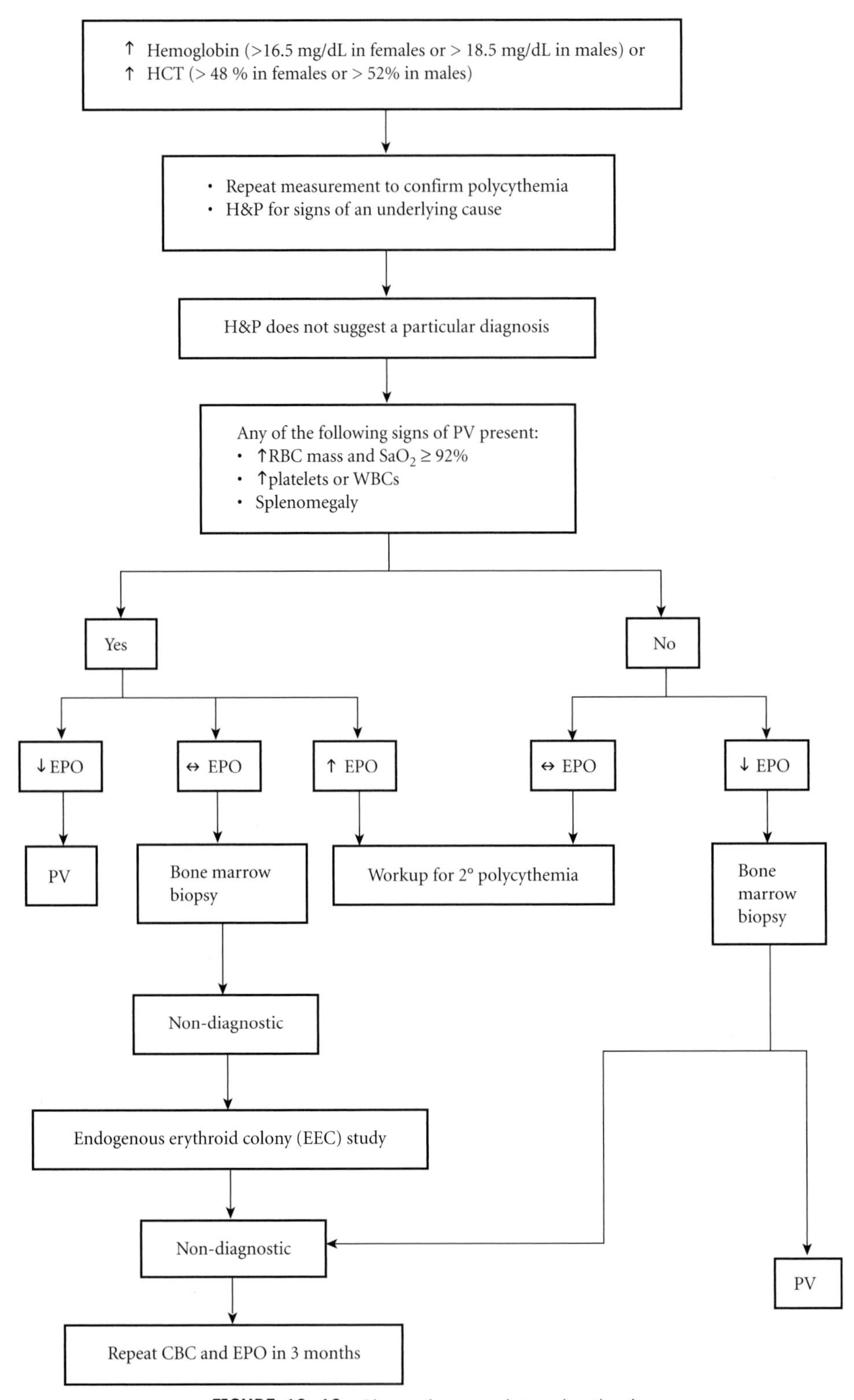

FIGURE 10–18 Diagnostic approach to polycythemia.

What is the next step in management?

Obtain RBC mass, serum EPO, and ambulatory pulse oximetry (Fig. 10-18). Increased EPO indicates second-degree polycythemia, whereas decreased EPO indicates PV.

Increased RBC count but decreased Hb, HCT, and MCV: Suspect thalassemia minor.

RBC mass is high, and EPO is low.

Does this patient meet diagnostic criteria for PV?

Major PV criteria are:

1. Increased RBC mass
2. Ambulatory oxygen saturation $\geq$92%
3. Splenomegaly

Minor PV criteria are:

1. Thrombocytosis
2. Leukocytosis
3. Increased or normal serum LAP
4. Serum vitamin B12 >900 pg/mL

Diagnosis of PV requires a patient to meet all three major criteria or two major criteria plus at least two minor criteria. This patient with all three major criteria meets the requirements for diagnosis of PV.

How is PV treated?

First-line therapy for PV is repeated phlebotomy to lower HCT (target HCT is $\leq$45% in men and $\leq$42% in women). Also, administer aspirin unless contraindicated to prevent thrombosis. Other therapies are as follows:

1. **Hydroxyurea**: Administer to patients with increased risk of thrombosis (prior thrombosis, platelets >1.5 million, age >70 years, or multiple CV risk factors).
2. **Anegrelide**: Consider for refractory thrombocytosis.
3. **Interferon-A**: Consider in patients with refractory pruritus.
4. **Allopurinol**: Consider for urine uric acid >1100 mg/day or symptomatic hyperuricemia.

What would have been the diagnosis if the patient with fatigue, headache, blurry vision, erythromelalgia, and splenomegaly had a normal RBC count but platelet count was 700,000/μL?

Isolated thrombocytosis can cause signs and symptoms of hyperviscosity, including thrombosis and bleeding. Increased platelets on CBC can be caused by:

1. Pseudothrombocytosis: Caused by laboratory error. Patient does not have signs of hyperviscosity. Platelets are normal on repeat testing.
2. Reactive thrombocythemia: The most common causes of increased platelets are IDA, splenectomy, infections, and inflammatory disorders (malignancies, autoimmune disorders).
3. Essential thrombocythemia (ET): In this rare idiopathic myeloproliferative disorder, diagnostic criteria are platelet count consistently >600,000/μL and no evidence of reactive thrombocytosis. Patients may also have increased RBCs and WBCs. The first step is to rule out pseudothrombocytosis and reactive thrombocytosis. Then obtain cytogenetics and bone marrow biopsy to confirm the diagnosis and rule out the other three myeloproliferative disorders (myelofibrosis, CML, and PV). First-line therapy for symptomatic patients is hydroxyurea plus aspirin (no therapy is necessary in asymptomatic patients).

JAK-2: A few cases of PV and ET are the result of JAK-2 mutation.

Unlike PV, ET and reactive thrombocytosis do not cause pruritus.

chapter **11**

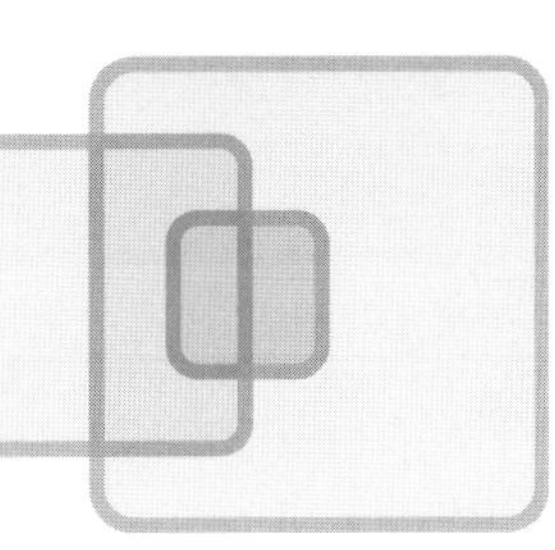

HIV and AIDS

CASE 11–1 HIV DIAGNOSIS AND INDICATIONS FOR ANTIRETROVIRAL THERAPY

A 21-year-old man presents with a 2-day history of fatigue, headache, sore throat, and myalgia. There are tender mouth ulcers. Temperature is 38.6°C. He is concerned that his symptoms may be caused by HIV because he participated in unprotected anal intercourse 3 weeks ago.

How is HIV infection acquired?

The three main modes of HIV transmission are:

1. Unprotected sex: Risk with anal intercourse > vaginal intercourse > oral sex. Risk is greater with receptive intercourse than insertive intercourse.
2. Maternal-fetal transmission: Can occur before birth, during childbirth, or after birth via breast milk.
3. Infected blood: Blood transfusions (especially before widespread screening was initiated in 1985), needle sharing (common in intravenous (IV) drug users), and needle sticks (health-care workers).

Urine, tears, and saliva contain low concentrations of HIV in infected patients. There are no documented cases of transmission via these bodily fluids.

Male circumcision: Greatly reduces HIV risk in the circumcised man. May serve as a primary preventive measure in the developing world. There is, however, increased risk with unprotected intercourse in the first 4 weeks after circumcision (before wound has healed).

What are the different types of HIV?

1. **HIV-1** causes the vast majority of HIV infection in the United States. HIV-1 is divided into three groups (M, N, and O); group M has at least nine subtypes (A to K).
2. **HIV-2**, largely restricted to Western Africa, is primarily spread through infected blood. Unprotected sex and mother–fetus transmission is less common.

How does HIV spread systemically after unprotected genital intercourse?

1. The genital mucosa (particularly the uncircumcised penis foreskin) is rich in dendritic Langerhans cells. HIV has a high affinity for these Langerhans cells.
2. Langerhans cells fuse with helper T lymphocytes (CD4 cells).
3. Glycoprotein 120 on the HIV cell surface binds to chemokine receptor 5 (CCR-5) on the CD4 cell surface. This allows HIV RNA and enzymes to enter CD4 cells.
4. HIV enzyme reverse transcriptase mediates transcription of HIV RNA to DNA.
5. HIV DNA integrates into CD4 DNA (mediated by the viral enzyme integrase).
6. HIV enzyme protease aids transcription of HIV DNA into multiple RNA copies.
7. CD4 cells travel throughout the body via lymph nodes.
8. Newly formed HIV RNA cells lyse the CD4 cells and infect other cells.

> **CCR-5 deletion mutation**: occurs in approximately 20% of white Europeans. Homozygotes are relatively resistant to HIV infection. Heterozygotes have a slower rate of progression.

What are the clinical manifestations of recently acquired HIV infection?

Acute HIV is infrequently diagnosed because symptoms are nonspecific and self-limited. Most patients experience constitutional symptoms 2 to 4 weeks after initial infection. Symptoms typically develop over 1 to 2 days and persist for 1 to 2 weeks. The most frequently reported symptoms are headache, sore throat, gastrointestinal (GI) symptoms (nausea, vomiting, and diarrhea), myalgia, and arthralgia. Common physical findings are low-grade fever, lymphadenopathy, hepatosplenomegaly, painful mucocutaneous ulcers, and a maculopapular truncal rash.

> **Infectious mononucleosis**: Clinical features are very similar to acute HIV. However, mucocutaneous rash and maculopapular truncal rash are uncommon. Patients with acute HIV can have atypical lymphocytes and a false-positive monospot test.

Why are symptoms of acute HIV infection transient?

Symptoms of acute HIV are caused by high levels of viral replication, which leads to a very high viral load. Viral replication activates a delayed cytotoxic T lymphocyte (CD8) response. Cytotoxic T cells contain viral replication, which helps resolve symptoms of acute HIV. After symptoms resolve, patients enter a latent phase of asymptomatic infection. This latent phase usually lasts for years to decades.

What tests should you order to detect HIV infection in this patient?

Obtain the following serological tests if you suspect acute HIV (Fig. 11-1):

1. **HIV-1 antibody**: Use this test to establish a baseline. Initial antibody test is enzyme immunoassay (EIA). EIA is negative in the first 3 to 6 weeks after infection.
2. **HIV-1 viral load**: The preferred diagnostic test is reverse-transcriptase polymerase chain reaction for HIV RNA. A less expensive but less sensitive alternative is p24 antigen.

EIA is negative. HIV-1 viral load is 800,000/mL.

What are the next steps in management?

The patient has acute HIV-1 (see Fig. 11-1). The next steps are genotype resistance testing and counseling to prevent transmission to other persons. Repeat HIV-1 antibody

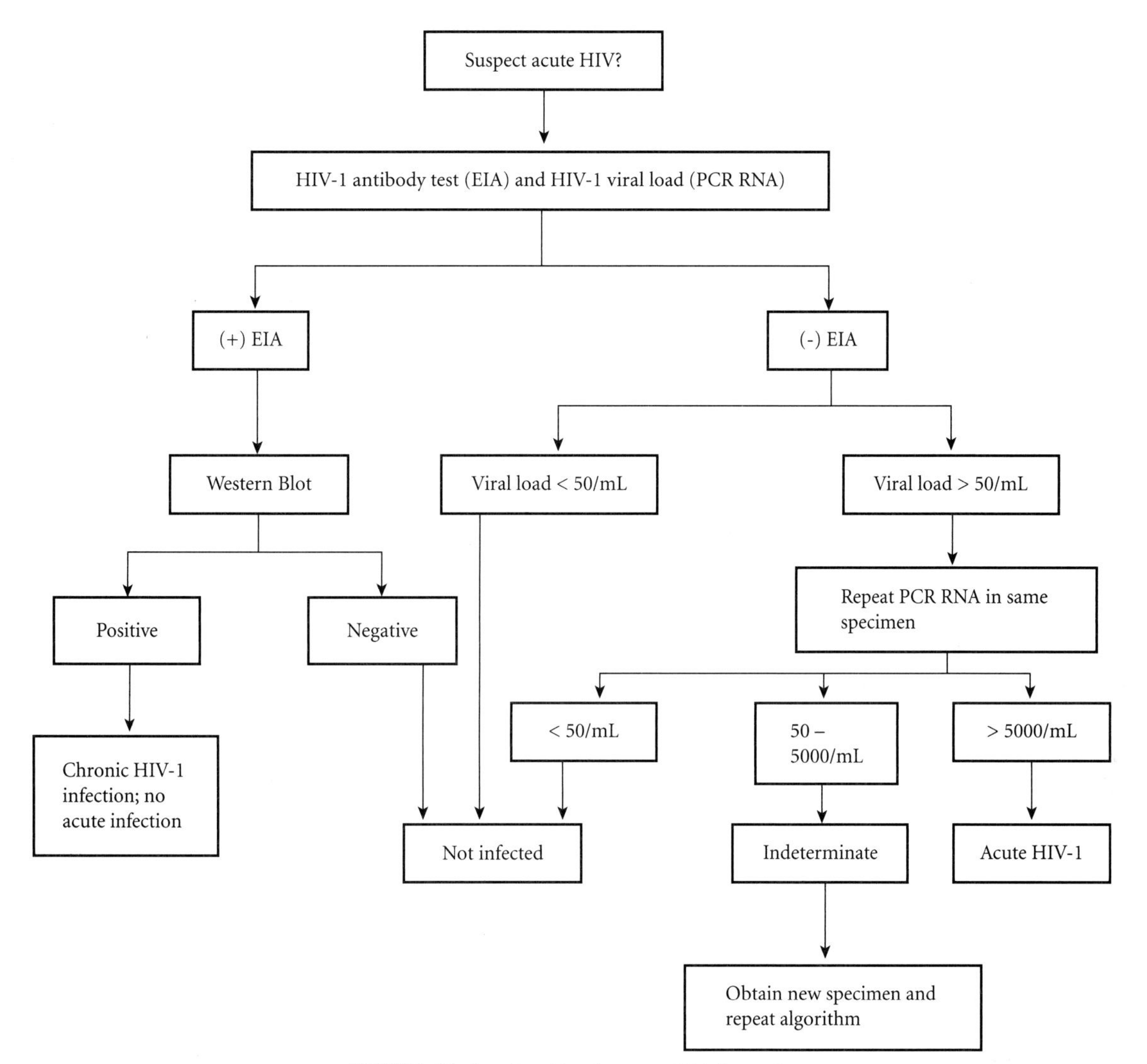

FIGURE 11–1 Algorithm for acute HIV diagnosis.

measurement a few weeks later to confirm seropositive status. Also, test all recent sexual partners for HIV-1 using EIA and PCR for HIV RNA.

> Whether or not to initiate antiretroviral therapy for acute HIV is controversial.

EIA is positive 4 weeks later (seropositive).

What tests are used to monitor severity and rate of disease progression in patients with documented HIV infection?

Obtain CD4 count and HIV viral load routinely to monitor disease severity and rate of progression. CD4 count is drastically reduced in acute HIV, but it increases to normal levels ($>500/mm^3$) as CD8 cells contain viral replication. On average, CD4 count declines at a rate of $50/mm^3$ every year in HIV-positive patients.

> CD4 percentage:
>
> **CD4 count $>$ 500/mm^3:** $>$29%
> **CD4 count 200 to 500/mm^3:** 14% to 28%
> **CD4 count $<$ 200/mm^3:** $<$14%

Acquired immunodeficiency syndrome (AIDS): End-stage HIV disease. Patients must have CD4 count <200 or an AIDS-defining illness (Table 11-1). AIDS causes increased susceptibility to opportunistic infections (OIs).

What other tests should you routinely obtain in all HIV-positive patients?

- Complete blood count (CBC), serum chemistry, and liver function tests (LFTs): Obtain at initial diagnosis and repeat annually.
- Pap smear: Obtain at initial diagnosis and repeat every 6 to 12 months.
- Tuberculosis screening: Obtain a purified protein derivative (PPD) test (to test for tuberculosis) and chest x-ray (CXR) at initial diagnosis. Repeat PPD annually. Repeat CXR if ≥5 mm of induration on PPD.
- Syphilis screening: Obtain baseline Veneral Disease Research Laboratory (VDRL) test or rapid plasma reagin (RPR) test. If test is positive, confirm with fluorescent treponemal antibody absorption (FTA-ABS). If either test is negative, repeat VDRL or RPR every 12 months.
- Toxoplasma screening: Obtain baseline IgG; repeat when CD4 <100/mm^3.
- Cytomegalovirus (CMV) screening: Obtain baseline IgG; repeat when CD4 <50/mm^3.
- Hepatitis B and C virus (HCB, HCV) screening: Obtain HbsAg and anti-HCV antibodies. If HBsAg is negative, measure HBsAb. If HBsAb is negative, administer HBV vaccine. Even if anti-HCV antibodies are negative, obtain repeat anti-HCV antibodies if the patient has abnormal LFTs in the future.

What vaccinations are generally recommended in HIV-positive patients?

1. All patients: Pneumococcal and annual influenza vaccine.

TABLE 11–1 AIDS Defining Illnesses

INFECTIONS

CNS	Eyes	Lungs	Genitals, Mouth, and Esophagus	Intestines	Others
• *Toxoplasma gondii* • *Cryptococcus neoformans* • JC virus	• Cytomegalovirus	• Bacterial pneumonia (>1 episode/year) • PCP	• *Candida albicans* • Cytomegalovirus • Herpes simplex virus lesions >1 month	• Cryptosporidiosis (>1 month) • Isosporiasis (>1 month)	• Tuberculosis (pulmonary or extrapulmonary) • Other mycobacterial infections (*M. avium* complex, *M. kansasii*) • Salmonella septicemia • Extrapulmonary histoplasmosis, coccidiomycosis

MALIGNANCIES

- Kaposi's sarcoma
- Cervical cancer
- CNS lymphoma
- Non-Hodgkin's lymphoma

OTHER

- AIDS wasting syndrome
- AIDS dementia complex (includes HIV encephalopathy)

Abbreviations: CNS, central nervous system; JC virus, John Cunningham virus; PCP, *Pneumocystis carnii* pneumonia.

2. HbsAb-negative patients: Administer hepatitis B vaccine.
3. Age-appropriate killed virus vaccines.

Avoid live virus vaccines in HIV-positive patients. The exception is MMR.

The patient's sexual partner is located. He is asymptomatic. Serum EIA is positive. Confirmatory Western blot test is positive. CD4 count is 900/mm^3. HIV viral load is 2000/mL. CBC, serum chemistries, LFTs, PPD, CXR, and infectious disease serologies are negative.

What antiretroviral therapy (ART) is indicated at this time?

The patient has chronic HIV-1 infection. No antiviral therapy is indicated in asymptomatic patients with CD4 count >500/mm^3.

The sexual partner has a history of IV heroin use. He used to share needles with his neighbor Tom. Tom is asymptomatic. On physical exam, there is oral candidiasis. EIA and Western blot are positive. CD4 count is 600/mm^3 and viral load is 70,000/mL.

Is ART indicated for this patient?

Absolute indications for initiating ART are:

1. All symptomatic patients (AIDS-defining illness) regardless of CD4 count
2. CD4 count <200/mm^3 regardless of symptoms

This patient with an AIDS-defining illness should initiate ART despite the normal CD4 count. Most highly active ART regimens (HAART) consist of a base (a protease inhibitor or a non-nucleoside reverse-transcriptase inhibitor) and a backbone (two nucleoside/nucleotide reverse-transcriptase inhibitors) (Table 11-2). Four-drug combinations are not any more effective than three-drug combinations.

Asymptomatic patients with CD4 count between 200 and 500/mm^3:
CD4 count <350 or viral load >100,000: Most clinicians begin ART.
CD4 count >350 and viral load <100,000: Most clinicians defer ART.

TABLE 11–2 Antiretroviral Drugs Used in the Treatment of HIV/AIDS

Drug class	Notes	Examples
NRTIs	• A nucleoside analog "***DAZZLES***" reverse transcriptase • Avoid the following combinations: ***STA-ZI*** (**STA**vudine and **ZI**dovudane), ***STA-DI*** (**STA**vudine and **DI**danosine), and ***EM-LA*** (**EM**tricabine and **LA**mivudine) • Zalcitabine is rarely used because of side effects	**D**idanosine (ddI) **A**bacavir (ABC) **Z**idovudine (ZDV) **Z**alcitabine (ddC) **L**amivudine (3TC) **E**mtricabine (FTC) **S**tavudine (d4T)
NRTIs	• nucleo**T**ide **A**nalogs inhibit reverse transcriptase	**T**enofovir **A**defovir
NNRTIs	• NNRTIs **DEN**y movement of protein domains needed by reverse transcriptase. • Delavirdine is rarely used	**D**elavirdine **E**favirenz **N**eviparine
PIs	• Protease inhibitors (end in "-navir" = "never") let viral DNA become RNA.	Saqui**navir** Rito**navir** Indi**navir**
Fusion inhibitor	• Enfurtivide (Fuzeon) blocks fusion of HIV cell with CD4 cell.	Enfurtivide (Fuzeon)

Abbreviations: NRTI, nucleoside reverse-transcriptase inhibitor; NNRTI, non-nucleoside reverse transcriptase inhibitor; PI, protease inhibitor.

Strict compliance with HAART is essential to minimize drug resistance. Perform psychosocial evaluation in all patients to determine whether they have any issues that may reduce compliance (e.g., homeless, substance abuse, or psychiatric illness).

Tom's CD4 count rises to 1000/mm^3 and viral load is undetectable after starting HAART. Six months later the viral load is 7000/mL.

What is the next step?

Repeat drug resistance testing. Alter the treatment regimen if the virus is resistant. Suspect noncompliance if tests show that the virus is sensitive to the current regimen.

Tom's girlfriend Emily finds out she is pregnant. EIA is positive. Western blot confirms the diagnosis.

Is any ART indicated?

ART is indicated in all HIV-positive pregnant patients after the first trimester to reduce maternal–fetal transmission. Continue ART until delivery. Consider elective cesarean section if the patient's viral load is >1000/mL. After delivery, advise the patient not to breast-feed. Continue ART in the child for 6 to 12 weeks after delivery. Risk of transmission is approximately 25% in untreated patients and <1% in patients who received ART ± cesarean section.

"*Avoid **ET***" (**E**favirenz and **T**enofovir) because use of these drugs can cause the baby to look like E.T. (i.e., birth defects).

Resource-poor nations: Infant formula is often not widely available. Consider postpartum ART in the mother as well to reduce viral load in breast milk.

Emily's roommate Jamie presents to the clinic after she learns of Emily's recent HIV diagnosis. Jamie is asymptomatic. She is in a monogamous relationship with her boyfriend. She denies IV drug use. She has never had an HIV test.

Is HIV testing indicated in the roommate?

Even though Jamie's risk of HIV is low, she should undergo HIV screening because the Centers for Disease Control (CDC) recommends universal screening of all persons ≥13 years of age. If the test is negative, she does not require further screening as long as she continues to remain at low risk. The most commonly used screening test for HIV-1 is serum EIA (standard blood test). Other less invasive options are EIA of urine or oral mucosa. EIA is almost 100% sensitive, so a negative result rules out non-acute infection. EIA is not 100% specific, so a positive test must be confirmed by Western blot.

Rapid HIV-1 Test: Turnaround time is approximately 20 minutes, whereas the EIA test takes days. Sensitivity and specificity is similar to EIA. Negative result rules out non-acute HIV. Positive test requires confirmation with Western blot.
Home Access Test: This is the only over-the-counter test approved by the U.S. Food and Drug Administration as of March 2007. Patient takes blood samples at home and sends it in the mail to a laboratory, which performs EIA analysis for HIV-1.

Jamie has a positive EIA but indeterminate Western blot. There is a single band against p24.

How should you interpret this result?

Western blot is considered positive if it detects at least two antibodies (gp120/160 plus p24 or gp41). The test is negative if it does not detect any antibodies. All other results are classified as indeterminate (e.g., no antibodies against gp120/160 or only one positive antibody). HIV infection is unlikely in this asymptomatic person with no risk factors and an indeterminate Western blot. The next step is to repeat EIA in 6 months.

Three groups of HIV proteins:

1. **Envelop proteins (env)**: glycoproteins 120, 160, and 41
2. **Polymerase proteins (pol)**: p66 (reverse transcriptase) and p31 (integrase)
3. **Core proteins (gag)**: p24, p18, p7, p55

Jamie's EIA is positive 6 months later. Western blot shows the same indeterminate pattern.

What is the next step in management?

The next step is reassurance, because a stable indeterminate pattern on Western blot for ≥6 months indicates that Jamie is not HIV-positive.

CASE 11–2 HIV TESTING AND PROPHYLAXIS AFTER NEEDLE-STICK INJURY

A 41-year-old HIV-positive man undergoes cardiac catheterization. His initial hepatitis serologies were negative, but current hepatitis status is unknown. The patient's last viral load and CD4 counts were 450,000/mL and 350/mm^3. During the procedure, the 32-year-old cardiac nurse is stuck deeply by a needle that had been placed in the common femoral artery. Blood was visible on the needle. She has no known medical conditions. She has been immunized against HBV.

What is the risk of HIV transmission after a needle-stick injury?

As of 2002, 57 healthcare workers had acquired HIV infection via occupational exposure. The two modes of transmission were needle-sticks (1 in 300 risk) and mucous membrane exposure (1 in 1000 risk). The following situations increase the overall risk of transmission after a needle-stick injury:

1. High viral load (acute HIV or AIDS)
2. Needle placed in a central artery or vein
3. Visible blood on the needle
4. Deep injury

What are the initial steps in management?

1. Wash exposed area with soap, water, and an alcohol-based agent.
2. Test the nurse for HIV antibody, HBsAg, anti-HBsAb, and anti-HCV antibody.
3. Test the source patient for HBsAb and HCV antibody (because current status unknown).
4. Initiate three-drug postexposure prophylaxis (PEP) within the first 2 hours (Fig. 11-2).

Do not delay PEP while waiting for the results of antibody tests. PEP is usually not effective if initiated >72 hours after exposure.

Obtain β-hCG in all women of childbearing age before starting PEP.

The nurse's labs are as follows: HIV EIA (+), Western blot (+), HbsAg (–), HBsAb (+), HCV antibody (–), and β-hCG (–). The source patient has similar hepatitis laboratory results.

How should you interpret these results?

The nurse acquired HIV infection prior to the needle-stick injury and currently has chronic HIV infection. She is immune to HBV infection. She does not have HCV infection.

What if the source patient's hepatitis serologies were negative and the nurse's labs were as follows: HIV EIA (–), HBsAg negative, (+) HBsAb, HCV antibody (–), and β-hCG (–)? Is any further testing indicated?

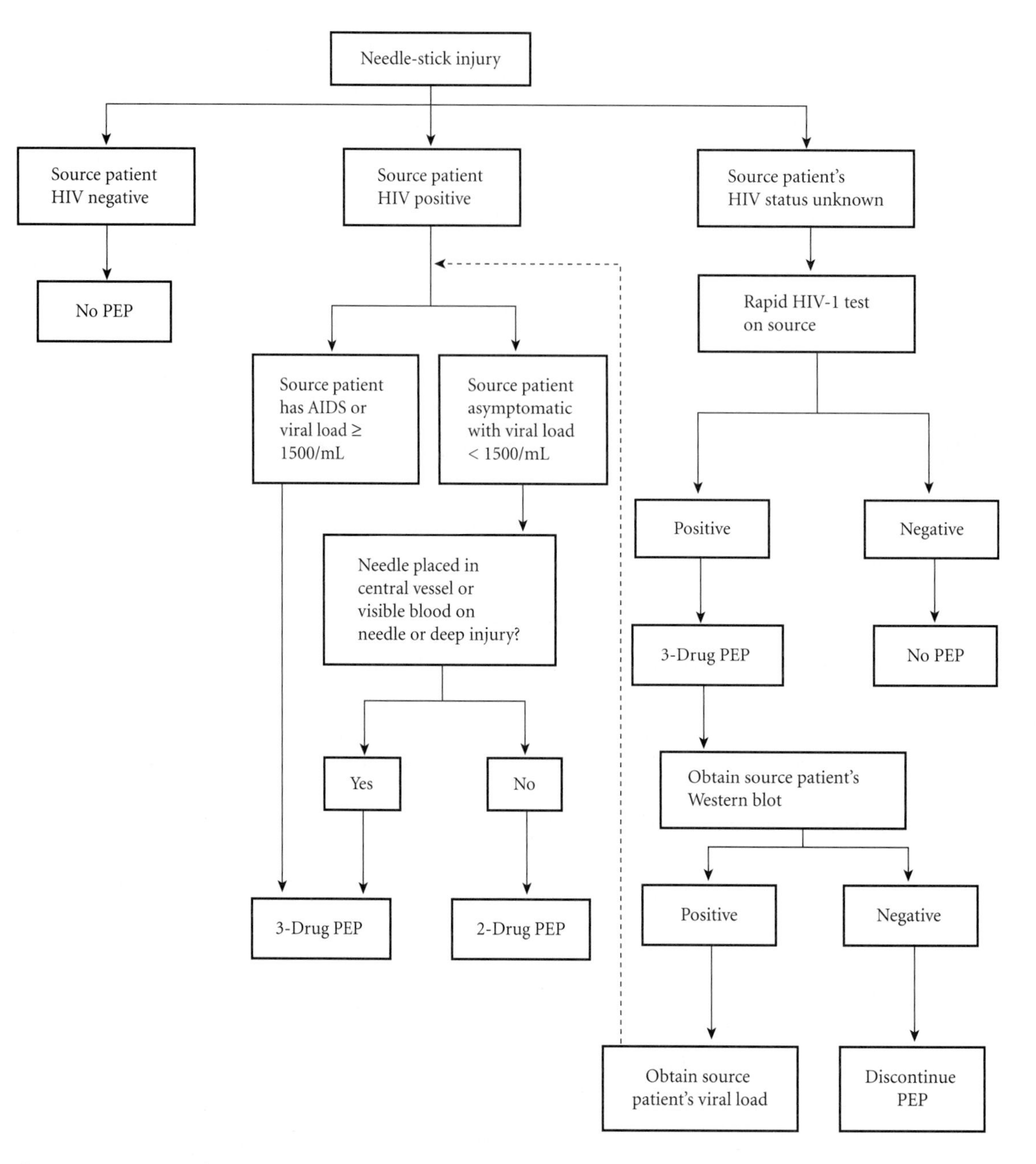

2-Drug PEP: Two NRTIs; 3-Drug PEP: 2NRTIs plus a PI or NNRTI

FIGURE 11–2 HIV postexposure prophylaxis (PEP) after needlestick injury.

Recheck the nurse's HIV antibodies at 6 weeks, 12 weeks, and 6 months after exposure. Although the optimal duration of PEP is unknown, current CDC guidelines recommend a 4-week course.

What if the source patient's hepatitis serologies were negative and the nurse's labs were as follows: HIV EIA (–), HBsAg (–), HBsAb (+), HCV Ab (+), and β-hCG (–)? Is any further HIV testing indicated?

The nurse has HCV infection, which increases the risk of delayed HIV seroconversion. Recheck the nurse's HIV antibodies at 6 weeks, 12 weeks, 6 months, and 12 months after exposure. As recommended earlier, if HIV serology remains negative, continue PEP for 4 weeks.

During the cardiac procedure, a few drops of blood splash on the physician's eyes. He is wearing contact lenses.

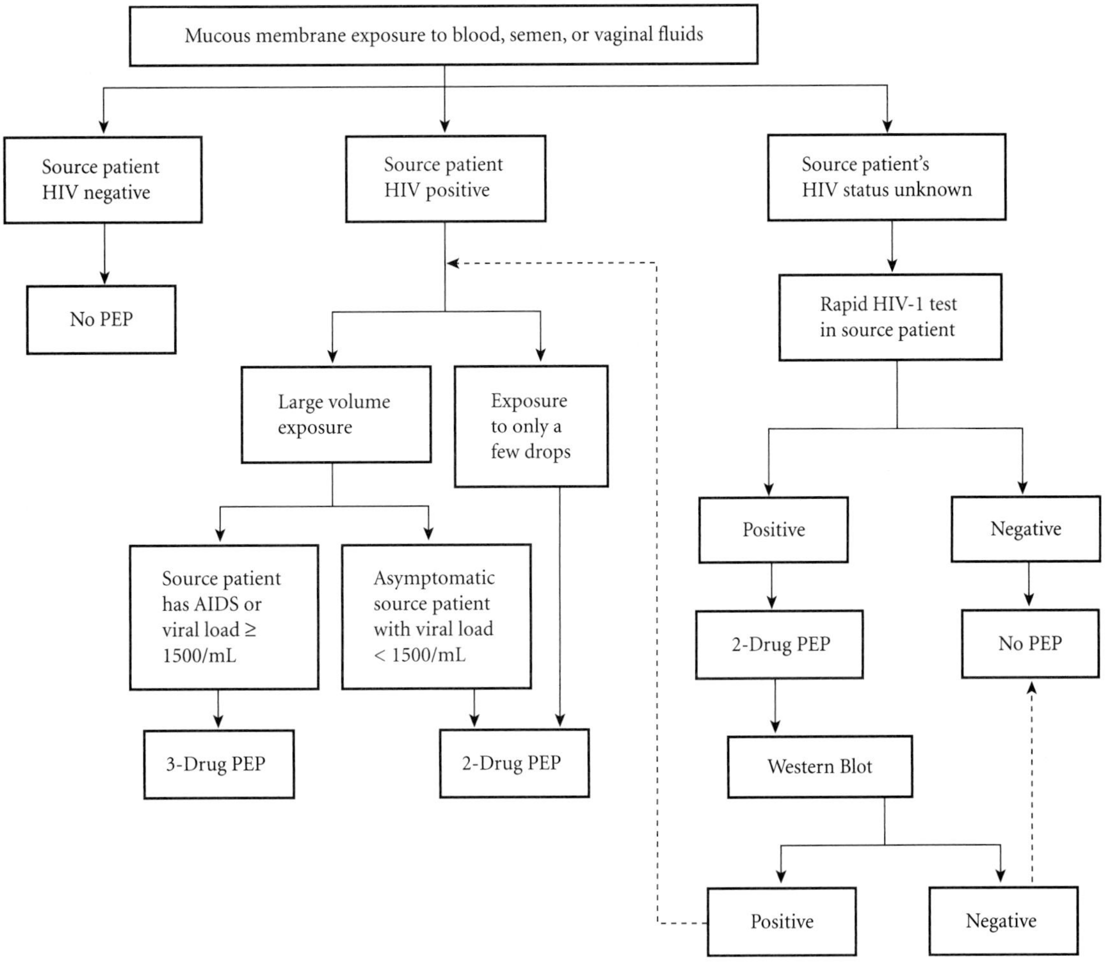

FIGURE 11–3 HIV PEP after mucous membrane exposure to HIV.

What are the next steps in management?

1. Remove contact lenses and wash the exposed area with copious water or saline.
2. Test the physician for HIV antibody, HBsAg, anti-HBsAb, and anti-HCV antibody.
3. Test the source patient for anti-HBsAb and anti-HCV antibody.
4. Initiate two-drug PEP within the first 2 hours (Fig. 11-3).

CASE 11-3 PRIMARY PROPHYLAXIS IN HIV-POSITIVE PATIENTS

A 37-year-old man is diagnosed with Kaposi's sarcoma (KS). He lives in Mississippi. He undergoes HIV testing, which is positive. Viral load is 650,000/mL. CD4 count is 30/mm^3. CBC, serum chemistries, and LFTs are normal. PPD is negative. CXR is normal. Toxoplasma and CMV IgG are positive. HBV and HCV serologies are negative.

In addition to initiating HAART, what primary prophylactic measures should you recommend to prevent OIs in this patient with AIDS?

This patient should initiate TMP/SMX to prevent *Pneumocystis carnii* pneumonia (PCP) and toxoplasmosis, azithromycin to prevent *Mycobacterium avium* complex (MAC), and itraconazole to prevent histoplasmosis (Table 11-3). Primary prophylaxis against the numerous other AIDS-related OIs (e.g., cryptococcosis, coccidiomycosis, cryptosporidiosis) is not recommended because mortality benefit is unclear.

Table 11–3 Primary prophylaxis against opportunistic infections in patients with AIDS

CD4<200/mm3:
Pneumocystis carnii pneumonia (PCP): 1st line is TMP-SMX. 2nd line is dapsone. 3rd line is atovaquone. Avoid TMP-SMX during 1st trimester of pregnancy (aerosolized pentamidine is 1st line during this period).
CD4<100/mm3:
Toxoplasma encephalitis: Initiate prophylaxis if patient has positive toxoplasma serology. 1st line agent is TMP-SMX. 2nd line is dapsone + pyrimethamine + leucovorin. 3rd line is atovaquone. Avoid pyrimethamine in pregnancy.
Disseminated histoplasmosis: Initiate prophylaxis with itraconazole if patient lives in an endemic area.
CD4<50/mm3:
Mycobacterium Avium Complex (MAC): 1st line is azithromycin, 2nd line is clarithromycin, and 3rd line is rifabutin. Avoid clarithromycin in pregnancy.

CD4 $<200/mm^3$: **PCP**: First-line drug is trimethoprim-sulfamethoxazole (TMP-SMX), second-line drug is dapsone, and third-line drug is atovaquone. Avoid TMP-SMX during the first trimester of pregnancy (aerosolized pentamidine is first-line drug during this period).

CD4 $<100/mm^3$:

- **Toxoplasma encephalitis**: Initiate prophylaxis if the patient has positive toxoplasma serology. First-line drug is TMP-SMX, second-line drug is dapsone + pyrimethamine + leucovorin, and third-line drug is atovaquone. Avoid pyrimethamine in pregnancy.
- **Disseminated histoplasmosis**: Initiate prophylaxis with itraconazole if the patient lives in an endemic area.

CD4 $<50/mm^3$: **MAC**: First-line drug is azithromycin, second-line drug is clarithromycin, and third-line drug is rifabutin. Avoid clarithromycin in pregnancy.

> **Eye exam**: Recommended every 3 to 6 months in AIDS patients with CD4 <50 to screen for CMV retinitis.

> **Coccidiomycosis (Valley Fever)**: endemic to southwestern US and northwestern Mexico.
> **Histoplasmosis**: endemic to **M**issouri, **O**hio, and **M**ississippi river valleys ("***MOM***").

CASE 11–4 ORAL LESIONS IN AN HIV-POSITIVE PATIENT

A 48-year-old HIV-positive man presents with mouth pain. On physical exam, there are white plaques on the buccal mucosa, palate, and tongue. The lesions easily scrape off with a tongue depressor, but they bleed a little in the process. CD4 count is $150/mm^3$.

What is the most likely cause of these white plaques?

The patient has oral infection by the fungus *Candida albicans* ("thrush"). The lesions present as diffuse white plaques in the oropharynx that scrape off easily with a little bleeding. Oral thrush is often asymptomatic. Others may experience symptoms such as a "cottony" sensation in the mouth, altered taste, and mouth pain, particularly while eating.

> **Oral thrush in HIV-negative patients**: Due to diabetes mellitus, inhaled steroids, antibiotics, poor denture hygiene, dry mouth (e.g., head and neck radiation), and immunosuppression (e.g., transplant, chemotherapy, etc.).

What is the next step in management?

Perform a potassium hydroxide (KOH) preparation of the scrapings, and analyze them under a microscope. *C. albicans* appears as budding yeast with or without pseudohyphae (Fig. 11-4).

KOH preparation confirms the diagnosis.

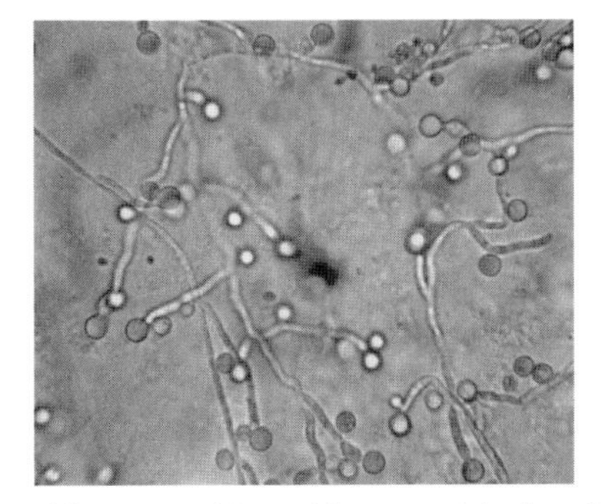

FIGURE 11–4 Candida KOH prep: Budding yeast with or without pseudohyphae. From *Goodheart's Photoguide of Common Skin Disorders*, 2nd ed. Lippincott Williams & Wilkins, 2003.

How should you treat this patient?

First-line therapy for the initial episode of oral thrush in patients with CD4 $>100/mm^3$ is topical clotrimazole. Topical nystatin is a cheaper alternative. If infection persists or recurs, treat with oral fluconazole.

What antimicrobial would you recommend as the first-line treatment if CD4 count were $<100/mm^3$?

First-line therapy for oral thrush in patients with CD4 $<100/mm^3$ is oral fluconazole.

What would have been the initial step if the patient presented with dysphagia, odynophagia, and no oral lesions?

Suspect infectious esophagitis when an AIDS patient presents with dysphagia and odynophagia. *C. albicans* is the most common cause of esophagitis in patients with CD4 $<200/mm^3$. Patients with candida esophagitis may or may not have concurrent oral thrush. Initial management is to treat empirically with oral fluconazole. If symptoms persist after 3 days, perform upper endoscopy with biopsy to rule out other infections:

1. **Herpes simplex virus esophagitis**: vesicles and erosions in the esophagus. Tzanck smear of vesicular fluid shows multinucleated cells. Treatment is oral acyclovir.
2. **CMV esophagitis**: less common. Occurs when CD4 $<50/mm^3$. Appearance is multiple large and shallow ulcers in the distal esophagus. Biopsy shows intranuclear inclusion bodies. First-line treatment is ganciclovir. Foscarnet (equally effective) is not a first-line drug because of increased cost and increased renal toxicity.

> **Oral herpes simplex virus**: prodrome of oral pain and burning followed by oral vesicles and erosions.

Alternative 11.4.1

A 37-year-old HIV-positive woman presents for a routine evaluation. On physical exam, there are white plaques on the lateral portion of the tongue. The plaques do not scrape off with a tongue depressor. CD4 count is $280/mm^3$.

What is the most likely diagnosis?

Oral hairy leukoplakia appears as painless white plaques on the lateral tongue. Unlike oral thrush, the lesions do not scrape off easily. This condition occurs almost exclusively in HIV-positive patients as a result of Epstein-Barr virus. No specific therapy is necessary.

CASE 11–5 SKIN LESIONS IN AN HIV-POSITIVE PATIENT

A 54-year-old homosexual patient presents with six painless purple papules on his face and legs (Fig. 11-5). He is HIV-positive. Last CD4 count was $100/mm^3$.

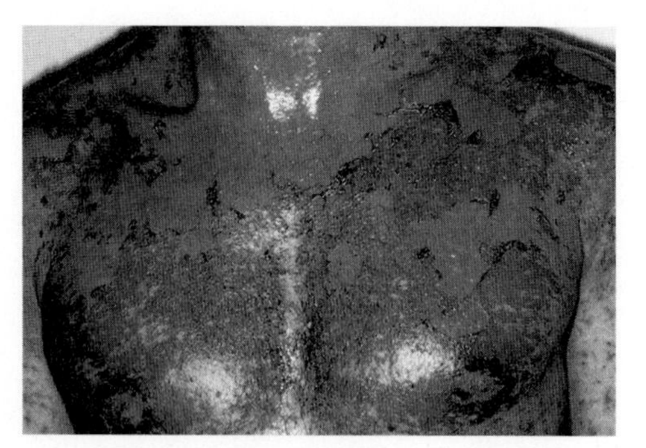

FIGURE 11-5 Kaposi's sarcoma image. From *Goodheart's Photoguide of Common Skin Disorders*, 2nd ed. Lippincott Williams & Wilkins, 2003.

What is the most likely diagnosis?

The most likely diagnosis is AIDS-related KS. AIDS-related KS occurs most frequently in HIV-positive homosexual or bisexual men. This neoplasm typically presents with purple, red, or pink papules on the face, lower extremities, mouth, and genitalia. The papules are not painful or pruritic.

> KS can affect any organ system. The GI tract and lungs are commonly affected viscera.

What causes Kaposi's sarcoma?

Kaposi's sarcoma results from infection by human herpes virus 8 (HHV8).

> **Classic KS**: occurs in immunocompetent Jewish or Mediterranean patients.
> **Endemic KS**: occurs in immunocompetent patients in sub-Saharan Africa.
> **Transplant-associated KS**: occurs due to immunosuppression after organ transplant.
> **Epidemic KS**: occurs due to immunosuppression in AIDS patients (AIDS-related KS).

What is the next step in management?

Biopsy any purple lesion occurring in an AIDS patient to differentiate between KS, bacillary angiomatosis (BA), and other lesions. If biopsy shows KS, check stool for occult blood to screen for GI involvement.

Skin biopsy confirms the diagnosis of KS. Stool is positive for guaiac. Endoscopy confirms the presence of GI lesions.

How is KS treated?

All HIV-positive patients with KS should receive HAART. In addition, patients with visceral involvement should receive chemotherapy (doxorubicin or daunorubicin).

Alternative 11.5.1

A 51-year-old HIV-positive woman presents with numerous purple nodules on her face. The nodules bleed profusely even with minor trauma. She also reports a 2-week history of fever and malaise. CD4 count is 30/mm^3.

What diagnosis should you suspect?

Purple nodules that bleed easily along with constitutional symptoms in an AIDS patient with CD4 <100/mm^3 should raise suspicion for BA. This condition results from infection with *Bartonella henselae* (spread by flea-infested cats) or *Bartonella quintana* (spread by the human body louse).

> BA lesions can also occur in mucosa, submucosa, bones, and the central nervous system (CNS).

> *Staphylococcus aureus* is the most common cause of skin infections in AIDS patients.

What is the next diagnostic step?

Obtain the following tests: biopsy with Warthin-Starry staining, IgG IFA, PCR, and blood culture on chocolate agar. None of these tests are extremely sensitive. Culture is often negative even in infected patients because Bartonella species (Gram-negative bacilli) are very fastidious organisms.

How is BA treated?

First-line antibiotic is oral erythromycin. Second-line is oral doxycycline. BA is often fatal without treatment.

> **Cat-scratch disease**: A cat scratch can spread *Bartonella henselae* to immunocompetent children and teenagers. Initial sign is a painless wound at the site of the scratch. Later, patients develop tender lymphadenopathy ± constitutional symptoms.

Alternative 11.5.2

A 64-year-old woman with CD4 count of 170/mm^3 is started on zidovudine, lamivudine, and saquinavir. She presents 4 months later with central obesity, buffalo hump, facial wasting, and lower extremity atrophy. There are lipomas on the trunk and legs. Fasting glucose is 200 mg/dL. Total cholesterol is 220 mg/dL, and low-density lipoprotein is 180 mg/dL. Serum cortisol is normal.

What is the most likely cause of her symptoms?

The patient most likely has lipodystrophy, a disfiguring side effect of HAART (occurs within 3 to 6 months of starting therapy). Clinical manifestations are similar to Cushing syndrome (peripheral atrophy, central obesity, and metabolic syndrome). Patients may also have facial wasting and lipomas. The antiretroviral drugs most frequently implicated are protease inhibitors and the nucleoside reverse-transcriptase inhibitors zidovudine and stavudine.

How can you manage this patient's symptoms?

Consider switching from zidovudine to abacavir or tenofovir. Also, treat lipid abnormalities and diabetes mellitus (glitazones are first-line agents). Consider injectable temporary fillers if the patient finds facial atrophy intolerable.

> Always obtain baseline fasting glucose and lipid profile before starting HAART, and reassess every 6 to 12 months.

Alternative 11.5.3

An asymptomatic, 31-year-old, HIV-positive woman has a CD4 count of 300/mm^3 and viral load of 120,000/ml. She begins to take abacavir, lamivudine, and efavirenz. Three months later, CD4 count is 600/mm^3 and viral load is 800/mL. Six months later, CD4 count is 160/mm^3. She admits that she has not been compliant with her regimen. She restarts her previous regimen and also begins PCP prophylaxis with TMP-SMX. Two weeks later, she presents with fever, nausea, and a diffuse pruritic maculopapular rash.

What is the cause of her symptoms?

TMP-SMX hypersensitivity occurs with increased frequency in HIV-positive patients. Common clinical manifestations are fever, malaise, nausea, vomiting, and a diffuse pruritic maculopapular rash approximately 2 weeks after initiation. The next step is to minimize symptoms with an antihistamine and/or diphenhydramine (Benadryl). Unless the patient has a severe hypersensitivity reaction such as Stevens-Johnson syndrome or toxic epidermal necrolysis (see Chapter 13: Dermatology), try not to discontinue TMP-SMX. HAART can also cause a similar reaction, but is less likely because the patient did not have any such signs earlier.

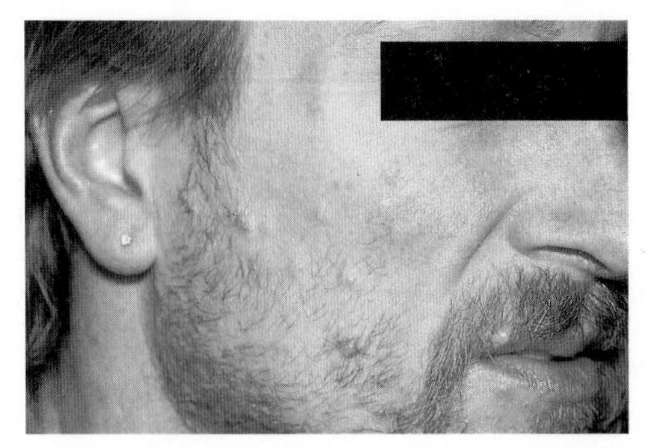

FIGURE 11–6 *Molluscum contagiosum*. From *Goodheart's Photoguide of Common Skin Disorders*, 2nd ed. Lippincott Williams & Wilkins, 2003.

> **HAART hypersensitivity**: Many antiretroviral drugs (particularly non-nucleoside reverse-transcriptase inhibitors and abacavir) can cause an erythematous maculopapular rash in the first 8 weeks. Unless symptoms are severe, continue the drug because the rash often resolves spontaneously.

> **Neutropenia**: possible complication of both TMP-SMX and HAART (especially zidovudine).

Alternative 11.5.4

A 37-year-old HIV-positive man presents with painless facial lesions (Fig. 11-6). He does not have any other symptoms. CD4 count is 70/mm^3.

What is the diagnosis?

Flesh-colored papules with an umbilicated center are the characteristic lesion of *Molluscum contagiosum*. This poxvirus spreads by direct skin-to-skin contact. Lesions can occur anywhere on the body. They are usually small and self-limited in immunocompetent patients but can be large, widespread, and refractory in immunocompromised patients. HIV-positive patients with severe or refractory Molluscum should initiate HAART.

> Histoplasmosis, cryptococcosis, and penicillinosis are opportunistic systemic fungal infections that can also cause a Molluscum-like rash.

> **Immunocompetent patients**: Use curettage, cryotherapy, or laser therapy to remove any Molluscum lesion in the genital area to prevent genital spread. Remove lesions in other areas if the patient finds them cosmetically intolerable.

CASE 11–6 COUGH AND DYSPNEA IN AN HIV-POSITIVE PATIENT

A 36-year-old HIV-positive man presents with a 5-day history of progressive dyspnea and non-productive cough. CD4 count 2 weeks ago was 150/mm^3. He does not take any prophylactic antibiotics or HAART. There are bilateral crackles on lung auscultation. Vital signs are temperature 38.1°C, pulse 110 bpm, respirations 24/min, and blood pressure 130/80. Oxygen saturation is 98%. CXR is obtained (Fig. 11-7).

What respiratory infections commonly occur in patients with HIV/AIDS?

The following respiratory infections occur with increased frequency in HIV-positive patients at any level of immunosuppression (incidence increases as CD4 count declines):

1. Acute bronchitis
2. *Mycobacterium tuberculosis* pneumonia
3. Community-acquired pneumonia: Causative pathogens are similar to those in HIV-negative individuals. *Pseudomonas aeruginosa* infection is also common in this population. Workup and management is similar to HIV negative patients.

The following respiratory infections are rare in immunocompetent patients but occur frequently in patients with low CD4 counts:

1. PCP: typically occurs only after CD4 $<200/\text{mm}^3$.
2. Other fungi: Histoplasma, Cryptococcus, and *Coccidioides pneumonia.*
3. MAC: Acid-fast organism; infection typically occurs after CD4 count $<50/\text{mm}^3$.
4. Other acid-fast organisms: Nocardia, Rhodococcus, and *Mycobacterium kansasii.*

> **Community-acquired pneumonia**: most common cause of pneumonia in HIV-positive patients.
> **PCP**: most common AIDS-defining illness in the United States.
> **Tuberculosis**: most common AIDS-defining illness in the developing world.

What noninfectious respiratory conditions should you consider in the differential diagnosis of a patient with HIV/AIDS?

KS, non-Hodgkin's lymphoma, and non-specific interstitial pneumonia can occur at any level of immunosuppression, although the frequency increases as CD4 count declines. Pulmonary KS usually occurs after cutaneous KS.

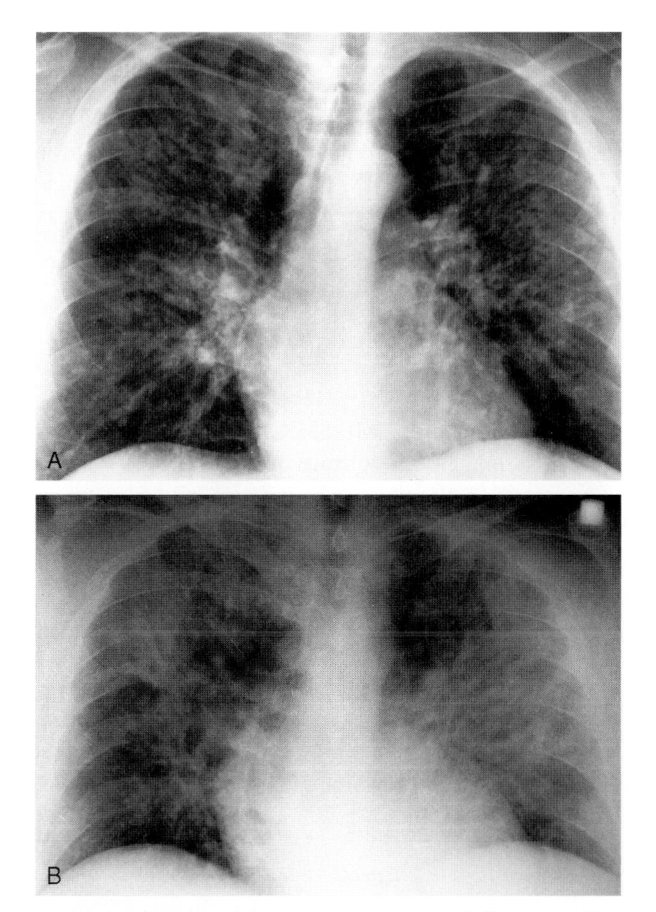

FIGURE 11–7 Chest x-ray showing *Pneumocystis carnii* pneumonia. From Daffner, RH. *Clinical Radiology: The Essentials*, 3rd ed. Lippincott Williams & Wilkins, 2007.

On the basis of his clinical features and CXR pattern, what is the most likely diagnosis?

PCP is the most likely diagnosis in this patient with CD4<200/mm^3, signs and symptoms of pneumonia, and characteristic CXR (bilateral diffuse perihilar infiltrates). Another common laboratory abnormality in PCP is increased lactate dehydrogenase (LDH).

> **Early PCP**: CXR often normal in the first few days.
> **Late PCP**: Bilateral perihilar infiltrates progress to airspace consolidation.
> **Atypical PCP**: CXR is atypical in almost 20% (e.g., lobar consolidation).

LDH is elevated.

What is the next step in management?

1. **Confirm the diagnosis**: First-line confirmatory test is IFA of induced sputum (noninvasive and specific but not sensitive). If induced sputum IFA is nondiagnostic or unobtainable, perform bronchoscopy with bronchoalveolar lavage (more invasive but also more sensitive).
2. **Obtain arterial blood gas**: Patients with PCP frequently have hypoxemia and hypercapnia. Arterial blood gas helps decide which PCP patients require steroids.

> Do not empirically treat patients for PCP without confirming the diagnosis. PCP treatments can harm patients who actually have other conditions (e.g., steroids are harmful in tuberculosis).

IFA of induced sputum confirms the diagnosis. PaO_2 is 80 and alveolar-arterial (A-a) gradient is 15. The patient does not have any GI symptoms.

What treatment is indicated?

Treat with a 21-day course of oral TMP-SMX. If symptoms fail to improve after 5 to 7 days, switch to IV TMP-SMX. If symptoms continue despite IV TMP-SMX, treat with IV pentamidine.

> Dead fungi cause an inflammatory reaction, so symptoms worsen in the first 2 or 3 days after starting TMP-SMX. Steroids help decrease this inflammatory response.

What additional treatment would you institute if PaO_2 was 62 on room air?

In addition to TMP-SMX, treat all PCP patients who have PaO_2 <70 or A-a gradient >35 with a 21-day course of oral or IV corticosteroids.

In addition to steroids, how would you tailor therapy if PaO_2 was 57 on room air?

Initiate IV rather than oral TMP-SMX if PaO_2 <60 or A-a gradient >45. Another indication for IV therapy is inability to tolerate oral intake.

When should you start HAART for this patient?

This patient should start HAART after the she recovers from the episode of PCP. Patients who are already on HAART should continue with their regimen even during the acute episode of PCP.

CASE 11–7 CNS SYMPTOMS IN AN AIDS PATIENT

A 36-year-old HIV-positive man presents with a 2-day history of headache, nausea, vomiting, blurry vision, and confusion. He has not been adherent with antibiotic prophylaxis or HAART. He is alert to person but not to place and time. Temperature is 38.1°C. CD4 count is 80/mm^3.

What diagnoses should you suspect?

Suspect increased intracranial pressure due to mass effect when a patient presents with a combination of the following signs and symptoms: altered mental status, focal neurological deficits, headache, nausea, vomiting, blurry vision, and papilledema (see Chapter 12: Neurology). The main causes of mass effect among AIDS patients in the United States are toxoplasma encephalitis and CNS lymphoma. Brain abscesses caused by other infections are also possible but less frequent. In the developing world, neurocysticercosis and CNS tuberculosis are important diagnostic considerations.

What is the next step in management?

Obtain computed tomography (CT) scan or magnetic resonance imaging (MRI) scan of the brain with contrast. Lesions that cause mass effect typically enhance with contrast administration (enhancement represents edema). Toxoplasmosis typically causes multiple small intracerebral ring-enhancing lesions. Intracerebral lesions of CNS lymphoma can be single or multiple and are often large.

CT scan with contrast shows multiple, small, ring-enhancing lesion. There is no midline shift, ventricle, chiasma, or cistern obliteration.

What tests could help distinguish toxoplasmosis from CNS lymphoma?

Obtain the following tests:

1. **Toxoplasma serology (serum IgG)**: The vast majority of toxoplasma encephalitis is caused by reactivation of prior infection. Negative serology makes this diagnosis far less likely. Positive serology does not rule out lymphoma.
2. **Lumbar puncture**: PCR often identifies whether toxoplasma is present.

> **Single ring-enhancing lesion on CT scan**: Consider MRI, SPECT (single-proton emission computed tomography), or PET (positron emission tomography) imaging to confirm whether the patient truly has a solitary lesion.

Serum IgG is positive. Cerebral spinal fluid (CSF) results are pending.

What is the next step in management?

Empirically treat patients who meet all four of the following criteria for toxoplasmosis:

1. CD4 $< 100/mm^3$
2. No primary prophylaxis for toxoplasma
3. Multiple ring-enhancing lesions on brain imaging
4. Positive serum IgG for toxoplasma

First-line therapy for cerebral toxoplasmosis is pyrimethamine plus sulfadiazine. If the patient cannot tolerate sulfadiazine, switch to pyrimethamine plus clindamycin. Typical treatment duration is 6 weeks. Patients taking pyrimethamine should also take folic acid.

When is brain biopsy indicated?

Perform brain biopsy in the following situations:

1. All four criteria not met (e.g., single ring-enhancing lesion or negative serology).
2. Patient does not respond to empiric therapy.

How would management differ if the patient had signs of impending herniation on brain imaging?

Patients with signs of impending herniation should receive steroids first to reduce edema. Obtain toxoplasma serology but avoid lumbar puncture in these patients.

Alternative 11.7.1

A 27-year-old man is brought to the emergency department after a seizure. He reports headache, blurry vision, nausea, and vomiting. He recently emigrated from China. MRI demonstrates three ring-enhancing lesions. One of the lesions contains an eccentric bright nodule. The other lesions contain calcifications. Rapid HIV-1 test is positive. CD4 count is 20/mm^3, and viral load is 900,000/mL.

What is the next step in management?

An eccentric bright nodule within a ring-enhancing lesion is the pathognomic finding of neurocysticercosis. The bright nodule represents the scolex of the pig tapeworm *Taenia solium.* Treat with albendazole plus corticosteroids. Also, administer anticonvulsants (phenytoin or carbamazepine) to prevent recurrent seizures. Prior to starting corticosteroids, perform the following:

1. Administer ivermectin (because increased likelihood of strongyloides infection).
2. Administer PPD. If PPD is positive, initiate INH.

Alternative 11.7.2

A 32-year-old HIV-positive man presents with fever, headache, left-sided weakness, and left-sided cranial nerve 3 palsy. He takes HAART and TMP-SMX. CD4 count last month was 40/mm^3. MRI is obtained (Fig. 11-8).

What is the most likely diagnosis?

The most common causes of CNS lesions without mass effect in patients with AIDS are progressive multifocal leukoencephalopathy (PML) and HIV encephalopathy. This patient with multiple areas of white matter demyelination most likely has PML, caused by John Cunningham (JC) virus infection. Demyelination occurs because JC virus attacks oligodendrocytes. The next step is lumbar puncture. Positive PCR for JC virus in a patient with compatible neuroimaging findings confirms the diagnosis. There is no specific therapy for PML. The most important measure is to decrease immunosuppression with HAART.

> Negative PCR does not rule out PML in a patient with compatible neuroimaging.

Alternative 11.7.3

A 41-year-old woman presents with fever and headache. She is HIV-positive. CD4 count 2 months ago was 92/mm^3. She takes HAART and TMP-SMX. There are no intracerebral lesions. CSF findings are: opening pressure 25 cm, leukocytes 200/mm^3 (predominantly lympocytes), glucose 40 mg/dL, and protein 200 mg/dL. Cultures and PCR antigen assays are pending. Figure 11-9 is the patient's India ink stain of CSF.

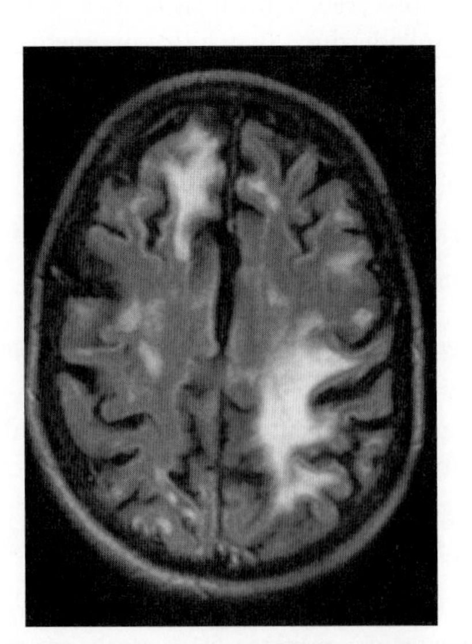

FIGURE 11–8 MRI showing demyelination due to progressive multifocal leukoencephalopathy. From Castillo M. *Neuroradiology Companion: Methods, Guidelines, and Imaging Fundamentals,* 3rd ed. Lippincott Williams & Wilkins, 2006.

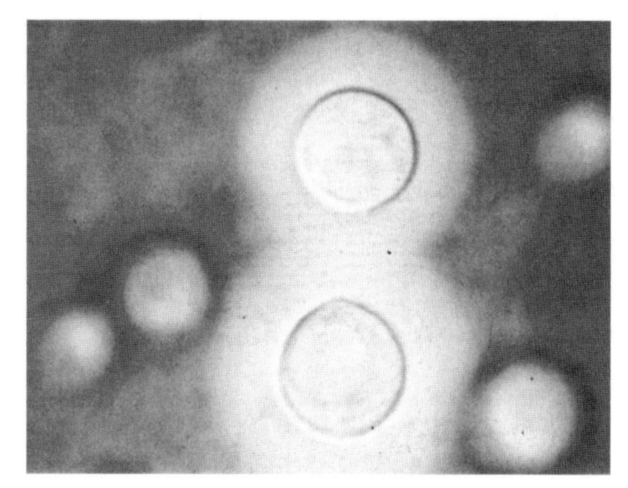

FIGURE 11–9 India ink stain for Cryptococcus. From Crapo JD, Glassroth J, Karlinsky JB, et al. *Baum's Textbook of Pulmonary Diseases,* 7th ed. Lippincott Williams & Wilkins, 2004.

How should you treat this patient?

CSF analysis indicates fungal meningitis. India ink stain reveals the characteristic appearance of *Cryptococcus neoformans* (dimorphic yeast surrounded by a capsule). Initiate treatment with IV amphotericin B and oral flucytosine. If the patient improves after 14 days, switch to oral fluconazole and continue treatment for 8 months.

> **Positive India ink stain:** CSF culture is required to confirm diagnosis.
> **Negative India ink stain**: Obtain cryptococcal antigen assay (rapid, sensitive, and specific).

Alternative 11.7.4

A 50-year-old HIV-positive man presents to the clinic for a routine evaluation. He takes HAART, TMP-SMX, and itraconazole. His sister reports that he has become increasingly depressed and withdrawn over the last 2 months. There is bilateral positive Babinski reflex and brisk deep tendon reflex on physical exam. Vital signs are normal. CD4 count is 80/mm^3. MRI shows bilateral diffuse subcortical demyelination. India ink staining, antigen assays, and CSF culture are negative.

What is the most likely diagnosis?

HIV encephalopathy is the most likely diagnosis in this patient with CD4 $<$200/mm^3, gradual onset of neuropsychiatric symptoms, and bilateral subcortical atrophy. Infection is less likely given the gradual onset and the fact that he is on appropriate primary prophylaxis. PML is less likely because demyelination is confined to the subcortical area and CSF findings are negative. There is no specific therapy, except to use antiretrovirals with high CNS penetration such as zidovudine, lamivudine, neviparine, or indinavir.

> **HIV myelopathy**: normal cognitive function but neurological signs of HIV encephalopathy (spasticity, positive Babinski reflex, erectile and sphincter dysfunction).

CASE 11–8 FEVER AND CONSTITUTIONAL SYMPTOMS IN AN AIDS PATIENT

A 34-year-old man presents with a 2-week history of fever, chills, night sweats, and a 5-lb weight loss. His last CD4 count was 25/mm^3. He has not been adherent with HAART or prophylactic antimicrobial therapy. Temperature is 39.1°C.

What are the chief causes of fever and constitutional symptoms in an AIDS patient?

The three main causes of fever and constitutional symptoms in AIDS are infections (approximately 90% of cases), lymphoma, and drug side effects. The latter is unlikely in this noncompliant patient.

What tests should you obtain initially to determine the cause of this patient's symptoms?

1. Laboratory tests: CBC, serum chemistry, LFTs, urinalysis, blood culture, LDH.
2. Imaging tests: CXR and sinus radiographs.

What tests would you order if initial tests were nondiagnostic?

1. Abdominal CT scan.
2. Sputum, urine, and stool cultures for Mycobacteria.
3. Serology for Toxoplasma and Cryptococcus antigen. Also obtain serology for Histoplasma, Coccidioides, Leishmaniasis, etc., based on local prevalence.
4. Eye exam by an ophthalmologist to screen for CMV or Candida retinitis.
5. Head CT (if the patient has any CNS symptoms).
6. Bone marrow biopsy (if the patient has peripheral blood cytopenias).
7. Liver biopsy (if the patient has abnormal LFTs).
8. Fecal leukocytes, culture, ova, and parasites (if the patient has diarrhea).
9. Skin or lymph node biopsy (if the patient has skin findings or lymphadenopathy).

What antimicrobial therapy is indicated if cultures demonstrate MAC?

The acid-fast bacillus MAC typically causes disseminated infection in patients with CD4 <50/mm^3. Treat MAC with a 12-month course of clarithromycin and ethambutol. Also add rifabutin if the patient is not taking a protease inhibitor (combination increases side effects).

How would you tailor antibiotic therapy if serology showed histoplasma instead?

First-line therapy for severe infection is a 4 to 6 week course of IV amphotericin B (meningitis, acute renal failure, acute liver failure, severe hypoxemia, etc.). First-line therapy for less severe disseminated histoplasmosis is oral itraconazole. All patients require maintenance itraconazole.

Blastomycosis: First-line treatment for severe infection is amphotericin B. First-line treatment for less severe infection is itraconazole.
Coccidiomycosis: First-line treatment for severe infection is amphotericin B. For less severe infection, either itraconazole or fluconazole are acceptable choices.

Alternative 11.8.4

A 27-year-old patient is found to have oral candidiasis. HIV EIA and Western blot are positive. CD4 count is 20/mm^3. He initiates HAART. Four weeks later, CD4 count is 600/mm^3. Six weeks after starting HAART, he develops fever and constitutional symptoms. CD4 count is now 900/mm^3. Initial laboratory and imaging tests are nondiagnostic.

What is the most likely cause of his symptoms?

The most likely cause of his symptoms is immune reconstitution inflammatory syndrome (IRIS), which can occur weeks to months after starting HAART. To diagnose IRIS, the patient must have pre-HAART CD4 count <100/mm^3, post-HAART CD4 count increase 200% to 400%, and exclusion of OIs. Continue HAART in patients with IRIS unless symptoms become life-threatening. Some clinicians prescribe corticosteroids to select patients with IRIS.

CASE 11–9 DIARRHEA AND WEIGHT LOSS IN AN AIDS PATIENT

Over the last month, a 40-year-old HIV-positive man reports increasing fatigue and a 30-lb weight loss. He also reports four or five episodes of profuse watery diarrhea. He takes TMP-SMP but is not on HAART. Temperature is 38.4°C. CD4 count is 100/mm^3. Fecal leukocytes, culture, O&P (ova and parasites) are negative. He undergoes colonoscopy, which is negative. All tests to evaluate fever and constitutional symptoms are negative.

What is the most likely diagnosis?

The patient most likely has AIDS-wasting syndrome. This diagnosis of exclusion presents with fever, fatigue, profuse diarrhea, and unexplained weight loss (primarily due to loss of lean body mass).

How is AIDS-wasting syndrome treated?

Treatment is challenging. In addition to initiating HAART, first-line measures include caloric supplements and exercise. If wasting persists, measure and correct any steroid hormone deficiencies.

> **Cryptosporidium**: In this common cause of profuse watery diarrhea in AIDS, stool studies are usually diagnostic. Treatment is HAART and supportive measures.

chapter 12

Neurology

CASE 12-1 TYPES OF ALTERED MENTAL STATES

A 64-year-old woman undergoes cholecystectomy on Monday morning. She is an otherwise healthy college professor. On Tuesday night, she seems confused. She does not remember where she is or who her family members are. She does not always answer questions, and she looks away from the examiner. She is oriented to person but not to place or time.

How would you categorize her mental status?

Delirium is characterized by sudden and fluctuating confusion and/or agitation, hallucinations, and illusions. Delirium is precipitated by an underlying medical condition. Remember important causes of delirium with the mnemonic "***I STOP HEAD MUSH***":

- **I**nfections
- **S**troke
- **T**raumatic brain injury (TBI)
- **O**peration (postoperative state)
- **P**sychiatric disorders
- **H**ypertensive encephalopathy (Chapter 2: Cardiology)
- **E**lectrolytes and fluids (Chapter 7: Fluids and Electrolytes): Dehydration, hyponatremia, and hypernatremia
- **A**lcohol overdose and withdrawal (Chapter 7: Fluids and Electrolytes)
- **D**rug overdose and withdrawal

- **M**etabolic/endocrine: hypoglycemia, DKA (Chapter 7: Fluids and Electrolytes), hyperosmolar nonketonic state, hypoglycemia, Addisonian crisis, myxedema coma, thyroid storm, and hypercalcemia (Chapter 8: Endocrinology).
- **U**remic encephalopathy (Chapter 6: Nephrology)
- **S**eizure
- **H**epatic encephalopathy (Chapter 5: Hepatology)

Note: A helpful way to categorize causes of delirium is:

1. **Focal neurological signs**: Suspect space-occupying lesion (e.g., abscess, hemorrhage).
2. **No focal signs**: Suspect diffuse brain injury (e.g., drug toxicity, metabolic disorder).

How does delirium differ from stupor, obtundation, and coma?

Delirium is a continuum that ranges from intact consciousness to obtundation, stupor, and coma. Consciousness is the ability to perceive the external environment, as assessed by response to verbal and noxious (e.g., painful) stimuli:

1. **Obtundation**: decreased response to verbal stimuli; normal response to noxious stimuli.
2. **Stupor**: no response to verbal stimuli; intact response to noxious stimuli.
3. **Coma**: no response to verbal or noxious stimuli (unconscious).

> Comatose patients can progress to recovery, persistent vegetative state, or death.

How would you characterize the mental status of a 32-year-old woman who was found lying sprawled in her apartment with the following findings: no response to verbal commands or light nudging, eyes remain closed despite painful stimuli, extremities withdraw in response to painful stimuli, and occasional incomprehensible sounds?

Stupor and obtundation are relatively subjective terms, so an objective measure such as the Glasgow coma scale (GCS) is preferred to describe states of decreased consciousness (Table 12-1). This woman has a GCS of 7 (E1, M4, and V2).

What score would you assign for the motor response portion of the GCS if her arms, wrists, and elbows were flexed, legs were extended, and feet were rotated inward?

The position described is termed decorticate posturing ("mummy baby"). Decorticate posturing indicates damage above the midbrain. Motor response is M3 on the GCS.

> **Decerebrate posturing**: Arched head and extended arms, wrists, and legs; feet rotated inward. This posturing indicates brainstem damage (more severe than decorticate posturing). Progression from decorticate to decerebrate posturing suggests brainstem herniation.

What are the initial steps when evaluating a person with acute decline in consciousness?

Figure 12-1 outlines a step-wise approach to patients with acute decline in consciousness. Brain imaging is not necessary if the patient meets all of the following criteria:

1. Step 2: Patient follows commands and there is no history of trauma.
2. Step 4: There are no focal neurological signs.
3. An obvious underlying cause is detected.

> **Focal neurological signs**: behavioral or perceptual impairments that indicate damage to a particular part of the central nervous system (CNS) (Tables 12-2 and 12-3).

> **Rapid sequence intubation (RSI)**: a commonly used technique for emergency intubation of conscious patients. Administer a fast-acting sedative (e.g., propofol, etomidate, or midazolam) followed by a fast-acting paralytic drug (e.g., succinylcholine) and then quickly intubate. RSI is unnecessary if the patient is comatose or in cardiac arrest.

TABLE 12–1 Glasgow Coma Scale

ACTIVITY	SCORE
Eye opening (E)	
Does not open eyes	1
Opens to painful stimulus	2
Opens to verbal command	3
Opens spontaneously	4
Verbal response (V)	
No sounds	1
Incomprehensible sounds	2
Inappropriate words	3
Appropriate but confused	4
Appropriate and oriented	5
Motor response (M)	
No movement	1
Decerebrate posture	2
Decorticate posture	3
Withdraws from pain	4
Localized painful stimulus	5
Obeys commands	6

Abbreviation: GCS, Glasgow coma scale.
Note: GCS $\leq$ 8 = severe coma; GCS 9–13 = moderate coma; GCS > 13 = minor coma.

Alternative 12.1.1

A 69-year-old man is found collapsed in his apartment. The paramedics detect ventricular fibrillation. They are able to hemodynamically stabilize him, but he remains unconscious. Over the next 4 months, there is no response to verbal or noxious stimuli. His eyes stay open for a few hours and close for a few hours. He occasionally moves his limbs for a few seconds. Brainstem reflexes are intact. He is mechanically ventilated through a tracheostomy and fed through a gastrostomy tube.

How would you describe his mental status?

The patient is in a persistent vegetative state, often described as "wakefulness without awareness." Patients do not respond to verbal or noxious stimuli, although they have normal sleep–wake cycles and intermittently move their limbs. Brainstem reflexes are sufficiently preserved to permit survival with life support measures. Some patients may regain consciousness, although recovery is rare after 3 months of persistent vegetative state.

What diagnosis should you suspect if the patient responds to "yes" and "no" questions by blinking his eyes but does not make any sounds or move any other part of his body, even in response to noxious stimuli?

The clinical description is characteristic of locked-in-syndrome. This rare condition results from a stroke or lesion at the base of the pons. Although patients cannot generate a verbal or motor response to stimuli, they are actually completely conscious. Patients are limited to communicating by blinking their eyes.

Alternative 12.1.2

A 75-year-old woman is found unconscious in her apartment. The paramedics and emergency physicians are able to hemodynamically stabilize her with vasopressors and mechanical ventilation, but she remains comatose. Head CT reveals a large middle cerebral artery (MCA) infarct.

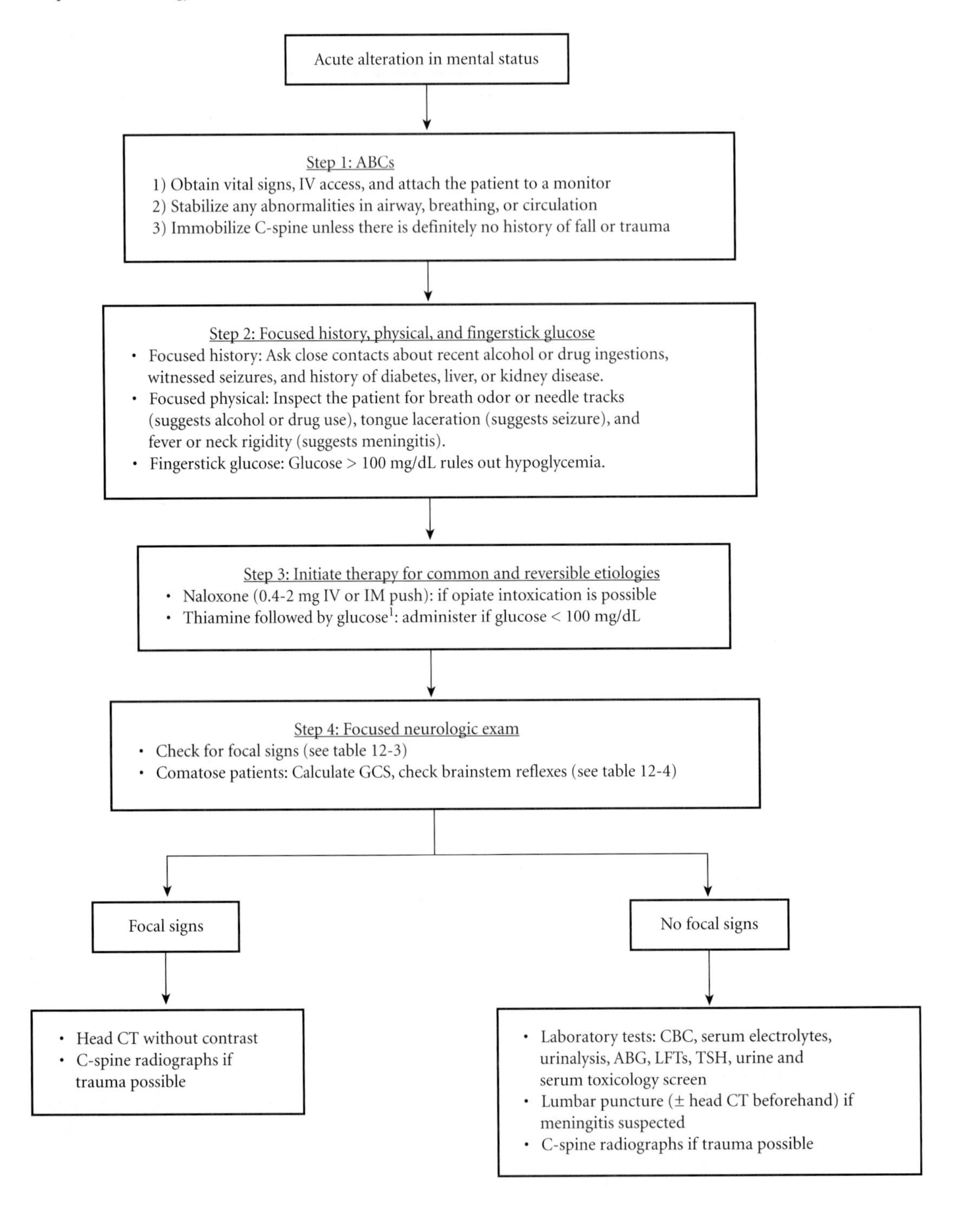

Acute alteration in mental status
Step 1: ABCs
1) Obtain vital signs, IV access, and attach the patient to a monitor
2) Stabilize any abnormalities in airway, breathing, or circulation
3) Immobilize C-spine unless there is definitely no history of fall or trauma
Step 2: Focused history, physical, and fingerstick glucose
• Focused history: Ask close contacts about recent alcohol or drug ingestions, witnessed seizures, and history of diabetes, liver, or kidney disease.
• Focused physical: Inspect the patient for breath odor or needle tracks (suggests alcohol or drug use), tongue laceration (suggests seizure), and fever or neck rigidity (suggests meningitis).
• Fingerstick glucose: Glucose > 100 mg/dL rules out hypoglycemia.
Step 3: Initiate therapy for common and reversible etiologies
• Naloxone (0.4-2 mg IV or IM push): if opiate intoxication is possible
• Thiamine followed by glucose[1]: administer if glucose < 100 mg/dL
Step 4: Focused neurologic exam
• Check for focal signs (see table 12-3)
• Comatose patients: Calculate GCS, check brainstem reflexes (see table 12-4)
Focal signs
No focal signs
• Head CT without contrast
• C-spine radiographs if trauma possible
• Laboratory tests: CBC, serum electrolytes, urinalysis, ABG, LFTs, TSH, urine and serum toxicology screen
• Lumbar puncture (± head CT beforehand) if meningitis suspected
• C-spine radiographs if trauma possible
[1]If the patient can swallow appropriately, give oral glucose. Otherwise, give D5W (if IV access not available, give IM glucagon).

FIGURE 12–1 Approach to acute alteration in mental status.

GCS is 3 (E1, M1, V1). Her pupils are fixed and dilated (absent papillary reflex). Corneal, gag, and oculocephalic reflexes are absent. A nurse mentions that she saw the patient moving her arms towards her chest for a few seconds as if she wanted to pray (Lazarus sign).

How would you characterize her mental status?

A comatose patient with no verbal or motor responses and absent brainstem reflexes is brain dead. Brain dead patients may demonstrate movements originating from the spinal cord or peripheral nerves such as finger flexion, positive Babinski sign, and Lazarus sign. Their heart

TABLE 12–2 Focal Neurological Signs

Frontal Signs (*"MP3 Brain Jam"*)	• ↑ **M**uscle tone: muscle rigidity; resistance to passive motion • **P**aresis: paralysis of limb, head, eye, or entire side of body • **P**ersonality changes: e.g., apathy, loss of inhibitions, akinetic mutism (patient doesn't move or speak) • **P**rimitive reflexes (frontal release signs): e.g., grasp reflex, snout reflex, unilateral loss of smell • **B**roca's aphasia: ↓ ability to verbally express thoughts despite normal comprehension • **J**acksonian seizure: focal seizures that spread to adjacent areas
Parietal Signs (*"Pariahs are able but Neglected"*)	• **Ability**: Loss of abilities such as reading (dyslexia), writing, (dysgraphia), calculating (dyscalculia), and identifying objects based on touch (astereognosia) • **Neglect:** lack of awareness of one side of body (sensory neglect) or a particular visual field (visual neglect)
Temporal Signs (*"SMAC"!!*)	• **S**ensory (Wernicke's) aphasia: comprehension and speech preserved but language content is incorrect • **M**emory disorders: short-term or long-term memory loss (e.g., déjà vu) • **A**uditory symptoms: tinnitus, auditory hallucinations, and cortical deafness (deafness in the absence of structural ear damage) • **C**omplex partial seizures (temporal lobe epilepsy)
Occipital Signs	• Visual illusions, visual hallucinations, or visual loss
Cerebellar Signs (*"NADIR"*)	• **N**ystagmus • **A**taxia: limb and torso unsteadiness • **D**isdiadochokinesis: can't perform rapid alternating movements • **I**ntention tremor: detected using finger to nose test • **R**omberg sign: limb and torso unsteadiness when eyes are closed

Information from Wikipedia: http://en.wikipedia.org/wiki/Focal_neurologic_signs. (Original source not listed).

can continue beating for months with hemodynamic support. By definition, there is no possibility of recovery.

How is brain death confirmed in mechanically ventilated patients?

The apnea test is required to confirm brain death in mechanically ventilated patients:

1. Maintain systolic blood pressure (SBP) $\geq$90, temperature $\geq$36.5°C, and discontinue sedative or paralytic drugs.
2. Stop mechanical ventilation and visually observe for spontaneous breaths.
3. If she does not take any breaths for 8 minutes, reconnect to the ventilator and measure $PaCO_2$. No spontaneous breathing despite $PaCO_2$ >60 confirms the diagnosis.

Alternative 12.1.3

A 60-year-old man is brought to the physician by his daughter. She says that over the last few months, he seems to be forgetting things easily. He often gets lost in his neighborhood, where he has lived for 30 years. He remembers distant events such as his wedding and his first job, but he cannot remember what he did yesterday. He does not take any medications.

How would you characterize his mental status?

Insidious onset of cognitive difficulties should raise suspicion for dementia. Unlike delirium, onset is gradual and consciousness is generally preserved.

Cognition: ability to think, reason, and remember.

TABLE 12–3 Brainstem Reflexes

Test	Description	Normal Response
Pupillary reflex	Shine light in each pupil and observe ipsilateral and contralateral eye.	Both ipsilateral and contralateral eye should constrict (direct and consensual reflex).
Oculocephalic reflex ("doll's eye maneuver")	Forcibly turn head horizontally and vertically. Contraindicated if C-spine injury not ruled out.	Both eyes deviate away from direction that head is turned (contralateral).
Caloric testing	Perform if "doll's eye maneuver" is contraindicated. Inject 50 mL of cold water into each ear.	Both eyes deviate towards ipsilateral ear; nystagmus to the contralateral side.
Corneal reflex	Touch lateral cornea with cotton tip.	Direct and consensual blink.
Gag reflex	Push cotton tip into posterior pharynx.	Patient gags or coughs.

Adapted from Frank Drislane, Juan Acosta, Michael Benatar, et al. *Blueprints in Neurology*. Blackwell Publishing. 2002.

How can you screen for cognitive impairment in a person with suspected dementia?

Use the Mini Mental Status Exam (MMSE) to quickly screen for cognitive impairment (Table 12-4). MMSE score <24 suggests that the patient may have dementia. Always interpret the MMSE in the context of the individual patient. For example, an illiterate person may find it difficult to score highly on the MMSE despite intact cognition. A highly educated person may have a score >24 despite a decrease in the baseline level of cognition.

CASE 12–2 ACUTE ONSET OF FOCAL NEUROLOGICAL SIGNS

A 65-year-old man is brought to the emergency department for evaluation of altered mental status. His wife reports that he began "talking weird" while watching television 2 hours ago. There is no history of trauma. There is no history of recent alcohol or drug ingestion. He has a

TABLE 12–4 Mini Mental Status Exam (*"ORARL"*)

Orientation	What is the (year) (season) (date) (day) (month)?	1 point for each correct answer (total 5 points)
	Where are we (country) (city) (part of city) (house number) (street name)?	1 point for each correct answer (total 5 points)
Registration	Name three objects and ask patient to repeat all three immediately.	1 point for each correct answer (total 3 points)
Attention	Spell "WORLD" backwards OR serial 7's.	Total 5 points
Recall	Ask patient what the three objects mentioned during registration portion of the MMSE were.	1 point for each correct answer (total 3 points)
Language	Point to a pencil and a watch and ask patient what it is.	1 point for each correct answer (total 2 points)
	Ask patient to repeat "No ifs, ands, or buts."	1 point
	Ask patient to take a paper in right hand, fold it, and put it on the floor (three-step command).	1 point for each correct task (total 3 points)
	Write "close your eyes" on a piece of paper. Ask patient to read and obey the command.	1 point
	Ask patient to write a sentence.	1 point
	Ask patient to copy a design.	1 point

history of hypertension and type 2 diabetes mellitus. Fingerstick glucose is 120 mg/dL. His right arm is weaker than his left. There is decreased pain, temperature, and vibration sensation in his right arm. He has a right-sided facial droop. His speech is slurred. Stool is guaiac-negative. Cardiovascular (CV) examination is normal. Vital signs are temperature 37.5°C, pulse 90 bpm, respirations 12/min, and blood pressure 160/100. Oxygen saturation is 99% on room air.

What is the differential diagnosis?

Acute onset of focal neurological deficits can result from "***STAT CT***":

1. **S**troke: focal neurological deficits due to ischemic or hemorrhagic damage to one or more regions of the brain (Fig. 12-2).
2. **T**ransient ischemic attack (TIA): also causes focal neurological deficits due to brain ischemia, but symptoms resolve within 1 hour (usually <5 minutes) and no tissue damage is detected on imaging.
3. **A**bscess or encephalitis
4. **T**raumatic brain injury (TBI)
5. **C**onversion disorder: rare psychiatric condition (diagnosis of exclusion).
6. **T**odd's palsy: focal paresis ± aphasia or visual loss up to 48 hours after a seizure.

On the basis of clinical findings alone, what diagnosis is most likely?

The clinical findings suggest an ischemic stroke involving the left MCA (Table 12-5).

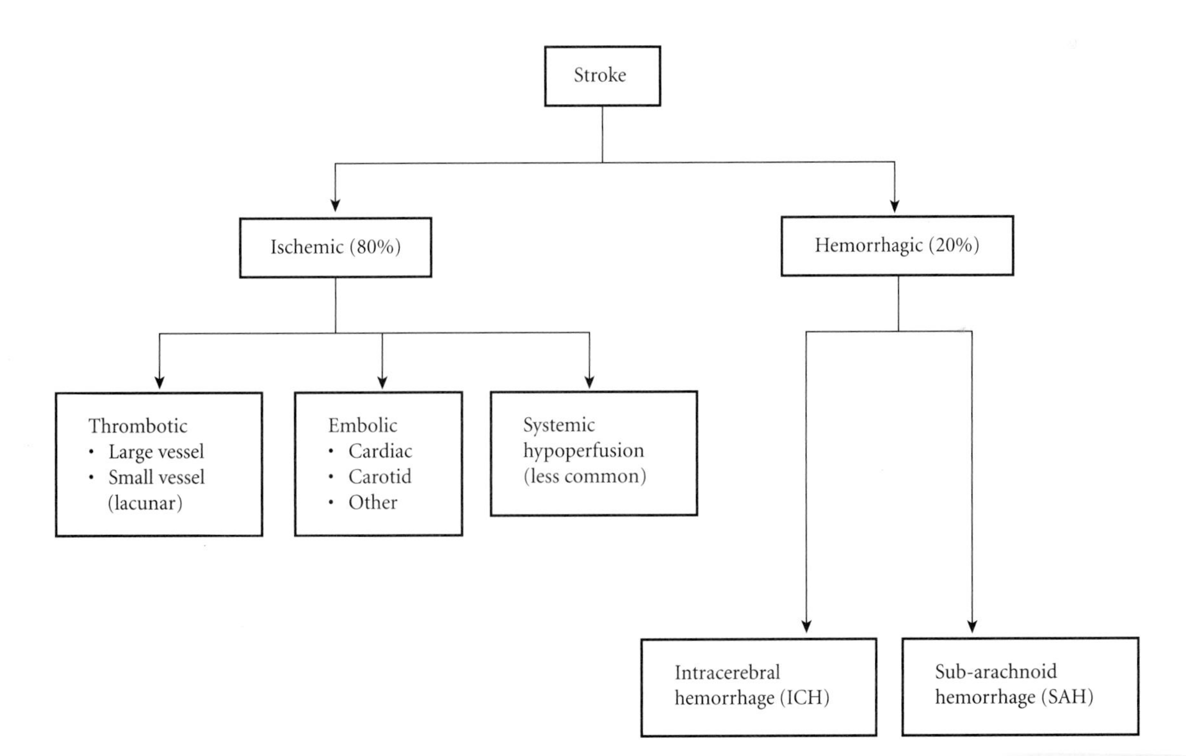

Classic presentations (not reliable!!)

Thrombotic	Fluctuating neurologic deficits
Embolic	Sudden onset of neurologic deficits (maximal at onset)
SAH	Sudden onset of extremely severe headache, vomiting ± focal deficits
ICH	Gradually worsening focal deficits ± headache, nausea, and vomiting

FIGURE 12–2 Classification of ischemic stroke.

TABLE 12-5 Focal Deficit Clues to Localize Ischemic Stroke

Artery	Motor Deficits	Sensory Deficits	Visual Deficits	Other
ACA	Contralateral lower extremity	Contralateral lower extremity	–	Incontinence and frontal signs
MCA	Contralateral upper extremity and lower quadrant of face	Contralateral face and upper extremities	Homonymous hemianopsia	Left-sided lesion: aphasia Right-sided lesion: apraxia and neglect
PCA	–	Contralateral half of body	Homonymous hemianopsia	Aphasia
ICA	Quadriplegia	Sensory loss in all extremities	Monocular blindness	Deficits of ACA, MCA, and PCA stroke
Vertebral artery	Contralateral hemiplegia	Contralateral extremities; ipsilateral face	IL Horner syndrome and diplopia	Aphasia
Basilar artery	Quadriplegia, cranial nerve paresis	Sensory loss in all extremities	Homonymous hemianopsia and diplopia	Pinpoint pupils
Lacunar stroke	Pure hemiplegia (internal capsule lesion)	Pure hemisensory loss (thalamus lesion)	–	Dysarthria, clumsy hand (pons lesion)

Abbreviations: ACA, anterior cerebral artery; ICA, internal carotid artery; IL, ipsilateral; MCA, middle cerebral artery; PCA, posterior cerebral artery.

Cincinnati Prehospital Stroke Scale: Suspect stroke if patient has any of the following (mnemonic: "***FAST***"): **F**acial droop, **A**rm drifts down when held out straight, **S**lurred **T**alk.

What is the most important next step in management?

Although clinical findings are suggestive, they do not reliably rule out hemorrhage. The most important next step is urgent head CT without contrast. Magnetic resonance imaging (MRI) is also very accurate, but it is not the first-line test at most centers because it takes longer and is more expensive.

Blood appears white (hyperdense) on CT scan; infarct appears black (hypodense). The right side of the image is the left lobe of the patient and vice versa.

Other basic tests in all persons with suspected stroke are EKG, complete blood count (CBC), serum chemistry, type and crossmatch, prothrombin time (PT), partial thromboplastin time (PTT), and International Normalized Ratio (INR).

EKG is normal. CT scan is performed and interpreted within 25 minutes. There is no hemorrhage or infarct. Laboratory studies are pending.

What is the next step?

Normal CT rules out hemorrhage but not ischemic stroke (CT is often negative in the first 24 to 48 hours after ischemic stroke). The next step is thrombolytic therapy in this patient without any contraindications (Table 12-6). Thrombolytics are only effective within 3 hours of symptom onset, so don't delay treatment to obtain the laboratory results (unless the patient is on anticoagulation or you strongly suspect a bleeding disorder). Intravenous (IV) alteplase (reverse-transcription tissue plasminogen activator (rt-tPA)) is the only thrombolytic approved for ischemic stroke.

TABLE 12-6 Contraindications to Thrombolytic Therapy for Ischemic Stroke

PAST MEDICAL HISTORY	
Any Prior History	**Intracranial Hemorrhage**
<3 months ago	Stroke, head trauma, or MI
<3 weeks ago	Gastrointestinal or genitourinary bleeding
<2 weeks ago	General surgery
<7 days ago	Lumbar puncture

CURRENT H&P

Duration > 3 hours
Rapidly improving symptoms
Pregnant or breastfeeding
Risk factors for hemorrhage:
- SBP > 185 or DBP > 110 despite antihypertensives
- Active bleeding (e.g., guaiac-positive stool, trauma)
- Warfarin anticoagulation and INR > 1.7
- Symptoms suggest SAH (even if CT scan is normal)

HEAD CT SCAN

Hemorrhage
Diffuse swelling
Infarction of > 30% of MCA territory

LABORATORY TESTS

INR > 1.7 and patient is taking warfarin
↑ PTT and patient received heparin in the last 48 hours
Platelets < 100,000
Glucose <40 mg/dL or >400 mg/dL

Abbreviations: DBP, diastolic blood pressure; INR, International Normalized Ratio; MI, myocardial infarction; PTT, partial thromboplastin time; SAH, subarachnoid hemorrhage, SBP systolic blood pressure.

Stroke is the third leading cause of death and the leading cause of disability.

Only 5% of stroke patients meet inclusion criteria for rt-tPA.

Would you administer rt-tPA if the patient had presented 5 hours after symptom onset, CT scan showed a small area of MCA infarct, and blood pressure were 160/100?

Most centers do not administer thrombolytics after the therapeutic window. Instead, administer aspirin (aspirin within the first 48 hours reduces mortality and disability).

Select, specialized centers obtain additional noninvasive imaging (MRI and magnetic resonance angiography) 3 to 6 hours after symptom onset and administer intraarterial rt-tPA if there is sufficient viable tissue. Many studies show that this practice reduces 3-month mortality.

MERCI device: a coiled wire that is threaded through the femoral artery to dislodge the cerebral clot. At present, it is unclear if this device improves outcomes.

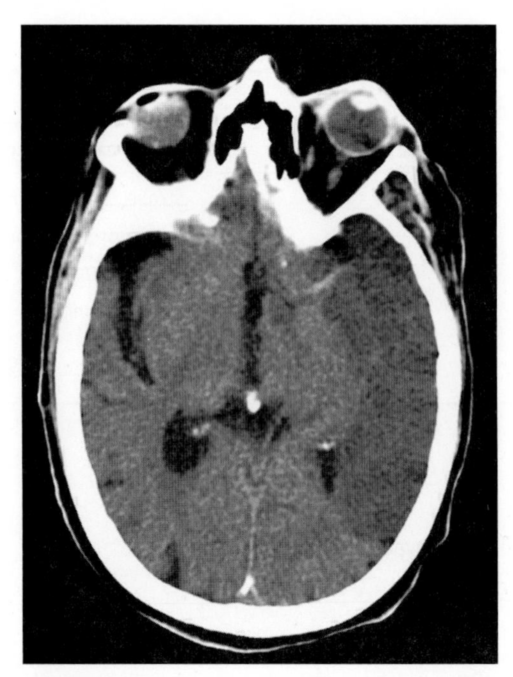

FIGURE 12–3 CT scan showing MCA infarct >30%. From Castillo M. *Neuroradiology Companion: Methods, Guidelines, and Imaging Fundamentals, 3rd ed.* Lippincott Williams & Wilkins, 2005.

Would you administer thrombolytics if the patient woke up with stroke symptoms and Figure 12-3 was the CT scan?

Patients who wake up with symptoms are not candidates for rt-tPA because the time of symptom onset is uncertain. Also, CT scan shows >30% MCA infarction, which is a contraindication to rt-tPA (increased risk of intracerebral hemorrhage (ICH)). Treat with aspirin instead.

> Never give aspirin and thrombolytics together in ischemic stroke (increased risk of ICH).

What other measures are recommended in the initial management of ischemic stroke?

1. **Monitor airway and breathing**: Administer O_2 if SaO_2 <92%. Consider intubation if GCS <12 (to decrease risk of aspiration pneumonia).
2. **Monitor blood pressure**: Treat hypotension with fluids ± vasopressors. Do not correct hypertension except in certain instances (Fig. 12-4) because increased mean arterial pressure is necessary to maintain cerebral perfusion pressure (CPP).
3. **Monitor temperature**: Maintain normothermia with acetaminophen if the patient has fever.
4. **Monitor glucose**: Maintain blood glucose between 60 and 150 mg/dL.
5. **Cardiac telemetry**: Arrhythmias (e.g., atrial fibrillation) and myocardial infarction (MI) are common complications of stroke. Continuously monitor EKG in the first 24 hours and treat any abnormalities. Arrhythmia prophylaxis is not recommended.
6. **Serial neurological exams**: Common neurological complications are ICH (increased risk with thrombolytics) and cerebral edema. Obtain repeat head CT if the patient develops new or worsening neurological deficits.

> The practice of correcting fever and hyperglycemia are based on animal studies and not human studies.

> Consider transthoracic echocardiography (TTE) or transesophageal echocardiography (TEE) during the acute period if initial EKG detects atrial fibrillation.

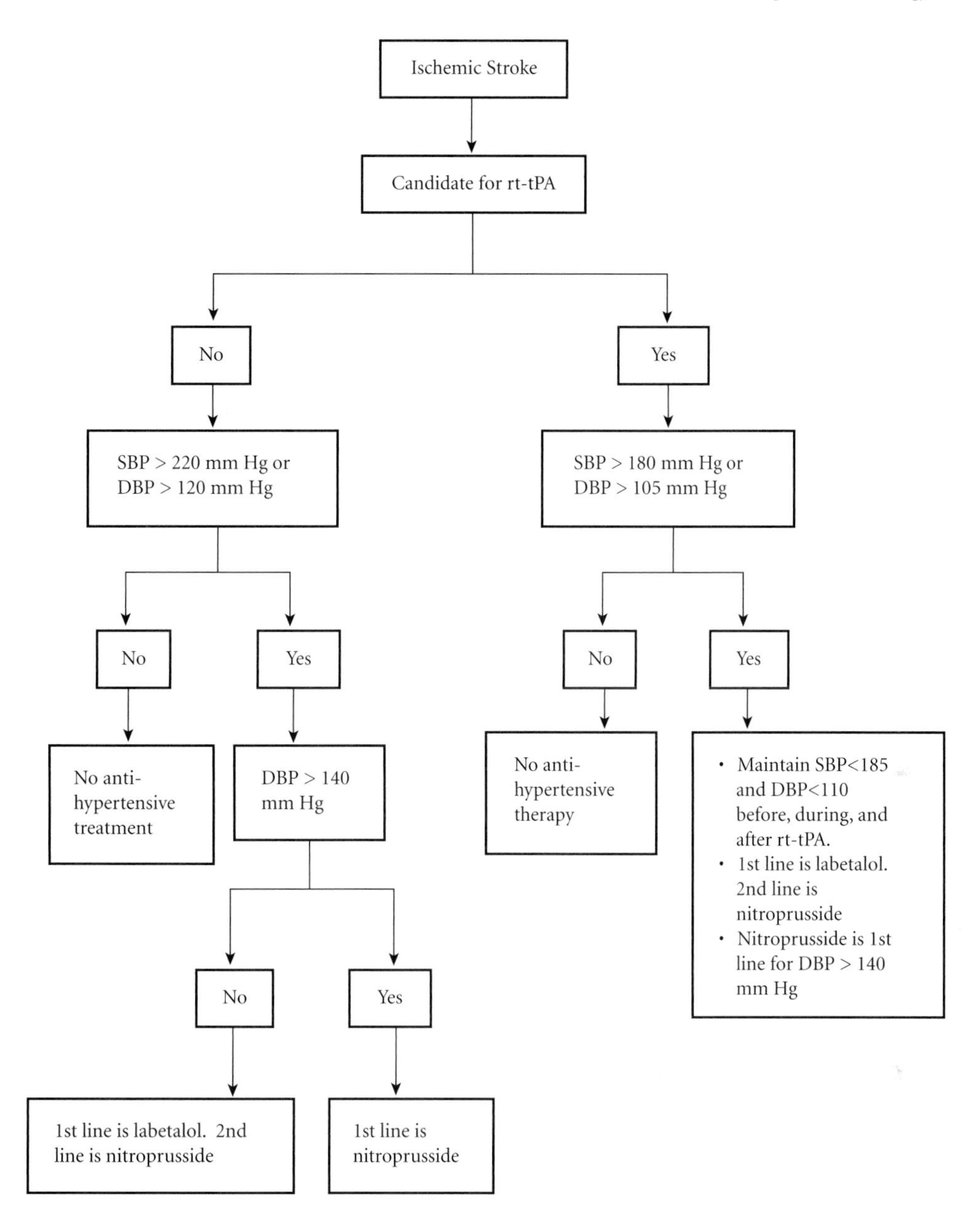

SBP = systolic blood pressure, DBP = diastolic blood pressure

FIGURE 12–4 Blood pressure control in ischemic stroke.

What measures are generally recommended after the acute period?

1. **Antiplatelet therapy**: First-line therapy is aspirin plus dipyridamole. The second-line option is clopidogrel alone (if dipyridamole is too expensive).
2. **Reduce CV risk factors**: Aggressive control lowers the risk of recurrent stroke. Target blood pressure is 130/80, and target low-density lipoprotein is ≤100 mg/dL.
3. **DVT prophylaxis**: Consider low-dose subcutaneous heparin for immobile patients. Pneumatic compression stockings are an alternative if heparin is contraindicated.
4. **Imaging**: Obtain cardiac imaging (TTE or TEE) and cerebrovascular imaging to determine the source of thrombus or embolism. Choice of cerebrovascular imaging depends on whether the infarct is in the internal carotid artery distribution (e.g., MCA, anterior cerebral artery) or vertebrobasilar (VB) distribution.

> **Internal carotid artery distribution**: Obtain duplex ultrasound of the neck plus transcranial Doppler ultrasound. Alternatives are CT angiography or magnetic resonance angiography.
> **VB distribution**: Obtain duplex ultrasound of vertebral and subclavian arteries.

Do focal neurological deficits ever resolve after an ischemic stroke?

Deficits in the core ischemic region are never regained. Deficits resulting from ischemia of the surrounding ischemic but viable tissue (penumbra) should resolve over the next few months. Physical therapy and rehabilitation are extremely important components of long-term management.

Alternative 12.2.1

A 65-year-old man had an episode of visual loss in his left eye 24 hours ago. He describes the symptom as a "curtain coming down and covering my eye." The visual loss resolved after 3 to 5 minutes. He is currently asymptomatic. He has a history of hypertension. Physical exam and vital signs are normal.

What is the most likely diagnosis?

Suspect TIA if a patient presents with focal neurological deficits that resolve completely within 1 hour. Unilateral visual loss (amaurosis fugax) is a common presentation and indicates an embolus from the internal carotid to the ophthalmic artery. TIA is a neurological emergency because it carries a 10% to 20% risk of stroke within the next 90 days.

> **Classic TIA definition**: Neurological symptoms last <24 hours. Irreversible tissue damage usually occurs after 1 hour, so classic definition is inadequate.

What is the next step in management?

The next step in this patient with amaurosis fugax is urgent carotid duplex ultrasound (CDUS). If CDUS detects >50% stenosis, refer for carotid endarterectomy (CEA). If CDUS detects <50% stenosis, treatment is aspirin and CV risk factor control.

> **Women**: CEA is only indicated in symptomatic women with carotid stenosis >70%.

The patient's 62-year-old brother is very worried about his risk of stroke. He asks if he should undergo CDUS as well. He has a history of hypertension and peripheral vascular disease that causes calf pain at rest. There are no carotid bruits.

What should you tell this patient?

Screening CDUS is not warranted in most asymptomatic patients (no history of TIA or stroke symptoms). Exceptions are "***Porsche & Corvette* = *RAD CAR***":

1. **P**eripheral vascular disease: Obtain CDUS only if symptomatic.
2. **C**ABG: Obtain CDUS prior to CABG if age >65 and ≥1 CV risk factor.
3. **RAD**iation: Obtain annual CDUS 10 years after head and neck radiation.
4. **CAR**otid bruit: Obtain CDUS if physical exam detects a carotid bruit.

> Carotid bruits can result from heart murmurs (referred sound) or carotid stenosis.

The brother with symptomatic peripheral vascular disease undergoes CDUS. There is 55% stenosis in the left carotid artery.

How should you manage carotid stenosis in this patient?

CEA is not indicated in asymptomatic men unless carotid stenosis >60%. Manage this patient with CV risk factor control, aspirin, and annual CDUS.

> CEA is not beneficial in asymptomatic women with carotid stenosis.

What diagnosis should you suspect if the 65-year-old man presented with bilateral blurry vision, diplopia, dizziness, and ataxia that resolved completely in 20 minutes?

The symptoms suggest a VB TIA. The next step is duplex ultrasound of the vertebral and subclavian arteries. Treatment is aspirin and CV risk factor control.

What syndrome should you suspect if the patient had recurrent symptoms of VB TIA after exercise, weak pulse in the left arm, and blood pressure in the left arm less than blood pressure in the right arm?

Subclavian steal syndrome is characterized by recurrent symptoms of VB TIA (especially after exercise) and unequal pulse and blood pressure in each arm. The syndrome results from severe atherosclerosis of the subclavian artery, which creates a low-pressure zone distal to stenosis. As a result, blood flows from the contralateral vertebral artery to the basilar artery to the ipsilateral vertebral artery (instead of brainstem). Duplex ultrasound of the subclavian artery can confirm the diagnosis. Treatment is surgical revascularization.

Alternative 12.2.2

A 70-year-old man presents with a 2-hour history of gradually increasing headache, nausea, and vomiting. He has a history of hypertension and atrial fibrillation and is on warfarin anticoagulation. On physical exam, there is right-sided weakness and sensory loss. Vitals signs are temperature 37.2°C, pulse 120 bpm, respirations 12/min, and blood pressure 165/95. Figure 12-5 is the patient's CT scan.

What is the diagnosis?

CT scan demonstrates ICH, which results from rupture of an intracerebral blood vessel. ICH classically presents with gradually progressive neurological deficits. Large hemorrhages can cause signs of increased ICP.

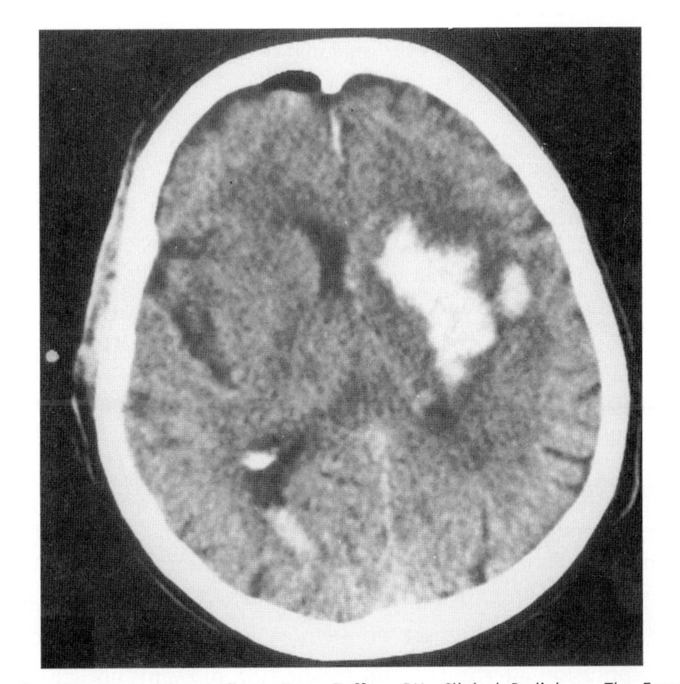

FIGURE 12–5 CT scan showing intracerebral hemorrhage. From Daffner RH. *Clinical Radiology: The Essentials, 3rd ed.* Lippincott Williams & Wilkins, 2007.

ICH locations: basal ganglia (two-third) > pons = cerebellum > other areas.

What are the most common underlying causes of ICH?

The most common causes are "*HIT A BAT*": **H**ypertension (this is the leading cause and accounts for >50% of ICH), **I**schemic stroke, **T**rauma, **A**myloid angiopathy, **B**leeding disorders (including anticoagulation), **A**rteriovenous malformation, and **T**umor in the brain.

Amyloid angiopathy: idiopathic β-amyloid deposition in cerebral blood vessels. Increased risk in Alzheimer's and Down's syndrome. Main complications are ICH and dementia.

Hemoglobin is 9.1. INR is 1.7. Serum chemistries are normal.

How is ICH treated?

- Measures similar to ischemic stroke:
  1. Stabilize airway, breathing, and circulation (ABCs).
  2. Maintain serum glucose <150 mg/dL, and treat fever with acetaminophen.
  3. Perform serial neurological exams.
- Measures that differ from ischemic stroke:
  1. Hypertension: maintain SBP <160 and diastolic blood pressure <105. Labetalol and nitroprusside are both first-line antihypertensive drugs.
  2. Reverse anticoagulation: Stop warfarin and administer vitamin K and fresh frozen plasma. For patients on heparin, stop heparin and administer protamine.

Resuming anticoagulation: Consider 3 to 4 weeks after acute event if anticoagulation is necessary. Initially, initiate anticoagulation with heparin and not warfarin.

Recall that hemorrhage is an absolute contraindication to thrombolytics.

When is surgery indicated for ICH?

Refer for decompressive surgery if imaging detects cerebellar hemorrhage >3 cm. In other instances, the role of surgery is controversial.

CASE 12–3 TRAUMATIC BRAIN INJURY

A 25-year-old man is hit on the head while playing football. He was unconscious for approximately 1 minute after impact, and seemed confused for approximately 5 minutes after recovering consciousness. He presents for evaluation to the emergency department 2 hours later. He does not have any known medical conditions or take any medications. He is alert and oriented. There is no impairment in short or long term memory. Physical exam, including neurological exam, is normal. Vital signs are normal.

What is the most likely type of head injury?

Concussion is a milder subset of mild TBI (GCS > 13). Concussion causes temporary confusion and amnesia. Patients may or may not lose consciousness for a brief period. Other early signs are nausea, vomiting, headache, and dizziness. Concussion is classified as:

1. Grade 1: confusion after impact; no memory loss; no loss of consciousness (LOC).
2. Grade 2: confusion after impact; no recollection of event; no LOC.
3. Grade 3 (classic concussion): brief LOC; no recollection of the event.

Is any imaging indicated in this patient?

Remember indications for non-contrast head CT after TBI with the mnemonic "***Vomiting = BAD, BAD SIGN***" (Table 12-7). These indications are based on the New Orleans and Canadian decision rules. This patient does not have any indications for head CT.

> MRI is also very sensitive but is not the first-line imaging test because of cost and increased false-positive tests (detects many clinically insignificant signs).

> New Orleans criteria are more sensitive, but Canadian head CT rule is more specific.

> Imaging is normal in uncomplicated concussion.

Would you obtain head CT if he had a bruise and scratches on his forehead?

Superficial contusions (bruises) and lacerations are not an indication for head CT unless they are located in a region that is suspicious for basilar skull fracture. This man would not require any imaging even if he had a bruise and scratches on his forehead.

The patient asks when he can start playing football again.

What should you tell him?

An athlete who experienced LOC for any period of time or other symptoms of concussion for >15 minutes should not return to play for at least 1 week. Athletes who have more than one such concussion should not return to play for the entire season.

> **Post-concussion syndrome**: Headache, dizziness, and personality changes can occur a few days after concussion. They generally resolve over the next few weeks to months.

TABLE 12-7 Indications for Head CT After Blunt Head Trauma

Obtain head CT if patient has any of the following criteria ("*Vomiting* = ***BAD, BAD SIGN***"):

- **V**omiting (≥2 episodes)
- **B**leeding disorder or anticoagulation
- **A**ge > 65 years
- **D**epressed or open skull fracture suspected
- **B**asilar skull fracture signs

1. Hemotympanum: appears as dark blue TM discoloration
2. Raccoon eyes: periorbital bruising
3. CSF otorrhea or rhinorrhea: clear fluid drips out of ear
4. Battle's sign: bruising behind the ear (postauricular)

- **A**mnesia of events ≥30 minutes before impact
- **D**angerous mechanism

1. Occupant ejected from a motor vehicle
2. Fall from elevation of ≥3 feet or ≥5 stairs
3. Pedestrian struck by a motor vehicle

- **S**eizure
- **I**ntoxication with drugs or alcohol
- **G**CS <15 at 2 hours after injury
- **N**eurological signs (focal)

Abbreviations: CSF, cerebrospinal fluid; TM, tympanic membrane.

Alternative 12.3.1

A 75-year-old man falls from his bed. His wife brings him to the emergency room 2 hours later. There is a bruise on his lateral forehead. GCS is 14 (E4, V4, and M6). Figure 12-6 is the non-contrast head CT scan.

What is the diagnosis?

Head CT demonstrates a crescent-shaped (concave) hematoma, which is characteristic of subdural hematoma (SDH). SDH results from a tear in the bridging veins that run from the cerebral cortex to the dural sinuses. Bleeding disorders, anticoagulation, and cerebral atrophy (e.g., elderly and alcoholics) increase the risk of SDH. SDH is three times more common in men than women.

> **Cerebral atrophy**: increased risk because bridging veins must traverse a greater distance.

How is acute SDH treated?

First stabilize ABCs. Then, refer for emergent neurosurgery if there is >5 mm midline shift on CT scan. If there is <5 mm midline shift, perform serial neurological exams. Consider neurosurgery if the patient develops new or worsening neurological signs or other signs of increased ICP.

What imaging test should you obtain if the elderly man with altered mental status presented for evaluation 72 hours after head trauma?

SDH is often difficult to detect on CT scan 2 to 10 days after the injury (subacute SDH) because it appears isodense. Consider contrast-enhanced CT scan or MRI instead. Subacute SDH appears hyperdense (white) on T1-weighted MRI.

> **Chronic SDH**: SDH appears hypodense (black) on non-contrast CT after approximately 3 weeks. Chronic SDH can cause dementia.

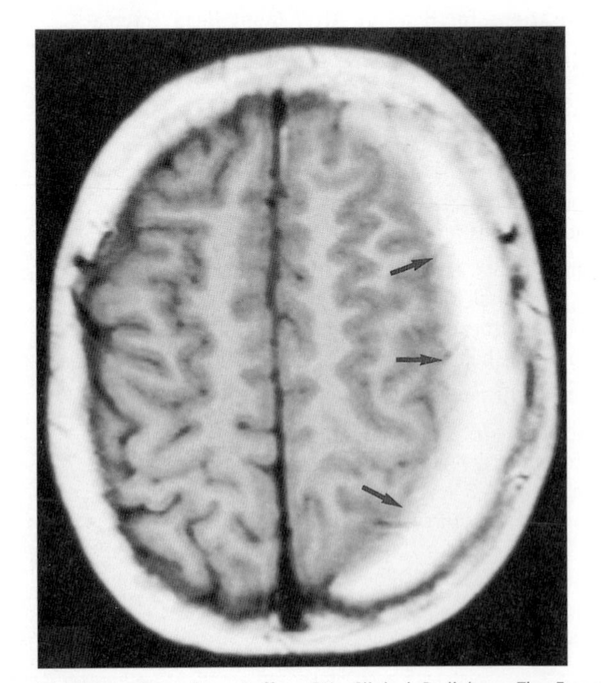

FIGURE 12–6 CT scan showing subdural hematoma. From Daffner RH. *Clinical Radiology: The Essentials, 3rd ed.* Lippincott Williams & Wilkins, 2007.

Alternative 12.3.2

A 49-year-old race car driver is involved in a motor vehicle accident during the Daytona 500. He is unconscious for about 5 minutes and then regains consciousness. The paramedics notice ecchymoses (bruises) behind the left ear and around the left eye. In the ambulance, he again loses consciousness. GCS is 11.

What is the most likely injury?

"Battle sign" (postauricular ecchymoses) and "raccoon eyes" (periorbital ecchymoses) are signs of basilar skull fracture. Brief LOC followed by a lucid interval followed again by LOC is the classic feature of epidural hematoma (EDH). EDH occurs when temporal bone fracture causes laceration of the middle meningeal artery. EDH appears as a convex (lens-shaped) hematoma on imaging (Fig. 12-7).

> Only 20% of EDH presents with the classic lucid interval.

In the ambulance, blood pressure rises to 220/80. Heart rate falls to 40 bpm. Respirations are irregular. The left pupil is fixed and dilated, and there is bilateral papilledema.

What are the next steps in management?

The patient has late signs of increased intracranial pressure (ICP), indicative of impending herniation. The initial steps in the ambulance are supportive: hyperventilation, reverse Trendelenburg, sedation, and mannitol (if available in the ambulance). When the patient reaches the hospital, obtain an emergent CT scan to confirm the diagnosis followed by emergent decompressive craniotomy. Details about ICP follow:

- **Background**: The intracranial compartment is a closed space that contains brain parenchyma, blood vessels, and cerebrospinal fluid (CSF). Normal ICP is <15.
- **Causes**: Increased ICP can result from increased brain parenchyma volume (e.g., tumors, cerebral edema, abscess), increased blood volume (ICH, subarachnoid hemorrhage (SAH), SDH, and EDH), or increased CSF (e.g., meningitis, choroid plexus tumor).

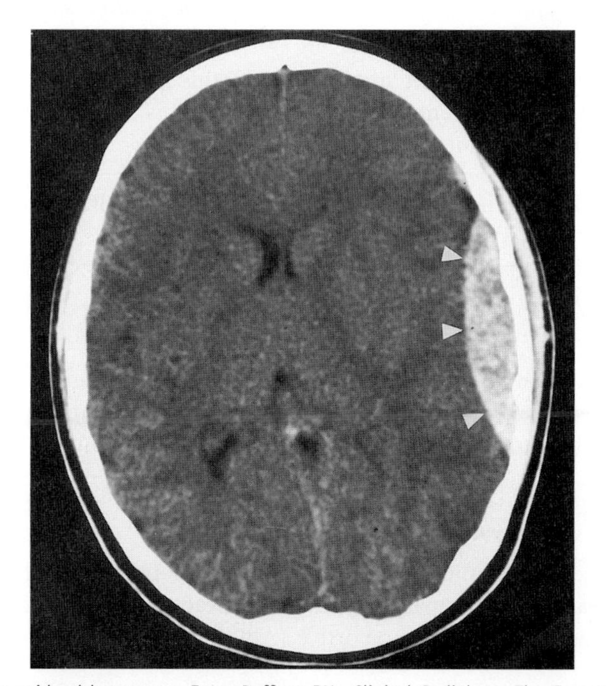

FIGURE 12–7 CT scan showing epidural hematoma. From Daffner RH. *Clinical Radiology: The Essentials, 3rd ed.* Lippincott Williams & Wilkins, 2007.

- **Clinical manifestations**: Early signs of increased ICP are nausea, vomiting, headache, and new or worsening neurological deficits. Late signs are papilledema, blown pupil (fixed, dilated pupil), and Cushing's triad (hypertension with wide pulse pressure, bradycardia, and irregular respirations).
- **Pathophysiology**: Intracranial ICP is dangerous for two reasons:
  1. Herniation: Increased ICP can precipitate brain herniation, which puts extreme pressure on parts of the brain and is rapidly fatal.
  2. CPP = MAP – ICP. Therefore, increased ICP leads to decreased cerebral blood flow. If ICP = MAP, then cerebral blood flow will stop completely and the patient will die.
- **Diagnosis**: Non-contrast CT scan is usually obtained to confirm the diagnosis.
- **Management**: The most important component of management is to treat the underlying cause (e.g., decompressive craniotomy of SDH or EDH). Other supportive measures to decrease ICP are:
  1. Hyperventilation: lowers $PaCO_2$ → vasoconstriction → decreased ICP. Rapid but transient effect.
  2. Reverse Trendelenburg: Head elevation helps increase cerebral venous outflow.
  3. IV Mannitol: This osmotic agent draws water out of brain cells.
  4. Reduce metabolic demand: acetaminophen for fever and morphine for sedation.
  5. Corticosteroids: Used to reduce edema; only useful for tumors or infections (not hemorrhage!).
- **ICP Monitoring**: Consider ICP monitoring if imaging detects a midline shift and the cause is not immediately treatable. There are four methods of ICP monitoring:
  1. Intraventricular catheter: most accurate and also allows for excess CSF drainage but increased risk of infection.
  2. Intraparenchymal device: low risk of infection, but accuracy decreases with time.
  3. Subarachnoid bolt: rarely used because it is unreliable (easily clogged).
  4. Epidural sensor: least invasive but also least accurate.

How would management differ if increased ICP with midline shift occurred as a result of cerebral edema on hospital day 2 after an ischemic stroke?

Decompressive neurosurgery is not possible in this situation. Admit this patient to the intensive care unit (ICU) and monitor ICP. Treatment is supportive. Try to maintain ICP <20 and MAP >80 (i.e., maintain CPP >60).

> **Seizures**: a common complication of increased ICP; prophylaxis is sometimes warranted.

Alternative 12.3.3

A 34-year-old woman is involved in a motor vehicle collision. She was ejected from her motorcycle. When the paramedics arrive, GCS is 8. There are no focal neurological signs. At the emergency department 30 minutes later, she is still comatose. Non-contrast head CT is normal.

What diagnosis should you suspect?

Suspect diffuse axonal injury (DAI) when a patient presents with coma after traumatic brain injury but head CT is normal. In DAI, rapid head acceleration or deceleration leads to white matter shearing. Treatment is supportive (ABCs and limit increased ICP).

> **MRI**: more sensitive than CT but still not very sensitive for DAI.

CASE 12-4 HEADACHE

A 22-year-old woman presents with a 2-year history of headaches that occur almost every week. She often feels tired and irritable a few hours before the headache. The headache increases in intensity over a few hours and is described as dull, throbbing, left-sided pain. During these episodes, she cannot stand loud noises or light, so she lies in a dark, quiet room. She often experiences nausea and sometimes even vomits. The headaches typically resolve over 6 to 24 hours. Acetaminophen and aspirin do not relieve her symptoms. Physical exam and vital signs are normal.

What is the differential diagnosis of headache?

There are numerous causes of headache, but the three most common causes are the primary headache syndromes: tension type headache, cluster headache, and migraine headache (Table 12-8). Other secondary causes of headache are listed below ("***VOMIT Three Times @ 4PM***"):

- **V**ascular: ICH and SAH (Case 12-3), and EDH and SDH (Case 12-4)
- **O**ther: connective tissue disorders (Chapter 9: Rheumatology), glaucoma (Chapter 16: Primary Care Ophthalmology), and chronic analgesic use
- **M**alignant hypertension (Chapter 2: Cardiology)
- **I**nfections: meningitis, encephalitis, and brain abscess (Case 12-5), sinusitis (Chapter 3: Pulmonary)
- **T**rauma (head injury)
- **T**umor: pituitary adenoma (Chapter 8: Endocrinology), brain metastases, and other first-degree brain tumors
- **T**emporal arteritis (Chapter 8: Endocrinology)
- **4P**: pituitary apoplexy and pheochromocytoma (Chapter 8: Endocrinology), pseudotumor cerebri (PTC), and post-lumbar puncture
- **M**edications or drugs

TABLE 12-8 Primary Headache Syndromes

Type of Headache	Migraine	Tension	Cluster
Onset	Gradual (hours)	Gradual (hours)	Rapid (minutes)
Duration	4 to 72 hours	Hours	15 min to 3 hours
Quality	Dull, throbbing	Waxing and waning pressure or tightness	Deep, burning, and stabbing pain
Location	70% unilateral, 30% bilateral	Bilateral	Unilateral; around eyes and temple
Severity	Moderate to severe	Mild to moderate	Extremely severe
Autonomic symptoms	Yes	No	Yes[a]
Nausea or vomiting	Yes	No	No
Photophobia	Yes	No	No
Phonophobia	Yes	No	No
Triggers	Yes	No	No
Other	Premonitory symptoms (30%) and aura (15%)	No	No

[a] Eyes: ipsilateral redness, lacrimation, and Horner's syndrome; nose: rhinorrhea and nasal congestion; other: sweating and pallor.

What is the most likely cause of this patient's headaches?

The most likely cause is migraine. There are three characteristic phases:

1. **Premonitory phase**: Nonspecific symptoms such as fatigue, decreased concentration, nausea, irritability, etc., precede the headache by a few hours to a couple of days in 30% of cases.
2. **Aura**: Neurological deficits occur 30 to 60 minutes before headache in 15% of cases. The most common aura is visual: flickering zigzag lines followed by scotoma (blind spot). Sensory symptoms (numbness and tingling) or speech deficits are less frequent. Aura typically resolves when the headache begins.
3. **Headache**: Migraines cause moderate to severe dull and throbbing pain. 70% of cases are unilateral while 30% of cases are bilateral or bifrontal. The headache usually lasts for 4 to 72 hours. Migraines are frequently accompanied by nausea, vomiting, photophobia, and phonophobia, so patients often lie down in a dark, quiet room. Many patients also have autonomic symptoms such as rhinorrhea and lacrimation.

> **Migraine without aura (85%)**: previously referred to as common migraine.
> **Migraine with aura (15%)**: previously referred to as classic migraine.
> **Aura without migraine** (<**1%**): uncommon migraine variant.

What causes migraines?

The exact mechanism of migraines is unclear. Genetics, serotonin, and trigeminal nerve stimulation have all been implicated. Predisposed patients develop migraine headaches from otherwise innocuous triggers such as behavioral disturbances (e.g., stress, hunger, fatigue, and lack of sleep), foods (e.g., cheese, chocolate, and monosodium glutamate), menstrual irregularities, odors, or medications (e.g., nitrates and oral contraceptives).

> **Menstrual migraines**: Suspect if migraines occur at the onset of the menstrual cycle.
> **Basilar migraine**: Suspect if aura consists of vertigo, tinnitus, ataxia, or dysarthria.
> **Hemiplegic migraine**: Suspect if aura consists of fully reversible hemiplegia.

> **Migraine epidemiology**: Women > men. Onset is typically in teens or early twenties.

She asks if she needs any "brain scan to check out her head."

Is any imaging indicated?

This patient with typical migraine symptoms does not require neuroimaging. Obtain imaging if any of the following "red flags" are present in a patient with headache:

1. Sudden onset of "worst headache ever" (suspect SAH)
2. Progressive and persistent headache over days to weeks (suspect tumor)
3. Headache wakes patient up from sleep (suspect tumor)
4. Headache severity increases on bending or Valsalva (suspect tumor)
5. Vomiting routinely precedes headache (suspect tumor)
6. Visual field defects (suspect stroke or pituitary lesion)
7. Focal neurological signs, new onset seizure, or papilledema (signs of increased ICP)

> **Papilledema**: swelling of the optic disk due to increased ICP (Fig. 12-8).

How should you treat this patient?

The initial measure to prevent future attacks is to identify and avoid triggers. During an acute attack, first-line therapy is a triptan (administer early). Metoclopropamide or prochlorperazine are adjunctive treatments for acute attacks with significant nausea.

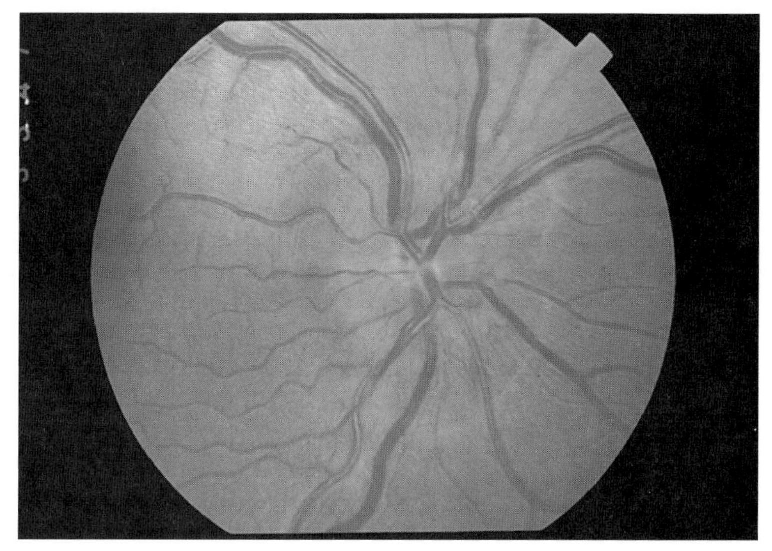

FIGURE 12–8 Eye image: papilledema. From Tasman W, Jaeger E. *The Wills Eye Hospital Atlas of Clinical Ophthalmology, 2nd ed.* Lippincott Williams & Wilkins, 2001.

> Do not use triptans more than once or twice a week.

How would management differ if she had never taken any drug to treat an acute attack?

Consider acetaminophen, aspirin, or another nonsteroidal anti-inflammatory drug (NSAID) as the initial therapy for an acute attack. If these cheap medications are not effective, switch to a triptan for subsequent attacks.

Sumatriptan effectively aborts acute attacks, but she continues to have weekly disabling migraines despite eliminating triggers. She was recently diagnosed with essential hypertension.

What measures can help prevent future attacks?

Consider prophylactic medications if headaches occur at least once a week and last ≥12 hours or cause significant subjective disability. Tricyclic antidepressants, β-blockers, and anti-convulsants are all effective options. Because this patient also has hypertension, a β-blocker is the preferred option.

> **Menstrual migraines:** NSAIDs are the first-line therapy for migraine prophylaxis.

The patient's episodes initially decrease in frequency with propranolol. After a few months, she presents with daily severe headaches. She ran out of sumatriptan a month ago, so she is taking acetaminophen everyday.

What is the next step in management?

The most likely cause of the increased headache frequency is medication overuse headache syndrome (MOHS). MOHS can result from overuse of any analgesic (acetaminophen is most frequently implicated in epidemiological studies). The next step is to discontinue acetaminophen. If the patient has a severe migraine soon after discontinuing acetaminophen, consider IV dihydroergotamine for the acute attack.

> Triptans and dihydroergotamine are both serotonin-1 agonists, but triptans are more selective.

Alternative 12.4.1

A 38-year-old man presents with a 2-year history of headaches. The headaches occur approximately once every other week. He describes the pain as diffuse bilateral pressure or tightness that waxes or wanes in severity and resolves completely after a few hours. He denies any nausea, vomiting, photophobia, phonophobia, or autonomic symptoms. He continues daily activities during the headaches. He does not take any analgesics because he likes to avoid medications as much as possible. Physical exam and vital signs are normal.

What is the most likely diagnosis?

The patient most likely has chronic tension type headaches (see Table 12-8). Unlike migraines, tension type headaches do not cause nausea, photophobia, phonophobia, or autonomic symptoms. First-line therapy is acetaminophen or NSAIDs. Consider prophylactic tricyclic antidepressants for patients with daily headaches to prevent MOHS.

> Some patients with tension headaches also have features of migraine headaches but do not meet diagnostic criteria. This has led investigators to suggest that chronic tension headaches and migraines represent a continuum.

Alternative 12.4.2

A 46-year-old man presents with a 2-week history of severe headaches. The headaches are localized to his left temple and left periorbital region. They reach their maximum severity in a few minutes and resolve within 15 to 60 minutes. The pain is so severe that he sometimes finds himself banging his head on the wall. He reports that his left eye becomes become red and tearful during the headache episodes. He also has a runny nose, nasal congestion, and sweating during the episodes. Physical exam and vital signs are normal.

What is the most likely diagnosis?

The most likely diagnosis is cluster headache (see Table 12-8). Symptoms typically occur in 15-minute to 3-hour episodes. The episodes occur frequently for weeks to months followed by a long period of remission.

> Approximately 10% of patients do not experience any period of remission.

How are cluster headaches treated?

1. **Acute attacks**: First-line therapy is intranasal or subcutaneous triptans.
2. **Prophylaxis**: Initiate in all patients until remission. First-line drug is verapimil.

Alternative 12.4.3

A 52-year-old man presents for evaluation after a seizure. Over the last 3 weeks, he mentions that he has had an increasingly worsening headache that does not respond to ibuprofen or aspirin and is accompanied by nausea. The headache is bilateral and worsens when he bends down or coughs. On physical exam, there is 3/5 strength in his right arm and legs and 5/5 strength in his left arms and legs. Vital signs are normal.

What is the next step in management?

Headache and seizures are the two most common presenting symptoms of brain tumors. The likelihood of a tumor is particularly high in this patient with focal neurological signs, progressively worsening headache, nausea, and increased severity on bending and Valsalva. The first-line test for suspected brain tumor is MRI with gadolinium contrast. CT is not a first-line imaging modality because it can miss posterior fossa and low-grade non-enhanced tumors.

> The classic "headache that awakens" is actually infrequent in patients with brain tumors.

What are the most common primary brain tumors in adults?

The three most common primary brain neoplasms in adults (in descending order) are glioblastoma multiforme (grade IV astrocytoma), meningioma, and schwannoma (acoustic neuroma). Glioblastoma multiforme is an extremely aggressive neoplasm with a poor prognosis. Meningioma and schwannoma are benign, resectable tumors. Other important tumors in adults are pituitary adenoma and oligodendroglioma.

> Approximately 50% of brain neoplasms are metastases from distant sites and approximately 50% are first-degree brain tumors.

> **CNS lymphoma (non-Hodgkin's lymphoma)**: common primary brain tumor in AIDS patients.

Alternative 12.4.4

A 32-year-old woman presents with a 3-month history of persistent and progressive headache and blurry vision. The headaches are accompanied by nausea and vomiting but not photophobia or phonophobia. On physical examination, there is horizontal diplopia, cranial nerve 6 palsy, and papilledema. Visual fields are normal. Vital signs are normal. Body mass index is 42. MRI does not reveal any space-occupying lesion. Lumbar puncture (LP) reveals opening pressure of 26 mm Hg. Cytology, protein, white blood counts (WBCs), and glucose are normal.

What diagnosis should you suspect?

PTC is an uncommon idiopathic disorder that predominantly affects obese women of childbearing age. The disorder is also called idiopathic intracranial hypertension or benign intracranial hypertension. The most common symptoms are headache and papilledema, but MRI does not reveal any space-occupying lesion. Opening pressure is usually >25 mm Hg but other findings on LP are normal. PTC is a diagnosis of exclusion, so first rule out connective tissue disorders (see Chapter 9: Rheumatology), Lyme disease (in endemic areas), and inherited or acquired thrombophilias (Chapter 2: Cardiology).

> The main complication of PTC is blindness due to progressive papilledema.

> Increased ICP can result from thrombophilias (due to increased risk of cerebral venous thrombosis) and connective tissue disorders or Lyme disease (due to increased risk of vasculitis).

How is PTC treated?

Initial treatment is conservative measures (weight loss) plus medications. The most commonly prescribed drug for PTC is acetazolamide (decreases CSF production). Other medications are diuretics, steroids, and topiramate. Treatment of severe or refractory PTC is neurosurgical shunting to drain excess CSF to other parts of the body (e.g., ventriculoperitoneal shunt or ventriculoatrial shunt).

Alternative 12.4.5

A 54-year-old man presents with a chief complaint of "the worse headache of my life." The headache began 1 hour ago, reached its maximum intensity within minutes, and is accompanied by nausea. He has a history of hypertension and smokes two packs of cigarettes every day. There are no focal neurological abnormalities. Temperature is 37.2°C, pulse 110 bpm, respirations 15/min, and blood pressure 130/80.

What diagnosis should you suspect?

Suspect SAH any time a patient presents with sudden onset of extremely severe ("thunderclap") headache. The headache causes LOC in one third of cases, and one third of sufferers experience a minor headache hours before the acute headache ("sentinel headache"). After a few hours, 75% of sufferers develop meningismus (neck stiffness, etc.). Unlike other types of stroke, focal neurological signs are often absent.

What causes SAH?

The majority of SAH results from rupture of an intracranial aneurysm. Saccular aneurysms at the circle of Willis (Berry aneurysms) are most frequently involved. Other common causes are trauma, cocaine, and bleeding disorders (and anticoagulation). Infrequent causes include amyloid angiopathy, arteriovenous malformations, and vasculitides.

> Hypertension and cigarette smoking are the main risk factors for cerebral aneurysms.

What is the next step in management?

The next step is urgent CT scan without contrast to rule out hemorrhage (avoid contrast if you suspect intracranial bleeding). CT scan detects SAH in 95% of cases.

Head CT scan does not reveal any hemorrhage.

What is the next step in management?

CT scan can miss 5% of SAH. The next step is LP. Normal CT scan and normal LP rule out SAH.

There is mildly elevated opening pressure and xanthochromia (increased red blood cells (RBCs)) on CSF analysis. The number of RBCs is the same in all four bottles.

What is the next step?

Xanthochromia and increased opening pressure are diagnostic of SAH. The next step is cerebral angiography to localize the bleeding aneurysm. First-line treatment of ruptured aneurysms is neurosurgery (place a clip across the ruptured vessel to stop the bleeding).

> **Endovascular coiling**: In this increasingly popular alternative to surgical clipping, place a coil into the ruptured vessel. A thrombus forms around the coil and stops the bleeding.

> **Traumatic LP**: Trauma from the needle can cause xanthochromia. Unlike SAH, opening pressure is normal and number of RBCs progressively declines from bottle 1 to bottle 4.

What other measures are recommended in patients with SAH?

1. Measures similar to intracerebral hemorrhage:
   - **i.** Stabilize ABCs.
   - **ii.** Maintain serum glucose <150 mg/dL, and treat fever with acetaminophen.
   - **iii.** Consider stool softeners because straining increases ICP.
   - **iv.** Perform serial neurological exams.
   - **v.** Reverse anticoagulation: Stop warfarin and administer vitamin K and fresh frozen plasma. For patients on heparin, stop heparin and administer protamine.
2. Measures that differ from intracerebral hemorrhage:
   - **i.** Hypertension: Maintain SBP <140 with labetalol in alert and cognitively intact patients. If the patient has decreased consciousness, withhold antihypertensives unless pressure is very high (exact number undefined).
   - **ii.** Nimodipine: May decrease vasospasm (improves outcomes).

> Seizure prophylaxis and glucocorticoids in patients with SAH is controversial.

> Hypertension worsens hemorrhage whereas decreased blood pressure can lower CPP.

CASE 12–5 CENTRAL NERVOUS SYSTEM INFECTIONS

A 37-year-old man presents with an 8-hour history of fever and headache. He does not have any known medical conditions or take any medications. He appears confused on examination, and GCS is 13 (E4V3M6). Full neck flexion or extension is difficult (nuchal rigidity). There are no focal neurological signs. Vital signs are temperature 39.1°C, pulse 110 bpm, respirations 12/min, and blood pressure 130/85.

What is the most likely diagnosis?

The classic triad of acute meningitis is "*FAN*" (**F**ever, **A**ltered mental status, and **N**uchal rigidity). Although many patients do not have all three features of the triad, almost all patients have at least one or two features. Other common findings are headache and photophobia. Seizures and focal neurological deficits are infrequent because meningitis causes diffuse brain injury. Symptoms typically develop over hours to days.

> Classic physical findings in meningitis:
> 1. **Nuchal rigidity**: 30% sensitive and approximately 70% specific
> 2. **Kernig sign**: Lay patient supine with hips and knees at 90°. Then passively extend leg. Resistance to passive extension is a positive test. Specific but only 5% sensitive.
> 3. **Brudzinski sign**: Lay patient supine and passively flex neck. Involuntary hip or knee flexion is a positive test. Specific but only 5% sensitive.

> Elderly patients may have hypothermia rather than fever.

What causes acute meningitis?

Acute meningitis results from meningeal inflammation. Acute meningitis is classified as either acute bacterial meningitis (due to bacterial infection) and aseptic meningitis (due to viruses, fungi, parasites, tuberculosis, intracranial tumors, or medications). Acute bacterial meningitis is a medical emergency (approximately 100% mortality if left untreated), whereas aseptic meningitis is usually self-limiting. It is difficult to differentiate bacterial from aseptic meningitis on the basis of clinical findings alone.

How do the clinical features of acute meningitis differ from chronic meningitis?

Chronic bacterial meningitis also classically presents with the FAN triad, headache, and photophobia, but symptoms occur over weeks to months. Chronic meningitis is also divided into chronic bacterial and chronic aseptic meningitis.

How do the clinical features of meningitis differ from encephalitis?

Encephalitis is diffuse inflammation of the brain parenchyma due to infectious or noninfectious causes. Like meningitis, encephalitis can cause fever, altered mental status, headache, and seizures. Seizures and focal neurological deficits are more common in encephalitis, whereas neck stiffness and photophobia are uncommon.

> **Meningoencephalitis**: Meningeal infection commonly spreads to brain parenchyma and vice versa. Meningoencephalitis presents with signs of meningitis and encephalitis.

What organisms are most frequently implicated in acute bacterial meningitis?

Streptococcus pneumoniae causes approximately 60% of acute bacterial meningitis. Other frequently implicated pathogens are *Neisseria meningitis* (second leading pathogen in adults <60 years), *Listeria monocytogenes* (second leading organism in adults >60 years), *H. influenza*, and group B streptococcus.

What are the next steps in management?

Although LP is the most helpful diagnostic test, it is contraindicated in patients with a mass lesion (e.g., abscess, tumor, etc.). Obtain head CT before attempting LP in the following patients ("*CT* ***F****irst, CSF* ***P****uncture Second*"):

1. Decreased **C**onsciousness
2. **F**ocal neurological deficits
3. **I**mmunocompromised
4. **C**NS disease (history of stroke, tumor, or CNS infection)
5. **P**apilledema
6. **S**eizure

The next steps in this patient with decreased consciousness are blood cultures followed by empiric IV antibiotics followed by non-contrast head CT scan (Fig. 12-9). The recommended antibiotic regimen in this young adult is ceftriaxone plus vancomycin (Table 12-9).

> Order head CT before LP in any patient with risk factors for increased ICP because CSF removal in a patient with increased ICP can precipitate brain herniation.

The patient is started on ceftriaxone and vancomycin. CT scan does not reveal any mass lesion.

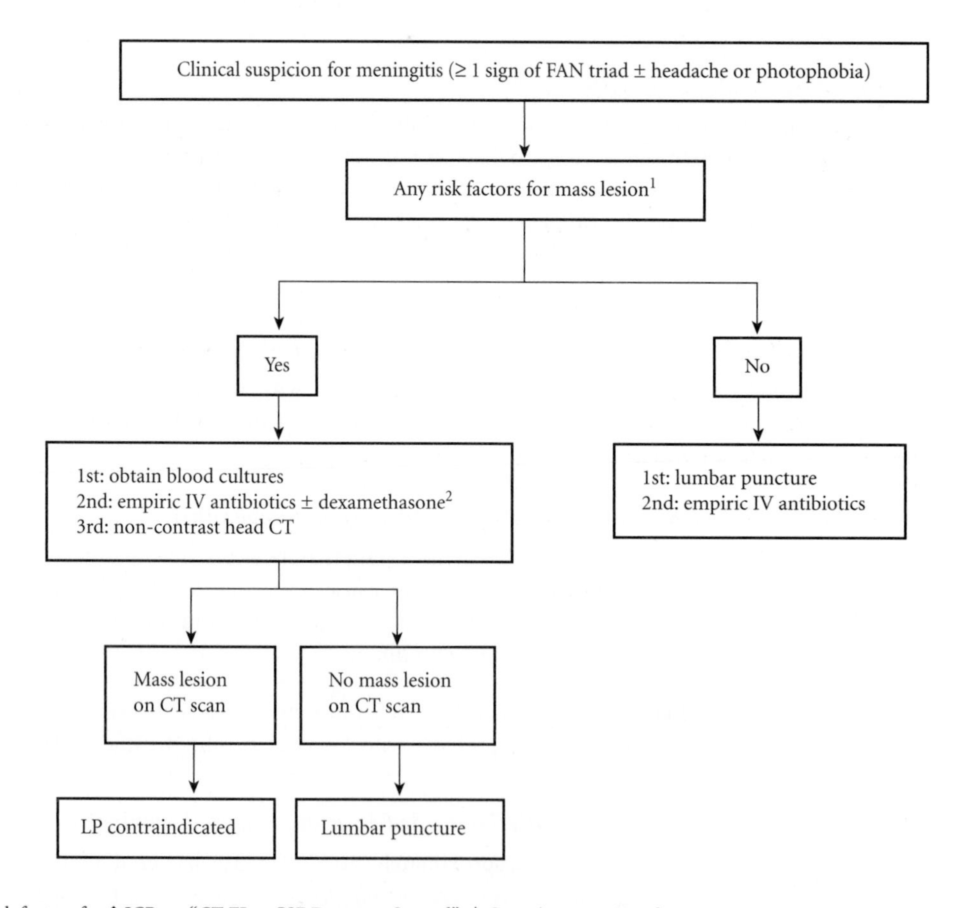

[1]Risk factors for ↑ ICP are "CT **FI**rst CSF **P**uncture **S**econd": ↓ **C**onsciousness, **F**ocal neurologic signs, **I**mmunocompromised, **C**NS disease (history of stroke, tumor, or other mass lesion), **P**apilledema, or **S**eizure

[2]Give dexamethasone if patient has signs of acute bacterial meningitis and GCS 8-11

FIGURE 12–9 Initial approach to suspected meningitis.

TABLE 12-9 Empiric IV Antibiotic Regimens for Suspected Bacterial Meningitis

Clinical Scenario	Empiric IV Antibiotic Regimen
Adult < 50 years	Ceftriaxone + vancomycin
Adult > 50 years	Ceftriaxone + vancomycin + ampicillin
Immunocompromised	Ceftazidime + vancomycin + ampicillin + acyclovir
Nosocomial meningitis	Ceftazidime + vancomycin
CSF shunt or recent neurosurgery	Ceftazidime + vancomycin
Head trauma	Ceftazidime + vancomycin

Abbreviation: IV, intravenous.
Ceftriaxone covers most organisms implicated in meningitis except listeria. Vancomycin covers cephalosporin resistant *S. pneumoniae*. Ampicillin covers *Listeria monocytogenes*. Ceftazidime covers pseudomonas as well as organisms covered by ceftriaxone. Acyclovir covers herpes simplex virus.
Adapted from Sabatine M. Pocket Medicine, 2nd ed.

What is the next step in management?

The next step is LP. Always measure the opening pressure and note the color of CSF obtained. Then, send the fluid for analysis of WBCs and differential, glucose, protein, Gram stain, culture, ± cytology (Table 12-10).

Immunocompromised patients: CSF analysis should also include acid-fast stain (for TB), India ink stain (for cryptococcus), fungal cultures, and polymerase chain reaction (PCR) for herpes simplex virus (HSV).

Antibiotics do not usually affect the results of LP in the first 4 to 6 hours. After that time, there is increased likelihood of false-negative Gram stain and culture.

Meningeal carcinomatosis: Cancer that metastasizes to meninges can cause signs of meningitis. LP findings are positive cytology, decreased glucose, increased protein, and increased lymphocytes.

TABLE 12-10 CSF Findings in Various Causes of Meningitis

Type of Meningitis	Opening Pressure[a]	Protein[b]	WBC Count	Differential	CSF Glucose[c]	Other Possible Findings
Bacterial	↑	↑ or ↑↑	>1000/mm^3	Predominant neutrophils	↓ or ↓↓	Positive Gram stain and culture
Viral	↔	↑/↔	<100/mm^3	Predominant lymphocytes	↔	Positive PCR in HSV
Fungal	Variable	↑	Variable	Predominant lymphocytes	↓	Positive fungal cultures or India ink stain
Tuberculosis	Variable	↑	Variable	Predominant lymphocytes	↓	Positive acid-fast stain
Metastasis[d]	↔	↑	↔	Predominant lymphocytes	↓	Positive cytology

Abbreviations: HSV, herpes simplex virus; PCR, polymerase chain reaction; WBC, whole blood count; ↑, increase; ↓, decrease; ↔, stable.
[a] Normal CSF opening pressure is <20 mm with the patient in lateral recumbent position.
[b] Normal CSF protein is typically 18 to 58 mg/dL.
[c] Normal CSF glucose is about two thirds that of serum glucose.
[d] Cancer that metastasizes to the meninges is termed meningeal carcinomatosis.

CSF analysis is as follows: cloudy appearance, opening pressure 22 cm (↑), WBCs 5000/mm^3 (↑), WBC differential mostly PMNs, glucose 38 mg/dL (↓), and protein 500 mg/dL (↑). Gram stain demonstrates Gram-positive bacilli.

What is the next step?

The CSF findings are consistent with bacterial meningitis. Gram-positive bacilli suggest *L. monocytogenes.* The next step is to add ampicillin to the regimen. If culture confirms the presence of listeria, discontinue ceftriaxone and vancomycin.

> **Opening pressure** >25: Increased risk of herniation. Only remove CSF in manometer.

How would you tailor therapy if Gram stain and culture demonstrate N. meningitides?

N. meningitides (Gram-negative diplococci) often causes a diffuse erythematous maculopapular rash. If culture confirms the diagnosis, discontinue empiric antibiotics and treat with penicillin G.

How would you tailor therapy if Gram stain and culture revealed S. pneumoniae?

S. pneumoniae appears as Gram-positive cocci in chains. The next step is to continue the initial regimen until sensitivities are available. If the organism is sensitive to cephalosporin, discontinue vancomycin and treat with ceftriaxone alone. Otherwise, discontinue ceftriaxone and treat with vancomycin.

> **Dexamethasone**: indicated if increased risk of mass lesion and GCS 8 to 11. Start at the same time as initial empiric therapy. Continue only if Gram stain or culture indicates *S. pneumonia.*

How would you tailor therapy if CSF analysis revealed the following: clear appearance, opening pressure 12 (normal), WBCs 80/mm^3 (mostly lymphocytes), glucose 85 mg/dL, proteins 80 mg/dL, and negative Gram stain?

The CSF findings indicate aseptic meningitis (see Table 12-10). The next step is to discontinue antibiotics, treat supportively (control fever, pain, etc.) and observe.

Alternative 12.5.1

A 58-year-old man is brought to the emergency department after a seizure. His wife mentions that he has had a headache for the last 8 hours. He appears confused during the evaluation. Temperature is 39.2°C. Head CT does not demonstrate any mass lesion.

What is the next step in management?

Fever, altered mental status, headache, and seizures are suggestive of encephalitis. The next step after CT scan rules out a mass lesion is LP. In addition to tests ordered routinely for meningitis, order culture and PCR for HSV and PCR for West Nile virus. Then, initiate empiric therapy with acyclovir (ACV). Discontinue ACV only if culture and PCR for HSV are negative.

> **West Nile virus**: Symptoms are usually nonspecific. This virus may present with encephalitis plus maculopapular rash and flaccid paralysis. Treatment is supportive.

What diagnosis should you suspect if the patient presents with signs and symptoms of encephalitis as well as hydrophobia and aerophobia?

Hydrophobia, aerophobia, pharyngeal spasms, or hyperexcitation should raise suspicion for rabies virus encephalitis. The most common sources of transmission in the United States are bat, raccoon, skunk, and fox bites. The most common source of transmission worldwide is dog bites. Diagnosis requires analysis of specimens from multiple sites. Only one nonimmunized patient has ever survived from rabies. The treatment regimen was drug-induced coma, mechanical ventilation, and IV ribavirin.

> Administer rabies immunoglobulin plus rabies vaccine to any person with mucous membrane or non-intact skin exposure to infected fluid or tissues.

> **Brain abscess:** a challenging diagnosis. Suspect if headache + focal neurological signs but negative non-contrast CT. Risk factors are recent dental procedure or decreased immunity. First-line test is MRI. CT scan with contrast is an alternative. Abscess appears as mass lesion(s) with ring enhancement. Treat with IV antibiotics and surgical drainage.

CASE 12–6 SEIZURES

A 75-year-old man's sister notices her brother's body stiffen for about 30 seconds. The stiffening is followed by rhythmic jerking of his arms and legs. He does not respond when she asks him "What's wrong?" She immediately calls her physician for advice. She has never noticed this kind of behavior in the patient before.

On the basis of this description, what is the most likely abnormal movement?

Seizures (ictus) are temporary, hypersynchronized, electrical impulses from the cerebral cortex. Seizures that affect a single part of the cortex are termed partial seizures, whereas those that affect the entire cortex are termed generalized seizures (Fig. 12-10). This patient's symptoms suggest a generalized tonic-clonic seizure.

> **Epilepsy:** recurrent epileptic seizures; more common in children and elderly.

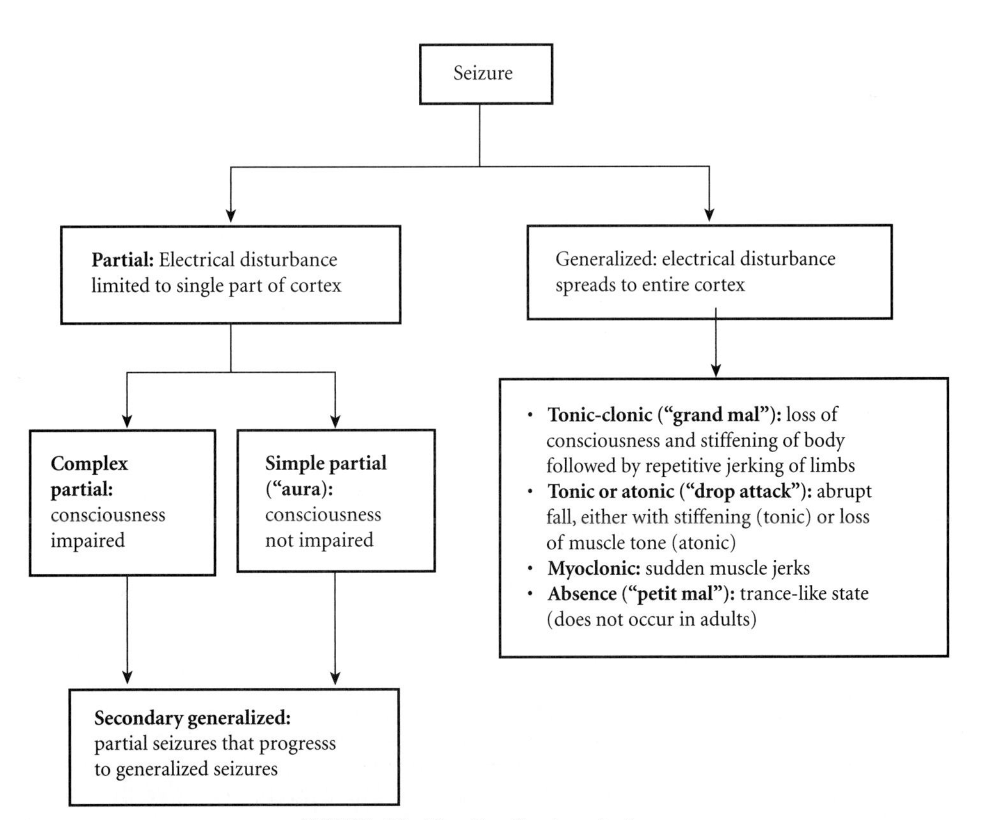

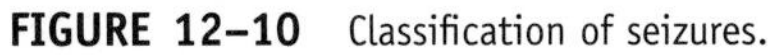
FIGURE 12–10 Classification of seizures.

Aura: Many patients experience automatisms (e.g., lip smacking) or hallucinations (abnormal smells or tastes) before the actual seizure. Aura before a generalized seizure suggests a partial seizure with secondary generalization.

What advice should you give the patient's sister?

Most seizures resolve within a few minutes. First-line measures outside a medical setting are:

1. Prevent injury: Move all sharp objects away from the patient's vicinity.
2. Recovery position: After the seizure, move the patient to the left side with his head tilted down (to prevent aspiration of vomit).
3. Persistent seizure: If the seizure persists >5 minutes, call emergency services.

Do not restrain the patient or put anything in his mouth during the seizure.

The patient continues to seize for 5 minutes. Paramedics arrive 5 minutes after the sister calls emergency services. He is still seizing.

What are the initial steps in management?

The patient is in status epilepticus, defined as a single seizure lasting >5 minutes or multiple seizures with no inter-ictal return to baseline. Status epilepticus is a medical emergency. Figure 12-11 outlines an algorithm for management of status epilepticus. When the patient reaches the hospital, try to determine the underlying cause. If history and physical do not suggest an obvious cause, obtain the following initial studies:

1. **Laboratory tests**: Obtain serum chemistries, LFTs, and urine toxicology screen to evaluate for electrolyte and metabolic disturbances.
2. **Imaging**: CT scan without contrast is the first-line test if the patient is unstable or has deficits suggestive of a stroke. MRI is more sensitive at identifying mass lesions (tumor, hemorrhage, etc.).
3. **EEG**: This is the most helpful test to confirm the diagnosis of seizures and identify the type of seizure. A normal EEG does not rule out seizure. Also, many EEG abnormalities are nonspecific.

Remember the important causes of seizures in adults with the mnemonic "***I'M MOE WHITE***":

- **I**schemia: TIA and ischemic stroke
- **M**ass lesions: e.g., tumors and metastases, hemorrhage and hematoma
- **M**etabolic derangements: hepatic and uremic encephalopathy, hypo- and hyperthyroidism, and hyperthermia
- **O**verdoses: e.g., cocaine and lithium
- **E**lectrolyte abnormalities: hyponatremia and hypocalcemia
- **W**ithdrawal: e.g., alcohol, sedative-hypnotic, or anticonvulsant withdrawal,
- **H**ypertensive encephalopathy
- **I**nfections: septic shock, meningitis, encephalitis, and brain abscess
- **T**raumatic brain injury: even in the absence of a space-occupying hematoma
- **E**clampsia

Placing an IV is often challenging in a seizing patient. In such a situation, consider intramuscular midazolam or rectal diazepam instead of IV lorazepam as initial therapy.

Fosphenytoin has fewer infusion site reactions but is more expensive than phenytoin.

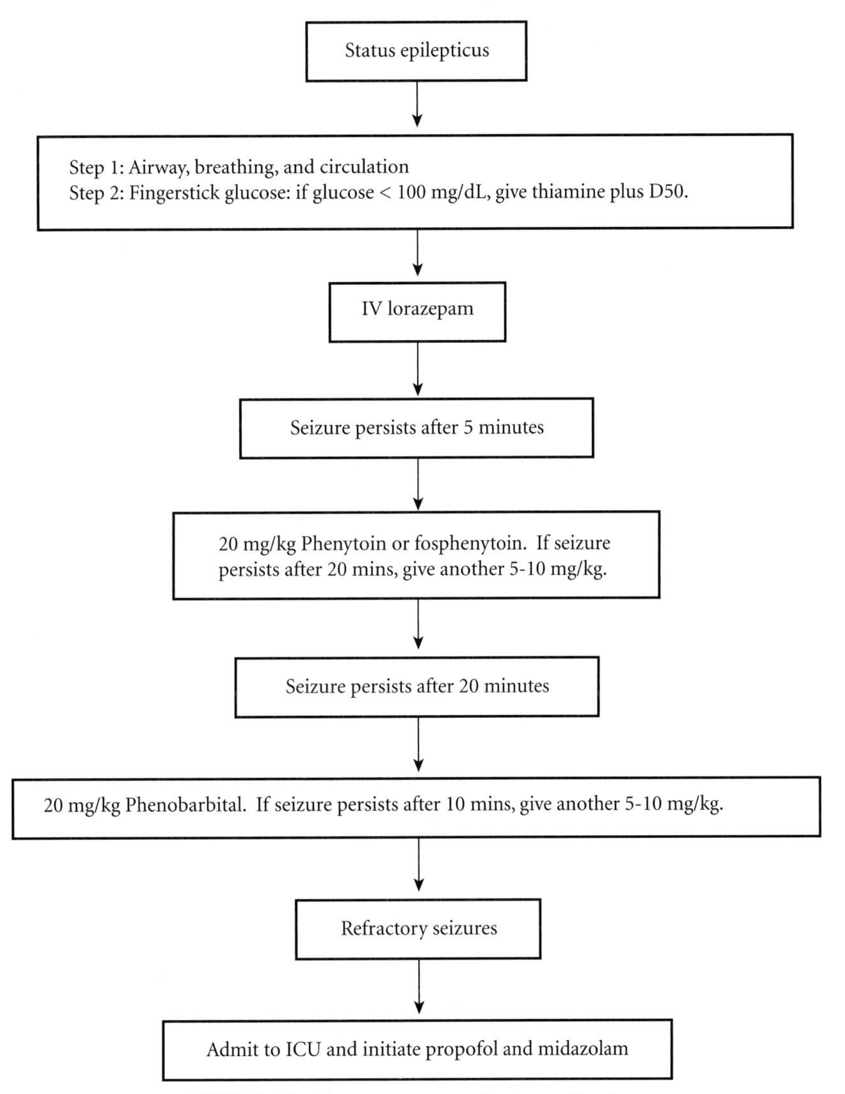

FIGURE 12–11 Management of status epilepticus.

The patient receives supplemental oxygen. The paramedic is able to place an IV and administers lorazepam. The seizure persists, so the patient receives fosphenytoin. Ten minutes later, the seizure resolves. Immediately after the seizure, the patient appears confused. His right arm and leg are weak. Initial laboratory tests and head CT are negative.

What is the most likely cause of these post-ictal symptoms?

Immediately after a partial complex or generalized seizure, most patients have a period of confusion that lasts for seconds to hours. Some patients may have focal deficits such as weakness on one side of the body that resolves within 48 hours (Todd's palsy).

> Normal EEG is associated with a lower incidence of recurrent seizures.

No underlying cause is detected. The patient asks if he needs to take any medicine to prevent another seizure.

What should you tell the patient?

In general, anti-epileptic drugs (AEDs) are not indicated until a person has two unprovoked seizures. Neurologists often consider AEDs to prevent recurrences after a single seizure in the following instances:

1. Status epilepticus or Todd's palsy
2. Abnormal EEG
3. Risk factors like Alzheimer's disease

Fully reversible underlying cause: Do not initiate AED if seizure is caused by alcohol withdrawal, infection, hypertensive encephalopathy, etc.
Underlying cause that is not immediately reversible: Consider AED if the patient has an unresectable mass lesion, stroke, recent traumatic brain injury, etc.

What AED should the patient with a single episode of status epilepticus initiate?

Studies have not found any one AED superior to others. Older AEDs such as phenytoin, carbamazepine, and valproate are cheaper but have more side effects and require frequent monitoring. Second-generation AEDs such as gabapentin, lamotrigine, and oxcarbazepine are more expensive but have fewer side effects. In general, initiate treatment with a single drug. "Start low and go slow" until you reach the lowest dose that prevents seizures. Increase the dose of the first AED until the patient develops side effects. Then add a second AED if seizures continue to recur.

A single AED is sufficient to prevent recurrent seizures in 70% of patients.

Young women: AEDs reduce the effectiveness of oral contraceptives. Other modes of contraception are preferred. AEDs also increase risk of fetal malformation, so women on AEDs should take folic acid.

The patient asks when he can stop taking the AED.

What should you tell him?

Discontinuation is an option if he remains free of seizures after 2 years with a single AED and EEG is normal. AEDs are discontinued by tapering the dose over 2 to 6 months.

Each state has different rules regarding how long a person must remain seizure-free to drive a vehicle. These laws often influence duration of therapy.

The patient initiates phenytoin. He remains seizure-free for 13 months but then has another seizure.

What is the next step in management?

The most common cause of recurrence in a patient with previously well-controlled seizures is noncompliance. After controlling the seizure, the most important step is to check serum AED levels.

Alternative 12.6.1

A 32-year-old man has a 2-minute episode of smacking his lips repeatedly. He is aware of the symptoms but cannot control them.

What diagnosis should you suspect?

Suspect a simple partial seizure in this patient with a single temporary neurological abnormality and no LOC. Automatisms such lip smacking are common symptoms of partial seizures. Other common disturbances include déjà vu and olfactory or gustatory hallucinations.

Partial complex seizure: automatism plus LOC.

What diagnosis would you suspect if the patient's symptoms continue for >20 minutes and consist of turning his head side to side, large thrusting movements of his pelvis, and he repeatedly cries out "Bobby, save me!"?

Side-to-side head turning, large amplitude movements such as pelvic thrusting, and talking during the episode are uncommon in true seizures. Suspect a psychogenic seizure (pseudo-seizure), which is caused by psychosocial issues and not neuronal hyperexcitation.

CASE 12–7 DEMENTIA

A 60-year-old man is brought to the physician by his daughter. She says that over the last 12 months he seems to be forgetting things easily. He often asks her the same questions, and he gets lost in the neighborhood where he has lived for 30 years. He remembers distant events such as his wedding and his first job but cannot remember what he did yesterday. He does not take any medications. He denies any depression. Physical exam and vital signs are normal. MMSE is 23.

What is the most likely cause of dementia?

The most likely diagnosis is Alzheimer's disease (AD), which accounts for 60% to 80% of dementia. AD is an incurable disease that that causes progressive cognitive decline. AD patients typically die within 8 to 10 years of diagnosis. The stages of AD are:

1. Early: Difficulties with short-term memory are the earliest symptom in 80% of AD patients. Many patients are unaware of the memory loss (anosognosia). Commonly reported symptoms are forgetting appointments, leaving the stove on, repeating questions, and getting lost in the local area.
2. Middle: In addition to worsening memory loss, patients develop progressive visual, spatial, and language deficits (e.g., aphasia and apraxia) as well as visuospatial deficits. At this stage, patients require daily supervision.
3. Late: Delusions, hallucinations, and personality changes are common. Eventually, the patient cannot perform any activity of daily living.

> There are five activities of daily living ("***DEATH***"): **D**ressing, **E**ating, **A**mbulating, **T**oileting, **H**ygiene

> Physical exam is usually normal in early and middle stage AD.

What are risk factors for AD?

The most important risk factor for AD is older age (prevalence is 20% to 40% in persons >85 years old). Another important risk factor is family history.

> **Chromosome 21 and AD**: Many cases of early onset autosomal dominant AD result from point mutations in the APP gene on chromosome 21. Early-onset AD is also very common in Down's syndrome (chromosome 21 trisomy).

What is the next step in management?

Consider the following tests in all patients with dementia to rule out reversible causes due to underlying medical illnesses: vitamin B12 level, serum chemistry, thyroid-stimulating hormone (TSH), VDRL, and a neuro-imaging study (usually MRI). Remember that AD is a clinical diagnosis, and there are no specific tests to diagnose this disorder. Clinical diagnosis is accurate in 90% of patients (in studies that compared clinical diagnosis to the brain biopsy at autopsy).

As AD progresses, CT or MRI will show diffuse cerebral atrophy and dilated ventricles.

AD pathology: Brain biopsy at autopsy (gold standard) demonstrates neurofibrillary tangles and senile β-amyloid plaques. Clinical diagnosis is 90% accurate in studies that compared clinical diagnosis to the gold standard.

Laboratory tests are negative. MRI demonstrates mild cerebral atrophy and dilated ventricles.

What is the next step in management?

Initiate the following medications at diagnosis:

1. **Cholinesterase inhibitors**: Donepezil, rivastigmine, and galantamine are first-line agents because AD patients have decreased cerebral acetylcholine production. These drugs are associated with small improvements in cognition and activities of daily living. It is unclear if they reduce mortality or long-term disability.
2. **Vitamin E**: Vitamin E is an adjunctive therapy that is frequently initiated at diagnosis because studies have shown that this antioxidant can delay symptom onset. Patients with a history of CV disease should not take vitamin E (increased risk of mortality).

AD prevention: Consider vitamin E only in patients with AD in multiple family members. Do not recommend vitamin E to other groups (may increase risk of mortality).

Avoid anticholinergic drugs in patients with AD.

Tacrine: cholinesterase inhibitor. Rarely used because of side effects and four times/day dosing.
Donepizil: popular because it has the least liver toxicity of the cholinesterase inhibitors.

Over the next four years, the patient has progressive cognitive decline.

Are there any other medications that can slow cognitive decline in this patient?

Memantine (NMDA-antagonist) may slow cognitive decline in moderate to severe AD.

Cholinesterase inhibitors are ineffective in severe AD.

Six months later, the family decides to place the patient in a nursing home. They feel he is doing relatively well there. He recognizes his daughter and remembers some distant events. He follows most commands. After 2 months, the family members mention that they are troubled by a pattern they have noticed over the last 2 weeks. In the evening, he becomes confused and agitated. He does not recognize his daughter and often wanders the hallways aimlessly. During the daytime hours, his behavior returns to baseline. Physical exam and vital signs are normal.

What is the most likely cause of his symptoms?

Sun-downing is a poorly understood phenomenon that tends to occur in elderly demented patients in hospitals or long-term care facilities. Patients become increasingly agitated during the evening hours, but return to baseline during the day. Symptoms frequently occur during shift changes. Avoid restraints, sedatives, and neuroleptics to control agitation. Instead, first-line measures are conservative:

1. Minimize confusion: structured activities, frequent calming and re-orientation.
2. Environment: increased sunlight, increased clocks, and decreased ambient noise in the room.
3. Minimize use of catheters and IV lines.

Rule out delirium in patients who do not follow the classic pattern of sun-downing.

Postoperative delirium: symptoms similar to sun-downing except that they occur postoperatively. First-line therapy is conservative (similar to sun-downing).

Alternative 12.7.1

A 72-year-old man is brought by his daughter for evaluation of cognitive difficulties. About 2 years ago, she noticed that he was finding it difficult remember recent events and to balance his checkbook. About 6 months ago, the memory deficits worsened, and about 2 weeks ago he began to have aphasia. Past history is significant for a TIA and an ischemic stroke 3 years ago. Physical exam is normal. Blood pressure is 160/90; MMSE is 22. Vitamin B12 level, serum chemistry, and TSH are normal. VDRL is negative. MRI shows multiple old infarcts.

What is the most likely diagnosis?

The most likely diagnosis is multi-infarct dementia (vascular dementia). As the name suggests, dementia results from multiple small infarcts and is more common in patients with a history of TIA or stroke. Although MRI is suggestive, the diagnosis is clinical. Unlike AD, multi-infarct dementia tends to cause step-wise rather than gradual decline in cognition. Control of CV risk factors (especially hypertension) is the primary treatment to prevent further decline in cognition. Many neurologists also use donepezil and memantine, although studies have not demonstrated a clear benefit from their use.

The distinction between AD and vascular dementia is often difficult, even using neuropsychiatric scales such as the Hachinski score. AD and vascular dementia frequently coexist in the same patient (which is one rationale for using donepezil + memantine).

Alternative 12.7.2

A 58-year-old man is brought by his wife for evaluation of inappropriate behavior over the last 8 months. He often makes crude and disparaging remarks in social situations. He was arrested last month for shoplifting. She has been married to him for 30 years, and she says, "This is not the man who married me and raised our children." The patient does not feel like anything is wrong. MMSE is 23. Vitamin B12 level, serum chemistry, and TSH are normal. VDRL is negative. MRI demonstrates diffuse and asymmetric atrophy in the frontal and temporal lobes.

What is the most likely diagnosis?

The most likely diagnosis is frontotemporal dementia (FTD). This uncommon disorder presents with gradual onset of inappropriate behavior and language difficulties. Patients often have poor insight regarding their condition. Diagnosis is clinical, although imaging often demonstrates diffuse and asymmetric atrophy of the frontal and temporal lobes. FTD is often misdiagnosed as AD. Like AD, FTD is incurable and follows a progressive course of cognitive decline and death.

FTD versus AD:

1. Early disease: Socially inappropriate behavior is uncommon in early AD. Memory loss that affects daily functions is uncommon in early FTD.
2. Imaging: AD causes symmetric atrophy in the temporal lobe around the hippocampus.
3. Treatment: Cholinesterase inhibitors are ineffective in FTD.

FTD is a collective term for a number of disorders. The prototype FTD is Pick's disease.

Alternative 12.7.3

A 67-year-old woman present with an 8-month history of memory difficulties. She finds it difficult to balance her checkbook. She recently lost her job because she couldn't stay organized. Over the last 7 years, her movements have "slowed down" a lot, which she attributes to aging. She also mentions worsening tremor over the last 6 years. On physical exam, there is an oscillating tremor at rest that disappears with activity. Her muscles feel stiff. She walks in small, shuffling steps. Her arms do not swing as she walks. On passive flexion and extension, her wrists give way in a series of ratchet-like jerks. MMSE is 23.

What is the most likely diagnosis?

The woman has the classic clinical manifestations of Parkinson's disease (PD):

- Tremor: "pill rolling" (oscillating) resting tremor that disappears with activity.
- Rigidity: Increased muscle tone leads to:
  1. Lead-pipe rigidity: muscles feel stiff on physical exam.
  2. Bradykinesia: slow movements.
  3. Festination: small shuffling steps.
  4. Decreased arm swing during walking.
  5. Cogwheel rigidity: "ratchet-like" jerks in rapid succession on passive flexion or extension; caused by rigidity plus tremor.
  6. Mask-like facies, dysarthria, and dysphagia; caused by facial muscle rigidity.
  7. Dysgraphia: handwriting is small as a result of decreased muscle movements.
- Postural instability: difficulty maintaining balance. The combination of postural instability and rigidity lead to episodes of "freezing" (inability to initiate a movement).
- Personality changes and dementia: Apathy and withdrawal may occur early but dementia is typically a later finding.

Dementia is usually a late feature in many but not all patients. Tremor, rigidity, and postural instability occur as a result of decreased dopamine-producing neurons in the substantia nigra of the basal ganglia. Most cases are idiopathic (genetics and environmental factors such as trauma have been implicated). Although PD can occur in younger people, most patients are >50 years old. Diagnosis is clinical (i.e., there are no laboratory tests for PD).

> **MPTP**: Improperly prepared MPPP (synthetic heroin) can form this byproduct. MPTP kills neurons in the substantia nigra and leads to abrupt onset of severe PD.

> Decreased dopamine leads to unopposed acetylcholine in the basal ganglia.

What treatment should you initiate in this patient?

First-line therapy in older patients (age > 65 years) with advanced PD is levodopa-carbidopa. Levodopa crosses the blood–brain barrier and is converted to dopamine in the CNS. Carbidopa prevents conversion to dopamine in peripheral tissues.

The patient initiates levodopa-carbidopa. After approximately 1 year, he complains that the effects wear off in 3 hours and then he has excessive tremor.

What is the next step?

Patients with advanced PD often experience "off phenomenon" (effects wear off in <4 hours). The first-line measure is to avoid taking levodopa with high-protein meals and to shorten the dose interval. The second option is to add a COMT inhibitor (entacapone) to the regimen. Alternative options are addition of a dopamine agonist (e.g., pramipexole or ropinirole) or an monoamine oxidase inhibitor (MAOI) such as selegiline or rasagiline to the regimen.

Five years later, the patient complains of uncontrollable, large amplitude movements. The symptoms are very troublesome.

What is the next step in management?

Abnormal involuntary movements (dyskinesia) occur in >50% of patients after 5 to 10 years of levodopa therapy. Minor dyskinesias (e.g., small, jerky movements) do not require any specific therapy. In this patient with troublesome symptoms, lower levodopa-carbidopa dose and add a dopamine agonist and/or amantadine (anticholinergic) to the regimen.

> **Pergolide and cabergoline**: These agents are dopamine agonists used to treat excess prolactin. Avoid in PD because they increase risk of valvular disease.

How would initial management differ if the patient were 45 years old and presented with mild resting tremor and bradykinesia but no signs of dementia?

Consider a dopamine agonist as a first-line agent in young patients (<65 years old) with early PD. The rationale is to delay levodopa and its concomitant side effects.

> Amantadine (anticholinergic) is an option for initial therapy in young patients with tremor as the predominant symptom with little or no rigidity.

Alternative 12.7.4

A 60-year-old man is brought by his daughter for evaluation of cognitive difficulties. The symptoms have been slowly progressing over the last few months. He recently lost his job because he was "unorganized." He has gotten lost driving on familiar roads. He sometimes thinks his daughter is an imposter (Capgras syndrome), and he sometimes sees his mother, who has been dead for 10 years. On examination, there is "pill rolling" resting tremor that resolves with activity, bradykinesia, cogwheel rigidity, and dysgraphia. MMSE is 22.

What is the most likely diagnosis?

Suspect dementia with Lewy bodies if cognitive decline appears before or at the same time as other symptoms of PD. Visual hallucinations and Capgras syndrome are common early findings in dementia with Lewy bodies but not PD.

> Capgras syndrome also occurs in 10% of cases of late AD.

> **Shy Drager syndrome**: autonomic instability plus symptoms of PD.
> **Progressive supranuclear palsy**: ophthalmoplegia + other PD symptoms except tremor.

How is dementia with Lewy bodies treated?

Treat movement symptoms with levodopa (tremor, rigidity, and postural instability). Treat cognitive difficulties with rivastigmine (anticholinergic). Consider a low-dose atypical antipsychotic for persistent hallucinations and delusions.

> **Essential tremor**: fine tremor; worse with certain postures (e.g., arms outstretched) or activities (e.g., writing), improved with alcohol. No other associated symptoms.
> **Cerebellar ("intention") tremor**: coarse tremor; worse with activity (e.g., pointing at objects), improved with rest. Associated symptoms are ataxia and nystagmus.

Alternative 12.7.5

A 37-year-old musician presents with a 12-month history of cognitive and movement disturbances. He initially began to have difficulties playing his guitar because of uncontrollable hand jerking. He also complains of memory impairment and depression. He was an adopted child. On examination, there are jerky, irregular limb movements (chorea). Gait is unsteady. He moves slowly and facial expressions are decreased. MMSE is 23.

What diagnosis should you suspect?

Suspect Huntington's disease (HD) in this adopted young person with dementia and chorea. HD can also cause bradykinesia, mask-like facies, and behavioral abnormalities (depression, anxiety, etc.). HD results from autosomal dominant inheritance of the HD gene (increased CAG trinucleotide repeats) on chromosome 4. Symptoms typically begin in the third or fourth decade. Genetic testing can confirm the diagnosis. Treatment is supportive. HD follows a progressive course and is uniformly fatal within a few years of diagnosis.

What is the risk that his 10-year-old daughter will develop HD?

Because HD is autosomal dominant, his offspring all have a 50% chance of inheriting the gene. If his daughter has inherited the gene, she has a 100% chance of developing HD.

> Genetic testing in family members is controversial. Most neurologists discourage testing in persons <18 years because of the psychosocial impact and lack of treatment options.

Alternative 12.7.6

A 43-year-old man is brought by his wife for evaluation of a 3-month history of progressive cognitive decline. He often has quick, small limbs jerks during the evaluation (myoclonus). MMSE is 18. Gait is ataxic. MRI reveals mild cerebral atrophy but is otherwise nonspecific.

What diagnosis should you suspect?

Progressive cognitive decline and myoclonus over the course of a few weeks to months should raise suspicion for Creutzfeldt Jacob disease (CJD). This rare disorder results from prion infection (prions are infectious protein particles). CJD is incurable and causes death within weeks to months of diagnosis.

What tests can help confirm the diagnosis?

Obtain EEG and perform LP. CJD diagnosis requires the following:

1. Abrupt onset of cognitive decline
2. Two of the following: myoclonus, akinetic mutism, visual or cerebellar symptoms, or Parkinsonian symptoms
3. EEG shows periodic synchronous bi- or triphasic sharp wave complexes or CSF 14-3-3 protein assay is positive.

> Brain biopsy at autopsy demonstrates spongiform vacuoles.

Alternative 12.7.6

A 78-year-old man presents with a 6 month history of cognitive decline and difficulty walking. Over the last 6 months, he has experienced new-onset urinary urgency and incontinence. MMSE is 24. On physical exam, he walks with a broad-based gait. Vital signs are normal.

What is the most likely diagnosis?

Dementia, ataxia, and urinary incontinence are the classic triad of normal pressure hydrocephalus (NPH). This uncommon and reversible disorder results from impaired CSF absorption into the systemic circulation.

What is the next step in management?

First, obtain MRI to rule out other causes, which will increase the likelihood of NPH. NPH typically causes enlarged ventricles but no sulcus thickening or cerebral atrophy.

MRI is suggestive of NPH.

What is the next step in management?

Perform the lumbar tap test (Fisher test). The test involves removal of 30 to 50 mL of CSF and measurement of cognition and gait 30 to 60 minutes later. If symptoms improve, the patient is likely to benefit from a ventricular shunt procedure.

Reversible dementias are high yield!: Hemochromatosis and WD (Chapter 5: Hepatology), hypothyroidism (Chapter 8: Endocrinology), chronic alcoholism and vitamin B12 (cobalamin) deficiency (Chapter 10: Hematology and Oncology), HIV encephalopathy (Chapter 11: HIV and AIDS), neurosyphilis (Chapter 14: Primary Care Gynecology and Urology), and chronic SDH.

False negative: Remember that normal vitamin B12 (cobalamin) level does not rule out deficiency in a patient with characteristic clinical features and blood smear.

Alternative 12.7.7

A 70-year-old man complains of memory difficulties. He sometimes forgets the names of people he met months ago. Occasionally, he cannot remember the word for a particular situation. He recently authored a book titled *Those Magnificent North Carolina Tar Heels and Their Basketball Machine.* MMSE is 29.

What is the most likely diagnosis?

Difficulty remembering words and people's names is a normal part of aging (benign senescent dementia). This patient with a MMSE of 29 who recently authored a book does not appear to have any cognitive decline. Reassure this patient and continue to monitor during regular visits.

Alternative 12.7.8

A 71-year-old woman is brought by her son to the clinic. Since her husband's death 2 months ago, she has become increasingly withdrawn. She does not remember to keep appointments. She left the stove on 3 times in the last week after cooking. She has told her son a couple of times that she can't wait to be with her dear husband again. MMSE is 23.

What is the next step in management?

The patient with symptom onset soon after her husband died most likely has depression rather than dementia. Elderly people with depression often present with cognitive deficits (pseudodementia). The next step in any patient with thoughts of suicide is urgent psychiatric referral. First-line therapy is a selective serotonin reuptake inhibitor (SSRI). Cognitive behavioral therapy may also benefit the patient. If she continues to have cognitive deficits despite adequate treatment for depression, consider detailed neuropsychiatric evaluation for true dementia.

CASE 12–8 DRUG INTOXICATIONS AND WITHDRAWAL

A 27-year-old man is brought to the emergency department 30 minutes after a seizure. His friend reports that he was "doing drugs" at a house party but is not sure what he took. The patient is agitated and in restraints. Pupils are dilated. There are no focal neurological signs. Blood pressure is 200/100, pulse 125 bpm, respirations 25/min, and temperature 38.2°C.

Is stimulant or depressant intoxication more likely in this patient?

This agitated patient with tachycardia, tachypnea, hypertension, and a seizure most likely has stimulant intoxication (Table 12-11).

A second friend arrives at the emergency room and tells you that the patient snorted multiple lines of cocaine.

What is the next step in management?

There is no specific therapy for cocaine intoxication. Benzodiazepines are the first-line drugs to control cocaine-induced agitation, hypertension, and seizures.

TABLE 12–11 Drug Intoxications

	Stimulants	Depressants
Behavior	Restless, aggressive, and hypervigilant	Labile mood
Pupils	Dilated pupils	Constricted pupils
Vital signs	Tachycardia, tachypnea, fever, and HTN	Bradycardia and bradypnea
Neurological	• ↑ Reflexes • Seizures • Tremor and sweating	• ↓ Reflexes and coordination • Slurry speech • Stupor and coma if severe
Examples	• Cocaine • Amphetamines • Arylhexamines (PCP, ketamine) • Psychedelics (LSD, psilocybin, etc.) • Anticholinergics (TCAs, atropine, etc.)	• Alcohol • Benzodiazepines • Barbiturates • Opiates (Chapter 7: Fluids and Electrolytes) • Cholinergics

Abbreviations: HTN, hypertension; LSD, lysergic acid diethylamide; PCP, phencyclidine; TCA, tricyclic antidepressants.

Haloperidol: This drug is not indicated unless the patient is psychotic (e.g., hallucinations or delusions).

How would management differ if the patient reported chest pain and palpitations?

Cocaine can cause CV complications (MI, myocarditis, and arrhythmias). Six percent of cocaine-intoxicated patients with chest pain have MI. In addition to benzodiazepines, obtain EKG and baseline cardiac biomarkers and administer oxygen, nitrates, and aspirin.

Cocaine can also cause stroke, pulmonary infiltrates, and rhabdomyolysis-induced acute renal failure.

Urine toxicology screen is positive for cocaine. EKG and initial cardiac biomarkers are negative for MI. The patient is much calmer after receiving lorazepam. Vital signs are normal. His girlfriend reports he has been using cocaine with increasing frequency over the last 6 months.

What symptoms do you expect over the next few hours to days?

Chronic cocaine users often experience a withdrawal syndrome. Some users experience an initial post-use crash within 15 to 30 minutes of cessation (intense craving for more cocaine, depression, and suicidal ideation). Over the next few hours, they experience hypersomnolence (sleepiness) and hyperphagia (hunger). Over the next few days, they experience fatigue and depression. No specific therapy is necessary because cocaine withdrawal (including post-use crash) does not cause any harmful physiological effects. Monitor for relapse because patients may self-medicate with cocaine to treat withdrawal.

Amphetamines and methamphetamines: Stimulant effect is caused by dopamine release from nerve endings. Clinical presentation and management of overdose and withdrawal is similar to cocaine. Unlike cocaine, overdose can also cause liver failure and DIC (disseminated intravascular coagulation).

Synthetic amphetamines: Drugs such as MDMA ("ecstasy") and MDEA ("eve") release dopamine and serotonin from nerve endings (leads to stimulant and hallucinogen effect).

Alternative 12.8.1

A 28-year-old man is brought to the emergency room after using an unknown drug. Emergency medical services restrained him because he was violent, aggressive, and paranoid. He tells you he doesn't know who he is and where he is from. Pupils are dilated and there is vertical nystagmus. Vital signs are temperature 38.9°C, pulse 120 bpm, blood pressure 210/120, and respirations 20/min.

What is the most likely drug ingested by this patient?

The most likely drug ingested by this patient is phencyclidine (PCP). PCP causes signs of stimulant intoxication plus ataxia, vertical nystagmus (classic finding), and dissociative amnesia, an inability to remember personal information. Severe overdose can cause hypertensive emergency and hyperthermia.

> Arylhexamines (PCP and ketamine) are NMDA-receptor antagonists.

How is PCP intoxication treated?

Treatment is supportive. Treat hypertension and hyperthermia if present. Consider haloperidol if the patient is psychotic. Consider urine acidification with ammonium chloride or ascorbic acid (to increase PCP excretion) as long as the patient has no signs of rhabdomyolysis or underlying liver or kidney disease.

> **Psychedelics**: These drugs cause stimulant symptoms plus psychotic symptoms (hallucinations and delusions). Some psychoses are those of extreme fear (known as a "bad trip"). Hold the patient's hands and reassure the patient repeatedly during a bad trip.

> PCP does not cause a withdrawal syndrome.

Alternative 12.8.2

A 54-year-old farmer is brought to the emergency department for evaluation of altered mental status. He was found lying in a pool of vomit. His son mentions that he had been very depressed after his farm was foreclosed and had mentioned that life was not worth living. GCS is 12. There are copious respiratory and salivary secretions. His pants are soiled from urine and loose stool. Pupils are constricted. His breath has a garlic-like odor. Occasional muscle fasciculations are detected. Vital signs are temperature 37.9°C, pulse 40 bpm, respirations 8/min, and blood pressure 100/60.

What is the most likely cause of his symptoms?

This patient has the classic manifestations of cholinergic excess (mnemonic: "***DUMBELS***"):

1. **D**efecation
2. **U**rination
3. **M**iosis, **M**uscle weakness, and fasciculations
4. **B**ronchorrhea, **B**radycardia, **B**ronchospasm
5. **E**mesis
6. **L**acrimation
7. **S**alivation

The most likely cause of cholinergic excess in this patient with garlic (or petrol-like) breath odor is organophosphate poisoning (found in pesticides, solvents, etc.). Organophosphates are often ingested in suicide attempts. Diagnosis is based primarily on clinical grounds.

> **RBC AChE**: This test can determine the degree of toxicity but is not widely available.

How is suspected organophosphate poisoning managed?

First, evaluate and stabilize the ABCs. Second, administer atropine (anticholinergic). Next consider pralidoxime. Also consider a benzodiazepine if the patient has a seizure.

Nasogastric lavage and activated charcoal do not reduce mortality.

Alternative 12.8.3

An 18-year-old college student presents 30 minutes late for a routine appointment. He eats three triple-patty hamburgers during the evaluation. His grade point average has dropped from 3.5 to 2.5 because he rarely goes to class. He denies any depression. On examination, both conjunctiva are red. He has bilateral gynecomastia. Pulse is 110 bpm.

What is the most likely cause of these findings?

Hypherphagia, conjunctival injection, and tachycardia are signs of marijuana intoxication. Social withdrawal and gynecomastia suggest he is a chronic marijuana user.

The patient admits to marijuana use. He asks if there are any long-term consequences of smoking marijuana.

What should you tell him?

Marijuana intoxication poses an increased risk of automobile accidents. Chronic users may have decreased ability to achieve life goals. The long-term risk of lung cancer, chronic lung disease, and schizophrenia is unclear.

The patient tells you that he has been smoking every day for the last 6 months. He asks if he will experience any symptoms if he quits.

What should you tell him?

Chronic users may experience restlessness, anorexia, irritability, and insomnia within 24 hours. Symptoms generally resolve in 7 to 10 days and do not require any specific therapy.

CASE 12–9 DEPRESSION

A 33-year-old woman presents to the clinic with a 6-month history of low energy. She does not feel like going out or having fun. She finds it difficult to fall asleep and often lies awake in bed until 5 am. She has lost 5 lbs over the last 6 months because she rarely feels hungry. She denies any feelings of depression or suicidal thoughts. Her affect is flat. She looks down during the entire interview. She does not have any other medical conditions or take any medications. She denies fever, chills, or night sweats. She does not drink alcohol or use illegal drugs. She smokes a pack of cigarettes every day and is not interested in quitting. Physical exam and vital signs are normal.

What is the most likely diagnosis?

The patient has major depression. To make this diagnosis, the patient must have at least 2 weeks of depression or anhedonia (decreased **I**nterest in activities) plus four or more of the following:

1. **S**leep: difficulty falling asleep or early morning awakening
2. **G**uilt: thoughts of worthlessness or guilt
3. Decreased **E**nergy
4. Decreased **C**oncentration
5. Decreased **A**ppetite
6. **P**sychomotor symptoms: agitation or withdrawal (e.g., flat affect)
7. **S**uicide: occasional thoughts, a well-formed plan, a suicidal gesture, or an attempt

A mnemonic device to remember the major depression criteria is "***SIG E CAPS.***"

Depressed mood is not required to make the diagnosis if the patient has anhedonia.

Rule out underlying medical causes of depression if the patient has suggestive symptoms or risk factors (Table 12-12).

How would you treat this patient?

Either psychotherapy or pharmacotherapy is an acceptable option for mild to moderate depression. Pharmacotherapy is preferred for severe depression. A number of drug classes are available to treat depression (Table 12-13). Although all of them are effective, SSRIs are generally the first-line choice because:

1. SSRIs have a better side effect and safety profile compared with older agents (tricyclic antidepressants (TCAs) and MAOIs).
2. SSRIs have a once-daily dosing.
3. SSRIs are cheaper than the newer agents (e.g., venlafaxine).

Depression severity: Beck depression inventory is a 21-question survey that assesses severity (a score >30 indicates severe depression). In general, depression accompanied by thoughts of suicide is considered severe.

Initial SSRI side effects: SSRIs can initially cause headache, gastrointestinal discomfort, and anxiety. These side effects generally resolve in 1 to 2 weeks.
Initial SSRI dosing: Start at a low dose. Increase once a week to full dose.

What antidepressant would you offer first if the patient were interested in smoking cessation?

Consider bupropion because it has also shown benefit for smoking cessation (Chapter 1: Health Maintenance and Statistics).

The patient who does not wish to stop smoking initiates sertraline. Ten days after starting therapy, she tells you the drug is not working and asks if she should try another medicine.

What should you tell her?

SSRI response typically takes 2 to 6 weeks. Switch to another SSRI only if there is no response after 8 weeks of therapy. If symptoms do not respond to 8 weeks of another SSRI, consider switching to another drug class (usually a serotonin and norepinephrine reuptake inhibitor (SNRI) or norepinephrine and serotonin antagonist (NASA)). Refer patients with refractory severe depression to a psychiatrist. Options for such patients are electroconvulsive therapy or addition of an older antipsychotic.

TABLE 12–12 Medical Conditions That Can Cause Depression

Cause	Examples
Chronic neurological conditions	Neurodegeneration (Alzheimer's and Parkinson's disease) Demyelination (Multiple sclerosis) Traumatic brain injury (chronic subdural hematoma) Brain tumors
Endocrine/metabolic	Hypothyroidism, uremia, cirrhosis, Cushing's disease, porphyria
Drugs	Chronic depressant use, stimulant withdrawal, steroids, cimetidine
Poisons	Lead poisoning
Infections	Neurosyphilis, HIV
Other	Cancer, heart failure

TABLE 12–13 Drugs Used to Treat Depression

Class	Examples	Notes
SSRIs	• Fluoxetine • Sertaline • Paroxetine • Citalopram	• Generally a first-line drug because: 1. Safer and better tolerated than older agents (TCAs, MAOIs) 2. Cheaper than newer drugs (e.g., SNRIs) • Serotonin syndrome: altered mental status, autonomic symptoms, and rigidity; rare complication of SSRIs; not dose-dependant.
TCAs	• Amitriptylene • Imipramine • Nortriptylene • Desipramine	• Not a first-line drug because of side effects and safety issues; overdose is often lethal
MAOIs	• Phenelzine • Tranylcypromine	• Not a first-line drug because of side effects and safety issues; can cause hypertensive crisis if combined with tyramine-rich foods (e.g., red wine, cheese)
SNRIs	• Venlafaxine • Duloxetine	• Side effect profile similar to SSRIs
NDRIs	• Bupropion	• First-line drug if patient also wants to quit smoking • Alternative if SSRIs cause sexual side effects • Avoid if history of seizures
SARIs	• Trazodone • Nefazodone	• Priapism is an uncommon but classic side effect (Chapter 14: Primary Gynecology and Urology)
NASAs	• Mirtazapine	• First-line drug if patient wants to gain weight

Abbreviations: MAOIs, monoamine oxidase inhibitors; NASAs, norepinephrine and serotonin antagonists; NDRIs, norepinephrine and dopamine reuptake inhibitors; SARIs, serotonin antagonist and reuptake inhibitors; SNRIs, serotonin and norepinephrine reuptake inhibitors; SSRIs, selective serotonin reuptake inhibitors.

Over the next 6 months, the patient switches to paroxetine and then to venlafaxine. She finally decides the drugs are useless and abruptly discontinues venlafaxine. The next day, she presents with myalgias, dizziness, and anxiety.

What is the next step in management?

Abrupt discontinuation of SSRIs or SNRIs causes SSRI discontinuation syndrome, characterized by flu-like symptoms and dizziness. The next step is to restart venlafaxine.

Over the next 2 years, the patient continues to have episodes of major depression and even entertains thoughts of suicide. She is referred to a psychiatrist. One year later, she is brought to the emergency room with decreased consciousness. GCS is 12. Pupils are dilated, skin is flushed, oropharynx is dry, and bladder is distended. She has hyperactive reflexes and positive Babinski sign. Temperature is 38.7°C, blood pressure is 90/70, and pulse is 120 bpm.

What is the most likely cause of her symptoms?

Her symptoms suggest either an accidental or intentional TCA overdose (presents with a combination of anticholinergic and other distinctive neurological signs):

1. **Anticholinergic signs**: Signs of anticholinergic overdose are urinary retention and intestinal ileus plus "mad as a hatter" (altered mental status), "dry as a bone" (dry oropharynx), "red as a beet" (flushed skin), "blind as a bat" (dilated pupils and visual disturbances), and "hot as a hare" (hyperthermia).
2. **Neurological signs**: Important signs are hyperactive reflexes and positive Babinski sign. Although they are anticholinergics, TCAs can cause profound respiratory depression leading to stupor and coma.

> **Cardiac toxicity**: TCA overdose can cause a number of arrhythmias. The most common rhythm is sinus tachycardia. The classic abnormality is wide QRS complex. Always obtain an EKG in suspected overdose.

How is TCA overdose treated?

The initial steps are to evaluate and stabilize ABCs. Also, administer sodium bicarbonate if the patient has hypotension or QRS >100 ms.

> **Suicide**: Women attempt suicide more often than men, but men are more likely to be successful because they tend to use more lethal methods (e.g., guns rather than pills).

Alternative 12.9.1

A 35-year-old man is diagnosed with major depression and is started on paroxetine. Eight weeks later, he is asked to switch to sertraline because of inadequate effect. Ten hours later, he is brought to the emergency room confused and agitated. On inspection, he is diaphoretic. Neurological exam demonstrates hyperreflexia, clonus, and muscle rigidity. Temperature is 40°C, blood pressure 160/90, pulse 120 bpm, and respirations 23/min.

What is the most likely cause of his symptoms?

Suspect serotonin syndrome when a patient on SSRIs presents with the triad of altered mental status, rigidity, and autonomic instability (sweating, hyperthermia, hypertension, tachycardia, and tachypnea). Clonus and hyperreflexia are common findings on neurological exam. This rare syndrome typically occurs soon after a new SSRI is started. SSRI syndrome commonly causes increased creatine kinase and WBC, but diagnosis is primarily clinical.

> SSRI syndrome is a spectrum that ranges from mild symptoms to the classic triad.

What are the next steps in management?

Treatment of this medical emergency is mostly supportive. The initial step is to discontinue all SSRIs immediately and stabilize ABCs. Additional important measures are to control autonomic symptoms (first-line drugs are benzodiazepines, second-line drug is the serotonin antagonist cyproheptadine) and treat hyperthermia (described below).

What is hyperthermia?

Although both hyperthermia and fever cause increased body temperature, they are different conditions. In fever, increased temperature results from cytokine release, which causes the hypothalamus to shift temperature set point to a higher level. In hyperthermia, an uncontrolled increase in body temperature results from failure of hypothalamic regulation. Hypothalamus regulation can be overwhelmed by:

1. Excessive exposure to ambient heat (sunstroke)
2. Excessive heat produced by rigid muscles: usually caused by medications. Classic triad is similar to SSRI syndrome. Elevated creatine kinase and leukocytosis are the most common laboratory abnormalities. Important causes other than SSRIs are typical antipsychotics (neuroleptic malignant syndrome) and general anesthetics like halothane or succinylcholine (malignant hyperthermia).

> Differentiating fever from hyperthermia is very important because management is different.

How is hyperthermia managed?

Treatment of hyperthermia is "***DiaPER Dandy***":

1. **D**iscontinue causative agent (SSRI, general anesthesia, or antipsychotic).
2. **P**assive cooling: Remove all clothing to promote passive cooling.

3. **E**vaporative cooling: First-line measure in the hospital is to place fans near the patient and spray lukewarm mist.
4. **R**apid sequence intubation: Consider this if temperature reaches >41°C to protect the airway.
5. **D**antrolene: This is a muscle relaxant that is always used for malignant hyperthermia and is occasionally used for neuroleptic malignant syndrome. Dantrolene is not used in cases of sunstroke or SSRI syndrome.

> Antipyretics (acetaminophen, NSAIDS, etc.) play no role in treating hyperthermia.

Alternative 12.9.2

During a routine evaluation, a 21-year-old woman tells you she has been depressed for the last 5 years. She can't remember a time when she was not sad for more than a month. She feels like she is "not as good as everyone else." She often cannot sleep until 4 am. She reports chronic fatigue and low energy. She is very involved in her local church, and she looks forward to their biweekly socials. She denies guilt, decreased concentration, loss of appetite, or thoughts of suicide.

What is the most likely diagnosis?

Chronic depression in a patient who does not meet criteria for major depression is classified as either minor depression or dysthymic disorder (Table 12-14). This patient meets diagnostic criteria for dysthymic disorder (rule of 2's):

TABLE 12–14 Variants of Major Depression

Atypical Depression

- Mood reactivity (mood readily improves or worsens)
- Leaden paralysis (extremities feel heavy and difficult to move)
- Reverse vegetative symptoms (hyperphagia, hypersomnolence)
- Hypersensitivity to rejection

Melancholic Depression

- Nonreactive mood (mood doesn't temporarily improve)
- Severe neurovegetative symptoms (e.g., waking very early in the morning)

Seasonal Affective Disorder

- Begins in fall, continues in winter, and resolves in spring
- Reverse vegetative symptoms (hyperphagia, hypersomnolence)
- Treatment: First-line treatment is phototherapy (unless the patient has suicidal thoughts, in which case SSRIs are the first-line drug choice)

Premenstrual Dysphoric Disorder

- Depression, anxiety, irritability, crying spells, and mood swings
- Begins approximately 2 weeks before the menstrual period
- Ends at the start of the menstrual period
- Symptoms must significantly impair daily activities (otherwise, the diagnosis is premenstrual syndrome (PMS))

Postpartum Depression

- Major depression within the first month of delivery
- Treatment: SSRIs are first-line drug choice
- Differentiate from "postpartum blues" (minor depression, irritability, and somatic complaints occurs in 80% of women)

Psychotic Depression

- Severe major depression plus hallucinations and mood congruent delusions (nihilism, worthlessness, etc.)
- Grossly disordered thought, tangentiality, and clang associations are not characteristic (suspect schizophrenia or bipolar disorder)

- Depressive symptoms that do not meet all criteria for major depression or dysthymic disorder.

- ≥2 years of depression
- ≤2 months of symptom-free intervals
- ≥2 associated symptoms (sleep disturbances, guilt, decreased energy, decreased concentration, increased or decreased appetite, low self-esteem, or feelings of hopelessness)

Dysthymia treatment: psychotherapy and/or SSRIs.

How would you categorize the patient if symptoms had been present for 6 months?

Depression for ≤2 years that never meets diagnostic criteria for major depression is classified as minor depression. First-line management is psychotherapy.

Adjustment disorder with depressed mood: minor depression that occurs within 3 months of an identifiable stressor (e.g., divorce, move to a new location, etc.) and resolves within 6 months. Counseling is usually sufficient to manage these patients.

Alternative 12.9.3

A 32-year-old woman presents with a 1-month history of sadness. The symptoms began soon after her 8-year-old son died of leukemia. Since then, she feels like she is just "going through the motions of life." She has periods where she feels normal and then experiences waves of sadness when she encounters something that reminds her of her son. She finds it difficult to sleep and does not feel like eating anything. She sometimes has hallucinations of seeing and hearing her son. She does not have any thoughts of suicide.

What diagnosis is most likely?

The most likely diagnosis is normal bereavement. Most people experience grief and sadness immediately after the death of a loved one. Symptoms typically occur in "waves" of grief interspersed with episodes of normal mood. Searching behaviors (hallucinations of seeing or hearing loved one) are common. Insomnia, anxiety, and other somatic complaints can also occur. Pharmacotherapy or psychotherapy is not recommended for normal bereavement. Instead, encourage patients to reach out to their loved ones for support.

Six months later, the patient says she feels sad all the time and does not want to live now that her son is gone. She often misses work because she lies in bed all day. She has lost 5 lbs because she does not feel like eating.

What is the next step in management?

Most people are able to move along with their life within a few months after the death of a loved one. Consider psychotherapy (complicated grief therapy) for patients who are unable to move along with their life after 6 to 8 weeks. Also, consider SSRIs if patients meet criteria for major depression after 6 to 8 weeks.

Antidepressants decrease symptoms of depression but not grief.

CASE 12–10 SYNCOPE

A 27-year-old man presents to the clinic for evaluation of a fainting spell. He reports that shortly after urinating in the morning, he began to feel nauseated, lightheaded, and diaphoretic and then fainted. His wife witnessed the event and says that he regained consciousness within moments. He does not have any other medical conditions or take any medications. Physical exam and vital signs are normal.

TABLE 12-15 Causes of Syncope

Category	%	Causes
Unknown origin	33	• Unknown
Neurocardiogenic (vasovagal)	25	• Prolonged standing or heat exposure • Painful or noxious stimuli • Fear of pain (e.g., prior to injection) • Exercise • Carotid sinus hypersensitivity • Situational syncope (micturition, coughing, defecation)
Cardiovascular	18	• Arrhythmia (most common cardiovascular cause) • Valve stenosis (causes outflow tract obstruction) • Hypertrophic cardiomyopathy (causes outflow tract obstruction)
Orthostatic hypotension	10	• **D**rugs: antihypertensives, antidepressants, diuretics • **A**utonomic insufficiency (e.g., diabetes mellitus), Age, or Alcohol • **D**ehydration
Seizures	5–15	Refer to Case 12-6.

How would you characterize the patient's symptoms?

Transient LOC and posture is called syncope. Syncope results from decreased cerebral perfusion. The most common causes are cardiac and neurocardiogenic (Table 12-15).

> **Coma**: LOC without spontaneous recovery
> **Drop attack**: loss of posture without LOC
> **Pre-syncope**: lightheadedness without actually fainting

What is the next step in management?

The initial steps in any patient with syncope are a thorough history, physical, and EKG.

EKG is normal.

What is the most likely cause of syncope?

Premonitory symptoms of nausea, diaphoresis, and lightheadedness immediately before fainting are characteristic of neurocardiogenic (vasovagal) syncope. Vasovagal syncope immediately upon standing after urination is called micturition syncope.

What causes vasovagal syncope?

Fear, pain, excess straining during defecation or coughing, etc., activates the sympathetic nervous system. Excess sympathetic stimulation triggers a paradoxical parasympathetic response. As a result, patients feel nauseated, lightheaded, and fatigued. Vasovagal syncope typically occurs in the standing position and often occurs in patients with orthostatic hypotension (which is also an independent cause of syncope).

> **Orthostatic hypotension**: standing position → blood pools in lower extremities → baroreceptors detect decreased cerebral blood flow → triggers sympathetic response.

How is vasovagal syncope managed?

The initial management of vasovagal syncope is conservative. Instruct patients to sit down and cross their legs when they experience premonitory symptoms. Prevent future episodes by avoiding triggers, decrease or discontinue drugs associated with orthostatic hypotension, and increase salt intake (to expand intravascular volume).

> Further diagnostic testing is not indicated for obvious vasovagal syncope.

β-Blockers are widely prescribed for recurrent vasovagal syncope, but randomized trials have not shown any benefit compared to placebo.

Alternative 12.10.1

A 75-year-old man presents with an episode of syncope. He was at a cocktail party and remembers that his collar felt particularly tight. A friend called his name from behind, so he rapidly turned his head. Within a few moments, he began experiencing premonitory symptoms and fainted. He has a history of hypertension and takes hydrochlorothiazide and amlodipine. Vital signs are normal. EKG is normal.

What is the most likely diagnosis?

Symptoms of vasovagal syncope precipitated by neck turning or a tight collar should raise suspicion for carotid sinus hypersensitivity. Unlike other causes of vasovagal syncope, this condition is more common in the elderly than in young patients. Diagnosis involves the following steps:

1. **Neck auscultation**: Do not perform the remaining steps if auscultation detects a carotid bruit (because carotid massage can dislodge an embolus).
2. **Position**: Place patient in a supine position with the neck slightly extended.
3. **Massage**: Rub the carotid artery at the level of the cricoid cartilage. At the same time, monitor blood pressure and EKG. Positive findings include reproduction of premonitory symptoms, a drop in blood pressure, bradycardia, or transient asystole.

How is carotid sinus hypersensitivity treated?

Initial management is conservative (similar to other types of vasovagal syncope). Cardiac pacing is an option for recurrent syncope caused by carotid hypersensitivity.

Alternative 12.10.2

An 18-year-old athlete presents to the clinic after an episode of syncope. The episode occurred during an intense basketball practice session. He did not experience any premonitory symptoms. Physical exam and vital signs are normal. EKG is normal.

What is the next step in management?

If history, physical exam, and EKG do not suggest a specific cause for exercise-related syncope, consider further testing in the following sequence: laboratory tests (CBC and serum chemistry), echocardiogram, and exercise stress test. If these tests are normal, the next step is reassurance.

What would have been the next step in management if physical exam detected a grade III systolic murmur that increased with Valsalva maneuvers (bearing down, coughing, etc.)?

Hypertrophic cardiomyopathy is an important cause of sudden cardiac death in younger patients. This disorder presents with the murmur described above (Chapter 2: Cardiology). The next step is echocardiography to confirm the diagnosis.

Alternative 12.10.3

A 35-year-old man presents with an episode of syncope while standing. He did not experience any premonitory symptoms before the events. He does not take any medications. EKG is normal. There is no orthostatic hypotension. Carotid sinus massage is negative.

What is the next step in management?

No further testing is indicated in young patients after a single episode of syncope with no obvious cause on history, physical exam, or EKG.

> **San Francisco syncope rule**: Consider hospital admission if any of the following are present (mnemonic: "***CHESS***"): **C**ongestive heart failure, **Hematocrit** <30% (if obtained), **E**KG abnormal, **S**hortness of breath, or **S**BP <90 mm Hg.

The 35-year-old patient has another three episodes of syncope over the next 6 months. Physical exam and EKG have been normal after each episode.

What test should you consider at this stage?

The initial test in a young patient with recurrent syncope and no cardiac risk factors is head-up tilt-table test (HUTT) to evaluate for vasovagal syncope.

> Simultaneous HUTT can increase sensitivity of carotid sinus massage.

What tests would you consider first if the patient reported palpitations during syncope episodes?

Consider cardiac testing in patients with cardiac risk factors (e.g., older age) or cardiac symptoms (e.g., palpitations). The exact order of testing is not specified, but initial options are echocardiography, stress test, and Holter monitoring. If initial tests are nondiagnostic, consider an implantable loop recorder (ILR).

> **Electrophysiology study**: Consider this test for patients with known cardiac disease (e.g., bundle branch block or prior MI) if noninvasive studies and implantable loop recorder are nondiagnostic.

> **Neurological testing**: EEG and brain imaging are often obtained in patients with syncope but are rarely helpful unless the patient has signs of seizures or focal neurological signs.

CASE 12–11 WEAKNESS

A 44-year-old woman complains of weakness and fatigue over the last 7 months. She often feels too tired to get out of bed and initiate routine activities. She is able to carry her grocery bags but feels tired performing this activity. She denies depressed mood or anhedonia. She does not have any other symptoms, and she does not take any medications. Physical exam and vital signs are normal.

Does this patient have weakness?

Exhaustion before, during, or after usual activities is termed fatigue. Patients with fatigue often complain of weakness as well. Physical exam can distinguish fatigue from true weakness (Table 12-16). This patient has fatigue and asthenia (feeling of weakness without actual loss of strength) but not true weakness.

> **Recent fatigue**: fatigue <1 month
> **Prolonged fatigue**: symptoms for 1 to 6 months
> **Chronic fatigue**: symptoms for >6 months

What workup is indicated in patients with prolonged or chronic fatigue/asthenia?

If history and physical (including review of medications and depression screen) do not suggest a specific cause, consider the following workup:

1. Monitor temperature and weight at home.
2. Laboratory tests: CBC with differential, serum chemistry, LFTs, and serum TSH.

Temperature and weight are consistently normal. Laboratory tests are normal.

TABLE 12–16 Grading of Muscle Weakness

Grade 0	No muscle contraction
Grade 1	Trace (flicker) muscle contraction
Grade 2	Movement only when gravity eliminated
Grade 3	Movement against gravity but not resistance
Grade 4	Decreased power of movement against resistance
Grade 5	Normal power of movement against resistance

How would you categorize her symptoms?

The patient has idiopathic chronic fatigue. No further workup is indicated at this time. The patient should continue to make regular scheduled appointments with her primary care physician. Consider further workup if symptoms worsen.

Chronic fatigue syndrome: This uncommon syndrome is identified by chronic unexplained fatigue with four or more symptoms such as low-grade fever, malaise, lymphadenopathy, arthralgias, myalgias, sore throat, headaches, or unrefreshing sleep.

Alternative 12.11.1

A 23-year-old man presents with a 7-day history of weakness. The symptoms began after an episode of abdominal pain and diarrhea. He initially experienced lower extremity weakness and tingling but he now reports upper extremity weakness as well. He also mentions severe back pain over the last 2 days. He does not have any other medical conditions or take any medications. On physical exam, there is 3/5 strength in both lower extremities and 4/5 strength in the upper extremities. Muscle tone and deep tendon reflexes are markedly decreased. Sensation is intact. Bladder is distended. Temperature is 37.1°C, pulse is 112 bpm, and blood pressure is 140/80 lying down and 110/60 standing.

What is the most likely diagnosis?

The patient has objective evidence of weakness. Decreased muscle tone and reflexes indicate weakness is the result of a lower motor neuron cause (Table 12-17). Acute onset of symmetric weakness that begins in the lower extremities and progresses to the upper extremities is suggestive of Guillain-Barré syndrome (GBS). GBS can eventually progress to the face and respiratory muscles (ascending paralysis). Back pain and autonomic symptoms are other common findings in this disorder.

GBS can progress from upper extremities to face and respiratory muscles.

What causes GBS?

Infection or inflammation (e.g., connective tissue disorders, malignancies) can activate an autoimmune response that targets peripheral nerves. The resulting demyelination causes flaccid paralysis and autonomic dysfunction.

Campylobacter jejuni causes abdominal pain and diarrhea and is a common cause of GBS.

How is the diagnosis of GBS confirmed?

Confirm the diagnosis with LP and neurophysiological studies such as repetitive nerve stimulation (RNS) or electromyelography. The characteristic abnormality on LP is albuminocytological dissociation (increased CSF protein but normal WBCs and glucose).

TABLE 12–17 UMN versus LMN Weakness

	UMN Lesions	LMN Lesions
Atrophy	No	Yes
Fasciculations	No	Yes
Reflexes	↑	↓
Muscle tone	↑ (spasticity)	↓ (flaccidity)
Babinski	Toe goes up (abnormal)	Toe goes down (normal)
Location of lesion	Brain or spinal cord	Anterior horn, peripheral nerve, neuromuscular junction, or muscles

Abbreviations: LMN, lower motor neuron; UMN, upper motor neuron.

CSF findings are often nondiagnostic before the first week.

How is GBS treated?

1. Supportive care: Admit patients with autonomic symptoms to the ICU. Consider intubation and mechanical ventilation if the patient has difficulty swallowing (pharyngeal muscle weakness) or has decreased forced vital capacity (respiratory muscle weakness).
2. Disease-altering therapy: The first-line agent is IV immunoglobulin (IVIG). If symptoms persist or IVIG is not available, consider plasmapheresis.

Steroids are not used anymore because studies have not shown any benefit.

What diagnosis should you suspect if the patient presented with acute onset of cranial nerve deficits and difficulty swallowing that progressed to symmetric flaccid weakness of the upper extremities followed by the lower extremities?

Acute onset of descending flaccid paralysis or weakness should raise suspicion for botulism. This rare condition results from a neurotoxin produced by *Clostridium botulinum.* Infection is usually acquired from food or a wound infection. Food-borne botulism (but not wound botulism) can also cause a prodrome of gastrointestinal symptoms.

Botulism: acute onset of descending weakness/paralysis.
GBS: acute onset of ascending weakness/paralysis.

How is botulism managed?

1. **Supportive care**: This is the initial and most important step in management (most patients require intubation and mechanical ventilation).
2. **Laboratory testing**: While supportive care is being initiated, obtain serum assay for the *C. botulinum* toxin. If food-borne botulism is suspected, analyze stool and recently consumed food for the toxin.
3. **Equine serum botulism antitoxin**: This medication is available from public health departments.

Antibiotics are not beneficial because symptoms are caused by the antitoxin. Also, antibiotics can increase toxin absorption in food-borne botulism.

Alternative 12.11.2

A 42-year-old woman presents with a 6-month history of gradually progressing weakness. She has difficulty climbing stairs and reaching for objects on a higher shelf. She needs to hold on to the side of her chair to stand from a sitting position (Gower's sign). There is a scaly erythematous plaque over the dorsal aspect of her left and right MCPs (Gottron's sign) and a reddish purple rash over both eyelids (heliotrope rash). There is 4/5 strength in both shoulders and quadriceps.

What is the most likely diagnosis?

Difficulty climbing stairs, reaching for overhead objects, and Gower's sign are suggestive of proximal muscle weakness. Gradually progressive proximal muscle weakness should raise suspicion for an inflammatory myopathy. The most likely diagnosis in this woman with Gottron's and heliotrope rash is dermatomyositis.

> Other skin findings of diabetes mellitus are:
> **Shawl sign**: erythematous patch over neck, chest, and shoulder.
> **Nailbed findings**: erythema and telangiectasias.
> **Mechanic's hands**: palms are rough and cracked.

How can you confirm the diagnosis?

Confirm the diagnosis with a combination of laboratory, EMG (electromyelography) and/or biopsy findings.

> **Laboratory findings**: increased muscle enzymes (serum creatine kinase, LDH, AST, ALT, and aldolase) and positive antibodies (antisynthetase, anti-M2, anti-signal recognition particles).

What are important complications of dermatomyositis?

Dermatomyositis increases the risk of interstitial lung disease and all types of cancers. Screen all dermatomyositis patients for cancer with laboratory tests (CBC, serum chemistry, LFTs, urinalysis, CA-125, and ESR), FOBT, and imaging tests (chest CT, mammography, and pelvic ultrasound).

How is dermatomyositis treated?

First-line therapy is glucocorticoids and azathioprine or MTX.

What diagnosis is likely if a patient with chronic, progressive, symmetric proximal muscle weakness with elevated muscle enzymes has no skin rash?

The absence of any rash suggests polymyositis rather than dermatomyositis. Diagnostic evaluation and treatment are similar to dermatomyositis. Polymyositis carries a lower cancer risk than dermatomyositis.

> **Inclusion body myositis**: This rare inflammatory myopathy has symptoms similar to polymyositis. Muscle biopsy showing filamentous inclusions differentiates this disorder from polymyositis. Treatment is glucocorticoids.

> **Critical illness myopathy**: Symmetric proximal muscle weakness, usually after a long course of steroids in the ICU, can delay liberation from the ventilator. There is no specific treatment except to correct the underlying cause.

> The most common cause of myopathy in primary care is a negative reaction to medications such as steroids and statins.

Alternative 12.11.3

A 29-year-old woman presents with episodes of fatigue and weakness. She has had the episodes for almost 1 year now. The episodes initially lasted a few days followed by weeks of symptom-free intervals, but now they last for weeks with symptom-free intervals lasting only a few days. During the episodes, she often experiences blurry vision. She gets tired chewing and finds it difficult to swallow food during the episodes. She is currently asymptomatic.

What diagnosis should you suspect?

Chronic episodes of muscle weakness should raise suspicion for myasthenia gravis (MG). The triad of episodic weakness in the skeletal, ocular, and bulbar muscles is characteristic of generalized MG. Skeletal muscle weakness is usually diffuse and generalized. Ocular weakness (eyelids and extraocular muscles) leads to blurry vision and binocular diplopia. Bulbar weakness (mouth and throat) leads to dysphagia and dysarthria. MG results from autoantibodies against the acetylcholine receptor.

> **Ocular MG**: weakness limited to eyelid and extraocular muscles.

How can you confirm the diagnosis?

Figure 12-12 outlines the diagnostic approach to MG. The initial test in this patient with ocular symptoms is the Tensilon test plus acetylcholinesterase antibodies (AChE Ab).

> **Tensilon test**: Tensilon (edrophonium) is an AChE inhibitor; IV Tensilon causes rapid but transient (seconds to minutes) improvement in weakness.

Tensilon test and AChE Abs are positive.

How is MG treated?

First-line treatment is pyridostigmine (AChE inhibitor). If symptoms persist, add an immunomodulator to the regimen (e.g., corticosteroids, azathioprine, and cyclosporine).

> **Thymus**: This organ may be involved in MG pathogenesis, because thymoma is very common in MG. Always obtain chest CT after MG diagnosis. Thymectomy is indicated if patient has a thymoma or is young (prophylactic surgery may improve long-term prognosis).

Over the next 10 years, this patient's symptoms are reasonably controlled with pyridostigmine and azathioprine. At the age of 40, she is diagnosed with essential hypertension. Her physician initially starts her on hydrochlorothiazide. Three months later, he adds metoprolol to the regimen. One week after starting therapy, she presents to the emergency department with increasing weakness and dyspnea. On evaluation, she has 3/5 strength and is diaphoretic and uncomfortable. Pulse is 120 bpm, and respirations are 28/min and shallow. Oxygen saturation is 88%.

What is the most likely cause of her symptoms?

Acute onset of profound weakness of the skeletal and respiratory muscles should raise suspicion for myasthenic crisis. Myasthenic crisis is a life-threatening complication (almost 5% risk of mortality). Common precipitants are infection, surgery, and drugs (most likely precipitant in this patient is the β-blocker). Treatment involves the following:

1. Supportive care: Measure forced vital capacity; consider elective intubation if forced vital capacity is <15 ml/kg.
2. Specific therapy: Plasmapheresis (first line) or IVIG.

> **Common drugs associated with myasthenic-crisis**: antibiotics (especially aminoglycosides), antihypertensives (calcium channel blockers, β-blockers), anticholinergics, and antipsychotics.

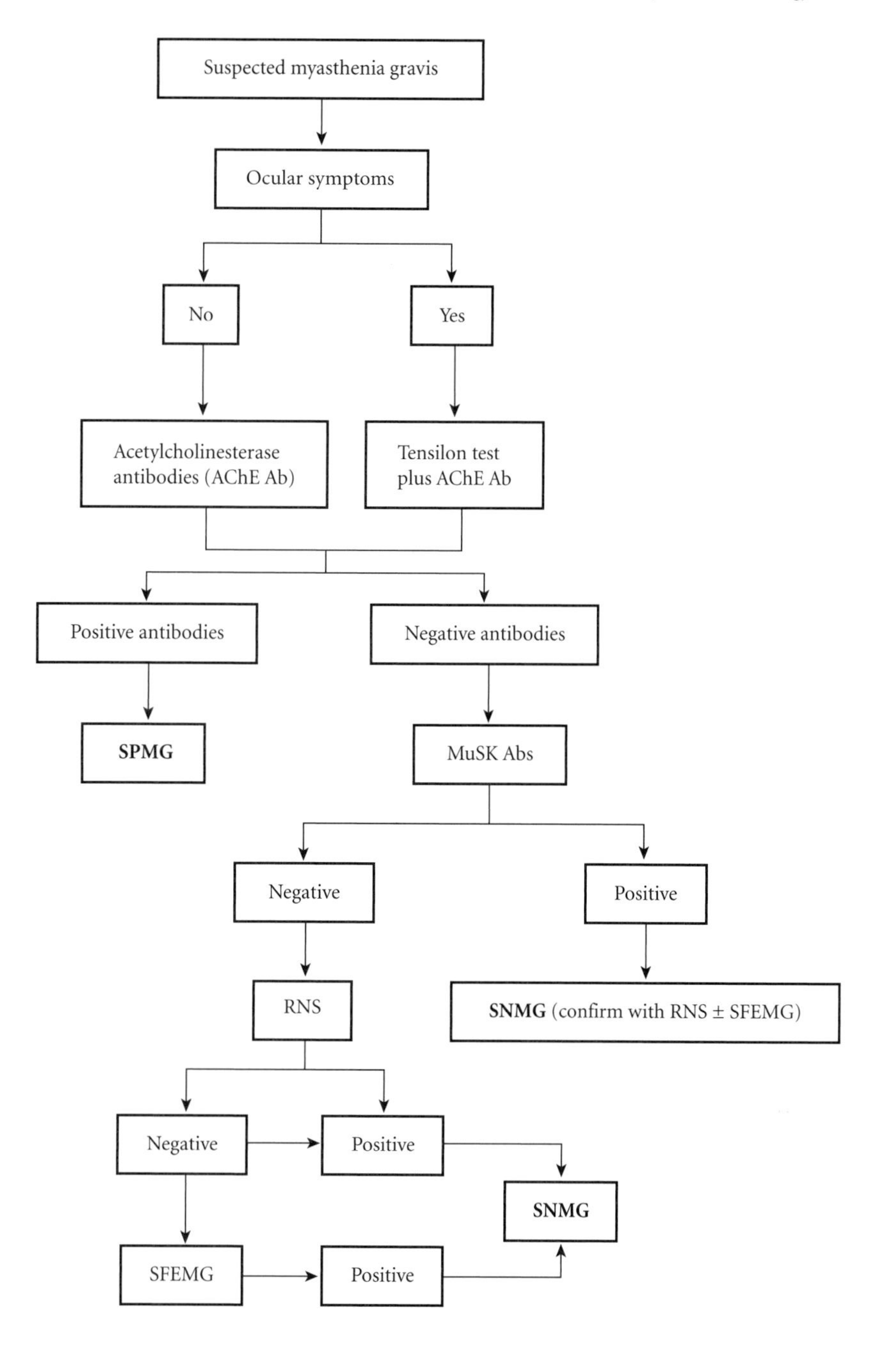

RNS = repetitive nerve stimulation; SFEMG = single fiber electromyelography
SPMG = seropositive myasthenia gravis; SNMG = seronegative myasthenia gravis

FIGURE 12–12 Diagnostic approach to myasthenia gravis.

Case 12.11.4

A 60-year-old man presents with a 4-month history of progressively worsening symmetric proximal muscle weakness. He also reports a troublesome blood-tinged cough. Review of systems is positive for a 6-month history of worsening cough, constipation, and dry mouth. He has a 30-pack/year smoking history. There are decreased breath sounds at the right lower base. Reflexes are decreased and strength is 4/5 at the proximal muscles. Chest CT shows a new irregular mass (4 cm in diameter).

What diagnosis should you suspect?

New onset of hemoptysis and an irregular mass in a long-time smoker is highly suspicious for lung cancer. A common paraneoplastic syndrome associated with small cell lung cancer is Lambert-Eaton myasthenic syndrome (LEMS). Like MG, the defect is at the neuromuscular junction, although the cause is decreased acetylcholine release rather than acetylcholine receptor destruction. Unlike MG, clinical presentation is similar to an inflammatory myopathy. Also unlike MG, symptoms improve with repetitive motion. Autonomic symptoms are common, whereas ocular and bulbar symptoms are less frequent.

> **Autonomic symptoms**: Examples are dry mouth, orthostatic hypotension, erectile dysfunction, constipation, urinary retention, and bowel or bladder incontinence.

How can you confirm and treat LEMS?

Voltage-gated calcium channel antibodies (VGCC Abs) and nerve conduction studies (RNS and EMG) confirm the diagnosis. Treating the underlying malignancy is the most important step in management.

> In rare cases, no underling malignancy is identified. In this case, first-line therapy of LEMS is pyridostigmine. Second-line therapy is diaminopyridine.

Case 12.11.5

A 40-year-old baseball player presents with a 6-month history of progressive weakness. He finds it difficult to grip his bat with his left hand. He also finds it difficult to raise his bat with his shoulder. He has recently begun to notice that his arm and hand muscles often twitch involuntarily (fasciculations). On physical exam, there is 4/5 strength in the left hand and right shoulder. There is marked atrophy in these regions. Reflexes are brisk, and there is increased tone. MRI of the brain and spinal cord is unremarkable.

What diagnosis should you suspect?

Suspect amyotrophic lateral sclerosis (ALS) in patients with gradually progressive asymmetric weakness and a combination of upper motor neuron signs (increased tone and reflexes) and lower motor neuron signs (atrophy and fasciculations). Symptoms initially begin in the upper or lower extremities in the majority of patients. Workup of this uncommon condition includes RNS and EMG as well as tests to rule out other conditions (MRI of the brain and spinal cord, LP, etc.). ALS is a uniformly fatal condition (average lifespan is 3 to 5 years after diagnosis). Riluzole is the only drug shown to improve mortality (exact mechanism unclear).

> **Progressive bulbar palsy**: This sub-type of ALS initially presents with isolated mouth and throat muscle weakness. Most patients eventually develop other features of ALS.

Case 12.11.6

A 32-year-old woman presents to the clinic for evaluation of muscle weakness and speech difficulties. Symptoms began 36 hours ago. She has had two similar episodes over the last 3 years. On physical exam, there is a blind spot in the center of her visual field, hyperreflexia, and spasticity. Brain MRI is obtained (Fig. 12-13).

What is the most likely diagnosis?

The most likely diagnosis is multiple sclerosis (MS). MS results from autoimmune myelin destruction, which leads to white matter destruction (Fig. 12-13). This disease presents with highly variable neurological symptoms. Common clinical features are:

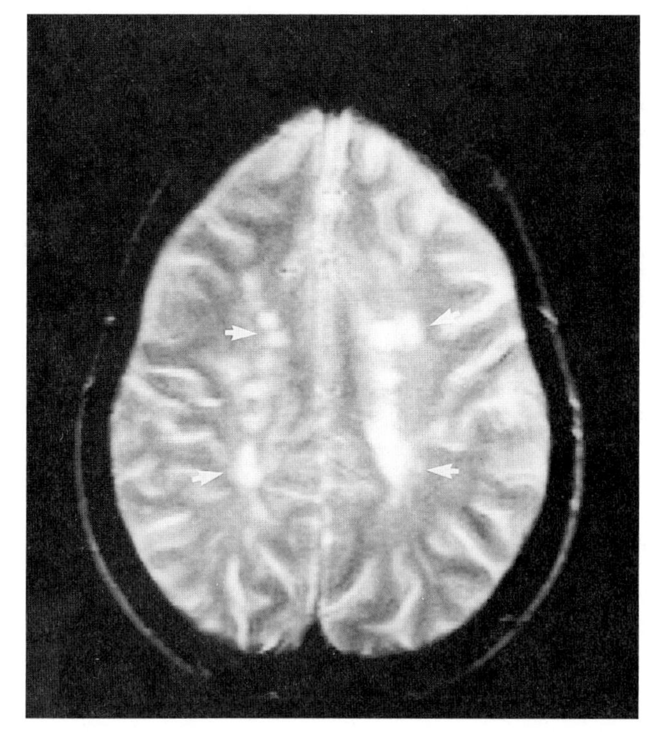

FIGURE 12–13 Multiple sclerosis. Contiguous T2-weighted MRI images show areas of ventricular plaques of high signals (arrows). From Daffner RH. *Clinical Radiology: The Essentials, 3rd ed.* Lippincott Williams & Wilkins, 2007.

1. Sensory symptoms: Numbness, tingling, and paresthesia are common initial symptoms. Many patients experience painful syndromes like trigeminal neuralgia or Lhermitte's phenomenon (neck flexion leads to shock-like sensation in spine and lower extremities).
2. Motor symptoms: Weakness with upper motor neuron signs (spasticity, increased deep tendon reflexes).
3. Ocular symptoms:
   - Marcus Gunn pupil: This is a unilateral lesion in the afferent visual pathway anterior to the optic chiasm. When light is shined in the ipsilateral pupil (damaged), both eyes constrict (normal). When light is shined in the contralateral pupil (normal), both eyes dilate (abnormal).
   - Internuclear ophthalmoplegia: Medial longitudinal fasciculus lesion leads to ipsilateral CN3 palsy and contralateral CN 6 palsy.
   - Pendular nystagmus.
   - Central scotoma.
4. Autonomic symptoms.
5. Other neurological symptoms include cerebellar symptoms (ataxia, intention tremor, dysarthria), nystagmus, and personality changes (due to frontal lobe lesions).

MS epidemiology: Affects more women than men; greater incidence at higher latitudes than at the equator.

What additional tests are needed to confirm the diagnosis?

No additional tests are needed in this patient with two or more attacks and two or more lesions on MRI. Helpful tests in patients with more than two lesions on MRI and/or more than two clinical attacks are LP (90% of patients have increased oligoclonal IgG bands on CSF analysis) and nerve conduction studies (demyelinated areas have slow evoked potentials).

The patient asks about her overall prognosis.

What should you tell her?

There are four general patterns of MS:

1. **Relapsing remitting (RR)**: Symptomatic episodes are interspersed with asymptomatic periods with no symptoms except possible residual defects from prior episode; 85% to 90% of patients have a RR pattern.
2. **Primary progressive (PP)**: Symptoms progressively worsen. Although patients may occasionally experience minor symptom improvement, there are no asymptomatic periods. PP disease has a greater likelihood of long-term disability than RR disease; 10% of patients have a primary progressive pattern.
3. **Secondary progressive (SP)**: RR MS progressing to progressive MS. Most patients with RR disease progress to SP disease eventually.
4. **Progressive relapsing (PR)**: Episodes of acute worsening are interspersed with progressively worsening disease (i.e., no asymptomatic episodes). PR disease carries the greatest potential for long-term disability.

How is MS treated?

1. **Relapsing remitting disease**: Treat acute attacks with IV corticosteroids. After the acute episode, treat with β-interferon or glatiramer acetate.
2. **Progressive disease**: The efficacy of treatment options is questionable. Options are monthly IV corticosteroid pulses and/or IV cyclophosphamide or oral MTX.

What are other causes of CNS demyelination in adults?

1. PML and HIV encephalitis: Suspect in HIV-positive patients.
2. Radiation and chemotherapy: Suspect if there is a history of cancer.
3. Migraines: Suspect if there is a history of typical migraine headaches.
4. Acute disseminated encephalomyelitis: Caused by autoimmune destruction after a viral infection, this condition presents with a single episode of severe neurological deficits (may require ICU admission). Prognosis is excellent with supportive care.

chapter 13

Dermatology

CASE 13–1 FACIAL PAPULES AND PUSTULES

An 18-year-old woman presents with multiple papules and pustules on her face, back, and upper arms (Fig. 13-1).

What is the diagnosis?

The presence of closed comedones (whiteheads) and open comedones (blackheads) in this patient with multiple red papules and pustules (Tables 13-1, 13-2, and 13-3) is diagnostic of acne vulgaris (in Latin, vulgar = common), referred to in lay terms as pimples. Lesions can occur on the face, neck, back, shoulders, and upper arms. No further tests are necessary.

Older adults: The lower jaw and neck are the most common sites of acne vulgaris.

What causes acne vulgaris?

During puberty, increased sex hormones stimulate sebum (oil) production. When the hyperactive sweat glands are blocked by desquamated keratinocytes (cause is unclear), microcomedones result. The skin bacterium propionibacterium acne grows excessively in these oil-filled comedones, which leads to inflammation of the microcomedones and formation of papules, pustules, and nodules.

How is acne vulgaris treated?

All patients should avoid occlusive clothing and repetitive scrubbing. Also, use water rather than oil-based soaps and oils. Treatment depends on acne severity (Table 13-4).

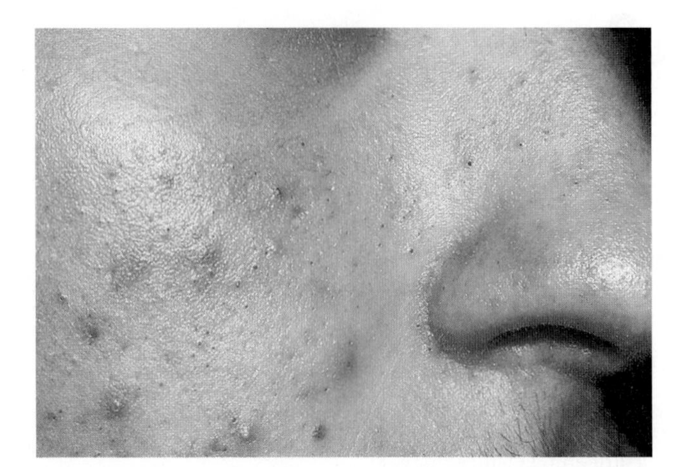

FIGURE 13–1 Acne vulgaris plus whiteheads and blackheads. From Goodheart HP. *Goodheart's Photoguide of Common Skin Disorders*, 2nd ed. Lippincott Williams & Wilkins, 2003.

> Consider oral contraceptive pills (OCPs) prior to oral isotretinoin in women with type 3 acne unresponsive to oral antibiotics (OCPs may reduce acne).

The patient does not respond to oral antibiotics, benzoyl peroxide, or azelaic acid. She decides to initiate therapy with oral isotretinoin.

How does this drug work? What are the most common side effects?

Oral isotretinoin decreases sebum production and reduces inflammation. The most common side effects are:

1. **Dry lips**: This is the most common side effect of oral isotretinoin (occurs in almost 100% of patients).
2. **Photosensitivity**: Minimal sunlight exposure causes sunburn (common side effect).

> **Depression**: Studies have not clearly linked oral isotretinoin to depression.

TABLE 13–1 Primary Skin Lesions

Macule	Flat, nonpalpable skin discoloration <1 cm in diameter
Papule	Elevated palpable skin discoloration <1 cm in diameter without any fluid
Patch	Flat, nonpalpable skin discoloration >1 cm in diameter
Plaque	Broad, elevated palpable lesion >1 cm in diameter without any fluid
Nodule	Dome-shaped elevated palpable lesion >1 or 2 cm in diameter without fluid
Tumor	Dome-shaped elevated palpable lesion >2 cm in diameter without fluid
Cyst	Dome-shaped elevated palpable lesion that contains clear fluid
Pustule	Any elevated palpable skin lesion that contains pus
Vesicle	Any elevated palpable skin lesion <1 cm that contains clear fluid
Bulla	Any elevated palpable skin lesion >1 cm that contains clear fluid
Wheal	Raised area of epidermal edema that quickly disappears
Ulcer	Depressed skin lesion with loss of epidermis and a portion of the dermis
Erosion	Depressed skin lesion with loss of epidermis but not dermis
Fissure	Linear cracks in skin
Burrow	Irregular line caused by scabies mite burrowing into skin
Atrophy	Loss of dermis ± subcutaneous fat but intact epidermis

TABLE 13–2 Secondary Skin Lesions

Scar	Fibrous tissue that replaces normal skin after injury
Erythema	Abnormally red skin
Hyperpigmentation	Area of skin that skin that is darker than surrounding skin
Hypopigmentation	Area of skin that is lighter than surrounding skin
Hyperkeratosis	Thickening of the stratum corneum
Crust	Dried plasma or exudates covering skin
Scale	Flakes covering skin due to shedding of stratum corneum
Lichenification	Plaques with exaggerated skin lines caused by excessive scratching
Excoriation	Scratch or abrasion in the skin due to excessive scratching
Exudate	Clear, cloudy, or purulent fluid surrounding area of inflammation

What laboratory testing is necessary before initiating oral isotretinoin?

1. β-hCG: Oral isotretinoin is teratogenic, so rule out pregnancy in all women of childbearing age before starting therapy. Women should also agree to OCPs for the duration of therapy.
2. Liver function tests, complete blood count, and fasting lipid profile: Obtain baseline values before starting therapy and check at regular intervals during therapy. These labs are obtained because oral isotretinoin can cause hepatitis, neutropenia, and hyperlipidemia.

Alternative 13.1.1

A 50-year-old white woman presents with episodes of facial rash and flushing. Alcohol worsens her symptoms. Figure 13-2 is a picture of the patient's rash.

What is the most likely diagnosis?

The patient has acne rosacea, which presets with papules, pustules, and telangiectasias on her cheeks, nose, and forehead on an erythematous base (Table 13-2). Unlike acne vulgaris, rosacea is most common in older patients (classically white women) and comedones are absent. Although the exact cause is unclear, the Demodex mite may play a role in pathogenesis. Alcohol, stress, and irritants often worsen symptoms.

TABLE 13–3 Skin Lesion Patterns and Configurations

Annular	Skin lesions are circular
Linear	Skin lesions along a line
Serpiginous	Skin lesions in a wavy pattern
Clustered	Skin lesions that are grouped together
Confluent	Clustered skin lesions that join with each other
Targetoid	Skin lesions in a bulls-eye shape
Dermatomal	Skin lesions distributed along a particular dermatome
Follicular	Skin lesions that involve hair follicles
Guttate	Skin lesions that appear as drops on the skin (in Latin, "gutta" = drop)
Koebner phenomenon	Skin lesions that appear at the site of an injury
Multiform	Skin lesions of different shapes and sizes
Reticular	Skin lesions in a net-like pattern
Scarlatiniform	Diffuse erythematous maculopapular rash
Morbilliform	Diffuse erythematous macules that may appear confluent
Satellite lesions	Erythematous macules surrounding main lesion

TABLE 13–4 Treatment of Acne Vulgaris

Type	Description	Medical Therapy
Type 1	Comedones and few facial papules and pustules	Topical retinoid ± benzoyl peroxide, azelaic acid, or salicylic acid. If there is no response after 3 months, treat as type 2 acne.
Type 2	More facial comedones, papules, and pustules but minimal scarring	Topical retinoid, benzoyl peroxide, azelaic acid PLUS a topical antibiotic (clindamycin, erythromycin, or metronidazole). If there is no response after 3 months, treat as type 3 acne.
Type 3	Many comedones, papules, and pustules on face, back, and shoulders with moderate scarring	Topical retinoid, benzoyl peroxide, or azelaic acid PLUS an oral antibiotic (first-line agent is tetracycline; other choices include minocycline, doxycycline, erythromycin, or TMP-SMX). If there is no response after 3 to 6 months, treat as type 4 acne.
Type 4	Many large cysts on face, back, and shoulders with severe scarring	Oral isotretinoin (accutane)

Abbreviation: TMP-SMX, trimethoprim-sulfamethoxazole.

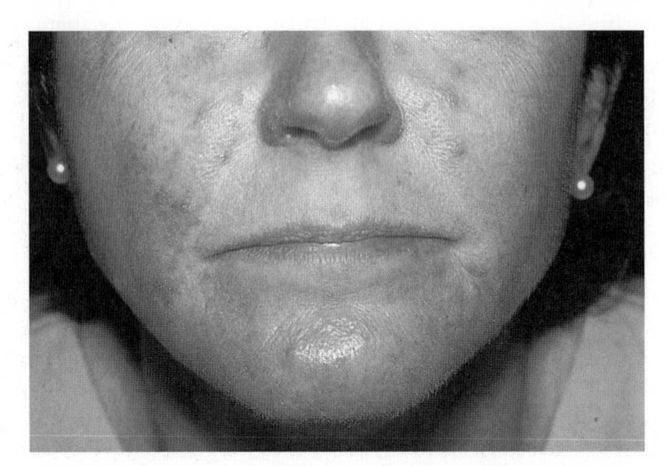

FIGURE 13–2 Rosacea. From Goodheart HP. *Goodheart's Photoguide of Common Skin Disorders*, 2nd ed. Lippincott Williams & Wilkins, 2003.

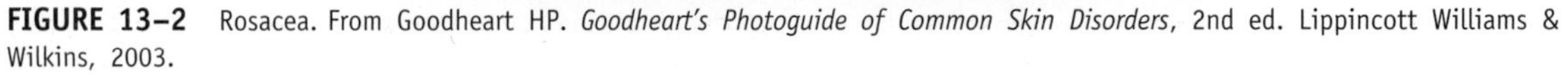

Rhinophyma: Bulbous erythematous nose enlargement can occur in rosacea patients.

How is rosacea treated?

First-line therapy is conservative measures (sunscreen, water-based soaps, and alcohol avoidance) and/or topical antibiotics (metronidazole, clindamycin, or erythromycin). If symptoms persist, consider oral antibiotics (e.g., tetracycline). Oral isotretinoin is an option for refractory acne rosacea.

CASE 13–2 FOLLICULAR LESIONS

A 58-year-old man presents with papules and pustules in the area of his moustache. The lesions are surrounded by erythema, and many of the lesions are pierced by the moustache hair.

What is the most likely diagnosis?

Papules and pustules pierced by hair suggest the patient has folliculitis (superficial infection of hair follicles). Causes include infection (bacterial, viral, or fungal), irritation (clothes rubbing against skin, sweating while exercising), and drugs (steroids).

> ***Staphylococcus aureus***: This is the bacteria most commonly associated with folliculitis.
> **Pseudomonas**: Suspect this organism if folliculitis occurs hours to days after being in a hot tub.

How is folliculitis managed?

1. Warm saline compress: Vasodilation promotes infection clearance.
2. Wash affected area thoroughly with soap and water.
3. Topical antibiotics.

> **Mupirocin ointment**: Consider this treatment for prevention of future episodes in patients with recurrent folliculitis (nasal application reduces carriage of *S. aureus*).

Alternative 13.2.1

A 30-year-old man presents with an underarm rash. The symptoms began with pustules on his axilla that coalesced to form a large painful pustule. Vital signs are normal.

What is the most likely diagnosis?

The patient likely had furuncles (deeper infection of the hair follicles) that coalesced to form a carbuncle. These lesions are typically caused by staphylococcus aureus. Treatment is incision and drainage of the lesion. Consider oral antibiotics (dicloxacillin) for patients with fever or other systemic findings.

Alternative 13.2.2

A 22-year-old man presents with a 7-year history of recurrent axillary lesions. The lesions have been diagnosed as furuncles in the past. On exam, there is a there is a solitary, deep, round, and painful lesion without central necrosis. In addition, there is axillary scarring, pitting, and induration.

What is the most likely diagnosis?

The most likely diagnosis is hydradenitis suppurativa, which is often misdiagnosed as furuncles. Hidradenitis suppurativa occurs in intertriginous areas (most commonly the axilla) and often begins during puberty. The pathophysiology most likely involves occlusion of hair follicles and overgrowth of Pseudomonas in the follicles. Key differences between hydradenitis suppurativa and folliculitis are:

1. Shape: Furuncle shape is pointed, whereas hydradenitis is round.
2. Central necrosis: Seen in furuncles but not hydradenitis suppurative.
3. Scarring, pitting, and induration: Occurs in hydradenitis as a result of recurrent painful episodes, but is uncommon with furuncles.

How is hydradenitis suppurativa treated?

1. Stage 1 disease (single abscess without scarring): First-line therapy is topical steroids and topical antibiotics (e.g., clindamycin and triamcinolone). Consider oral antibiotics (e.g., clindamycin or tetracycline) if lesions persist.
2. Stage 2 disease (recurrent abscesses with sinus tract or scarring): Administer topical steroids and oral antibiotics; unroof sinus tracts.
3. Stage 3 disease (diffuse disease with multiple sinus tracts and scarring): Treat with oral antibiotics, topical steroids, and excisional surgery.

> Consider zinc and spironolactone in all three stages.

CASE 13–3 PAPULES, NODULES, OR PLAQUES ON SUN-EXPOSED AREAS

A 70-year-old man presents with erythematous macules on his face. The tiny macules feel rough to the touch (like sandpaper). The lesions are painless and have developed over the past several months.

What is the most likely diagnosis?

A plaque of hyperkeratosis with surrounding erythema on a sun-exposed area is most likely an actinic keratosis (AK). Removal is necessary because AK has a high risk of progressing to cutaneous squamous cell carcinoma (SCC). Remove these few small lesions with cryotherapy (with liquid nitrogen). Consider chemotherapy with 5-FU or imiquimod for multiple AKs.

> **SCC**: Perform excisional biopsy of any large AK to rule out SCC. Treatment of SCC or large AKs is surgical removal.

> **Cutaneous horn**: This horn-shaped hyperkeratosis is benign but requires excisional biopsy to rule out SCC.

Alternative 13.3.1

A 70-year-old man presents with the facial lesion depicted in Figure 13-4. The lesion is painless and developed over the last 2 weeks.

What is the most likely diagnosis?

The most likely lesion is a keratoacanthoma. The appearance is a rapidly growing nodule with a central keratinaceous plug on a sun-exposed area. Most lesions spontaneously regress within months. Distinguishing keratoacanthoma from SCC is often challenging, so excision is usually necessary.

Alternative 13.3.2

A 70-year-old man presents with the lesion in Figure 13-5.

What is the likely diagnosis?

A pearly papule with telangiectasias is characteristic of basal cell carcinoma (BCC). The next step is to confirm the diagnosis with biopsy. Treatment is surgical excision. Although BCC has a very low risk of metastasis, local recurrence is common. Follow up every 6 months after removal to detect new lesions or recurrences.

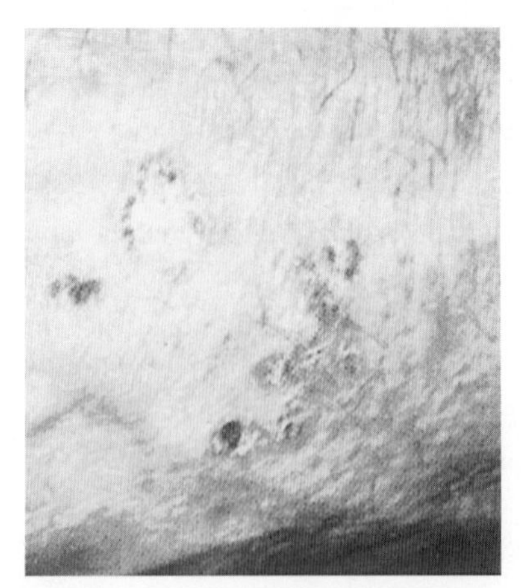

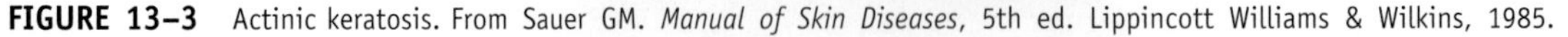

FIGURE 13–3 Actinic keratosis. From Sauer GM. *Manual of Skin Diseases,* 5th ed. Lippincott Williams & Wilkins, 1985.

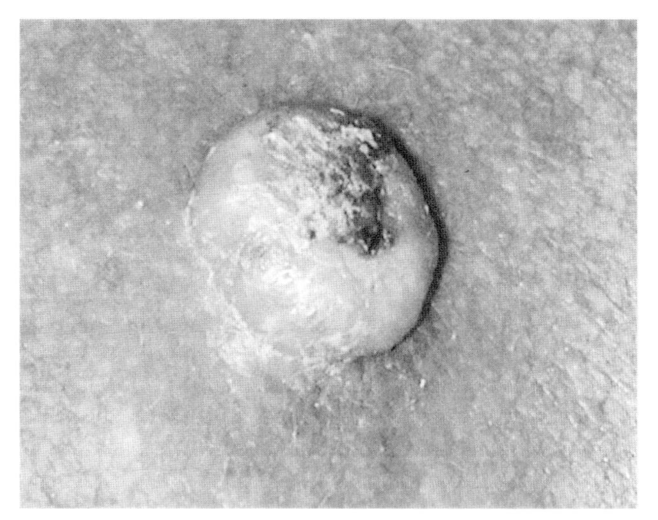

FIGURE 13–4 Keratoacanthoma. From Campen R. *Blueprints Dermatology*. Lippincott Williams & Wilkins, 2004.

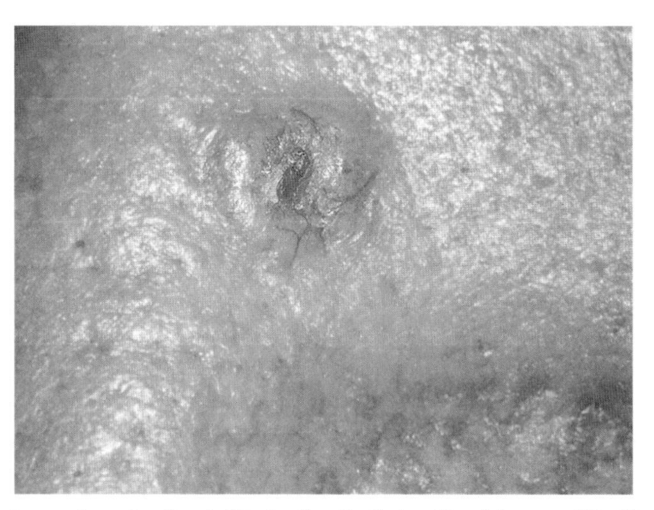

FIGURE 13–5 Basal cell carcinoma. From Goodheart HP. *Goodheart's Photoguide of Common Skin Disorders*, 2nd ed. Lippincott Williams & Wilkins, 2003.

> **MOHS surgery**: Step-wise tumor excision is indicated to remove SCC or BCC that is large or recurrent, or minimal cosmetic disfigurement desired (e.g., lip or eyelid lesion).

CASE 13–4 HYPERPIGMENTED PLAQUES

Routine physical examination of a 50-year-old white woman detects a 2-cm hyperpigmented patch on her back. Figure 13-6 is a picture of the lesion.

What is the most likely diagnosis?

Suspect melanoma when a hyperpigmented lesion has the following characteristics (mnemonic: "***ABCDE***"): **A**symmetry, **B**order irregularity, **C**olor variation, **D**iameter >6 mm, and **E**nlargement. The next step in management is full-thickness excisional biopsy.

> **Metastatic melanoma**: The most common sites of distant spread are lymph nodes, lungs, and liver. Obtain sentinel node biopsy if depth of invasion >1 mm. Obtain chest CT, lactate dehydrogenase, and liver function tests if melanoma invades the dermis.

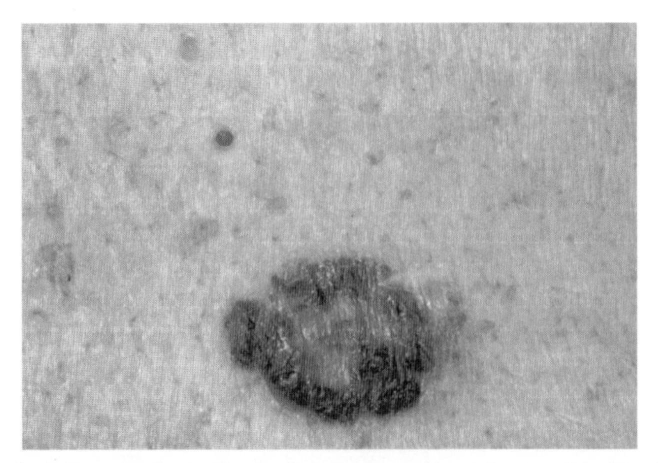

FIGURE 13–6 Melanoma on back. From Goodheart HP. *Goodheart's Photoguide of Common Skin Disorders*, 2nd ed. Lippincott Williams & Wilkins, 2003.

What is the most likely subtype in this patient?

Radially growing melanoma on an area of skin not exposed to the sun in a white woman usually represents superficially spreading melanoma (Table 13-5). Superficially spreading melanomas can occur anywhere on the body, but the back is the most frequent location.

Biopsy detects melanoma. There are no signs of metastasis.

How is melanoma treated?

First-line therapy for nonmetastatic disease is full-thickness excision. The extent of excision depends on the depth (thickness) of invasion:

1. Thickness >0.5 mm: 0.5 cm margin of normal skin
2. Thickness 0.5 to 1.9 mm: 1 cm margin of normal skin
3. Thickness ≥2 mm: 2 to 3 cm margin of normal skin

Metastatic disease: Chemotherapy and radiation may prolong survival.

What strategies are recommended to prevent melanoma, SCC, and BCC?

Sunlight exposure is the major preventable risk factor for melanoma, SCC, and BCC. Primary prevention strategies are:

1. Wear protective clothing and sunglasses.
2. Minimize sunlight exposure during peak hours of type B ultraviolet light (10 am to 4 pm).

TABLE 13–5 Melanoma Subtypes

Type	% of Cases	Description	Race	Prognosis
Superficial	70%	Enlarges radially for 1–5 years, then begins to grow vertically; occurs anywhere on body	White	Good if detected before vertical growth occurs
Nodular	20%	Presents as a vertically growing hyperpigmented nodule; occurs anywhere on body	White	Poor
Acral lentiginous	5%	Hyperpigmented patches on palms, soles, and nailbed	Dark-skinned	Poor
Lentigo maligna melanoma	5%	Presents as a single, slowly enlarging, hyperpigmented lesion on sun-exposed areas	White	Good if detected before vertical growth occurs

3. Use sunscreen with sun protection factor ≥15.
4. Avoid tanning beds.

What are the nonpreventable risk factors for melanoma?

1. Family history.
2. Race: Fair skin and blue eyes are a risk factor for melanoma, SCC and BCC.
3. Dysplastic nevi: Appearance is similar to melanoma. Monitor closely for increases in ABCDE because these lesions have increased risk of progressing to melanoma.

> **Dysplastic nevus syndrome**: multiple dysplastic nevi. Patients with this syndrome and a family history of melanoma have a nearly 100% risk of melanoma.

Alternative 13.4.1

A 55-year-old man presents with small brown macules on the backs of both hands. The lesions developed over a period of several months and cause no symptoms. There is no asymmetry, irregular borders, color variation, or elevation.

What is the most likely diagnosis?

The most likely diagnosis is solar lentigo ("sun spots"). These benign lesions occur as a result of exposure of melanocytes in older individuals to the sun, particularly on the backs of the hands. No specific therapy is necessary, except to biopsy any lesion that develops ABCDE (to rule out acral lentiginous melanoma and lentigo maligna melanoma).

Alternative 13.4.2

A 45-year-old man presents with a 1.5-cm hyperpigmented plaque. The lesion is rough and has a "stuck on" appearance. There is no asymmetry. The border is well defined. There is no color variation.

What is the most likely diagnosis?

The classic description of seborrheic keratosis is a rough, hyperpigmented plaque with a "stuck-on" appearance. No treatment is necessary for this benign condition. If the patient wishes to remove the lesion for cosmetic reasons, consider cryotherapy, shaving excision, or curettage.

CASE 13–5 PRURITIC ERYTHEMATOUS LESIONS

An 18-year-old man presents with the intensely pruritic lesions shown in Figure 13-7. He has had episodes with similar lesions since he was a child. Past medical history is significant for asthma.

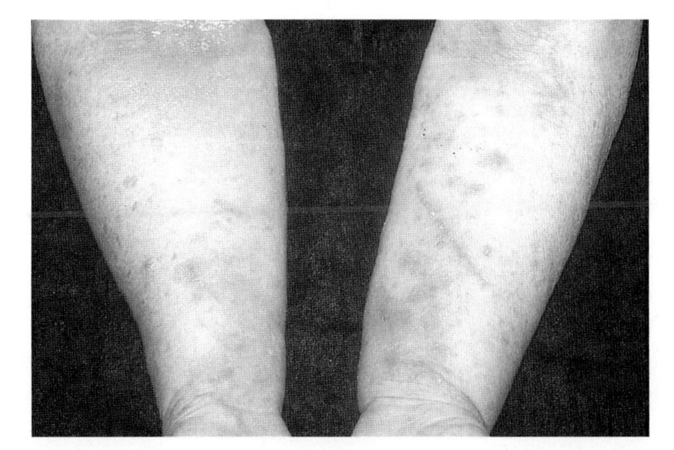

FIGURE 13–7 Eczema. From Goodheart HP. *Goodheart's Photoguide of Common Skin Disorders*, 2nd ed. Lippincott Williams & Wilkins, 2003.

What is the most likely diagnosis?

This patient with pruritic, erythematous papules, plaques, and vesicles has eczematous dermatitis (eczema). Excessive itching can cause the skin to develop scale, excoriations, and lichenification. There are many subtypes of dermatitis. Atopic dermatitis is the most likely diagnosis in this patient with asthma (another atopic condition) and episodic symptoms since childhood. Flexor areas are commonly involved.

> Atopic dermatitis often resolves spontaneously by young adulthood.

How is an acute episode of atopic dermatitis treated?

First-line therapy is topical corticosteroids and antihistamines (to control pruritus). Second-line therapy is topical pimicrolimus or tacrolimus (calcineurin inhibitors). If symptoms are severe and refractory to topical therapies, consider a short course of oral corticosteroids.

What measures should patients with atopic dermatitis adopt to prevent recurrent flares?

1. Avoid triggers such as heat, stress, sweat, and low humidity.
2. Hydrate skin with creams with low water content (e.g., petroleum jelly).

> **Nummular dermatitis**: Suspect this condition if the patient has coin-shaped eczema (in Latin, numma = coin). Most common location is extremities. Management is similar to atopic dermatitis.

Alternative 13.5.1

A 35-year-old woman presents with a pruritic rash on her left arm. The symptoms began after her left arm brushed against a plant while camping. There are erythematous papules, plaques, and vesicles localized to the left arm.

What diagnosis is most likely?

The most likely cause of this dermatitis is contact dermatitis. Causes include:

1. **Irritants**: These are the most common causes of contact dermatitis. Exposure to irritant detergents, alkalis, and solvents are common examples.
2. **Allergens**: Dermatitis is the result of type 4 hypersensitivity reaction (Table 13-6). The most common allergen is poison ivy. Others include nickel, fragrances, and topical antimicrobials (bacitracin and neomycin).
3. **Sun exposure (photosensitivity)**: Suspect if only sun-exposed areas are affected.

How are acute episodes of contact dermatitis treated?

First-line treatment of allergic contact dermatitis is topical corticosteroids. Consider oral steroids for severe cases. Once the acute episode has resolved, the most important component of management is to avoid the offending irritant or allergen.

Alternative 13.5.2

A 35-year-old man presents with a pruritic rash on his knees and elbows (Fig. 13-8). He has experienced similar episodes before.

What is the most likely diagnosis?

The most likely diagnosis is psoriasis. The most common form of psoriasis (plaque psoriasis) causes well-demarcated erythematous plaques with a silvery scale. If the scale is peeled off, minute capillary bleeding occurs (Auspitz sign). Although the extensor surfaces of the knees and elbows are the most frequent sites, any portion of the skin can be affected. Psoriasis lesions commonly occur at sites of skin trauma (Koebner phenomenon).

TABLE 13–6 Hypersensitivity Reactions

Type	Description	Examples
Type 1 (immediate)	Initial exposure sensitizes IgE antibodies; re-exposure causes IgE mediated release of histamines, leukotrienes, and prostaglandin.	Urticaria and the 5 A's (**A**ngioedema, **A**naphylaxis, **A**topic dermatitis, **A**sthma, and **A**llergic rhinitis)
Type 2	IgG or IgM antibodies bind to antigens on cell surface or foreign substances, which activates complement.	Rheumatic fever, AIHA and allergic transfusion reactions, *Pemphigus vulgaris* and *bullous pemphigoid*
Type 3	Antibody-antigen complexes deposit on tissues, which activates complement.	SLE, RA, immune complex glomerulonephritis
Type 4 (delayed)	T cells recognize incompatible antigens on macrophages, which stimulates cytokine release.	Contact dermatitis, transplant rejection, TB symptoms

Abbreviations: AIHA, autoimmune hemolytic anemia; RA, rheumatoid arthritis; SLE, systemic lupus erythematosus; TB, tuberculosis.

> **Other psoriasis subtypes**: pustular psoriasis, guttate psoriasis (strep throat is a common precipitant), nail psoriasis (nailbed discoloration and onycholysis), and psoriatic arthritis.

What causes psoriasis?

Psoriasis is most likely an immune-mediated disease that occurs in genetically predisposed individuals. Patients with psoriasis have accelerated, defective keratinization, which leads to the formation of plaques and scale.

> **Keratinocytes** arise in innermost (basal) layer of epidermis and differentiate as they travel to the outermost layer. Their function is to maintain structural integrity of skin.

How is psoriasis treated?

Initial therapy for localized disease is combination therapy with topical corticosteroids and topical calcipotriene (vitamin D analog that slows keratinization). If symptoms persist, add topical anthralin to the regimen (wood tar derivative). Consider intradermal steroid injections

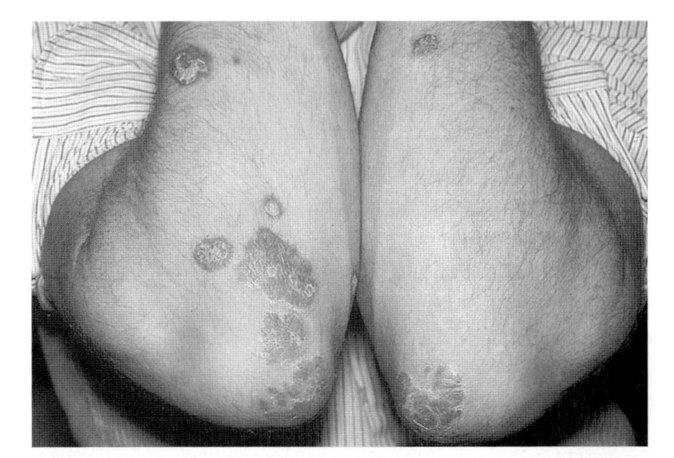

FIGURE 13–8 Psoriasis (on knee or ebow). From Goodheart HP. *Goodheart's Photoguide of Common Skin Disorders*, 2nd ed. Lippincott Williams & Wilkins, 2003.

for lesions that fail to respond to topical therapy. Options for refractory psoriasis are phototherapy and biological agents (methotrexate and cyclosporine).

Coal tar shampoo: helpful adjunctive therapy for scalp psoriasis.

Seborrheic dermatitis: Symmetric plaques with thick scale can occur on nasolabial folds or hairy areas (forehead near hairline, mustache, or beard area). Mild seborrheic dermatitis manifests as dandruff. The yeast *Pityrosporum ovale* may play a role in pathogenesis. This condition is typically treated with selenium sulfide or zinc shampoo.

Alternative 13.5.3

A 22-year-old medical student presents with episodes of pruritic rash. The episodes occur within minutes of exposure to cold water. The rash disappears within minutes. The patient has taken a photograph of the lesions, which appear as pink plaques with central pallor.

What diagnosis should you suspect?

Suspect urticaria when a patient presents with pruritic erythematous plaques with central pallor (wheals) that resolve within minutes. Severe cases may be accompanied by angioedema or anaphylaxis. Unlike contact dermatitis, urticaria appears within minutes to an hour of exposure and resolves within minutes of removing the offending allergen.

Chronic urticaria: urticaria that persists for >6 weeks.

What causes urticaria?

Urticaria results from type 1 hypersensitivity to an allergen (Table 13-6). Common allergens are:

1. Food: Peanuts, milk, and eggs are the most common offenders.
2. Drugs: Nonsteroidal anti-inflammatory drugs (NSAIDS), angiotensin-converting enzyme inhibitors, and antibiotics (β-lactams, cephalosporins, etc.).
3. Environmental exposures: Heat, cold, and water.
4. Other: Parasite infections (less common in the United States), latex, and insect bites.

Non-immune cutaneous drug eruptions: Examples are maculopapular rash (the most common drug-induced skin reaction) and fixed drug eruption (a single red plaque).

How is urticaria treated?

The most important step in management is to avoid exposure to the precipitant (in this case, cold water). Treat acute episodes with antihistamines.

Red man syndrome: Flushing and erythema on face, neck, and torso due to type 1 hypersensitivity is the most common side effect of rapid vancomycin infusion. Treat with drug discontinuation and antihistamines.

How does urticaria differ from angioedema and anaphylaxis?

Patients with angioedema have non-pitting edematous swelling of the subcutaneous tissues, larynx, or abdominal organs. Lesions are typically tender but, unlike urticaria, they are not pruritic. In anaphylaxis, a type 1 hypersensitivity reaction affects multiple organ systems and can progress to shock (Chapter 2: Cardiology).

What diagnosis should you suspect if the patient reports repeated episodes of angioedema lasting >12 hours and no offending allergen is identified?

Suspect C1 inhibitor deficiency if a patient has recurrent and unexplained angioedema lasting >12 hours or recurrent laryngeal edema. This disorder can be inherited or acquired. The next step is to obtain C4, C1q, and C1 inhibitor levels. No treatment is recommended for acute cutaneous attacks. Fresh frozen plasma is recommended for acute attacks of laryngeal edema.

Decreased C4, decreased C1q, and normal C1 inhibitor indicate acquired C1 inhibitor deficiency.
Decreased C4, decreaed C1 inhibitor, and normal C1q indicate hereditary C1 inhibitor deficiency.

Alternative 13.5.4

A 27-year-old man presents with a 5-day history of the pruritic and erythematous truncal lesion in Figure 13-9.

What is the most likely diagnosis?

An erythematous annular plaque with central clearing on the body is characteristic of tinea corporis, also known as ringworm infection (Table 13-7). Lesions result from superficial skin infection by dermatophyte fungi. The three principal types of dermatophytes are Epidermophyton, Trichophyton, and Microsporum.

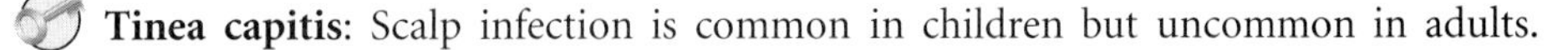

Tinea capitis: Scalp infection is common in children but uncommon in adults.

What is the next step in management?

Try to confirm suspected dermatophyte infections by examining KOH prepared scrapings under the microscope (look for characteristic segmented, branched hyphae). First-line therapy of dermatophyte infection is a topical antifungal (except for tinea capitis or tinea unguium, in which case oral antifungal drugs are preferred).

Tinea incognito: Steroids decrease inflammation, which modifies the appearance.

Alternative 13.5.5

A 37-year-old woman presents with a 4-day history of intensely pruritic erythematous papules on her wrist flexors and elbow extensors. Her children and husband have experienced similar lesions recently.

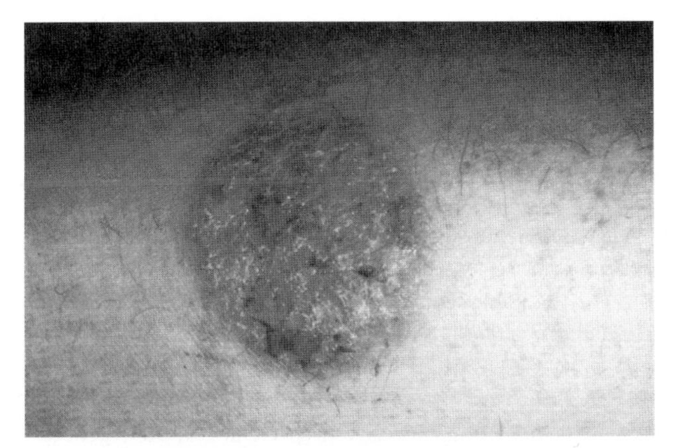

FIGURE 13–9 Tinea corporis. From Campen, Rebecca B. *Blueprints Dermatology*, 1st ed. Lippincott Williams & Wilkins, 2004.

TABLE 13–7 Dermatophyte Infections in Adults

Infection	Description
Tinea faciae	Pruritic erythematous annular plaque with central clearing on face.
Tinea barbae	Erythematous pustules and crust in the beard. Hair is easy to pull out. Lesions are often not very pruritic or painful.
Tinea manus	Erythema, hyperkeratosis, and scale on hands. Patients often have coexisting tinea pedis.
Tinea unguium	Hyperkeratosis and chalky appearing nail bed with or without nailbed separation (onycholysis). Feet are affected more frequently than hands.
Tinea corporis	Pruritic erythematous annular plaque with central clearing on trunk, arms, and legs.
Tinea cruris (jock itch)	Pruritic erythematous patch with partial central clearing on medial thigh near the groin.
Tinea pedis (athlete's foot)	Acute tinea pedis appears as intensely pruritic papules and vesicles on the feet. Chronic tinea pedis appears as pruritic erythema and scale between the digits.

What diagnosis should you suspect?

Suspect scabies when a patient presents with intensely pruritic papules in any of the following regions: wrist flexors or elbow extensors, genitalia, axilla, near nipples, or the periumbilical area (back and head are generally spared). Sometimes, characteristic burrows are also present. Lesions are caused by the highly contagious mite *Sarcoptes scabei* (spread by direct touch and sexual transmission).

> **Dyshidrotic dermatitis**: chronic and recurrent episodes of intensely pruritic vesicles on the palms and soles. First-line therapy is topical corticosteroids.

What is the next step in management?

Pruritic papules in the characteristic distribution are sufficient to establish the diagnosis. Treat with a single application of 5% permethrin cream applied all over the body. An alternative for patients with severe scabies (crusted or refractory lesions) is weekly use of 5% permethrin cream plus oral ivermectin. Also treat close contacts, and wash all clothing and linens to prevent repeat transmission.

> If the diagnosis is not obvious, examine scrapings of lesions for mites, eggs, or feces.

CASE 13–6 ERYTHEMA, WARMTH, AND SWELLING

A 30-year-old man presents with an erythematous patch on his arm. The patch is warm, swollen, and tender. Margins are not very distinct. Vital signs are normal.

What diagnosis should you suspect?

An erythematous patch that is warm, swollen, and tender should raise suspicion for cellulitis (infection of skin and subcutaneous tissues). Although any skin area can be affected, the lower extremity is the most common site. Patients may or may not have systemic signs of infections (fever, chills, etc.). Diagnosis is clinical.

How is cellulitis treated?

Treat cellulitis with a penicillinase-resistant β-lactam or first-generation cephalosporin to cover *Staphylococcus aureus* and *Streptococcus pneumoniae.* A 10- to 14-day course of oral cephalexin is sufficient for this patient with limited lesions and no systemic signs. If the patient is allergic to penicillin, treat with clindamycin instead.

> **Lymphangitis**: Lymph vessel infection appears as painful red streaks below the skin surface. Can occur as a complication of cellulitis.

What are the indications for intravenous antibiotics in the treatment of cellulitis?

Remember indications for intravenous antibiotics with the acronym "***PERMS***" (**P**ersistent symptoms despite oral antibiotics, **E**xtensive lesions, **R**ecurring cellulitis, **M**RSA (methicillin-resistant *S. aureus*) risk factors, or **S**ystemic signs).

> **MRSA risk factors**: multiple hospitalizations, intravenous drug use, or resident at a long-term facility.

What diagnosis should you suspect if the warm erythematous lesion had distinct borders?

Swelling, warmth, and erythema with distinct margins suggest erysipelas (infection of skin but not subcutaneous tissue). Like cellulitis, the most commonly implicated organism is group A Streptococcus. Treatment is intravenous antibiotics (penicillin G or cefazolin).

Alternative 13.6.1

A 34-year-old woman presents with an extremely painful leg rash. The rash began 3 days ago on her toe at the site of a minor cut. It now involves her entire foot and part of her leg. On physical exam, there is a large confluent erythematous patch that is warm to touch. Temperature is 39°C.

What diagnosis should you suspect?

Rapidly expanding cellulitis, severe pain, and systemic signs should raise suspicion for necrotizing fascitis. In otherwise healthy persons, this soft-tissue infection is most commonly caused by group A Streptococcus. Symptoms typically occur at sites of trauma because infection is acquired via a breach in skin integrity. Elevated creatine phosphokinase is the most common laboratory abnormality.

> **Type I necrotizing fascitis**: Suspect this polymicrobial infection if the patient has diabetes mellitus, cervical necrotizing fascitis, or perineal necrotizing fascitis (Fournier's gangrene).

Creatine phosphokinase is elevated.

What is the next step in management?

Necrotizing fascitis can rapidly progress to septic shock (streptococcal toxic shock syndrome). The next step is to perform emergent surgical exploration. Treatment is surgical debridement of all necrotic tissue and intravenous antibiotics.

CASE 13–7 BLISTERING DISORDERS

A 37-year-old man presents with a 3-month history of blisters. The blisters originally developed in his mouth, but he now has generalized lesions. On physical exam, there are numerous flaccid bullae that rupture easily when rubbed (Nikolsky sign). The underlying skin is tender. Vital signs are normal.

What is the most likely diagnosis?

Pemphigus vulgaris is the most likely diagnosis in this patient with flaccid bullae and positive Nikolsky sign. Symptoms typically begin on mucosal surfaces and then progress to the skin over the next few months. The skin under the ruptured bullae is usually very tender. The underlying mechanism is IgG antibodies against the adhesion protein desmoglein. The next step in management is a punch or a shave biopsy to confirm the diagnosis. First-line therapy is systemic corticosteroids.

> Pemphigus vulgaris can occur as a paraneoplastic syndrome.

Alternative 13.7.1

A 58-year-old man with hypertension, diabetes mellitus, and class I congestive heart failure presents with widespread tense bullae. He takes metformin, captopril, and furosemide. Nikolsky sign is negative.

What is the most likely diagnosis?

The most likely diagnosis is bullous pemphigoid. This disorder is less common than pemphigus vulgaris. The typical presentation is widespread tense bullae and negative Nikolsky sign in a middle-aged man. The underlying mechanism is antibodies against basement membrane proteins. If biopsy confirms the diagnosis, discontinue captopril and furosemide (frequently implicated in bullous pemphigoid). If symptoms persist despite drug discontinuation, treat with systemic steroids.

Alternative 13.7.2

A 37-year-old man receives a 10-day course of intramuscular procaine penicillin for primary syphilis. He then starts taking ibuprofen for back pain. Two weeks later, he experiences fever, chills, and skin tenderness. Three days later, he develops confluent erythematous patches and targeted lesions that progress to flaccid vesicles and bullae. At this point he presents to the clinic again. On examination, there is erosion and crust on his lips. Nikolsky sign is positive. Temperature is 39°C.

What is the diagnosis?

The description is characteristic for Steven Johnson syndrome (SJS) and toxic epidermal necrolysis (TEN). Both conditions are most frequently caused by reaction to medications, particularly penicillins, NSAIDS, and anticonvulsants. About 2 to 4 weeks after initiating a drug, patients experience a prodrome of fever, chills, and skin tenderness. Patients then develop confluent erythematous patches with or without target lesions that progress to flaccid bullae and vesicles. In SJS, <10% of the epidermis sloughs off, whereas in TEN >30% of the epidermis sloughs off. Mucous membrane lesions are almost always present.

> **Erythema multiforme (EM)**: painful, pruritic target lesions, macules, and papules of different shapes. Severe EM is called SJS. TEN is the most severe form of SJS.

> Infections (particularly herpes simplex virus) are a less common cause of EM, SJS, and TEN.

How are SJS and TEN treated?

The most important steps in management are to discontinue all offending drugs and correct fluid and electrolyte imbalances. Other measures include:

- Increase room temperature because patients lose heat through denuded skin.
- Topical antibiotics: Consider silver nitrate to prevent secondary skin infections.
- Culture: Routinely monitor skin, blood, and catheter site culture.
- IVIG is often administered to patients with TEN but the benefit is unclear.

> All patients with SJS require admission to the intensive care unit. Consider transfer to a burn unit if patients have TEN or severe SJS.

EM treatment: Discontinue drugs and administer antihistamines and analgesics as needed.

What diagnosis is more likely if the patient were a 23-year-old woman who did not take any medications, her prodromal symptoms began shortly after she used a tampon, and there is diffuse erythema with desquamation along with temperature of 39°C, blood pressure 90/70, and creatinine 2.7 mg/dL?

A more likely cause of desquamation in this patient is staphylococcal toxic shock syndrome. Symptoms result from toxic shock syndrome toxin-1 release by *S. aureus.* Almost 50% of cases result from infected tampons. Diagnosis requires the presence of septic shock and diffuse erythema ± desquamation. Treatment is to correct septic shock.

CASE 13-8 BURNS

A 30-year-old cook at a Chinese restaurant presents with a burn injury that occurred when hot oil from a wok spilled onto his arm. The burn involves his anterior forearm and biceps. The burned area appears moist and erythematous. It is exquisitely painful to touch and blanches with pressure. Vital signs are temperature 37°C, pulse 110 bpm, respirations 25/min, and blood pressure 110/80.

How would you classify this patient's burn on the basis of depth of involvement?

The patient has a superficial, partial thickness burn (Table 13-8).

What percentage of the total body surface area (TBSA) does the burn involve?

The rule of 9s is a quick method to estimate the TBSA involved (Table 13-9). This man with an anterior arm burn has <10% TBSA involvement.

Lund and Browder chart: more accurate method for estimating TBSA.

Should you manage this patient as an outpatient or admit him to the hospital?

Outpatient management is sufficient for this patient with a minor burn (Table 13-10). Moderate burns require hospital admission, and severe burns require admission to an intensive care unit (preferably a burn unit).

How are minor burns managed?

Remember the components of outpatient burn management with the "*6 Cs*":

1. **C**lothes: First remove any burned or hot clothing. If a piece of fabric is adherent, remove it during the cleaning phase.
2. **C**ooling: Next, place cool, saline-soaked gauze over the burned area. Avoid applying ice because this practice increases the risk of hypothermia.

TABLE 13-8 Classification of Burns on the Basis of Depth

Classification	Appearance	Painful	Blanches With Pressure	Pressure Sensation
Superficial	Dry and red	Yes	Yes	Intact
Superficial partial thickness	Moist and red	Yes	Yes	Intact
Deep partial thickness	Blisters with positive Nikolsky sign	No	No	Intact
Deep	Waxy white or leathery grey or black	No	No	Absent

TABLE 13–9 Rule of 9s for Estimating TBSA Involved in Burn

Head and neck (front and back)	9%
Each upper limb (front and back)	9%
Thorax and abdomen (front)	18%
Thorax and abdomen (back)	18%
Each lower limb (front and back)	18%
Perineum	1%
Hand (front and back)	1%

Abbreviation: TBSA, total body surface area.

3. **C**leaning: Clean the wound with soap and water. If the burned area is painful, consider injecting a local anesthetic first. If the wound contains tar or asphalt residue, remove with water and mineral oil. Finally, debride any necrotic tissue or ruptured blisters (do not unroof intact blisters).
4. **C**hemoprophylaxis: Administer a tetanus shot to all patients. Apply topical bacitracin or silver sulfadiazine to prevent infection (unless the burn is superficial). Avoid silver sulfadiazine in face burns and pregnant women.
5. **C**overing: Cover superficial burns with a lubricating cream. Cover other burns with strips of sterile gauze. Change dressings once they become soaked.
6. **C**omfort: Administer acetaminophen, NSAIDS, or opiates depending on pain severity.

What additional measures are necessary if a hemodynamically stable patient with a moderate burn is rescued from a burning building and has dark sputum?

Suspect inhalation injury if a burn patient is exposed to smoke in an enclosed space. The presence of dark sputum or a facial burn increases its likelihood. A high index of suspicion is necessary because symptoms are often absent for 24 to 72 hours after exposure. After rapidly completing the 6 Cs, perform fiberoptic bronchoscopy. If there is any sign of inhalation injury, intubate with the largest endotracheal tube possible and administer PEEP (positive end expiratory pressure). Also, administer maintenance fluids (normal saline or lactated ringers) to patients with moderate or severe burns.

How can you calculate the amount of maintenance fluids to administer?

Calculate maintenance fluid requirements in a burn patient using the Parkland formula:

Total fluids (mL) over 24 hours = 4 × body weight (kg) × % of TBSA burned

Administer half the total in the first 8 hours and the other half over the next 16 hours.

Example: 70 kg man with 20% TBSA burn: 24 hour requirement = 4 × 70 × 20 = 5600 mL. Administer 2800 mL over the first 8 hours (350 mL/hour) and 2800 mL over the next 16 hours (175 mL/hour).

TABLE 13–10 Criteria for Grading of Burn Severity

MINOR	MODERATE	SEVERE
• <10% TBSA • <5% TBSA if elderly • <2% TBSA if deep burn	• 10% to 20% TBSA • 5% to 10% TBSA if elderly • 2% to 5% TBSA if deep burn • Circumferential partial thickness burn • Medical condition that increases risk of infection (e.g., diabetes mellitus)	• >20% TBSA • >10% TBSA if elderly • >5% TBSA if deep burn • Burn affects face (including eyes and ears), genitals, or joints • Inhalation injury • High voltage injury • Associated injuries like fractures

How would initial management differ if the patient rescued from a burning building had difficulty breathing and oxygen saturation was 83% and falling?

Always tend to the ABCs (*A*irway, *B*reathing, *C*irculation) first in hemodynamically unstable patients. The initial step is to attempt endotracheal intubation. If intubation is not successful after the first attempt in a patient with inhalation injury, perform cricothyroidotomy (with conversion to tracheostomy later on). When stabilization measures are completed, attend to the 6 Cs.

CASE 13-9 HYPOPIGMENTATION

A 25-year-old man presents with clearly demarcated patches of hypopigmentation on his hands, eyes, and mouth. He is otherwise asymptomatic. The lesions are not painful or itchy. Sensation is intact.

What is the most likely diagnosis?

The lesions described are characteristic of vitiligo. Lesions most commonly occur on acral areas and around the mouth, eyes, and nose. Vitiligo results from autoimmune destruction of melanocytes. Pathogenesis is unknown, although genetics may play a role.

How is vitiligo treated?

First-line therapy for this patient with limited skin lesions is topical corticosteroids. Second-line therapy is topical calcineurin inhibitors. Surgical skin grafting is an option for refractory limited disease.

What options exist for patients with widespread vitiligo?

Options include oral corticosteroids, ultraviolet therapy, and depigmentation therapy.

> **Depigmentation therapy**: Consider sunscreen if the patient has widespread refractory vitiligo. Sunscreen prevents sunlight-induced skin darkening, which helps make the entire body uniformly hypopigmented.

Alternative 13.9.1

A 38-year-old man presents with a patch of hypopigmentation on his left arm. The lesion has diminished sensation. The patient recently emigrated from Brazil.

What diagnosis should you suspect?

Hypopigmented macules or patches with diminished sensation or anesthesia should raise suspicion for leprosy (Hansen's disease), particularly if the patient recently emigrated from a developing country (most commonly India and Brazil). Disease progression can damage nerves in the vicinity of the lesions leading to claw hand, foot drop, etc.

What causes leprosy?

Leprosy is caused by the acid-fast bacillus *Mycobacterium leprae.* Exposure to respiratory droplets is the most likely route of transmission.

What are the next steps in management?

Establish the diagnosis with a skin smear of the lesion (to detect acid-fast bacilli). Treat patients with five or fewer lesions (paucibacillary leprosy) with a 6-month course of dapsone and rifampin. Treat patients with six or more lesions (multibacillary leprosy) with a 2-year course of dapsone, rifampin, and clofazimine.

CASE 13-10 ULCERS AND ABRASIONS IN A BEDRIDDEN PATIENT

A 75-year-old woman is admitted to the hospital for treatment of pneumonia. Past history is significant for a stroke that has rendered her immobile. On physical examination, there are ulcers and abrasions over the ischial tuberosity, greater trochanter, and sacrum.

TABLE 13–11 Staging of Decubitus Ulcers

Stage	Skin Involvement	Appearance
1	Skin is intact	Erythema that may or may not blanch with pressure
2	Entire epidermis ± partial dermis	Abrasions, blisters, or superficial ulcers
3	Entire epidermis and dermis	Deep crater
4	Entire epidermis and dermis plus fascia (can affect bones, muscles, or tendons)	Deep crater and signs of muscle, bone, or tendon involvement (e.g., sinus tracts, osteomyelitis, and pathological fractures)

What is the most likely cause of these lesions?

Ulcers and abrasions on the skin over bony prominences in an immobile patient are most likely to be decubitus ulcers, also known as pressure ulcers or "bedsores." Ulcers result from ischemia and necrosis due to prolonged pressure from the weight of the patient.

How can you prevent the occurrence of decubitus ulcers?

Institute the following measures in all immobile patients to prevent pressure ulcers:

1. Position: Place patients at a 30° angle when lying on their side and elevate the head of the bed to minimize pressure over bony prominences.
2. Reposition: Move patients to a different position at least every 2 hours.
3. Pillows and mattresses: Place pillows between the ankles and knees. Place pillows under the legs (to raise heels). Consider specialized mattresses (e.g., air, foam, water, etc.) that reduce pressure over bony prominences.
4. Nutrition: Correct any deficiencies, if present.

How are decubitus ulcers treated?

Treatment varies depending on ulcer severity (Table 13-11):

1. Stage 1: Intensify preventive measures described earlier.
2. Stage 2: In addition to preventive measures, use occlusive or semipermeable dressings.
3. Stages 3 and 4: In addition to preventive measures, perform debridement of necrotic tissue. Options include mechanical debridement (with wet to dry dressings), surgical debridement (with scissors and scalpel), enzymatic debridement (e.g., topical collagenase), or autolytic debridement (with occlusive dressing).

The patient's stage 2 ulcers resolve with preventive measures and occlusive dressing. She returns 6 months later with increased pain in the ischial tuberosity. There are deep craters with a foul smell and a purulent discharge.

How should you treat this patient?

The patient most likely has an infected stage 3 decubitus ulcer. Treatment is surgical debridement and topical antibiotics (silver sulfadiazine). If the infection fails to resolve or if the patient develops signs of osteomyelitis, cellulitis, or septic shock, obtain deep tissue cultures and treat with systemic antibiotics.

CASE 13–11 MISCELLANEOUS SKIN LESIONS

A 32-year-old man presents with pain and swelling at the intergluteal cleft. On physical exam, there is a red patch over the coccyx.

What is the most likely diagnosis?

The most likely diagnosis is an infected pilonidal cyst (pilonidal abscess). This disorder is more common in men. The cause may involve trauma and/or ingrown hairs. Diagnosis is

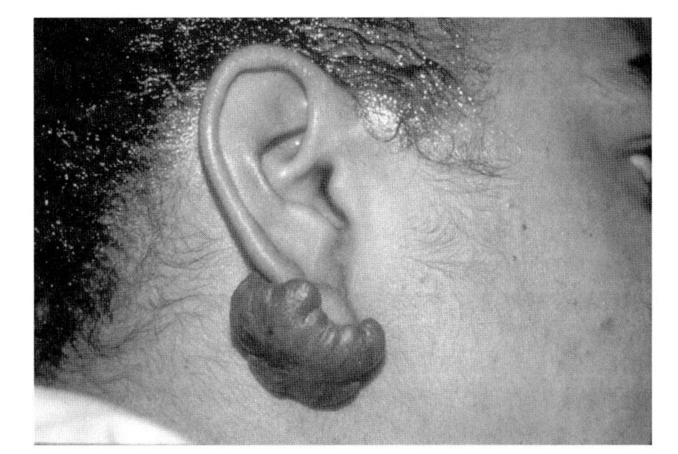

FIGURE 13–10 Keloid. From Rubin E, Farber JL. *Rubin's Pathology*, 3rd ed. Lippincott Williams & Wilkins, 2004.

clinical. Treatment is usually incision and drainage. Consider surgical drainage if the lesion persists or recurs after incision and drainage.

> Pilonidal cysts often contain tufts of hair.

Alternative 13.11.1

Within 2 weeks of getting her ears pierced, an African-American woman presents with the ear lesion in Figure 13-10.

What is the most likely diagnosis?

The patient has a keloid, a benign tumor-like growth in areas of trauma such as surgical scars, piercing sites, etc. Keloids are more common in African Americans. First-line therapy is intralesional corticosteroids. Therapeutic options for refractory keloids are surgical excision, cryosurgery, and pulsed dye laser therapy. Patients should also minimize piercings and surgeries to prevent recurrences.

Alternative 13.11.2

A 60-year-old man presents with a 3-day history of fever and arthralgias. On physical exam, there are tender erythematous papules and plaques throughout the body. Significant laboratory findings include increased white blood cell count with neutrophilia, increased erythrocyte sedimentation rate, and increased C-reactive protein. The physicians are unsure of the diagnosis, so they perform biopsy of the lesions, which demonstrates nonvasculitic neutrophil infiltration.

What is the most likely diagnosis?

The patient has the four key features required to make a diagnosis of Sweet's syndrome:

1. Abrupt onset of erythematous papules and plaques
2. Nonvasculitic neutrophil infiltration of skin lesions on biopsy
3. Fever
4. Peripheral neutrophilia

An underlying malignancy, infection, or autoimmune disorder is present in almost 50% of patients with this uncommon neutrophilic dermatosis. First-line therapy is oral corticosteroids.

chapter 14

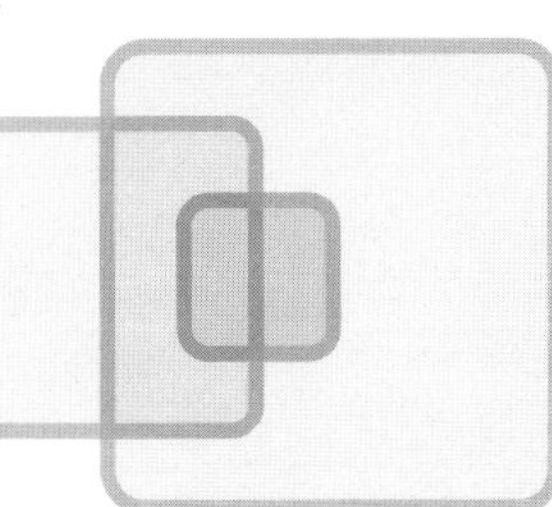

Primary Care Gynecology and Urology

CASE 14–1 VAGINAL DISCHARGE

A 22-year-old woman presents with a 7-day history of abnormal vaginal discharge. Symptoms are worse after intercourse. She denies abdominal pain, dysuria, or vaginal pruritus. She is in a monogamous relationship and has never had unprotected sexual intercourse. On examination, there is a foul-smelling, thin, gray, homogenous discharge. There are no signs of cervical inflammation. There is no cervical motion tenderness.

What are the most common causes of vaginal discharge?

In descending order, the three most common causes of vaginal discharge are bacterial vaginosis (BV), *Candida vaginitis*, and *Trichomonas vaginalis*. Allergens (e.g., latex condoms), irritants (e.g., spermicides and scented panty liners), and lower genital tract infection by *Neisseria gonorrhea* or *Chlamydia trachomatis* are other common causes.

What is the next step in management?

Laboratory testing is indicated in all women with abnormal vaginal discharge because clinical findings are suggestive but not specific. Obtain a sample of the discharge with a vaginal swab and perform the following tests (Table 14-1):

TABLE 14–1 Differentiating Features of Vaginal Discharge

Classic Findings	Bacterial Vaginosis	*Trichomonas vaginalis*	*Candida vaginitis*
Discharge	Thin, gray, and homogenous	Green-yellow and frothy	Thick, white and clumpy ("cottage cheese or curd-like")
Symptoms	None	Frequency, dysuria, and painful coitus	Pruritus ± dysuria and painful coitus
Physical exam	None	Vulvovaginal edema and erythema ± punctate hemorrhages	Vulvovaginal edema and erythema
Vaginal pH[a]	>4.5	>4.5	4–4.5
Microscopy (wet prep)	Clue cells	Motile trichomonads Increased PMNs	Pseudohyphae
KOH	Fishy odor ("whiff test")	Negative	Budding yeast, pseudohyphae

Abbreviations: PMN, polymorphonuclear neutrophils.
[a] Normal vaginal pH is 4–4.5.

1. **Vaginal pH**: This is the most important test.
2. **Wet prep**: Mix the sample with saline and examine under the microscope.
3. **KOH**: Mix sample with KOH and smell the specimen ("whiff test"). Then examine the specimen under the microscope (KOH test).

Normal discharge: 1 to 4 mL/day of thick, white, and odorless discharge.
Physiological leucorrhea: >4 mL of thick, white, odorless discharge and normal lab tests.

Vaginal pH is 5. A vaginal specimen is obtained and observed under the microscope (Fig. 14-1). Whiff test is positive.

What is the diagnosis?

Diagnosis of BV requires the patient to meet three of four Amsel criteria:

1. Discharge: thin, grey, homogenous, and foul-smelling.
2. Vaginal pH > 4.5.
3. Wet prep: clue cells (vaginal epithelial cells that are covered with bacteria).
4. Positive whiff test.

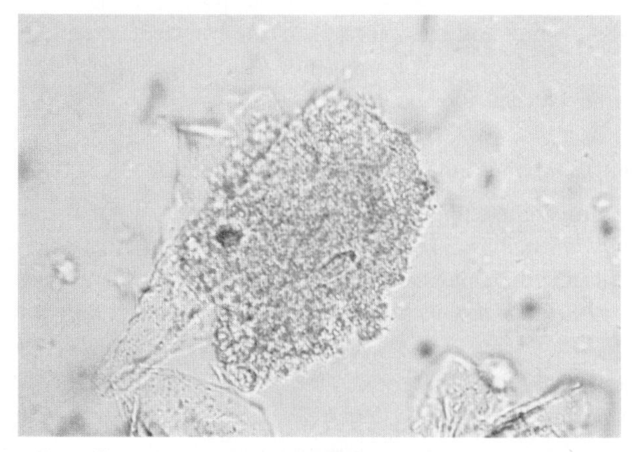

FIGURE 14–1 Vaginal wet prep: Clue cells. From McClatchey KD. *Clinical Laboratory Medicine*, 2nd ed. Lippincott Williams & Wilkins, 2002.

This patient meets all four criteria for BV, which results from alteration of normal vaginal flora, most commonly decreased Lactobacillus and increased *Gardnerella vaginalis.* Although BV is not considered a sexually transmitted disease (STD), symptoms are often worse after intercourse, and multiple sexual partners is a risk factor. Other risk factors are cigarette smoking and douching, which alters vaginal pH.

> Most patients with BV are asymptomatic.

How is BV treated?

Treat symptomatic patients with a 7-day course of oral metronidazole or topical clindamycin. No treatment is necessary for asymptomatic patients.

> Avoid alcohol consumption with metronidazole. The combination can cause flushing, headache, nausea, vomiting, dyspnea, and palpitations (disulfiram-like reaction).

Alternative 14.1.1

A 24-year-old woman presents with dysuria, urgency, frequency, painful coitus (dyspareunia), and vaginal discharge. There is vulvovaginal erythema and edema. Vaginal pH is 5.5. Wet prep is obtained (Fig. 14-2).

What is the diagnosis?

Wet prep demonstrates the flagellated parasite *T. vaginalis*, which is transmitted sexually. Almost 70% of women present with classic symptoms. The most common physical finding is vulvovaginal edema and erythema. Less than one third of patients have the characteristic frothy, green-yellow discharge. A small minority of patients demonstrate punctate cervical hemorrhages ("strawberry cervix").

How is T. vaginalis infection treated?

Administer a single dose of oral metronidazole or tinidazole to all patients (symptomatic and asymptomatic) as well as their sexual partners (to prevent re-infection).

> The majority of men with *T. vaginalis* infection are asymptomatic.

> *T. vaginalis* infection increases transmission risk of HIV and other STDs.

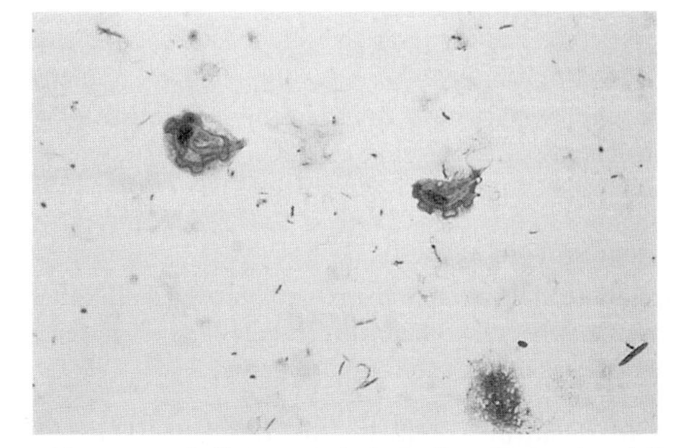

FIGURE 14–2 Vaginal wet prep: *Trichomonas vaginalis*. From Ayala C, Spellberg B. *Boards and Wards*, 3rd ed. Lippincott Williams & Wilkins, 2007.

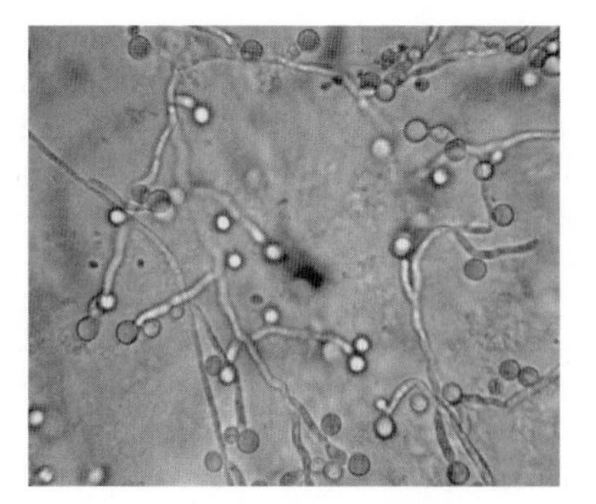

FIGURE 14–3 KOH: Pseudohyphae. From Goodheart HP. *Goodheart's Photoguide of Common Skin Disorders,* 2nd ed. Lippincott Williams & Wilkins, 2003.

Alternative 14.1.2

A 58-year-old woman presents with a 3-day history of vaginal discharge and pruritus. She also reports pain during coitus. The vulva and vagina are edematous and erythematous. The discharge looks like thick white clumps. Vaginal pH is 4.2. Whiff test is negative. KOH test is obtained (Fig. 14-3).

What is the diagnosis?

The patient has vulvovaginal candidiasis (i.e., yeast infection). Almost 90% of cases occur as a result of overgrowth of *Candida albicans* (part of normal vaginal flora). Important risk factors are diabetes, immunosuppression, and oral contraceptives.

How should you treat this patient?

First-line therapy of *C. vaginitis* is a single dose of oral fluconazole; 3- to 7-day courses of topical antifungals are equally effective but less convenient.

Three months later, the patient is diagnosed with type 2 diabetes mellitus (DM). Five months later, she has another episode of *C. vaginitis.* Glycosylated hemoglobin (HbA1c) measurement 3 weeks ago was 8.7%.

How should you treat this patient?

Administer two doses of oral fluconazole 72 hours apart to patients with DM, immunosuppressed patients, patients with severe signs and symptoms, and patients with recurrent infections (more than four infections per year).

The patient has 5 more episodes of *C. vaginitis* over the next 12 months.

What measures can she institute to prevent recurrent infection?

The most important measure is to minimize risk factors (maintain tight glycemic control, discontinue oral contraceptives, etc.). If the patient continues to have recurrent infections, consider weekly prophylactic doses of oral fluconazole.

Alternative 14.1.3

A 28-year-old woman presents with a 4-day history of excessive vaginal discharge and pruritus. The vulva is erythematous. Vaginal fluid is thick, white, and homogenous. Vaginal pH is 4.2. Wet prep is nondiagnostic. Whiff test is negative. KOH test is nondiagnostic.

What is the next step in management?

Obtain vaginal culture if clinical findings and initial laboratory tests are nondiagnostic. Culture can differentiate between vaginal candidiasis and lower genital tract infection with *N. gonorrhea* or *C. trachomatis* (urethritis or cervicitis).

> **Gonorrhea or chlamydia urethritis or cervicitis**: More than 50% of women are asymptomatic. Others have mucopurulent discharge, dysuria, or lower abdominal pain.

Vaginal culture is negative. The patient continues to have recurrent unexplained episodes of vaginal discharge with vaginal pH <4.5.

What is the next step?

Consider sequential discontinuation of possible irritants and allergens such as scented panty liners and latex condoms.

What if the patient with vaginal discharge had a vaginal pH of 5.5 but wet prep, whiff test, and KOH test were nondiagnostic?

In addition to standard cultures, obtain vaginal culture on Diamond's medium to rule out *T. vaginalis.* An alternative to Diamond's medium culture is the commercially available "in-pouch culture system" for *T. vaginalis.*

CASE 14–2 DYSURIA AND PENILE DISCHARGE

A 32-year-old man presents with dysuria and penile discharge. The symptoms began 5 days after he participated in a ménage-a-trois while on a business trip in Thailand. On examination, a green-yellow discharge is evident at the urethral meatus. Digital rectal exam (DRE) is unremarkable. Vital signs are normal.

What is the differential diagnosis?

Dysuria and penile discharge indicate the patient has urethritis. The two broad categories of urethritis are gonococcal urethritis (due to *N. gonorrhea*) and nongonococcal urethritis (NGU). NGU can result from *C. trachomatis* (most common), herpes simplex virus (HSV) and genital mycoplasmas (*M. genitalium* and *Ureaplasma urealyticum*).

> The classic teaching is that gonococcal urethritis causes a mucopurulent (green-yellow) discharge and NGU causes clear watery discharge. However, discharge characteristics are not a reliable method to distinguish between the two categories.

What is the next step in management?

The next step in any male patient with dysuria is to obtain urinalysis, urethral Gram stain, and urethral culture. To culture *N. gonorrhea,* use Thayer-Martin media. An alternative to urethral culture is urine nucleic acid amplification tests (NAAT) such as polymerase chain reaction (PCR), which are quicker, easier to obtain, and more sensitive (but more expensive).

Urinalysis demonstrates positive LE and 10 to 12 white blood cells per high-powered field (WBC/HPF). Gram stain is obtained (Fig. 14-4). Culture is pending.

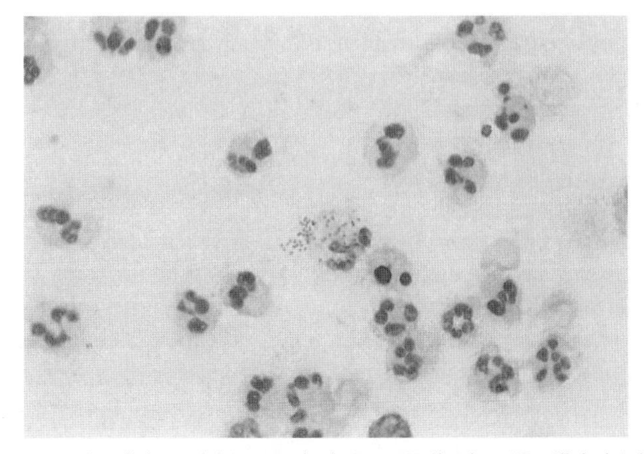

FIGURE 14–4 Gram stain: Gram-negative diplococci (*N. gonorrhea*). From McClatchey KD. *Clinical Laboratory Medicine,* 2nd ed. Lippincott Williams & Wilkins, 2002.

What is the next step in management?

Figure 14-4 demonstrates Gram-negative diplococci within polymorphonuclear neutrophils, which is sufficient to diagnose the patient with gonococcal urethritis. The next step is to treat with a single intramuscular (IM) dose of a third-generation cephalosporin (ceftriaxone or cefixime). Also, administer a single dose of azithromycin or a 7-day course of doxycycline because a large percentage of patients have concurrent chlamydia infection.

> Unlike women, >90% of gonococcal urethritis is symptomatic in men.

The patient had unprotected sexual intercourse with his wife after he returned from the business trip. He does not want her to find out about his sexual adventures in Thailand. He asks if the physician can prescribe him antibiotics for his wife, which he will then discreetly place into her food.

Should the physician comply with his request?

The current recommendation is to ask the patient to speak to his sexual partners about the need for medical evaluation and treatment. Do not prescribe any additional antibiotics for his wife at this time. Unfortunately, the current approach is a public health failure.

> A randomized trial in 2005 found that giving infected patients antibiotics for their sexual partners led to decreased re-infection and increased reporting of sexual partners.

How would you treat the patient if Gram stain did not reveal any intracellular Gram-negative diplococci and PCR demonstrated C. trachomatis?

C. trachomatis is the most common sexually transmitted bacterial infection. Treat with a single dose of azithromycin or a 7-day course of doxycycline.

> **Genital mycoplasmas**: First-line drug is erythromycin or tetracycline.

CASE 14–3 Acute Adnexal Pain

A 31-year-old woman presents with a 4-day history of bilateral lower abdominal pain. The pain began shortly after her menstrual period ended. She works as a prostitute in New York City. There is pain on palpation of both lower quadrants. Vital signs are temperature 38.5°C, pulse 85 bpm, respirations 25/min, and blood pressure 115/70.

What are the next steps in management?

Lower abdominal pain in women can result from abdominal or adnexal causes. Perform a pelvic exam and obtain the following tests in women with lower abdominal pain:

1. **Fecal occult blood test (FOBT)**: Guaiac-positive stool increases the likelihood of an abdominal cause.
2. **β-hCG**: Obtain this test to rule out ectopic pregnancy in all women of childbearing age.
3. **NAATs**: Urinalysis, wet prep, and urethral Gram stain and culture.
4. **Complete blood count (CBC)**: Decreased hematocrit increases the likelihood of an abdominal cause. Increased WBCs suggests an inflammatory or infectious cause (pelvic or abdominal).

> **Adnexa**: appendages of the uterus (ovaries, fallopian tubes, broad ligament).

There is cervical motion tenderness and a mucopurulent discharge. There are no palpable abdominal or adnexal masses. Stool is guaiac-negative. β-hCG is negative. There are 10 WBCs/HPF on wet prep. Gram stain is nondiagnostic. NAATs are pending. CBC shows leukocytosis with a left shift.

What is the most likely diagnosis?

Maintain a high index of suspicion for pelvic inflammatory disease (PID) if a sexually active woman with lower abdominal pain has a mucopurulent discharge or cervical motion tenderness (indicates adnexal inflammation). Other nonspecific findings in patients with PID are fever (occurs in 50% of cases), leukocytosis with a left shift (occurs in 50% of cases), and >5 WBCs/HPF on urinalysis (occurs in 80% of cases). Abdominal pain classically occurs during or after menstruation and is worse with coitus (not sensitive or specific).

> **Fitz-Hugh-Curtis syndrome**: In rare instances, inflammation from PID can spread to Glisson's capsule and cause right upper quadrant pain due to perihepatitis.

What causes PID?

PID results from adnexal infection by *C. trachomatis*, *N. gonorrhea*, or genital mycoplasmas. It occurs in 15% to 30% of untreated lower genital tract infections (recall that >50% of women with cervicitis and urethritis are asymptomatic).

> Positive Gram stain, culture, or NAAT can confirm PID. Negative tests do not rule out PID.

What are the next steps in management?

Perform transvaginal ultrasound to rule out tubo-ovarian abscess (TOA). If there is no TOA, treat empirically with a 14-day course of oral ofloxacin or levofloxacin ± metronidazole. An alternative is a single dose of IM ceftriaxone followed by a 14-day course of doxycycline ± metronidazole.

> TOA is much more likely if the patient has a palpable ovarian mass.

How would management differ if the patient had a history of noncompliance for treatment of prior sexually transmitted infections?

Indications for inpatient management with intravenous antibiotics (mnemonic: "**SHUNT**"):

1. **S**ymptoms persist despite oral antibiotics
2. **H**emodynamically **U**nstable
3. **N**oncompliance is likely
4. **T**OA

First-line antibiotic options are:

1. Clindamycin plus gentamycin.
2. Cefotetan (or cefoxitin) plus doxycycline.

> Major complications of PID are ectopic pregnancy, infertility, and chronic pelvic pain. These can occur because healing of tissues damaged by PID can cause scarring.

Twelve months later, the patient presents with acute onset of severe left lower quadrant pain and vaginal bleeding. She has not had a menstrual period in the last 7 weeks. On physical examination, there is left lower quadrant tenderness, cervical motion tenderness, and vaginal bleeding. Stool is guaiac-negative. β-hCG is 4000 mIU/mL. Vital signs are temperature 37.5°C, pulse 90 bpm, respirations 18/min, and blood pressure 110/75.

What is the most likely cause of her symptoms?

Positive β-hCG indicates that the patient is pregnant. Lower abdominal pain, amenorrhea, and vaginal bleeding compose the classic triad of ectopic pregnancy (pregnancy outside the uterus). Transvaginal ultrasound is the test of choice to evaluate for ectopic pregnancy.

> More than 50% of ectopic pregnancies do not present with the classic triad.

Transvaginal ultrasound confirms the diagnosis.

How should you treat this patient?

Both medical therapy with methotrexate or surgery are acceptable options in this hemodynamically stable patient with β-hCG <5000 mIU/ml.

How would management differ if β-hCG were 8000 or blood pressure were 85/70?

Patients with β hCG >5000 mIU/mL have an increased risk of developing a ruptured ectopic pregnancy, so treatment is surgery. Hemodynamic instability is highly suggestive of a ruptured ectopic pregnancy and indicates a need for emergent surgery.

How would management differ if the patient were stable and β-hCG were 700 mIU/mL?

Transvaginal ultrasound does not reliably distinguish the gestational sac until β-HCG is 1500 mIU/mL (discriminatory zone). Obtain serial β-HCG measurements over the next 3 days. After β-HCG reaches 1500 mIU/mL, perform transvaginal ultrasound to document whether the pregnancy is uterine or ectopic. If β-HCG does not double over a 3-day period, consider methotrexate because the pregnancy is unlikely to be successful.

Alternative 14.3.1

A 27-year-old woman presents with sudden onset of right lower quadrant pain, nausea, and vomiting. Vital signs are temperature 37.4°C, pulse 110 bpm, respirations 27/min, and blood pressure 110/70. There is no history of periumbilical pain. There is cervical motion tenderness but no discharge. β-hCG is negative. Urinalysis and urethral Gram stain are normal. CT scan demonstrates an intact ovarian cyst but no signs of appendicitis. Doppler ultrasound demonstrates decreased ovarian blood flow.

What diagnosis should you consider?

Consider the diagnosis of ovarian torsion when a woman of childbearing age presents with sudden onset of lower abdominal pain, nausea, and vomiting along with adnexal cysts or decreased ovarian blood flow. The next step in a patient with suspected ovarian torsion is prompt surgical de-torsion.

> Diagnosis of ovarian torsion is often clinical because ultrasound is not sensitive enough to detect this event consistently.

CASE 14–4 Chronic Adnexal Pain

An 18-year-old woman presents with cramp-like adnexal pain during menstruation. She has experienced these symptoms since she had her first menstrual period at age 13 years. The symptoms begin on the first day of her period and resolve over the next 24 hours. Abdominal and pelvic examination is normal.

What is the most likely diagnosis?

Cramp-like adnexal pain during menstruation ± nausea, vomiting, fatigue, and malaise are the characteristic symptoms of dysmenorrhea. Dysmenorrhea is common, and 75% of patients do not have any underlying cause. Primary dysmenorrhea is most likely in this young patient with a normal pelvic examination and recurrent symptoms that occur at the onset of menses and resolve within 12 to 72 hours.

What is the next step in management?

First-line therapy is nonsteroidal anti-inflammatory drugs (NSAIDs) ± oral contraceptive pills (OCPs). Consider evaluating the patient for secondary dysmenorrhea if symptoms do not improve after three cycles.

> **Heated pad**: An option for women with primary dysmenorrhea who wish to avoid medications.

What workup should you consider if a woman with apparent primary dysmenorrhea continues to have severe symptoms despite NSAIDs and OCPs?

Pelvic ultrasound is the first-line diagnostic test. Also obtain urethral Gram stain and culture (or NAATs) to evaluate for chronic PID in areas of high prevalence. If clinical findings, imaging, and laboratory tests do not reveal a particular cause, consider diagnostic laparoscopy.

Alternative 14.4.1

A 42-year-old woman presents with dysmenorrhea and excessive menstrual bleeding (menorrhagia). On pelvic exam, the uterus is diffusely enlarged (globular) and tender.

What diagnosis should you suspect?

Suspect adenomyosis when a woman with dysmenorrhea and/or menorrhagia has a tender and diffusely enlarged uterus on bimanual pelvic exam. In this disorder, ectopic endometrial tissue is located within the uterus. The only way to definitively diagnose and treat adenomyosis is hysterectomy. Magnetic resonance imaging (MRI) and ultrasound are less sensitive but are used increasingly to evaluate for adenomyosis because they are far less invasive than surgery.

> Obtain CBC and coagulation tests (prothrombin (PT), partial thromboplastin time (PTT), and International Normalized Ratio (INR)) to rule out a bleeding disorder in women with menorrhagia and no obvious pelvic cause.

What diagnosis should you suspect if the patient with dysmenorrhea and menorrhagia had an irregularly enlarged but mobile uterus?

Pregnancy and adenomyosis cause uniform uterine enlargement. The finding of irregular uterine enlargement in a patient with menorrhagia ± dysmenorrhea should raise suspicion for uterine leiomyomas (i.e., fibroids). Pelvic ultrasound is typically used to confirm the presence of this benign tumor. MRI is also very accurate, but it is more expensive. Hysterectomy is the treatment of choice to definitively cure the disease. Myomectomy is an option for select patients who wish to become pregnant. If the tumor is large, administer GnRH agonists before surgery to reduce the size of the fibroid(s).

Alternative 14.4.2

A 48-year-old white woman presents with a 6-week history of lower abdominal pain and bloating. Pelvic exam demonstrates a fixed, irregular, solid adnexal mass on the left side.

What diagnosis should you suspect?

An adnexal mass on pelvic examination should raise suspicion for ovarian cancer. Primary ovarian cancer is frequently asymptomatic in the early stages. Initial symptoms are nonspecific and include lower abdominal pain, bloating, early satiety, constipation, and urinary frequency. As the disease progresses, patients may develop ascites and a fixed, irregular, solid adnexal mass.

> **Ovarian cancer risk factors**: white race, family history, nulliparity.
> **Ovarian cancer protective factors**: OCPs, multiple pregnancies.

What is the next step in management?

The next step in any woman with an adnexal mass is to obtain abdominal and transvaginal ultrasound. If ultrasound findings suggest cancer, obtain the following tests:

1. **FOBT**: to evaluate for metastatic gastrointestinal tract neoplasm (Krukenberg tumor).
2. **Bilateral mammography**: to rule out metastatic breast cancer.
3. **CA-125**: to establish a baseline before surgery.
4. **CT scan of the abdomen and pelvis**: to assess extent of invasion before surgery.

How would you manage this patient if ultrasound findings are nondiagnostic?

Surgery is indicated for an adnexal mass with any of the following characteristics:

1. Size: >10 cm if premenopausal or >3 cm if postmenopausal.
2. Ascites or other signs of metastatic disease (e.g., unintentional weight loss).
3. First-degree family history of ovarian or breast cancer.
4. Increased CA-125.

> Initial therapy of a cystic ovarian lesion without any of the above characteristics is OCPs. If size does not decrease within 4 to 6 weeks, perform surgery.

How is ovarian cancer treated?

Treatment for ovarian cancer is usually surgery and chemotherapy (Taxol and carboplatin). Overall survival is low because most patients are diagnosed at a later stage.

Alternative 14.4.3

A 32-year-old woman presents with chronic lower abdominal pain that is worse during her menstrual period. She also reports dyspareunia and deep pain on defecation (dyschezia). She mentions that she has been trying to become pregnant for the last 12 months without success. Rectal exam is normal. Stool is negative for occult blood. On pelvic exam, there is pain on palpation of the posterior fornix of the vagina. Vital signs are normal.

What diagnosis should you suspect?

Endometriosis (endometrial tissue outside the uterus) commonly presents with chronic adnexal pain (i.e., duration >6 months) that is worse during menstruation. Dyspareunia, dyschezia, and abnormal vaginal bleeding are other common symptoms. Endometriosis is the most common cause of infertility in women with no history of PID. Pain on palpation of the posterior fornix is the characteristic sign, although pelvic exam is frequently normal. Laparoscopy is the diagnostic test of choice. Endometriosis is the most common diagnosis in women who undergo laparoscopy for chronic pelvic pain.

> **Most common sites of endometriosis**: ovaries > cul-de-sac > broad ligaments.

How is endometriosis treated?

Treatment depends on disease severity. Consider medical therapy with a GnRH analog or progesterone for mild to moderate disease and surgery for severe or refractory endometriosis. Some gynecologists prefer surgery as first-line therapy for mild endometriosis in patients who wish to preserve fertility.

> CA-125 is often elevated in women with endometriosis.

What diagnosis would you suspect if laparoscopy did not detect any abnormalities except dilated ovarian veins?

Suspect pelvic congestion syndrome if the only abnormality on imaging or laparoscopy is dilated ovarian veins. Many patients have a history of varicose veins. This disorder causes chronic pelvic pain that may be worse during menstrual periods. Some patients may experience abnormal vaginal bleeding. Confirm the presence of ovarian varices with venography. Treatment options are surgery or ovarian vein embolization.

> **Chronic pelvic pain syndrome**: This is the diagnosis of exclusion after other causes are ruled out.

CASE 14–5 Nonmenstrual Bleeding

A 25-year-old G1P1OO1 woman presents with a small amount of pelvic bleeding between menstrual periods. She regularly has breast tenderness, bloating, and thin watery discharge approximately 14 days after her menstrual period begins (molimina). She is otherwise asymptomatic and has no other medical conditions. She recently began taking OCPs for birth control. Her last Pap smear 2 months ago was normal. There is no family history of cancer. Body mass index is 23. Pelvic exam is normal.

What is the most likely cause of her bleeding?

The most likely cause of intermenstrual bleeding is "breakthrough bleeding," which commonly occurs shortly after initiating or switching oral contraceptives. An intrauterine device or hormone replacement therapy can also cause breakthrough bleeding. In most women, bleeding is light ("spotting"), although sometimes heavy bleeding can occur.

> Incidence of breakthrough bleeding has increased as a result of decreased estrogen content in OCPs.

What is the next step in management?

The first step is to rule out pregnancy. If β-hCG is negative, discontinue the OCP and observe for a few cycles. Also, order a CBC if bleeding is significant.

> If hematocrit or platelet count is low, order PT, PTT, and INR to rule out bleeding disorders.

Alternative 14.5.1

A 22-year-old woman presents with recurrent episodes of intermenstrual bleeding. She also reports infrequent menstrual periods. On physical exam, there is acne and hair on her chin and above her lips. There is velvety brown discoloration at the crease of her neck (acanthosis nigricans). Body mass index is 34.

What diagnosis should you suspect?

Suspect polycystic ovarian syndrome (PCOS) in a young woman with any of the following:

1. **Decreased ovulation**: Suspect in patients with oligomenorrhea.
2. **Hyperandrogenism**: Signs include acne, hirsutism, and male pattern baldness.
3. **Refractory obesity**: More than 50% of PCOS patients are obese.

> **National Institutes of Health (NIH) criteria**: oligomenorrhea and hyperandrogenism in the absence of other causes.
> **Rotterdam criteria**: NIH criteria plus polycystic ovaries on ultrasound.

> **Insulin resistance**: common in PCOS (acanthosis nigricans is a characteristic sign).

What are signs of ovulation?

Ovulatory patients should have regular menstrual periods. Ovulation is indicated by any of the following traits midway through the menstrual cycle (approximately 14 days after onset of menses):

1. **Molimina**: breast tenderness, bloating, and clear watery discharge.
2. **Serum progesterone**: >9.5 nmol/L.
3. **Basal body temperature**: 0.3°F to 0.6°F increase in body temperature.
4. **Endometrial biopsy**: Secretory endometrium is indicative of ovulation.

What causes intermenstrual bleeding in women with PCOS?

Women with PCOS have adequate estrogen release, which stimulates endometrial proliferation. However, decreased ovulation leads to reduced progesterone release, which is required for differentiation of the thickened endometrium. The undifferentiated endometrium sloughs off and causes intermenstrual bleeding. Unopposed estrogen also leads to increased endometrial cancer risk in PCOS patients.

What diagnostic tests should you order to confirm the diagnosis?

1. Rule out other causes of oligomenorrhea: Order β-hCG, thyroid-stimulating hormone (TSH) (to rule out hypothyroidism), and serum prolactin (to rule out pituitary tumor).
2. Rule out other causes of hyperandrogenism: Order serum testosterone, DHEA, and DHEA-S (to rule out an adrenal neoplasm).
3. Consider pelvic ultrasound (not necessary for diagnosis using NIH criteria).

> Obtain fasting glucose and lipid profile in all patients with PCOS.

How is PCOS managed?

Correct hyperglycemia and hyperlipidemia if present. Treat intermenstrual bleeding and hirsutism with OCPs. OCPs also reduce risk of endometrial cancer.

The patient presents for evaluation 2 years later. She has tried to become pregnant for the last 12 months without success.

What measures should you recommend?

PCOS is one of the most common causes of infertility in women. The first-line measure is weight loss, which often restores ovulation. The second-line measure is clomiphene citrate. Add metformin to the regimen if clomiphene is unsuccessful.

> **Clomiphene** binds to estrogen receptors in anterior pituitary, preventing estrogen from binding to the gland. Anterior pituitary senses low estrogen and increases release of follicle-stimulating hormone, which induces ovulation.

Alternative 14.5.2

A 38-year-old woman presents with episodes of intermenstrual spotting. She regularly notices breast tenderness, mild bloating, and increased watery discharge midway through her menstrual cycle. She does not take any medications. She uses condoms for contraception. She has undergone regular Pap smears, which have all been normal. Pelvic exam is normal.

What is the next step in management?

Age >35 years is a risk factor for endometrial cancer; other risk factors include family history of breast or endometrial cancer; endometrial hyperplasia; obesity, DM, or PCOS; and unopposed estrogen therapy or nulliparity (increased lifelong unopposed estrogen). The first step

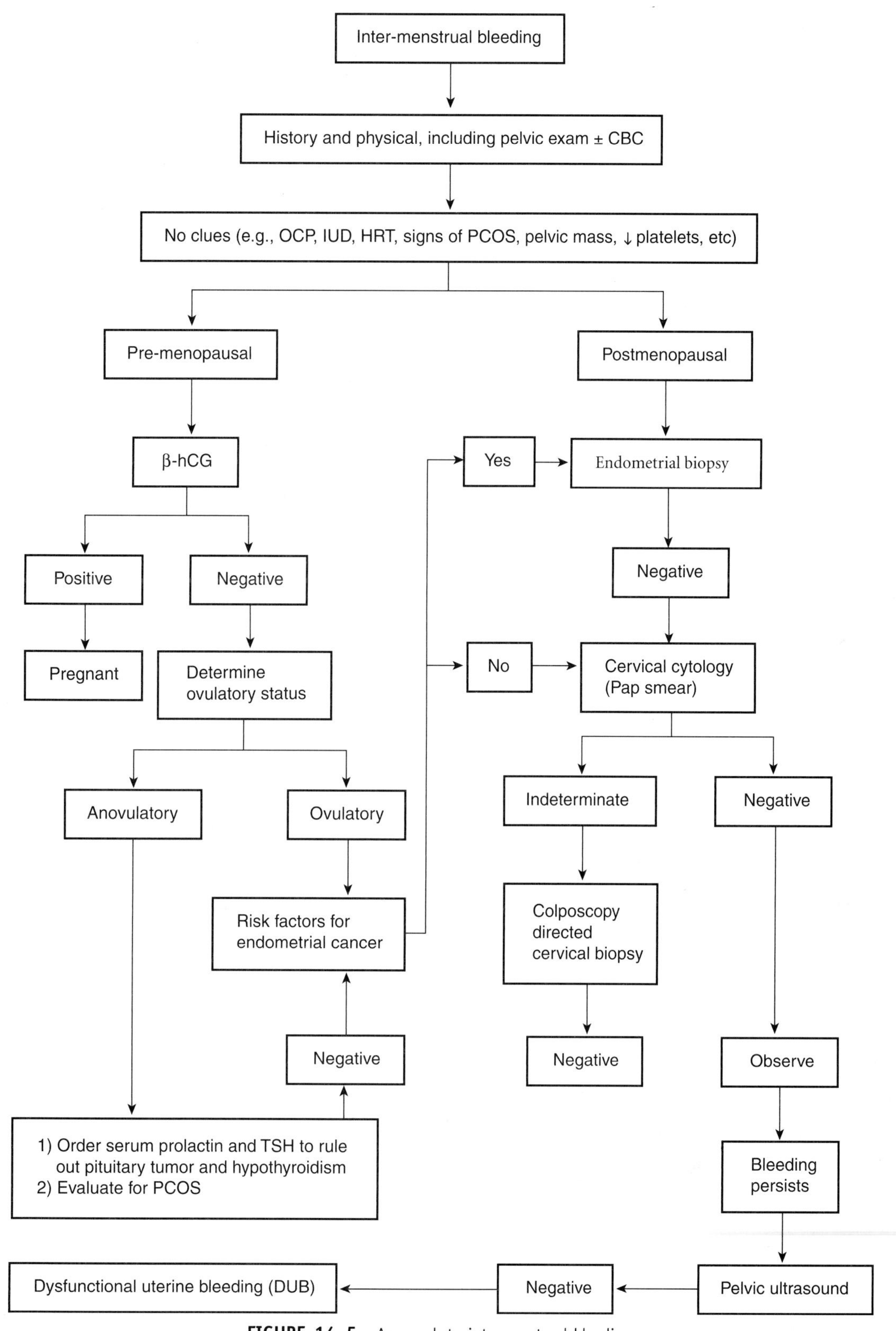

FIGURE 14–5 Approach to intermenstrual bleeding.

is to rule out pregnancy. If β-hCG is negative, obtain an endometrial biopsy (Fig. 14-5). Most women with endometrial cancer experience intermenstrual spotting at an early stage, which means that the neoplasm is often detected before metastatic spread occurs. As a result, overall prognosis is much better than ovarian cancer.

Alternative 14.5.3

A 47-year-old woman presents with intermenstrual spotting. Symptoms typically occur after sexual intercourse. She recently emigrated from Sierra Leone and has not visited a healthcare professional since she was a child. She occasionally uses condoms for contraception. Pelvic exam is normal.

What are the next steps in management?

Postcoital spotting should raise suspicion for cervical cancer or infection (cervicitis), particularly in a woman who has not had regular Pap smears. The major risk factor for cervical cancer is infection with the sexually transmitted human papillomavirus (HPV). Median age at presentation is 47 years. The first step is to rule out pregnancy. Then, perform a Pap smear (obtain cervical cytology and culture) and endometrial biopsy (because the patient is >35 years old).

> Many women with invasive cervical cancer have a visible cervical lesion, in which case biopsy of the lesion is the first step in management.

Pap smear is nondiagnostic. Endometrial biopsy is normal.

What is the next step?

This patient has a high risk of cervical cancer, so perform colposcopy-directed biopsy if Pap smear is nondiagnostic. If colposcopy-directed biopsy does not rule out the diagnosis, consider cold-knife conization or a loop electrosurgical excision procedure.

Alternative 14.5.4

A 46-year-year old woman presents with intermenstrual spotting. Her menstrual periods have become inconsistent. She does not take any medications. β-hCG is negative. Endometrial biopsy and Pap smear are normal. Bleeding persists, so she undergoes transabdominal and transvaginal ultrasound, which is normal. TSH and serum prolactin are normal. CBC, PT, PTT, and INR are normal.

What is the most likely diagnosis?

Abnormal uterine bleeding without any underlying cause is termed dysfunctional uterine bleeding (DUB). DUB is common among perimenopausal women with menstrual irregularities. First-line therapy is OCPs to regulate the menstrual cycle. If symptoms persist, consider endometrial ablation. Consider hysterectomy if the patient does not desire future pregnancies.

How would management differ if the 42-year-old woman with DUB smoked cigarettes?

OCPs are contraindicated in women >40 years old who smoke cigarettes (increases risk of myocardial infarction and thromboembolic events). Treat instead with cyclic progesterone therapy (5 to 12 days per month).

> **Massive intrauterine hemorrhage**: Administer 25 mg intravenous (IV) conjugated estrogen.

CASE 14–6 Urinary Incontinence in Women

A 33-year-old G3P3003 woman presents with a 2-month history of involuntary urinary leakage. Symptoms typically occur when she laughs, coughs, or lifts weights at the gym, and they greatly affect her daily activities. She denies frequency, urgency, or dysuria. She does not have any other medical conditions or take any medications.

What is the most likely cause of her symptoms?

Involuntary urinary leakage is termed urinary incontinence. There are six types of urinary incontinence (Table 14-2). Stress incontinence is most likely in this patient with symptoms

TABLE 14–2 Types of Urinary Incontinence

Type	Mechanism(s)	Causes/Risk Factors
Stress incontinence	Weakened pelvic diaphragm Failure of urethral closure (intrinsic sphincter deficiency)	Multiple childbirths Scarring after pelvic surgery Severe mucosal atrophy (in postmenopausal women)
Urge incontinence	Hyperactive detrusor muscle (bladder muscle)	Idiopathic (most common) Bladder irritation: UTI, kidney stones CNS diseases that damage nerves regulating detrusor: brain tumors, stroke, Alzheimer's disease, etc.
Overflow incontinence	Outlet obstruction causes full bladder; urine continuously dribbles from full bladder	Men (more common): BPH, prostate cancer, or urethral kink Women (less common): cystocele
	Underactive detrusor causes full bladder; urine continuously dribbles from full bladder	Peripheral neuropathy (diabetes mellitus, alcoholism, vitamin B12 deficiency, tabes dorsalis, etc.)
Mixed incontinence	Stress incontinence and urge incontinence	Causes of stress and urge incontinence
Anatomic deformity	Most frequently iatrogenic (pelvic surgery or radiation)	Most common cause is fistula (vesicovaginal or ureterovaginal)
Functional incontinence	Debilitated person unable to get to the toilet fast enough	Diagnosis of exclusion in patients with disabling disease

Abbreviations: BPH, benign prostatic hyperplasia; CNS, central nervous system; UTI, urinary tract infection.

that occur during periods of increased intra-abdominal pressure such as laughing, coughing, and lifting weights. Multiparity is an important risk factor because it weakens pelvic musculature.

> Stress incontinence is the leading cause of incontinence in young women. Screen all women who have had a child or are >65 years old for stress incontinence.

What diagnostic tests should you order at this time?

History, physical exam, urinalysis, and urine culture are usually sufficient in women with characteristic symptoms. Some clinicians also advocate measuring post-void residual (PVR) in all patients, but this is controversial.

> **PVR**: The patient must void as completely as possible. Then insert a catheter into the bladder to measure volume of residual urine. PVR >50 to 100 mL suggests overflow incontinence.

How is stress incontinence treated?

Treat in a stepwise fashion as follows:

1. Lifestyle measures: First steps are to avoid excessive fluids, minimize alcohol and caffeine, lose weight, stop smoking (to minimize cough), and discontinue medications that exacerbate incontinence (Table 14-3).
2. Behavioral therapy: Frequent voluntary voiding and pelvic muscle exercises (Kegel exercises) are indicated if symptoms persist despite lifestyle measures.
3. Medications: Third-line measure is topical estrogen (not very effective).
4. Surgery: Consider for refractory symptoms that affect daily activities.

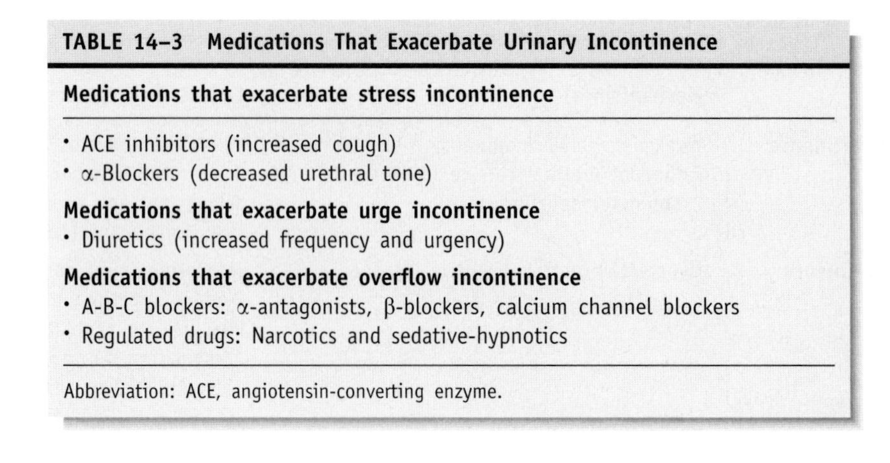

TABLE 14–3 Medications That Exacerbate Urinary Incontinence
Medications that exacerbate stress incontinence
• ACE inhibitors (increased cough) • α-Blockers (decreased urethral tone)
Medications that exacerbate urge incontinence
• Diuretics (increased frequency and urgency)
Medications that exacerbate overflow incontinence
• A-B-C blockers: α-antagonists, β-blockers, calcium channel blockers • Regulated drugs: Narcotics and sedative-hypnotics

Abbreviation: ACE, angiotensin-converting enzyme.

> **Vaginal pessary**: Consider in women who wish to avoid surgery. Many women find them unacceptably uncomfortable.

Alternative 14.6.1

A 77-year-old woman presents with urinary incontinence. She reports that she frequently has an urge to use the bathroom but often cannot make it in time. She has some symptoms for a number of years, but over the last 5 days frequency, urgency, and incontinence have gotten considerably worse. Her only medication is hydrochlorothiazide for hypertension. Urinalysis demonstrates positive leukocyte esterase (LE) and nitrites.

What is the most likely cause of her incontinence?

Frequency and urgency suggest that this patient has urge incontinence. Positive LE and nitrite indicate the recent worsening of symptoms is the result of bladder irritation by a urinary tract infection (UTI).

> Urge incontinence is the leading cause of incontinence in elderly women.

Acute symptoms resolve after treating the UTI with trimethoprim-sulfamethoxazole (TMP-SMX). Baseline symptoms persist.

What are the next steps in management?

The initial step is lifestyle measures as described earlier. In this particular patient, consider switching from hydrochlorothiazide to another antihypertensive. The second-line measure is behavioral therapy (frequent voluntary voiding and biofeedback). The third-line measure is antimuscarinic medications (e.g., oxybutynin and tolterodine) with or without topical estrogen.

> Medications are not very effective for stress incontinence.
> Surgery is not very effective for urge incontinence.

Alternative 14.6.2

A 62-year-old woman presents with urinary incontinence. Her undergarments are often wet, particularly in the morning. When she tries to use the bathroom, she has difficulty voiding. She denies frequency, urgency, or dysuria. She has a history of type 2 DM and diabetic neuropathy in her lower extremities. She takes insulin and gabapentin. HbA1c measurement 2 months ago was 9.1%. Urinalysis and urine culture are normal. PVR is 120 mL.

What is the most likely diagnosis?

Difficulty with voluntary voiding, dribbling, nocturnal bedwetting, and large PVR indicates that she has overflow incontinence. The most likely cause is neurogenic bladder due to uncontrolled DM. The most important step in management is to correct the underlying cause (in this case, improve glycemic control). Other measures are intermittent self-catheterization (most effective) and α-blockers.

CASE 14–7 Urinary Hesitation and Dribbling in Men

A 58-year-old man has multiple issues with urination. He frequently has the urge to urinate, but when he goes to the bathroom he has difficulty voiding. He says his urinary stream is considerably weaker than in his younger years. Symptoms have slowly progressed over the last few years.

What is the most likely cause of these symptoms?

Benign prostatic hyperplasia is the most common cause of slowly progressive frequency, urgency, hesitation, and weak urinary stream in middle-aged and older men. In this disorder, prostate enlargement causes outlet obstruction.

What is the next step in management?

Perform DRE and obtain urinalysis, serum creatinine, and fasting blood glucose to screen for other causes of overflow incontinence in men such as cancer (bladder or prostate), infection (UTI or prostatitis), stones, or DM (neurogenic bladder). Other optional tests are prostate-specific antigen (PSA) (to screen for prostate cancer) and PVR (to confirm overflow incontinence).

The prostate gland is symmetrically enlarged, smooth, and firm on DRE. Urinalysis and serum chemistry are normal.

What is the next step in management?

DRE findings are characteristic of benign prostatic hyperplasia. First-line therapy in symptomatic patients is α-blockers (offers immediate benefit). If symptoms persist, add a 5-α reductase inhibitor to the regimen (finasteride or dutasteride).

Alternative 14.7.1

A 58-year-old man presents with frequency, urgency, hesitation, and overflow incontinence. Urinalysis, serum creatinine, and serum glucose are normal. There is nodularity and irregularity on DRE.

What diagnosis should you suspect?

Prostate nodularity or asymmetry (irregularity) should raise suspicion for prostate cancer. Adenocarcinomas account for 95% of prostate cancers. Prostate cancer is the most common cancer in adult men (incidence increases with age). Initial stages are usually asymptomatic. Later, patients develop symptoms of urinary outflow obstruction. Sometimes, the initial symptom is that of metastasis to the bones (e.g., back pain).

> Some prostate adenocarcinomas remain well-differentiated and clinically insignificant, whereas others rapidly grow and metastasize.

What are the next steps in management?

The next step is to obtain PSA. Then, perform transrectal ultrasound (TRUS)-guided biopsy regardless of PSA level.

> Prostate manipulation (e.g., DRE, transrectal biopsy, and ejaculation) can falsely elevate PSA. Obtain PSA either before or at least 24 hours after prostate manipulation.

PSA is 11 ng/dL. The pathologist interprets the biopsy specimen as positive for adenocarcinoma with Gleason grade 7.

What additional tests are indicated?

The next step is to obtain radionuclide bone scan and CT scan of the abdomen and pelvis to evaluate for metastatic disease.

How would management differ if PSA were 4.4 ng/dL and the pathologist interpreted the biopsy specimen as adenocarcinoma with Gleason grade 3?

Imaging tests are not required if PSA is <10 and Gleason grade is <6 because risk of metastasis is low.

> **Gleason grade**: A pathologist grades histology in each of the two lobes of the prostate gland from 1 (well-differentiated) to 5 (poorly differentiated).

How would you manage an asymptomatic patient with normal DRE and PSA 5 ng/dL detected during routine screening?

Management of increased PSA with normal DRE is as follows:

1. **PSA > 10 ng/dL**: Perform TRUS-guided biopsy.
2. **PSA 4 to 10 ng/dL**: repeat PSA. If repeat PSA ≥4, perform TRUS-guided biopsy.
3. **PSA 2 to 4 ng/dL**: Monitor PSA annually. If PSA rises by ≥0.75 ng/dL, perform TRUS-guided biopsy.

How is prostate cancer treated?

1. **Early-stage disease**: Both surgery and radiation therapy are equally effective. An option in elderly patients is watchful waiting.
2. **Locally invasive disease**: Tumors that have invaded the capsule are typically treated with radiation therapy plus androgen deprivation therapy.
3. **Metastatic disease**: Treat with ADT (androgen deprivation therapy) (bilateral orchiectomy, GnRH agonists such as leuprolide or goserelin, or nonsteroidal anti-androgens such as flutamide). Most metastatic prostate cancers become resistant to androgen deprivation therapy within 2 years.

Alternative 14.7.2

A 28-year-old man presents with a 2-day history of fever, chills, dysuria, urinary hesitation, and dribbling. He can tolerate oral intake. The prostate is swollen and tender on DRE. Urinalysis reveals positive LE and nitrite. Urine cultures are pending. Vital signs are temperature 38.4°C, pulse 80 bpm, respirations 18/min, and blood pressure 130/80.

What is the most likely diagnosis?

Acute onset of fever, chills, dysuria, hesitation, or dribbling along with a tender prostate on physical exam is the characteristic presentation of acute bacterial prostatitis. The next step in this hemodynamically stable patient who can tolerate oral intake is empiric therapy with TMP-SMX or an oral fluoroquinolone until urine cultures return.

How would management differ if pulse were 120 bpm and blood pressure were 90/60?

Septic shock is not infrequent in patients with acute bacterial prostatitis. Treat with IV fluids and IV antibiotics (aminoglycosides plus fluoroquinolone). Tailor antibiotics when culture results are available.

> IV antibiotics are also indicated if the patient cannot tolerate oral intake.

The patient recovers from the episode of acute bacterial prostatitis. Over the next 12 months, he continues to have episodes of frequency and urgency. DRE during these episodes sometimes reveals mild tenderness but is often normal.

What diagnosis should you suspect?

Suspect chronic bacterial prostatitis when a man presents with multiple episodes of UTI-like symptoms, particularly if he has a history of acute bacterial prostatitis. DRE may or may not reveal prostate tenderness.

How can you confirm the diagnosis?

Consider the four-glass test to confirm the diagnosis:

1. **Glass 1**: Urinalysis and urine culture of first 10 mL of voided urine.
2. **Glass 2**: Urinalysis and urine culture of mid-stream voided urine.
3. **Glass 3**: Make the patient stop voiding; massage the prostate. Collect and culture any expressed secretions.
4. **Glass 4**: Urinalysis and urine culture of next 10 mL of urine after massage.

> Negative cultures do not rule out chronic bacterial prostatitis, so not all clinicians perform the four-glass test.

How is chronic bacterial prostatitis treated?

If the four-glass test identifies particular organisms, then tailor antibiotics towards those bacteria. Otherwise, consider a 4-week course of an oral fluoroquinolone.

> **Chronic prostatitis/chronic pelvic pain syndrome (prostatodynia)**: Suspect this diagnosis of exclusion if a man with frequent UTI-like symptoms with or without painful ejaculation and perineal pain has normal DRE, PSA, urinalysis, and persistently negative cultures.

CASE 14–8 Breast Complaints

A 30-year-old woman presents with a lump in her left breast. She noticed the lump 3 days ago. She also complains of mild left breast tenderness. On physical exam, there are two small nodules. The lumps are soft and mobile, with regular borders. The left breast feels nodular.

What is the most likely diagnosis?

Fibrocystic changes are the most common cause of breast lumps in premenopausal women. This benign condition usually causes diffuse "lumpiness" and nodularity in one or both breasts with or without breast tenderness. Some patients may have a single dominant breast mass. These changes are dependant on the menstrual cycle and often resolve.

What is the next step in management?

Observation for one to two menstrual cycles is the next step in this young woman with no physical signs of breast cancer (mnemonic: "***FISSH***": **F**ixed, **I**rregular borders, **S**ingle dominant mass, **S**ize ≥2 cm, and **H**ard). If symptoms persist, perform ultrasound or fine-needle aspiration biopsy (Fig. 14-6).

> **Mammography**: Low-dose x-rays to image the breast. Not used as a diagnostic test in women <35 years old because their breast tissue is very glandular (difficult to visualize). However, a single mammogram is recommended before the age of 35 years to obtain a baseline.

The patient's symptoms resolve. She presents 2 years later with a smooth, rubbery, freely mobile mass in her right breast. The mass is approximately 1.5 cm in size with regular margins. She has noticed the lump for 2 months now.

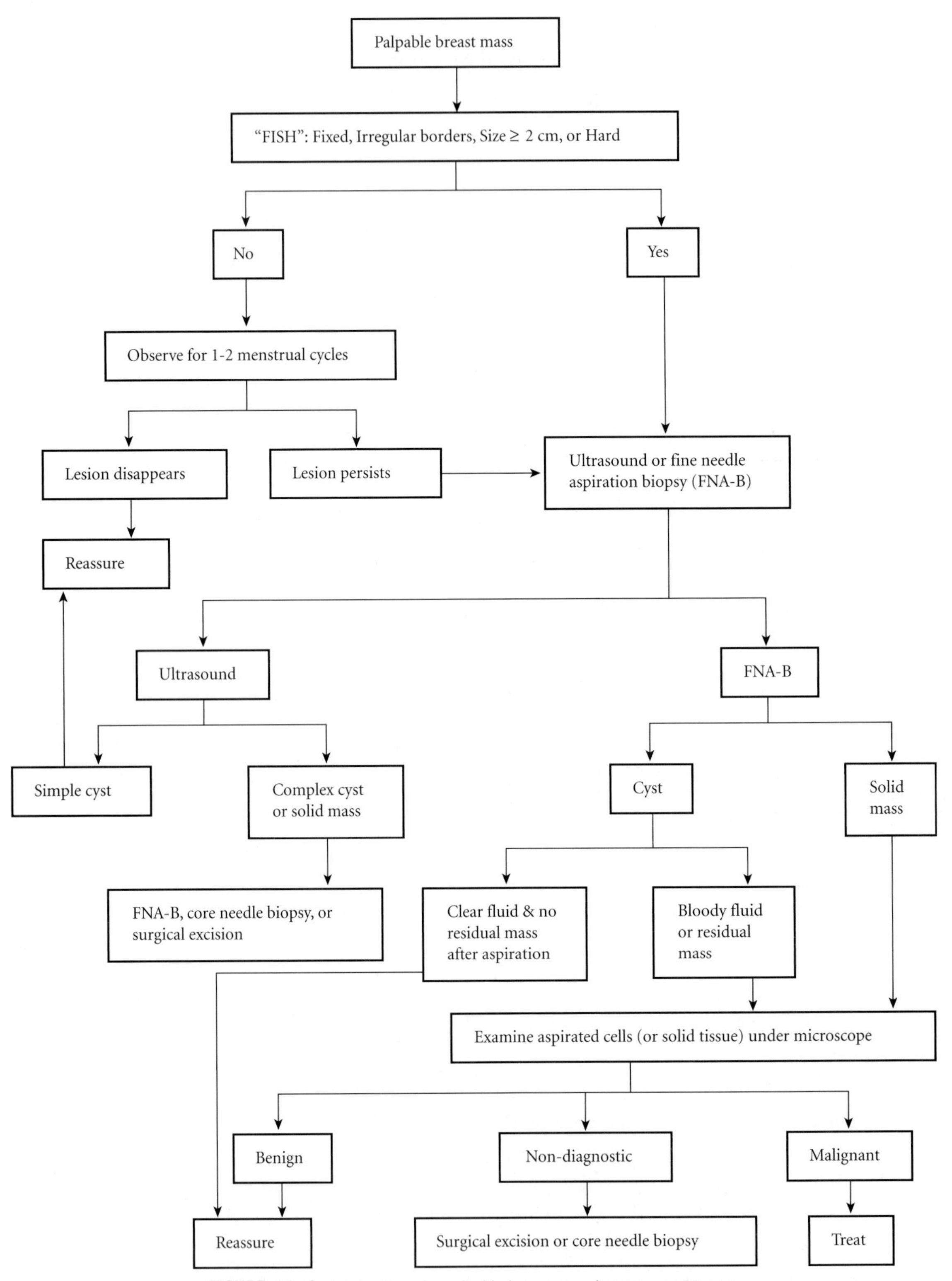

FIGURE 14–6 Evaluation of a palpable breast mass in women <35 years.

What is the most likely diagnosis?

A small, smooth, rubbery, well-circumscribed breast mass with regular margins in a premenopausal woman is most likely a benign fibroadenoma. Fibroadenoma is the most common cause of a dominant breast mass.

How should you manage this lesion?

Most physicians obtain ultrasound or fine-needle aspiration biopsy of this single dominant mass to rule out breast cancer (Table 14-6). Some physicians choose to observe a breast mass with classic features of fibroadenoma.

> Late breast cancer diagnosis is the leading cause of malpractice claims in the United States. More cases involve women <40 years old than older women.

After a careful discussion with her physician, the patient decides to observe the lesion. One year later, she presents with enlargement of the breast mass. She is in her third trimester of pregnancy. The smooth, rubbery, well-defined mass is now approximately 4 cm in diameter.

What is the next step in management?

Pregnancy and breast-feeding often stimulate fibroadenoma growth. In general, surgically excise fibroadenomas larger than 2 cm.

> Menopause causes fibroadenoma regression. Hormone replacement therapy stimulates fibroadenoma growth.

The fibroadenoma is successfully excised. The patient delivers a boy vaginally at term. She decides to breastfeed her baby. Two months after childbirth, she presents with a hard, red, tender area in her left breast. She also complains of fever and chills. Temperature is 38.3°C.

What is the next step in management?

The patient has mastitis (breast infection), which is common among nursing mothers. *Staphylococcus aureus* is the most commonly involved pathogen. First-line therapy is a 10- to 14-day course of dicloxacillin plus NSAIDs (for pain relief).

> **Plugged duct**: Localized area of milk stasis causes a tender lump but not fever or chills.

> **Breast abscess**: Symptoms of mastitis plus fluctuant mass. Treatment is antibiotics and drainage.

Alternative 14.8.1

A 52-year-old woman presents with a palpable lump in her right breast.

What is the next step in management?

The next step in any woman >35 years old with a palpable breast mass is mammography plus ultrasound or fine-needle aspiration biopsy (Fig. 14-7).

> **Risk factors for breast cancer**: age >40 years, female sex (breast cancer can occur in men), first-degree family history (consider testing for breast cancer genes BRCA 1 and 2 if early age at diagnosis in family members), increased endogenous estrogen (early menarche, late menopause, nulliparity, prolonged hormone replacement therapy, but not OCPs).

How would management differ if a suspicious lesion was detected on screening mammography but physical exam did not reveal a palpable mass?

Normal physical exam does not rule out cancer in women with a suggestive lesion on mammography (BI-RAD 4). The next step is core needle or excisional biopsy (Fig. 14-8).

Ultrasound detects a solid mass in the woman with a palpable lump. Mammography reveals microcalcifications suggestive of ductal carcinoma *in situ* (DCIS). Core needle biopsy confirms the diagnosis of DCIS.

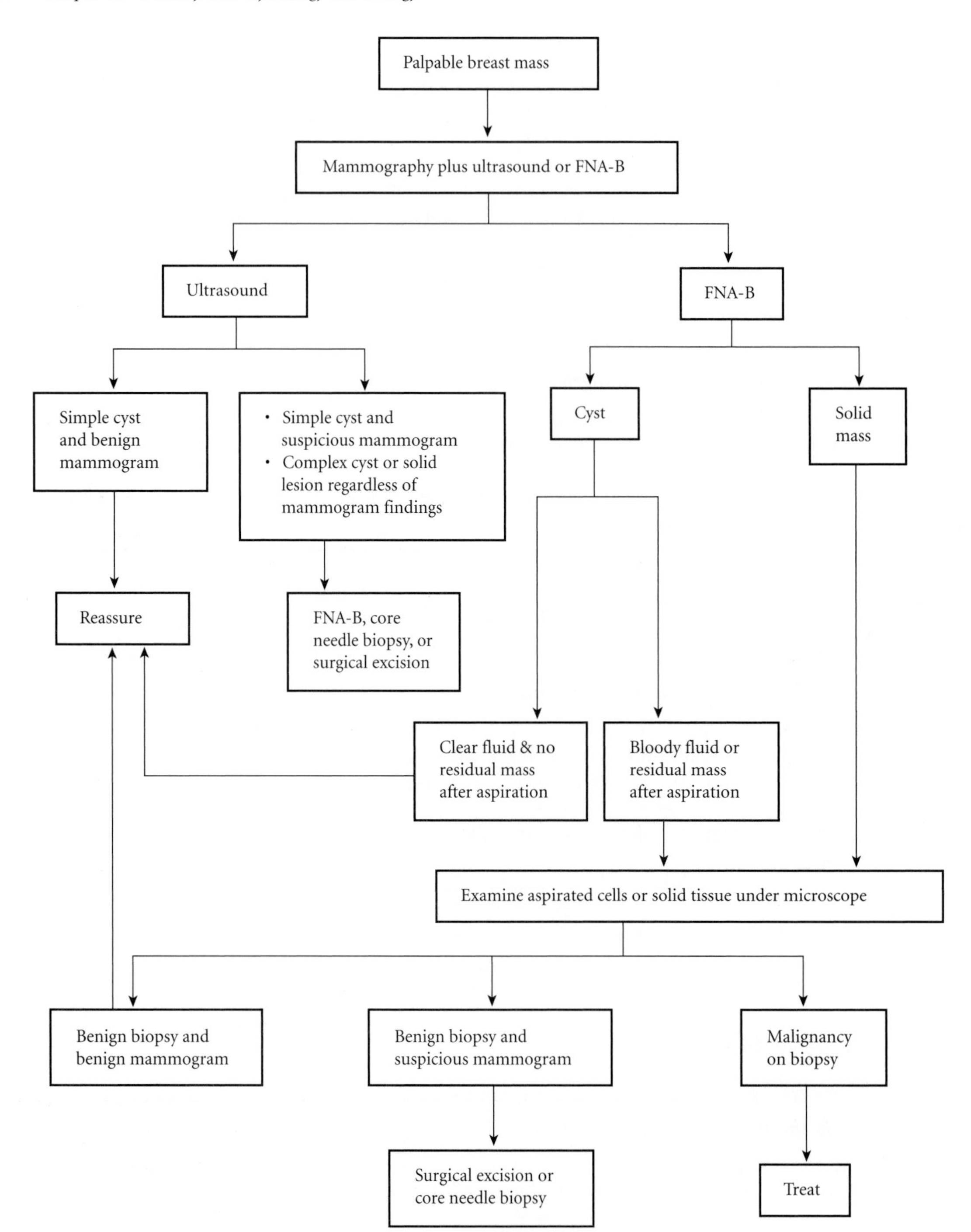

FIGURE 14–7 Evaluation of a palpable breast mass in women >35 years old.

How is DCIS treated?

DCIS typically appears as clustered microcalcifications on mammography. This precancerous lesion carries a high risk of progression to invasive breast cancer in the ipsilateral breast. Treatment options are:

1. **Lumpectomy**: Consider for small, low-grade lesion. At least 10-mm margins are recommended. If margins are <10 mm, consider radiation therapy as well.
2. **Mastectomy**: Preferred if size is >3 cm or high-grade lesion.

Lobular carcinoma *in situ*: Difficult to identify on physical exam or mammography. Increases risk of invasive carcinoma in both breasts by 1% per year. Treatment options are intensive surveillance, tamoxifen, or bilateral mastectomy.

How would management differ if the patient had invasive breast cancer?

First, use sentinel node biopsy to determine whether the tumor has spread to lymph nodes. Then, determine whether the tumor cells express estrogen receptors, progesterone receptors, or HER2-neu receptors. In general, treatment of nonmetastatic breast cancer (may or may not involve local lymph nodes) is as follows:

1. **Induction (neo-adjuvant) chemotherapy**: Decreases tumor burden prior to surgery.
2. **Surgery**: Perform mastectomy or lumpectomy plus radiation depending on patient preference (both have equivalent outcomes).
3. **Adjuvant therapy**: Consider chemotherapy for tumors ≥1 cm. Consider tamoxifen or an aromatase inhibitor (e.g., anastrazole) for tumors positive for estrogen or progesterone receptors. Consider trastuzumab (monoclonal antibody) for tumors positive for HER2-neu.

Inflammatory breast cancer: In this aggressive type of breast cancer, a lump is often absent. Initial presentation of this cancer is similar to mastitis. Later, patients may develop nipple retraction and red-orange, dimpled breast ("peau d'orange"). Prognosis is poor.

Breast cancer is the most common cancer in women.
Breast cancer is the second leading cause of cancer death in women.

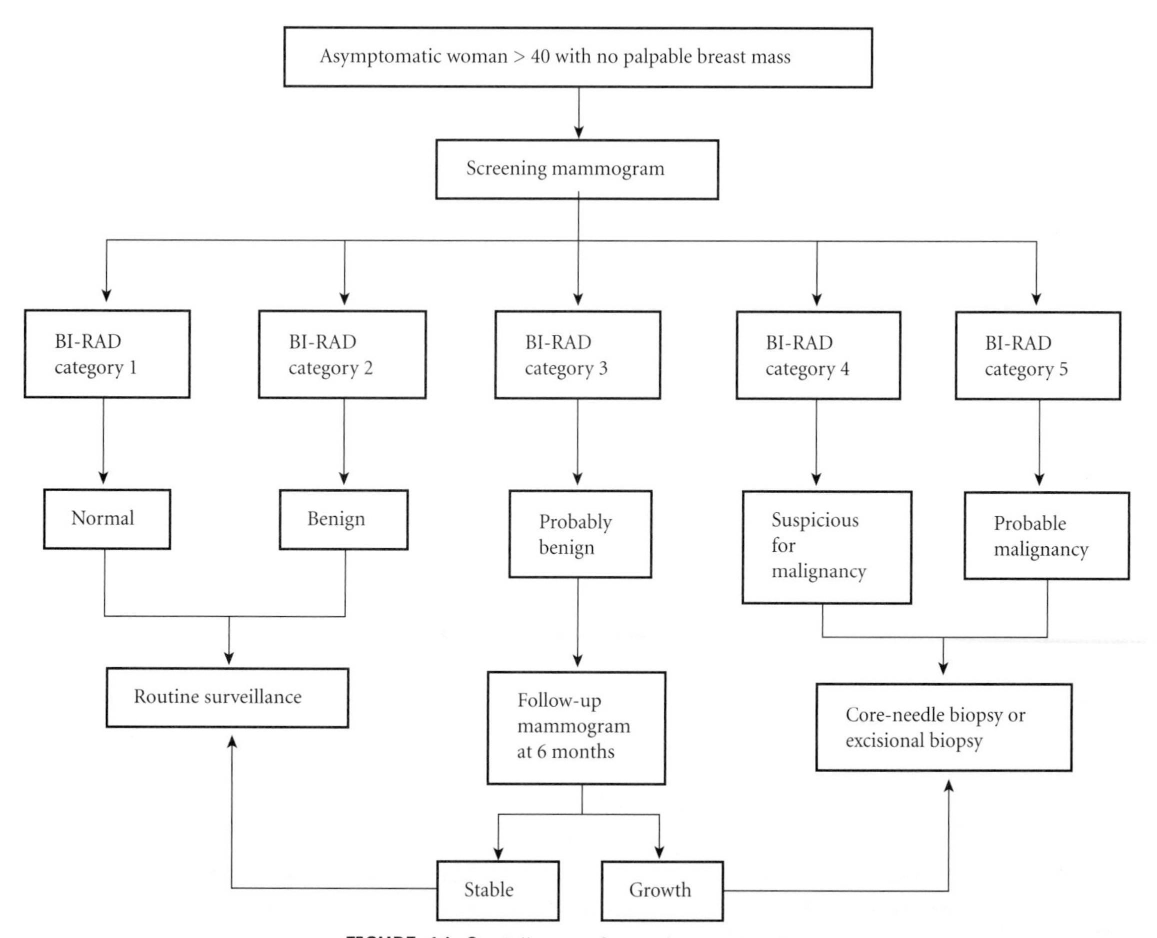

FIGURE 14–8 Follow-up of screening mammogram.

Alternative 14.8.2

A 36-year-old woman presents with unilateral clear nipple discharge. There is no palpable lump.

What is the next step in management?

Intraductal papilloma (benign neoplasm) is the most common cause of unilateral clear nipple discharge. The next step in any patient with unilateral discharge is mammography (ultrasound if <35 years old) and surgical exploration to rule out breast cancer.

How would management differ if she presented with bilateral clear nipple discharge?

Check the discharge for occult blood using a guaiac card. Evaluate any bloody nipple discharge (gross or occult) with cytology, mammography (ultrasound if <30 years old), and surgical exploration to rule out breast cancers. Evaluate non-bloody, bilateral nipple discharge with serum TSH and prolactin (to rule out endocrine causes).

> **Mammary duct ectasia**: Suspect this benign condition in women with unilateral or bilateral green-black nipple discharge. First-line therapy is hot compresses.

What diagnosis would you suspect if the woman presented with bloody staining of her bra without any obvious discharge and physical exam was significant for scale and erosions below the nipple?

Paget's disease presents with eczematous breast lesions with or without spotting of the bra with blood. This disorder results from *in situ* or invasive cancer, so cytology, mammography (ultrasound in women <35 years old), and surgical exploration are necessary.

CASE 14–9 Genital Lesions

A 27-year-old man presents to an STD clinic with a 7-day history of a painless lesion on his penis (Fig. 14-9). The lesion began as a painless papule that began to ulcerate. He has had unprotected sexual intercourse with three men and four women in the last 3 months. There is firm, painless, and bilateral inguinal adenopathy on physical exam.

TABLE 14–4 Inguinal Adenopathy and Constitutional Symptoms in Diseases With Genital Ulcers

Disorder	Lymph Node Timing	Lymph Node Appearance	Lymph Node Pain	Unilateral versus Bilateral	Constitutional Symptoms
Primary syphilis	Same time as ulcer	Firm lymph nodes	No	Usually bilateral	Absent
Lymphogranuloma venereum	~1 month after ulcer	Large fluctuant lymph nodes (bubo) ± lymphangitis	Yes	2/3 unilateral	Common
Granuloma inguinale	Varies	Pseudobuboes[a]	Yes	Varies	Uncommon
Chancroid	Same time as ulcer	Large fluctuant lymph nodes (bubo)	Yes	2/3 unilateral	Uncommon
HSV	Same time as ulcer	Firm lymph nodes	Yes	Usually bilateral	Common

Abbreviations: HSV, herpes simplex virus.
[a] Not true adenopathy. Lymph node swelling and pain is caused by infection of the lymph nodes by *Klebsiella granulomatis*.
Adapted from Stoller JK, Ahmad M, Longworth DL. *The Cleveland Clinic Intensive Review of Internal Medicine*, 3rd ed. Lippincott Williams & Wilkins, 2002, p. 168 (Table 14.3).

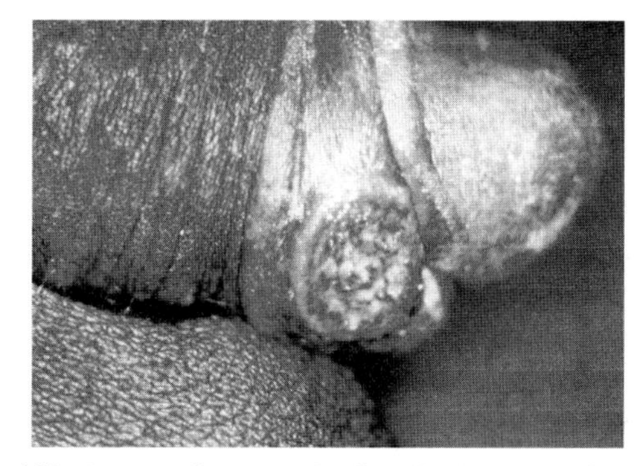

FIGURE 14–9 Chancre of primary syphilis. From Goodheart HP. *Goodheart's Photoguide of Common Skin Disorders*, 2nd ed. Lippincott Williams & Wilkins, 2003.

What is the most likely diagnosis?

The most likely diagnosis is primary syphilis (Tables 14-4 and 14-5). The classic chancre typically appears approximately 3 weeks after infection by the spirochete *Treponema pallidum.* The chancre is often absent or ignored, so first-degree syphilis often goes undiagnosed.

What is the next step in management?

The next step is to confirm the diagnosis. First-line test in this patient with a suggestive chancre is dark-field microscopy. *T. pallidum* appears as a spiral-shaped organism that moves back and forth. If dark-field microscopy is nondiagnostic, consider PCR or direct fluorescence antibody testing. Treatment is a single dose of IM benzathine penicillin G.

> **Syphilis screening**: Nontreponemal serological tests (RPR (rapid plasma reagin) and VDRL (venereal disease research laboratory)) are most commonly used to screen high-risk asymptomatic persons for syphilis. If the test is positive, confirm with a treponemal serological test (FTA-ABS (fluorescent treponemal antibodies) or MHA-TP (microhemagglutinationassay)).

TABLE 14–5 Differential Diagnosis of Genital Ulcers

Disease	Pathogen	Ulcer Description	Number of Ulcers	Pain	Duration
Primary syphilis	*Treponema pallidum*	Papule that progresses to clean, firm ulcer with a raised border	Single	No	3–6 weeks
Lymphogranuloma venereum	*Chlamydia trachomatis* L1–L3	Very small ulcer	Usually single	No	3–12 days
Granuloma inguinale	*Klebsiella granulomatis*[a]	Small nodules that burst and form an oozing ulcer	Single or multiple	No	Progressive
Chancroid	*Haemophilus ducreyi*	Soft ulcer with irregular, sharply defined border ± purulent material	Single or multiple	Yes	Progressive
HSV	HSV2 > HSV1	Grouped vesicles that progress to multiple shallow ulcers	Usually multiple	Yes	1–3 weeks

[a] Formerly called *Calymmatobacterium granulomatis*.

Adapted from Stoller JK, Ahmad M, Longworth DL. *The Cleveland Clinic Intensive Review of Internal Medicine*, 3rd ed. Lippincott Williams & Wilkins, 2002, p. 168 (Table 14.3).

One of the patient's sexual partners is identified at a primary care clinic. The 40-year-old man has fatigue, malaise, and a maculopapular rash on his palms, soles, and extremities. There is firm, rubbery, painless adenopathy in the cervical and axillary regions. There is no genital lesion.

What is the most likely cause of his symptoms?

Untreated primary syphilis can progress to secondary syphilis weeks to months after the chancre disappears. Secondary syphilis presents with constitutional symptoms and one or more of the following:

1. **Maculopapular rash**: This is the most common finding. Rash typically appears on palms, soles, and extremities (wear gloves because this rash is highly infectious!).
2. **Lymphadenopathy**: Painless, rubbery adenopathy in the cervical, axillary, and inguinal regions. Epitrochlear lymphadenopathy is highly suggestive.
3. **Laboratory abnormalities**: Increased LFTs or increased serum creatinine.
4. **Other**: Condyloma acuminata (smooth and moist outwardly growing genital lesions), synovitis, uveitis, and patchy alopecia ("moth-eaten alopecia").

> **Pityriasis rosea**: Idiopathic episodes of maculopapular rash on trunk and upper arms ± pruritus ± constitutional symptoms. Palms and soles are usually spared. "Herald patch" (initial, larger, salmon-colored patch) and "Christmas tree pattern" (seen in back lesions) are characteristic. Consider ultraviolet light therapy and topical steroids for severe symptoms.

How can you confirm that the 40-year-old man has secondary syphilis?

Serological tests are preferred to diagnose secondary syphilis (RPR and VDRL followed by FTA-ABS or MHA-TP). Treatment is similar to primary syphilis.

> **Jarisch-Herxheimer reaction**: Self-limiting fever, headache, and myalgias within 24 hours of penicillin administration. Treatment is NSAIDs.

Four months later, another sexual partner is located. This 27-year-old woman did notice a maculopapular rash a couple of months ago but is currently asymptomatic. RPR, VDRL, and FTA-ABS are positive.

Is any treatment necessary for this patient?

Positive syphilis serology in the absence of clinical signs and symptoms is termed latent syphilis. Latent syphilis in a person who acquired the infection <12 months ago is called early latent syphilis. Treatment with IM benzathine penicillin G is recommended to prevent transmission of infection and tertiary syphilis.

> **Late latent syphilis**: Infection was acquired >12 months ago. There is low risk of transmission.

What is tertiary syphilis?

Untreated latent syphilis can involve central nervous system (CNS), heart, or cause gummas years to decades later. With the advent of antibiotics, tertiary syphilis has become extremely rare.

1. **CNS**: Initially, spirochetes invade the cerebrospinal fluid and cause meningitis (often asymptomatic). Prolonged CNS infection can cause tabes dorsalis (posterior column invasion causes ataxia and sharp pain in the extremities) and general paresis (progressive dementia, difficulty speaking, and intention tremors).
2. **Cardiac**: Spirochetes invade the ascending thoracic aorta and cause aortic regurgitation. Long-term regurgitation can slowly progress to left heart failure.
3. **Gummas**: Large granulomas appear on the skin, bones, viscera, or subcutaneous tissues.

Tertiary CNS syphilis: treat with IV penicillin G for 10-14 days.
Cardiac tertiary syphilis or gummas: treat with weekly IM penicillin G for 3 weeks.

Alternative 14.9.1

A 28-year-old man presents with a 3-day history of painful penis ulcers. On examination, there are multiple grouped vesicles and shallow painful ulcers. He has tender bilateral inguinal adenopathy.

What is the most likely diagnosis?

The presentation is suggestive of genital HSV infection. Culture of vesicular fluid is recommended to confirm the diagnosis. Alternatives to culture are PCR or direct fluorescence antibody.

Tzank smear: Multinucleated giant cells indicate HSV or *Varicella zoster* virus. This test is less useful than culture of vesicular fluid, PCR, or direct fluorescence antibody.

What other organs can HSV affect?

1. **Oral herpes**: Painful vesicles or ulcers on the lips (associated with oral sex).
2. **Herpes proctitis**: More common in men who have sex with men.
3. **Whitlow**: Vesicles and pustules on the fingers ± lymphadenopathy.
4. **Herpes aseptic meningitis**: Occurs in 10% to 20% of primary HSV.
5. **Herpes autonomic nephropathy**: Occurs in 2% to 10% of primary HSV.
6. **Bell's palsy**: See Chapter 15: Primary Care Otolaryngology.

Disseminated HSV: Pneumonia, esophagitis, encephalitis, keratitis, and chorioretinitis can occur in immunocompromised patients.

Most genital herpes is caused by HSV Type 2. Most oral herpes is caused by HSV Type 1.

How is genital herpes treated?

Antiviral drugs can shorten symptom duration. Unfortunately, these drugs cannot completely eliminate the virus, so recurrent symptoms and viral shedding by asymptomatic patients is common. First-line therapy for primary and recurrent HSV is oral acyclovir. Valacyclovir is equally effective but more expensive.

HSV meningitis or disseminated HSV: Consider IV acyclovir instead.

HSV recurrences are usually less painful than primary HSV infection.

Alternative 14.9.2

A 32-year-old woman presents with a large and painful genital ulcer. The ulcer has sharp irregular borders. The base appears yellowish and bleeds when scraped. She also has large, fluctuant, painful inguinal lymph nodes on the left side. She emigrated from Senegal 2 weeks ago.

What is the most likely diagnosis?

The clinical presentation is characteristic of chancroid (Tables 14-4 and 14-5). This sexually transmitted infection is rare in the United States, but it is common in sub-Saharan Africa. Unlike syphilis, the ulcer and lymphadenopathy are painful. Unlike HSV, ulcers are not multiple and shallow. You must rule out syphilis and HSV with laboratory testing to make this diagnosis. Treatment is azithromycin or ceftriaxone.

> Appearance alone does not accurately distinguish between the different causes of genital ulcers, so some diagnostic tests are always indicated.

What diagnosis is more likely if the patient presents with large, fluctuant, painful lymph nodes but did not notice any ulcer?

The ulcer of *Lymphogranuloma venereum* is often not noticed because it is small. PCR is the first-line diagnostic test for this uncommon STD. First-line therapy is a 21-day course of doxycycline. Large buboes (fluctuant lymph nodes) may require needle aspiration.

> **Granuloma inguinale**: Perform ulcer biopsy if you suspect this rare STD. Classic finding is Donovan bodies (chromatin in mononuclear cells). Treatment is doxycycline.

> **Circinate balanitis**: Suspect if genital ulcer occurs in patient with signs of reactive arthritis (see Chapter 9: Rheumatology). Treat the ulcer with topical steroids.

Alternative 14.9.3

A 60-year-old Nigerian immigrant presents with an 8-month history of a painless penile ulcer. He has a history of genital warts. He smokes two packs of cigarettes every day. He is uncircumcised. The foreskin is difficult to retract and he says it has always been that way. There is painless inguinal adenopathy.

What diagnosis should you suspect?

Penis cancer is an uncommon neoplasm that can appear as an ulcer or as an exophytic mass (outwardly growing). Unlike other causes of painless ulcers (syphilis, *L. venereum*), the lesion is persistent. More than 50% of patients have painless inguinal adenopathy. The likelihood of penis cancer is increased in this patient with multiple risk factors: uncircumcised penis, phimosis (foreskin is difficult to retract), older age, African immigrant, smoker, and genital warts.

> Because presentation is nonspecific, consider biopsy of any persistent penile lesion.

What are genital warts?

Genital warts (condyloma acuminata) result from HPV infection (sexually transmitted). Like condyloma lata of secondary syphilis, they are pink and exophytic. Unlike condyloma lata, they are dry and verrucous (cauliflower-shaped). HPV infection increases the risk of penis cancer in men and cervical cancer in women. Diagnosis is clinical. Treatment options are:

1. **Topical chemicals**: podophyllin, trichloroacetic acid, or 5-FU gel.
2. **Immune modulators**: topical imiquimod or oral interferon.
3. **Excision**: cryotherapy, laser therapy, or surgical excision.

> **Pubic lice ("crabs")**: *Pthirus pubis* infection (STD) causes severe pubic itching. Lice are usually detected on visual inspection. Treat with 1% permethrin cream.

CASE 14–10 Hot Flashes

A 47-year-old woman complains of daily episodes of intense sensations of heat on her face and upper chest that lasts for a few minutes. The episodes are followed by shivering and perspiration. She also reports occasional night sweats. Her menstrual periods have been irregular for the last 6 months. She has no other medical conditions.

What treatment can you recommend to control her symptoms?

Episodes of night sweats, irregular vaginal bleeding, and hot flashes are characteristic symptoms of perimenopause (transition period to menopause). First-line therapy is a short, continuous course of estrogen (controls symptoms in 80%). Unless the patient has had a hysterectomy, prescribe concurrent progesterone to prevent endometrial hyperplasia. When she is ready to discontinue therapy, taper down the estrogen slowly because abrupt cessation leads to recurrence of symptoms.

> **Menopause**: No menstrual period for 12 months in a middle-aged woman. Vaginal dryness and osteoporosis are complications.

How would management of hot flashes differ if she had a history of breast cancer?

Breast cancer is a contraindication to estrogen replacement. First-line therapy for women with a contraindication to estrogen is venlafaxine. Other selective serotonin reuptake inhibitors and gabapentin have also demonstrated benefit.

CASE 14–11 Testicular pain

An 18-year-old man presents with a 2-hour history of severe right testicular pain. The symptoms began immediately after he played basketball. On physical exam, the right testis is diffusely swollen and exquisitely tender. The right testis is much higher than the left (high-riding testis) and oriented horizontally (bell clapper deformity).

What is the most likely diagnosis?

Acute onset of severe, diffuse testicular pain and swelling should raise suspicion for testicular torsion. High-riding testis and bell clapper deformity are classic findings on physical exam. The disorder results from twisting of the spermatic cord, which leads to testicular ischemia. Symptoms are often precipitated by vigorous physical activity. Testicular torsion is most common in young boys, although any age group is vulnerable. The next step in management of this patient with classic findings is emergent surgery.

> **Doppler ultrasound**: This method helps rule out testicular torsion if the diagnosis is equivocal.
> **Manual de-torsion**: Twist the testis laterally if surgery is not immediately available.

> **Cremasteric reflex**: Testis rises when the medial thigh is stroked. Absence of the reflex is a classic sign in young boys but an unreliable finding in adults.

Alternative 14.11.1

A 25-year-old man presents with a 7-day history of testicular pain. On physical exam, there is tenderness and blue discoloration localized to the anterior superior aspect of the right testis. There is no bell clapper deformity or high-riding testis. Cremasteric reflex is present.

What is the most likely diagnosis?

Subacute testicular pain localized to the anterior superior testis suggests torsion of the appendix testis (vestigial structure). Bluish discoloration in the tender area (blue dot sign) is the classic sign, although it is absent in 80% of patients. Like testicular torsion, this disorder is more common in young boys but can occur at any age.

What are the next steps in management?

The next step is to confirm the diagnosis with scrotal ultrasound. When ultrasound confirms the diagnosis, there are two treatment options: surgery or conservative therapy (rest, ice, NSAIDs, and scrotum elevation).

Alternative 14.11.2

A 23-year-old man presents with a 7-day history of testicular pain. On physical exam, the right testicle is tender. There is no high-riding testis, bell clapper deformity, or absence of the cremasteric reflex. There is no testicular or testicular appendix torsion on Doppler ultrasound of the scrotum.

What diagnosis should you suspect?

Subacute testicular pain with no evidence of testicular or testicular appendix torsion should raise suspicion for epididymitis (infection of the epididymis). Sexually transmitted infections are the most common cause in young men (especially *C. trachomatis*). Urinary tract pathogens such as *Escherichia coli* are more common in older men.

Noninfectious epididymitis: Prolonged sitting or vigorous exercise can cause reflux of urine into epididymis and result in chemical inflammation. Treatment is conservative.

What is the next step in management?

The next step is to obtain urinalysis and urine culture. Then treat empirically for gonorrhea and chlamydia while awaiting culture results.

Prehn's sign: Prehn reported that testicular elevation relieved testicular pain in epididymitis but not torsion. Later studies found that this finding was not reliable.

Alternative 14.11.3

A 37-year-old man presents with testicular pain and swelling. On examination, a hard and swollen mass can be traced up to the external inguinal ring. In the past he has often noticed a soft swelling at the inguinal ring that increased when he coughed and was easily reducible.

What is the most likely diagnosis?

An indirect inguinal hernia presents as a soft swelling at the inguinal ring that increases with Valsalva. The herniated bowel can migrate down the canal and into the scrotum. Normally, the patient should be able to push the bowel back into the abdomen easily (reducible). Inability to reduce the herniated bowel indicates that it is incarcerated (trapped) at the inguinal ring. Decreased blood supply to the incarcerated bowel can cause ischemia and necrosis of the incarcerated bowel (strangulation). Incarceration and strangulation present with pain and swelling. The next step in management is surgery.

Direct inguinal hernia: The bowel herniates through the triangle formed by the inferior epigastric artery (medial), inguinal ligament (inferior), and rectus muscle (medial).

Femoral hernia: The bowel herniates through empty space between the femoral vein and the lacunar ligament. This is less common than inguinal hernia but more likely to become incarcerated.

CASE 14–12 Painless Testicular Mass

A 32-year-old man presents with a painless testicular mass. On examination, there is a solid mass in the right testicle that does not transilluminate well. The man is a professional cyclist with no other symptoms or medical conditions.

What is the next step in management?

Rule out testicular cancer in any man with a solid testicular mass. The next step in management is scrotal ultrasound. If scrotal ultrasound is nondiagnostic, consider MRI. Also obtain serum alpha fetoprotein (increased in embryonal tumors) and β-hCG (increased in choriocarcinoma). If imaging is suggestive or if tumor markers are elevated, perform radical inguinal orchiectomy for histological confirmation. When the diagnosis is confirmed, perform retroperitoneal lymph node dissection, chest CT, and abdominopelvic CT scan for staging.

Do not perform scrotal biopsy because it increases risk of tumor seeding.

Testicular cancer is the most common solid tumor in men aged 18 to 40 years.

What diagnosis is more likely if the man with painless testicular swelling has a cystic scrotal sac on palpation that allows light to transilluminate well through the scrotum?

A hydrocele is an accumulation of peritoneal fluid between the parietal and visceral layers of the tunica vaginalis. Unlike testicular cancer, swelling is usually cystic and allows light to transilluminate. Most cases in the United States are idiopathic. Scrotal ultrasound is often performed to rule out reactive hydrocele (hydrocele that occurs in response to torsion or testicular cancer). No treatment is necessary for idiopathic hydrocele unless it is very uncomfortable (in which case, perform surgical excision).

Lymphatic filariasis: Lymphatic infection by the parasite *Wuchereria bancrofti* can cause massive thickening of the genitals (large hydroceles) and legs (elephantiasis). Diagnose with Giemsa-stained nighttime blood cultures. First-line therapy is diethylcarbamazepine.

What diagnosis is more likely if the patient reported a painless left testicular mass that increased on Valsalva and felt like "a bag of worms" on palpation?

The findings suggest that the patient has a varicocele. Varicoceles are dilations of the pampiniform plexus and are much more common on the left testis. They are a common cause of male infertility. Surgery is indicated if fertility is compromised and the man wishes to have a child. Otherwise, no specific therapy is necessary.

CASE 14–13 Erectile Dysfunction

A 58-year-old man presents with difficulty initiating and maintaining an erection.

What are common causes of erectile dysfunction (ED) in adults?

Remember causes of ED with the mnemonic "*Prince Albert Has Performance Anxiety*":

1. **Psychogenic**: Approximately 20% of cases of ED is caused by anxiety or interpersonal conflict.
2. **Atherosclerosis**: Cardiovascular disease and cardiovascular risk factors like DM, hypertension, and smoking.
3. **Hypogonadism**: Common causes are pituitary tumor and hypothyroidism.
4. **Perineal surgery, trauma, or lesions**: For example, fibrosis suggests Peyronie's disease.
5. **Alcoholism**

What features on history and physical exam would suggest that the man's ED is psychogenic in origin?

1. Rapid onset (symptoms seem to develop overnight).
2. Presence of spontaneous erections (e.g., during sleep).
3. No history or physical findings of organic causes.

The man says that he never has a spontaneous orgasm. He is in a healthy relationship with his wife. He does not smoke or drink alcohol. He does not have any other medical conditions or take any medications.

What further testing is indicated?

1. **Laboratory tests**: Consider CBC, serum chemistry, serum testosterone, TSH, and prolactin to rule out organic causes.
2. **Nocturnal penile tumescence (NPT)**: Devices are available that test the number and quality (e.g., rigidity) of erections during sleep. If NPT is abnormal, consider duplex ultrasound to search for areas of vascular obstruction. If NPT is normal, the patient likely has psychogenic ED.

How is ED treated?

The first-line measure is to correct any underlying psychogenic or organic dysfunction (e.g., marital counseling, smoking cessation, treatment of DM or hypogonadism). Second-line therapy is a 5-phosphodiesterase (5-PDE) inhibitor (e.g., sildenafil, vardenafil, or tadalafil). Third-line options are vacuum-assisted erectile devices or intracavernous injection of vasoactive drugs (alprostadil or papaverine). Consider surgical implantation of a penile prosthesis in motivated patients with refractory ED.

Contraindications to 5-PDE inhibitors: concurrent therapy with nitrates or α-blockers.

Premature ejaculation: First-line therapy is selective serotonin reuptake inhibitors. Second-line therapy is clomipramine.

chapter **15**

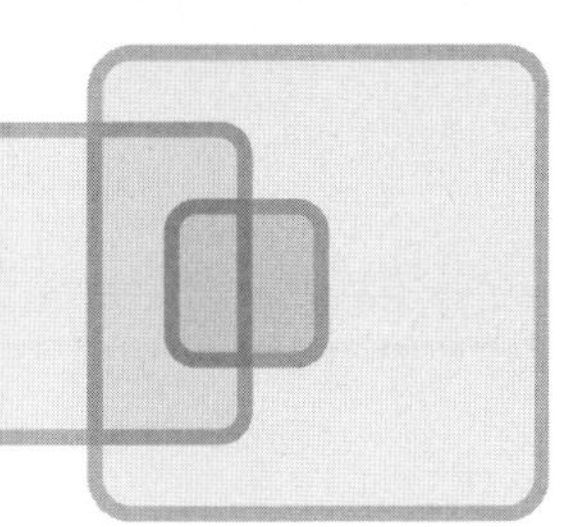

Primary Care Otolaryngology

CASE 15–1 PAINLESS HEARING LOSS

A 40-year-old woman reports a 4-week history of decreased hearing in her left ear.

What are the two broad categories of hearing loss?

Hearing loss (HL) is classified as conductive, sensorineural, or mixed:

1. **Conductive HL**: Sound is not transmitted effectively from the external auditory canal (EAC) and middle ear ossicles to the inner ear (Table 15-1).
2. **Sensorineural HL (SNHL)**: There is damage to the inner ear (cochlea) or to the nerve pathways between the inner ear and the brain (Table 15-2).

What physical exam test can document the presence of HL and distinguish between conductive HL and SNHL?

Physical examination of a patient with HL should include:

1. **Whisper voice test**: Whisper a series of letters and numbers into a patient's ear. The test is positive if the patient cannot repeat at least three consecutive characters.
2. **Rinne test**: Strike a 256- or 512-Hz tuning fork and place its base on the mastoid (sound is heard via bone conduction). When the patient no longer hears any vibration, place the tuning fork near the ear (sound is heard via air conduction). Normally, patients will hear vibrations of air conduction after the vibrations of bone conduction cease. In conductive HL, patients do not hear the vibrations of air conduction after those of bone conduction cease (i.e., in conductive HL, bone conducts better than air). In SNHL, Rinne test is normal.
3. **Weber test**: Place the struck tuning fork on the patient's forehead. Normally, patients hear sound equally in both ears. In conductive HL, sound lateralizes to the affected ear. In unilateral SNHL, sound lateralizes to the unaffected ear. The test is often normal in bilateral symmetric HL.
4. **Inspection**: Inspect the outer ear, EAC, and tympanic membrane (TM) for signs of obstruction, inflammation, or effusion.
5. **Pneumatic insufflation**: Perform this test to document whether the TM moves freely.

TABLE 15–1 Clues to the Diagnosis of Conductive Hearing Loss in Adults

Onset	Ear pain	Physical Exam	Suspected Diagnosis
Acute	Yes	EAC erythema; increased pain when auricle is pulled superiorly.	Otitis externa
Acute	Yes	Signs of middle ear effusion and inflammation.	Otitis media
Acute	No	Earwax completely occludes EAC.	Cerumen impaction
Gradual	No	Signs of middle ear effusion but no signs of middle ear or EAC inflammation.	TM effusion
Gradual	No	Retracted or perforated TM and drainage.	Cholesteatoma
Gradual	No	Bluish-red pulsating mass behind intact TM.	Glomus tumor
Gradual	No	Usually normal; 10% of patients have Schwartze's sign.	Otosclerosis

Abbreviations: EAC, external auditory canal; TM, tympanic membrane.
Adapted from Isaacson J. Differential diagnosis and treatment of hearing loss. *American Family Physician*. September 15, 2003, p. 1125–1132.

Remember the criteria of the Weber test with the mnemonic "***SUN CAFFE***": **S**ensorineural **UN**affected ear, **C**onductive **AFFE**cted ear.

Positive Rinne test is normal (air conduction > bone conduction). Negative Rinne test is abnormal (bone conduction > air conduction)

The patient is unable to distinguish characters whispered into her left ear. Hearing is normal in the right ear. Bone conduction is better than air conduction on the left. Sound lateralizes to the left ear when the tuning fork is placed on the patient's forehead. There is a large amount of earwax occluding the left EAC.

What is the most likely diagnosis?

Cerumen impaction is the most likely diagnosis in this patient with conductive HL and a large amount of earwax (cerumen). First-line therapy is EAC irrigation with normal saline at

TABLE 15–2 Clues to the Diagnosis of Sensorineural Hearing Loss in Adults

Onset	Symmetry	Other Clues on H&P	Audiogram	Suggested Diagnosis
Acute	Unilateral	Vertigo and tinnitus	Low frequency unilateral hearing loss	Ménière's disease
Acute	Unilateral	Vertigo, tinnitus, and nystagmus; recent facial trauma	Any unilateral abnormal test	Perilymphatic fistula
Acute	Bilateral	Fluctuating vertigo and hearing loss	Any abnormal test with poor speech configuration	Autoimmune hearing loss
Gradual	Bilateral	Elderly patient; chronic exposure to loud noise and cigarettes	Bilateral, symmetric high frequency loss	Presbycusis
Gradual	Bilateral	Exposure to loud noise; tinnitus	Bilateral, symmetric hearing loss at 4000 Hz	Noise-induced hearing loss
Gradual	Unilateral	May have vertigo, tinnitus, and facial nerve dysfunction	Any unilateral abnormal test	Acoustic neuroma (vestibular schwannoma)

Abbreviation: H&P, history and physical exam.
Adapted from Isaacson J. Differential diagnosis and treatment of hearing loss. *American Family Physician*. September 15, 2003.

room temperature. If impaction persists, consider instillation of a few drops of hydrogen peroxide, docusate sodium, or sodium bicarbonate into the EAC.

> Obtain formal audiological assessment (audiogram with tympanogram) if a patient exhibits no obvious cause for conductive HL.

Alternative 15.1.1

A 37-year-old woman presents with gradual onset of conductive HL and tinnitus. Family history is significant for HL in her maternal grandmother and maternal uncle. On ear examination, there is a reddish blush in the region of the promontory and oval window (Schwartze's sign).

What diagnosis should you suspect?

Suspect otosclerosis in this patient with gradual onset of conductive HL, tinnitus, family history of HL, and positive Schwartze's sign. This disorder results from fixation of the stapes to the oval window. Almost 70% of patients have a positive family history. Physical exam is normal except for conductive HL in most patients. Only 10% have positive Schwartze's sign.

What diagnostic tests are indicated in patients with suspected otosclerosis?

Patients with suspected otosclerosis should undergo audiological assessment, which typically demonstrates low-frequency HL with absence of stapedius reflex. Consider a CT scan (specific but not sensitive) if the diagnosis is still uncertain.

> **Human speech**: frequency ranges from 500 to 4000 Hz. Volume ranges from 40 to 60 dB.

How is otosclerosis treated?

First-line therapy for otosclerosis is stapedectomy. If the patient is not a surgical candidate or refuses surgery, options include fluoride and hearing aids.

What diagnosis would you suspect if the patient with gradual conductive HL had a negative family history and physical exam demonstrated a pulsating blue-red area behind the TM?

The physical findings suggest a glomus tumor. Magnetic resonance imaging (MRI) is the most reliable diagnostic test. Treatment of this benign neoplasm is surgical excision.

Alternative 15.1.2

A 75-year-old man presents with HL. The symptoms have progressed over the last 3 to 5 years. He does not take any medications. Whisper voice test is abnormal bilaterally. Rinne and Weber tests are normal.

What diagnosis should you suspect?

Presbycusis is the most common cause of SNHL in elderly patients. Risk factors include chronic exposure to loud sounds and cigarette smoking. Rinne test is normal because patients have SNHL. Weber test is often normal because HL is bilateral and symmetric.

> **MRI or CT scan**: initial diagnostic test for unilateral SNHL.
> **Audiologic assessment**: initial test for bilateral SNHL or unexplained conductive HL.

Audiogram demonstrates symmetric high-frequency HL.

How is presbycusis treated?

Treatment options include hearing aids, assisted listening devices, and cochlear implants.

> **Presbycusis screening:** Screen all elderly patients with the use of the whisper voice test.

What further tests should you consider if the patient with bilateral SNHL did not have typical findings on audiological assessment?

Obtain the following tests in patients with unexplained bilateral SNHL: complete blood count, fasting blood glucose, VDRL/RPR, and thyroid-stimulating hormone (because leukemia, diabetes mellitus (DM), syphilis, and thyroid disease can sometimes cause bilateral SNHL).

> **Drug-induced SNHL**: Loop diuretics, chemotherapy (cisplatin, 5-FU, and bleomycin), and antimicrobials (aminoglycosides, erythromycin, and tetracycline) can cause bilateral SNHL.

CASE 15–2 EAR PAIN AND CONDUCTIVE HEARING LOSS

Three days after recovering from an URI (upper respiratory infection), a 27-year-old man presents with a 2-day history of right ear pain (otalgia), discharge (otorrhea), and HL. On physical exam, the TM is erythematous and bulging. There is decreased TM mobility on pneumatic insufflation. Rinne test is abnormal. When a tuning fork is placed on the middle of the forehead, sound lateralizes to the right ear. Temperature is 39.1°C.

What is the most likely diagnosis?

Suspect acute otitis media (AOM) in this patient with acute onset of ear pain, ear discharge, conductive HL, and fever after an URI. This person meets all three diagnostic criteria for AOM:

1. Acute onset of ear symptoms
2. Signs of middle ear effusion (bulging TM, decreased TM mobility, or ear discharge)
3. Signs of middle ear inflammation (ear pain or ear erythema)

What is the next step in management?

Streptococcus pneumoniae, *Haemophilus influenza*, and *Moraxella catarrhalis* are the most common pathogens associated with AOM. Prescribe amoxicillin to this patient with all three diagnostic criteria and temperature >39°C.

How would management differ if the patient did not meet all three diagnostic criteria and temperature was 37.9°C?

Consider a 24 to 48 hour observation period if the diagnosis is uncertain and temperature is <39°C.

Two weeks later, the patient reports continued HL in his right ear. Physical exam demonstrates bulging TM and conductive HL. There is no ear pain or erythema.

What is most likely cause of these findings?

Effusion is a common complication of AOM. Patients have signs of ear effusion and HL, but no signs of ear inflammation. Most effusions resolve without any specific therapy.

The patient's HL resolves. One year later, he has another episode of AOM that is treated with amoxicillin. Two weeks after the episode of recurrent AOM, he presents with otalgia, otorrhea, and conductive HL. Physical exam demonstrates TM perforation.

What is the next step in management?

AOM is the most common infectious cause of TM perforation. Perform audiometry to confirm and establish a baseline for the degree of conductive HL. Treatment is usually supportive (avoid swimming or diving, use a petroleum jelly–coated cotton swab to cover the ear while bathing, and use analgesic ear drops). Consider surgery if the patient has severe conductive HL or persistent drainage.

Cholesteatoma: increased risk with TM perforation. Causes conductive HL and chronic drainage. Remove surgically because it can invade inner ear and facial nerve.

Alternative 15.2.1

A 52-year-old man presents with a 2-day history of left ear pain and drainage. On physical exam, the EAC is erythematous. There is conductive HL in the left ear. Pain increases when the auricle is pulled superiorly. The TM is not bulging. TM mobility is normal. Vital signs are normal.

What is the most likely diagnosis?

The most likely diagnosis is otitis externa. The classic sign is increased ear pain when the auricle is pulled superiorly. Patients may have otalgia, otorrhea, conductive HL, and EAC erythema, but no signs of a middle ear effusion. The most common cause is bacterial infection.

How is otitis externa treated?

Treatment involves the following steps:

1. Aural toilet (ear cleaning): This is the most important aspect of management. Use a cerumen wire loop or cotton swab with or without hydrogen peroxide irrigation to clean the EAC.
2. Topical ear drops: Use an acidic ear drop that contains an antimicrobial with coverage against *Staphylococcus aureus* and *Pseudomonas aeruginosa.* The solution should also contain steroids (to decrease ear pain). Fluoroquinolones (ciprofloxacin or ofloxacin) are the most commonly used antimicrobial in otic solutions.

How would management differ if the patient had type 2 DM?

Diabetics and immunosuppressed patients have an increased risk of necrotizing otitis externa (infection that spreads to cartilage, bone, or soft tissue). Add an oral fluoroquinolone to the regimen (to cover pseudomonas) if the patient has DM, immunosuppression, or any signs of inflammation extending beyond the ear canal. Also, obtain an MRI and consult a head and neck surgeon (otolaryngologist).

CASE 15–3 VERTIGO

A 32-year-old man presents with a 2-week history of dizziness. He describes his symptoms as a sensation of the room "spinning." The symptoms are provoked by moving around in bed, looking up or down, or moving from a upright or seated position to a horizontal position. He does not have any sensation that he is about to faint or any sensation of leg or trunk unsteadiness. He does not report any headaches, photophobia, or sonophobia. He does not take any medications. Neurological exam is normal. Vital signs are normal.

What type of dizziness do the patient's symptoms suggest?

Patients often describe a number of differing symptoms as "dizziness":

1. **Vertigo**: sensation of motion (of self or surroundings) when there is no motion.
2. **Dysequilibrium**: leg or trunk unsteadiness on standing or walking.
3. **Lightheadedness**: feeling that one is about to faint in a few moments.
4. **Mixed dizziness**: dizziness that does not fit into any of the above categories.

This patient with a sensation of spinning most likely has vertigo.

What is the differential diagnosis of vertigo?

1. Central vertigo originates in the central nervous system; causes include migraine-induced vertigo, multiple sclerosis, and brainstem or cerebellar stroke or transient ischemic attack.

2. Peripheral vertigo is caused by a defect in the vestibular nerve or cochlear apparatus. The most common causes are benign positional vertigo, vestibular neuritis, and Ménière's disease. Other important causes are endolymphatic fistula, medications, otosclerosis, cholesteatoma, acoustic neuroma (vestibular schwannoma), and Ramsay-Hunt syndrome.

> Constant (nonepisodic) vertigo for months is probably psychogenic.

Is central or peripheral vertigo more likely in this patient?

Peripheral vertigo is more likely in this patient. Patients with migraine-induced vertigo usually have other symptoms of migraine headaches. Other common causes of central vertigo usually exhibit/induce brainstem or cerebellar signs (see Chapter 12: Neurology).

The patient's head is tilted back approximately 20° and to the left approximately 45°. With his head tilted, he is quickly moved to a lying position, and eye movement is observed for 30 seconds. At approximately 15 seconds, there is vertical nystagmus.

What is the diagnosis?

The patient has benign positional vertigo, which is the most common cause of vertigo. The disorder results from calcium debris (otoconia) in the posterior semicircular canal. Patients have brief episodes (seconds) of vertigo provoked by head movement. The Dix-Hallpike maneuver described above is the key physical finding (positive in 50% to 80% of patients). First-line therapy is repositioning maneuvers such as Brandt-Daroff, Epley, or Semont maneuvers.

Alternative 15.3.1

Five days after an upper respiratory infection, a 32-year-old man presents with a 12-hour history of vertigo, nausea, and vomiting. On physical exam, gait is unstable. Dix-Hallpike maneuver is negative. When the head is turned rapidly to the right, his eyes cannot maintain visual fixation. Otherwise, neurological examination is negative. Vital signs are normal.

What is the most likely diagnosis?

The most likely diagnosis is vestibular neuritis (also called vestibular neuronitis). In this disorder, viral infection or postviral inflammation of the vestibular nerve leads to acute onset of vertigo, nausea, vomiting, abnormal gait, and nystagmus. The key physical finding is a positive head thrust test (when the head is turned toward the side of the lesion, the eyes cannot maintain visual fixation).

> **Vestibular labyrinthitis**: symptoms of vestibular neuritis + HL.

> **MRI**: Obtain in patients with dizziness and one or more focal neurological signs (e.g., abnormal gait) to rule out central vertigo.

Brain MRI is negative.

How is vestibular neuritis treated?

First-line therapy is oral corticosteroids. Also consider symptomatic treatment with antiemetics and vestibular suppressants (anticholinergics or antihistamines) in the first 24 to 48 hours. The disorder is usually self-limiting and resolves within a few days.

> Do not administer vestibular suppressants after 48 hours in vestibular neuritis (delays recovery).

Alternative 15.3.2

A 43-year-old woman presents with five episodes of vertigo, nausea, and vomiting over a 2-week period. She describes the episodes as the room rotating for 20 minutes to 1 hour. The episodes are preceded by loud ringing (tinnitus), HL, and a sensation of fullness in her left ear. There is no history of recent viral infection. She does not take any medications. Neurological exam is normal. Dix-Hallpike and head thrust maneuvers are negative. There are no brainstem signs.

What is the most likely diagnosis?

The most likely diagnosis is Ménière's disease. Patients experience tinnitus, SNHL, and aural fullness followed by vertigo, nausea, and vomiting. The usual pattern is a cluster of episodes interspersed with a long asymptomatic period.

> The three diagnostic criteria for Ménière's disease are:
> 1. Vertigo: at least two episodes of rotatory vertigo lasting ≥20 minutes.
> 2. Tinnitus (or aural fullness) in the affected ear.
> 3. SNHL in the affected ear.

What diagnostic tests should you order at this time?

All patients with suspected Ménière's disease should undergo audiometry to detect SNHL. Also, consider brain MRI to rule out central causes of vertigo.

What causes Ménière's disease?

Ménière's disease results from increased fluid buildup in the endolymphatic spaces of the inner ear. This disorder is usually idiopathic. In cases in which this disorder is caused by neurosyphilis, DM, thyroid disease, or a central nervous system disease, it is termed Ménière's syndrome.

Audiometry detects SNHL. MRI is negative. VDRL/RPR is negative. Fasting blood glucose and thyroid-stimulating hormone levels are normal.

How is Ménière's disease treated?

First-line therapy is effective in 90% of cases and includes lifestyle measures (dietary restriction of salt, caffeine, and tobacco) plus medications (diuretics ± betahistine). If symptoms persist, consider invasive procedures (e.g., instillation of gentamycin into the affected ear, endolymphatic decompression surgery, etc.).

> **Perilymphatic fistula**: Abnormal communication between fluid-filled inner ear and air-filled middle ear. Consider if the patient has symptoms similar to Ménière's disease immediately after head trauma or scuba diving, and symptoms worsen with Valsalva (coughing, sneezing, etc.). Treatment is stapedectomy.

CASE 15–4 SORE THROAT

A 22-year-old woman presents with a 3-day history of sore throat and malaise. She has pain on swallowing. She denies any cough. She has never had sexual intercourse or oral sex. She received all her childhood vaccinations. On physical examination, there is tender anterior cervical adenopathy and pharyngeal erythema but no exudates. Temperature is 38.2°C.

What is differential diagnosis of acute pharyngitis?

1. Viral infections: 90% of acute pharyngitis in adults is the result of viral infection. Common viral causes of acute pharyngitis are adenovirus and infectious mononucleosis (due to Epstein-Barr virus or cytomegalovirus). Primary HIV is an infrequent cause, but identification is important if this infection is suspected.
2. Bacterial infections: The most common bacterial cause of sore throat is group-A β-hemolytic streptococcus (GABHS), commonly referred to as "strep throat." *Neisseria gonorrhea* and *Corynebacterium diphtheria* are infrequent causes, but identification is important if these infections are suspected.

A viral cause is more likely if the patient has the ***3 Cs*** (**C**ough, **C**oryza, **C**onjunctivitis).

It is important to distinguish GABHS from viral pharyngitis because antibiotics are indicated in the management of the former but not the latter.

What is the next step in management?

Although no single clinical finding reliably distinguishes viral pharyngitis from bacterial pharyngitis, the Centor criteria are widely used to determine the likelihood of GABHS (Table 15-3). This 22-year-old patient with fever, tender cervical adenopathy, and absence of cough (3 points) should undergo testing for GABHS using the rapid strep test. If the test is positive, treat with penicillin V or amoxicillin. If the test is negative, antibiotics are not necessary.

Centor criteria mnemonic: "*FAT T.A.*" (**F**ever, **A**ge, **T**onsillar swelling or exudates, **T**ender cervical adenopathy, and **A**bsence of cough).

Rapid strep test is positive. The patient is allergic to penicillin.

What treatment is indicated?

If a patient with strep throat is allergic to penicillin, treat with erythromycin.

Treatment of streptococcal pharyngitis can prevent the complication of rheumatic fever but cannot prevent poststreptococcal glomerulonephritis.

What infection should you rule out if the patient with fever, tender cervical adenopathy, and absence of cough also had a history of recent oral sex and a greenish exudate was seen on physical exam?

Suspect gonococcal pharyngitis if the patient has a history of recent oral sex, multiple sexual partners, dysuria and discharge, or greenish pharyngeal exudates. Diagnose with Gram stain and culture nasopharyngeal swabs. Treat with a third-generation cephalosporin such as ceftriaxone or cefixime. Also administer azithromycin because the patient may have concurrent *Chlamydia trachomatis* infection.

What infection should you rule out if the patient with fever, tender cervical adenopathy, and absence of cough did not receive her childhood vaccinations and physical exam revealed an adherent, grayish-white pharyngeal membrane that bled when scraped?

Suspect *C. diphtheria* infection (pseudomembranous pharyngitis) if the patient has an adherent, grayish pharyngeal membrane that bleeds with scraping, unilateral serosanguinous nasal discharge, or appears toxic (i.e., signs of shock). The next step is to obtain nasopharyngeal swabs for culture and draw blood to test for diphtheria toxin antibodies. Then, initiate empiric

TABLE 15-3 Centor Criteria (a clinical decision rule for strep throat)

Criterion	Points
Fever (subjective or measured in office)	+1
Absence of cough	+1
Tender anterior cervical adenopathy	+1
Tonsillar swelling or exudates	+1
Age <15 years	+1
Age 15 to 45 years	0
Age >45 years	−1

Score: ≤0, infection ruled out; 1–3, order rapid test and treat accordingly; 4–5, initiate empiric antibiotics without testing.

therapy with antibiotics (penicillin G or erythromycin) and diphtheria antitoxin before laboratory results are available. Close contacts also require monitoring for signs of infection.

> With widespread DtaP vaccination, pseudomembranous pharyngitis has decreased dramatically.

Alternative 15.4.1

A 23-year-old man presents with a 3-day history of fever, sore throat, malaise, cough, and rhinorrhea (coryza). The pharynx is erythematous with petechiae and exudates. There is tender posterior cervical adenopathy and splenomegaly. Because he has fever, cervical adenopathy, and pharyngeal exudates, rapid strep test is performed; results are negative.

What diagnosis should you suspect?

Suspect infectious mononucleosis when a young patient with fever, sore throat, and malaise has posterior cervical adenopathy, palate petechiae, or splenomegaly.

> Sore throat is much more likely with Epstein-Barr virus than with cytomegalovirus infection.

What is the next diagnostic step?

Obtain white blood cell count and a heterophile antibody test (e.g., monospot test). Reactive heterophile antibodies are considered diagnostic of infectious mononucleosis.

> Leukocytosis with increased atypical lymphocytes is the most common laboratory abnormality in infectious mononucleosis.

The patient has leukocytosis with atypical lymphocytes but monospot test is negative.

What is the next step in management?

Heterophile antibodies are negative in up to 30% of patients during the first week of illness, but are very sensitive after the first week. Consider repeating the test if this patient with characteristic manifestations continues to have symptoms after 7 days.

> **False-positive monospot test**: Occasionally, disorders such as leukemia or first-degree HIV can cause reactive heterophile antibodies in the absence of Epstein-Barr virus or cytomegalovirus infection.

How is infectious mononucleosis treated?

Treatment of infectious mononucleosis is symptomatic. Treat fever and sore throat with acetaminophen or nonsteroidal anti-inflammatory drugs (NSAIDs). The patient should also avoid contact sports for 21 days after the onset of symptoms to prevent splenic rupture.

> **Ampicillin** causes a maculopapular rash in patients with infectious mononucleosis.

> **Airway obstruction** is a rare but serious complication of mononucleosis. If the patient has difficulty breathing, initiate corticosteroids and immediately refer to an otolaryngologist.

CASE 15–5 THROAT PAIN AND DYSPNEA

A 58-year-old man presents with a 10-hour history of severe throat pain, dyspnea, and odynophagia. He appears extremely uncomfortable. He is leaning forward and drooling. He has difficulty opening his mouth (trismus), and his tongue is pushed up. The submandibular area is swollen and tender. Vital signs are temperature 38.9°C, pulse 110 bpm, blood pressure 130/90, and respirations 25/min. Oxygen saturation is 98% on room air.

What is the most likely diagnosis?

Suspect a deep neck space infection in patients with fever, throat pain, and any of the following: dyspnea, odynophagia, neck swelling, or trismus. Most deep space infections are polymicrobial (caused by oral flora). Deep neck space abscesses that push the tongue posteriorly and threaten to strangle the patient are called Ludwig's angina. Ludwig's angina typically occurs as a result of the extension of mandibular molar infection into the submandibular space.

> Patients with Ludwig's angina often lean forward to increase airway patency and thereby reduce dyspnea.

What are risk factors for deep neck space infections?

Major risk factors are dental procedures, poor dental hygiene, and immunosuppression.

What are the next steps in management of this patient with Ludwig's angina?

1. Airway: Assess airway patency in all patients with dyspnea with the use of a flexible fiberoptic scope. If the airway is sufficiently patent, consider elective intubation. If the airway is not patent enough or if oxygen saturation is rapidly dropping, perform tracheotomy instead.
2. Empiric antibiotics: The first-line antibiotic choice in immunocompetent patients is ampicillin-sulbactam. If the patient is allergic to penicillin, use clindamycin.
3. Imaging: Obtain CT scan and lateral radiographs of the neck to assess the extent of infection after ensuring an adequate airway and initiating antibiotics.
4. Needle drainage: Consider this only if symptoms do not improve despite 2 to 3 days of antibiotics.

Alternative 15.5.1

A 23-year-old woman presents with a 6-hour history of throat pain, dyspnea, and odynophagia. She has difficulty opening her mouth. Her voice sounds as if there were a hot potato inside. On physical exam, the soft palate and anterior pillar of the left tonsil are swollen. The uvula is displaced to the right. Temperature is 38.6°C.

What is the most likely diagnosis?

Peritonsillar abscess (quinsy) is the most likely diagnosis in this patient with signs and symptoms of a deep space infection along with the characteristic "hot potato voice" and uvular deviation (due to unilateral tonsillar swelling). Most cases occur in patients aged 15 to 30 years.

What are the next steps in management?

First, perform needle drainage. Then, initiate ampicillin-sulbactam.

Alternative 15.5.2

A 50-year-old man is brought by a neighbor to the emergency department for evaluation of throat pain, dyspnea, odynophagia, and neck pain. There is swelling and erythema at the angle of the mandible. Temperature is 39°C. Oxygen saturation is 99%.

What diagnosis should you suspect?

Suspect a parapharyngeal abscess in this patient with signs and symptoms of a deep space infection and swelling at the angle of the mandible. The next step is to initiate ampicillin-sulbactam and quickly localize the infection with lateral radiographs and/or CT scan. When the infection is localized, perform needle drainage of the abscess.

Retropharyngeal abscess: Suspect if neck pain and other signs of deep space infection are present but there is no clear area of swelling. Diagnose with lateral radiographs and CT scan. Treat with needle drainage and ampicillin-sulbactam. This condition is more common in children.

The patient leaves the emergency department against medical advice before any treatment can be attempted. Two days later, he presents with bleeding from his nose, ears, and mouth.

What complication should you suspect?

Parapharyngeal space infections can spread to the carotid artery and cause carotid artery rupture. The initial presentation often includes "herald bleeds" (small amounts of bleeding from the ears, nose, and mouth). Emergent surgery is necessary to prevent impending death.

Necrotizing mediastinitis: This condition occurs if retropharyngeal or parapharyngeal abscess spreads to posterior mediastinum. This condition can cause empyema, pleural and pericardial effusions, and cardiac tamponade. Treatment is thoracotomy drainage and intravenous antibiotics.

CASE 15–6 FACIAL PAIN

A 54-year-old woman presents with recurrent episodes of severe facial pain. She describes the pain as "electric shocks" on her left cheek, left nose, and left jaw that last for approximately 20 to 30 seconds. Physical exam and vital signs are normal.

What is the most likely diagnosis?

Episodes of shock-like pain in the distribution of a particular nerve are called neuralgias. This patient with shock-like pain in the distribution of the trigeminal nerve has trigeminal neuralgia. Most cases result from compression of the trigeminal nerve root by an aberrant artery or vein. Diagnosis is usually clinical. Consider MRI to rule out a structural lesion such as a tumor compressing cranial nerve 5 if the patient is "***BUSY***" (**B**ilateral facial pain, **U**nresponsive to medical therapy, **S**ensory loss, **Y**ounger than 40 years old).

V2 and V3 are more commonly affected than V1 in trigeminal neuralgia.

How is trigeminal neuralgia treated?

First-line therapy for trigeminal neuralgia is the anticonvulsant carbamazepine. If the patient continues to have severe pain, consider a combination of anticonvulsants. If pain is unresponsive to medical therapy, consider a surgical procedure (e.g., microvascular decompression, radiofrequency rhizotomy, or gamma-knife radiosurgery).

Phenytoin can provide acute pain relief while oral medications are titrated.

Alternative 15.6.1

A 67-year-old man presents with a 2-day history of severe burning pain on the right side of his face. On physical exam, there is a vesicular eruption in the distribution of V1.

What is the diagnosis?

The patient has herpes zoster (i.e., shingles). This condition occurs most frequently in older patients as a result of reactivation of latent *Varicella zoster* virus, which travels along nerve fibers and causes a painful vesicular eruption along any unilateral dermatome.

How is herpes zoster treated?

Initiate antiviral therapy within the first 72 hours of symptom onset. First-line therapy is valacyclovir. Acyclovir is a less expensive but less effective alternative. Famciclovir is also effective in the treatment of symptoms of *Varicella zoster* virus.

What additional therapy is often administered to patients with shingles and why?

Many patients continue to experience pain months to years after the rash resolves. This complication is called postherpetic neuralgia (PHN) and is difficult to treat. In addition to antivirals, administer tricyclic antidepressants (TCAs) such as amitriptyline or nortriptyline during initial symptom onset to prevent PHN. Gabapentin is an alternative if a patient cannot tolerate TCAs.

> **Zoster vaccine (zostavax)**: Consider in all patients >60 years old to prevent zoster and PHN. Do not administer during a symptomatic episode. Contraindicated in immunocompromised and pregnant patients.

Alternative 15.6.2

A 67-year-old man presents with a 2-day history of severe burning pain on his left cheek, facial paralysis, and vertigo. On physical examination, he is unable to close his left eyelid or move the left side of his mouth. There are vesicles on the pinna of his left ear.

What is the most likely diagnosis?

Peripheral cranial nerve 7 paralysis along with ipsilateral facial pain and vesicles on the pinna of the ipsilateral ear are highly suggestive of Ramsay-Hunt syndrome. Patients with Ramsay-Hunt syndrome can also have vertigo, tinnitus, and HL. This disorder is caused by reactivation of *Varicella zoster* virus (or less frequently herpes simplex virus) along cranial nerve 7 (facial nerve). Treatment is as described for shingles.

> **Central versus peripheral lesions**: Upper motor neuron (central) lesions affecting cranial nerve 7 spare the eyelids, whereas lower motor neuron (peripheral) lesions typically do not.

What diagnosis would you suspect if the patient with acute onset of peripheral cranial nerve 7 paralysis did not have facial pain, vesicles, or any other symptoms?

Suspect Bell's palsy if a patient with acute onset of peripheral cranial nerve 7 paralysis does not have other findings suggestive of Ramsay-Hunt syndrome. The most likely cause of Bell's palsy is herpes simplex virus infection. Facial paralysis is generally less severe than Ramsay-Hunt syndrome, and a greater percentage of patients have a complete recovery. Bell's palsy is typically treated with steroids and valacyclovir (although studies have not clearly demonstrated that these drugs are effective).

> Lyme disease and HIV infection can also cause acute onset of cranial nerve 7 paralysis. Rule out these conditions if other findings/risk factors for HIV or Lyme disease are present.

How would management differ if the patient had gradual onset of facial nerve paralysis?

Gradual onset of cranial nerve 7 paralysis is more suggestive of a tumor than of Bell's palsy or Ramsay-Hunt syndrome. The next step in this case is CT scan or MRI of the brain.

Alternative 15.6.3

A 60-year-old man presents with a 2-week history of pain and swelling in the left submandibular area. The symptoms occur when the patient eats and resolve between meals. There is a hard "bump" in the region of Wharton's duct.

What diagnosis should you suspect?

Salivary gland pain and swelling that is worse with meals should raise suspicion for sialolithiasis (salivary gland stone). The stone is often palpable in Wharton's duct (for submandibular stones) or Stensen's duct (for parotid stones).

> Sialolithiasis occurs most frequently in the submandibular gland.

> Stones that completely obstruct the ducts can cause persistent pain and swelling.

What is the next step in management?

No further diagnostic testing is necessary in this patient with characteristic symptoms and a palpable stone. The next step is to advise conservative measures:

1. Promote stone passage: Increase fluid intake, massage the gland, and apply moist heat to the gland.
2. Increase salivation: Use sialogogues (e.g., lemon drops) and stop anticholinergics.
3. Analgesia: Use acetaminophen or NSAIDs.

> Confirm the diagnosis using CT scan without contrast if the stone is not palpable.

How would management differ if the patient had a painless solid salivary gland mass?

Consider fine-needle aspiration (with or without ultrasound guidance) of any solid salivary gland mass to rule out neoplasm. Important nonneoplastic causes of unilateral or bilateral salivary gland pain or swelling include autoimmune disorders (Sjögren's syndrome), infections (bacteria such as *S. aureus*, mumps, and HIV), stones, and sarcoidosis.

> Masses in larger glands have a larger likelihood of being benign (e.g., 75% of parotid masses are benign, but only 25% of submandibular masses are benign).

The patient begins conservative measures. One week later, he presents with increased and persistent pain, swelling, and erythema. There is pus draining from the duct. Temperature is 38.4°C.

What is the next step in management?

The patient has bacterial superinfection (sialadenitis) of the salivary gland. Treat with a 7- to 10-day course of antistaphylococcal antibiotics (dicloxacillin or cephalexin). Consider surgical removal after the infection resolves.

Symptoms persist despite 7 days of dicloxacillin.

What is the next step in management?

Consider urgent surgery if symptoms of superinfection persist despite a course of antibiotics (patient may have an abscess).

Alternative 15.6.4

A 34-year-old woman presents with aching facial pain that increases when she chews on food. She reports pain in her cheeks and ears. On physical exam, there is pain on palpation of the temporomandibular joint (TMJ).

What is the diagnosis?

The patient has TMJ syndrome, which presents with dull aching pain in the muscles of mastication while chewing. Pain may radiate to the ears and posterior cervix. TMJ tenderness is the key diagnostic finding. Ear and neck examination should be normal.

What causes TMJ syndrome?

The most common causes of TMJ syndrome are increased jaw clenching and bruxism (psychogenic grinding of the teeth). Other causes include degenerative joint disease, jaw malocclusion, trauma, and iatrogenic TMJ (dental manipulation, cervical traction, etc.).

There is no history of trauma or recent surgery. Dental examination does not reveal any malocclusion.

How is TMJ syndrome treated?

Treatment of TMJ syndrome usually involves conservative measures:

1. Avoid precipitating factors such as jaw clenching and bruxism.
2. Analgesia: NSAIDs are only effective in conjunction with jaw-opening exercises. If the patient does not wish to perform jaw-opening exercises, consider TCAs or muscle relaxants such as cyclobenzaprine.

CASE 15–7 MANAGEMENT OF NOSEBLEEDS

A 27-year-old man calls the urgent care clinic to find out what to do about a nosebleed (epistaxis) that has persisted for the last 10 minutes.

What should you tell the patient?

The initial step in controlling a nosebleed is to apply direct pressure to the nasal alae for at least 5 minutes. Also consider plugging the affected nostril with gauze or cotton and sit with the head bent forward (to prevent blood from pooling in the posterior pharynx).

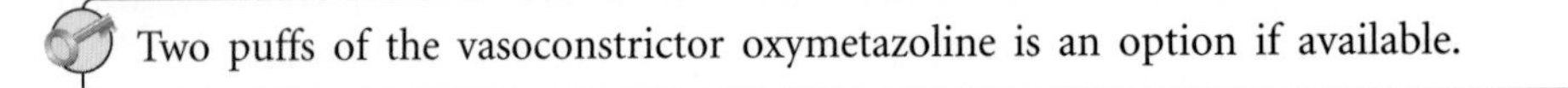

Two puffs of the vasoconstrictor oxymetazoline is an option if available.

The patient arrives to the urgent care clinic. The nosebleed has persisted despite 20 minutes of the initial recommended measures. He has no trouble speaking or breathing. Vital signs are normal.

What are the next steps in management?

If bleeding persists despite 20 minutes of initial measures, examine the nares using a nasal speculum. Anterior epistaxis is more common (particularly from Kiesselbach's plexus), but posterior epistaxis carries a much greater risk of significant hemorrhage.

Always assess hemodynamic status at initial presentation and initiate intravenous fluids if the patient is unstable.

Hypertension does not cause nosebleeds but can increase nosebleed severity. Studies have not shown a benefit from lowering blood pressure during an epistaxis episode.

An anterior source is identified.

What is the next step in management?

The next step is cautery (electrical or chemical cautery with a silver nitrate stick). If cautery is not successful, perform nasal packing with Xeroform gauze, nasal tampon, or nasal catheter. When bleeding has resolved, refer for follow-up in 24 to 48 hours. Always prescribe an oral antibiotic such as Augmentin or a topical antibiotic such as mupirocin in patients with nasal packing in place to prevent staphylococcal toxic shock syndrome.

If nasal packing does not stop the nosebleed, posterior epistaxis is likely. Treat with Foley catheter tamponade and admit to the hospital.

Alternatives to packing are surgical hemostatic products such as floseal gel.

When are laboratory studies indicated in the management of epistaxis?

1. **Complete blood count, type and crossmatch**: Obtain if the patient is hemodynamically unstable.
2. **Coagulation studies**: Obtain if the patient is on anticoagulation therapy (e.g., warfarin).

chapter **16**

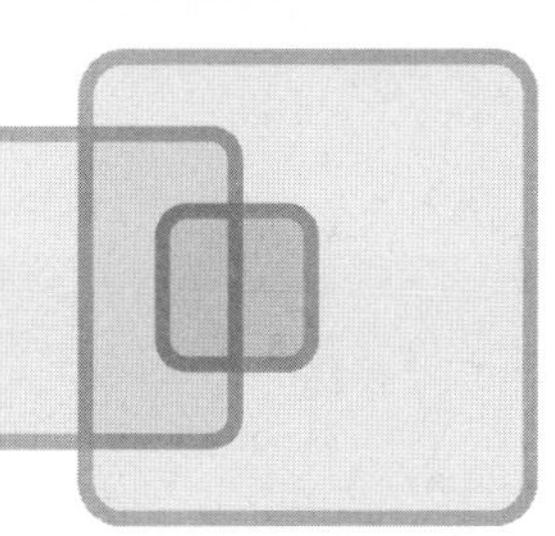

Primary Care Ophthalmology

CASE 16–1 GRADUAL LOSS OF VISUAL ACUITY

A 70-year-old man presents with 6 months of progressively worsening visual loss. He reports blurry vision, difficulty reading, and a blind spot in the center of the visual field. He denies any migraine headache. Visual acuity is 20/100 in both eyes. Pinhole test does not improve visual acuity. Ophthalmoscopy is performed (Fig. 16-1).

What does the finding of 20/100 visual acuity indicate?

Visual acuity is usually measured using a Snellen chart in the primary care setting. Normal visual acuity is described as 20/20 vision (patient can see at 20 feet what a person with normal vision can see at 20 feet). 20/100 visual acuity indicates the patient can see at 20 feet what a person with normal vision can see at 100 feet (Table 16-1). The most common cause of decreased visual acuity in all age groups is refractive error, also known as ametropia (error in focusing light that can be corrected with glasses or contact lenses).

> **E test**: An alternative to the Snellen test in illiterate or cognitively impaired patients.

> **Best corrected visual acuity**: Allow patients to wear their glasses or contact lenses when testing visual acuity.

What is the significance of the finding that pinhole mask does not improve visual acuity?

A pinhole mask test can be performed in the primary care setting. The patient covers his or her eyes with a dark mask that has small holes in front of the pupil. If visual acuity does not improve, suspect a nonrefractive cause.

What are the most common causes of chronic visual loss in the elderly?

The most common nonrefractive causes of chronic visual loss in the elderly are cataracts, glaucoma, age-related macular degeneration (ARMD), and diabetes mellitus.

What findings are evident on ophthalmoscopy?

Ophthalmoscopy reveals numerous yellow deposits in the macula (central area of retina). These deposits are termed drusen, and they are the earliest findings of ARMD. ARMD results from macular atrophy.

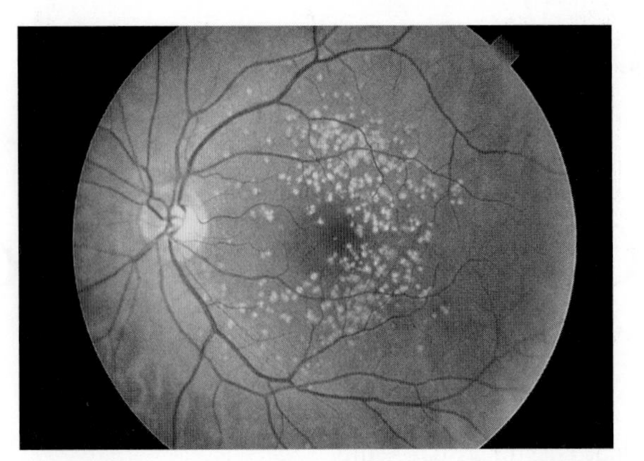

FIGURE 16–1 Eye image: Dry, age-related macular degeneration (drusen). From Tasman W, Jaeger E. *The Wills Eye Hospital Atlas of Clinical Ophthalmology,* 2nd ed. Lippincott Williams & Wilkins, 2001.

Ophthalmoscopy is performed in a dark room in the primary care setting. The test is more sensitive when the eye is dilated in an eye specialist's office.

Early ARMD (nonexudative or "dry" ARMD): Main finding is drusen.
Intermediate ARMD: Drusen coalesce; dark spot in macula (due to atrophy).
Advanced ARMD (exudative or "wet" ARMD): Subretinal fluid and hemorrhage.

What are common initial symptoms of ARMD?

Common initial symptoms are blurry vision, difficulty reading, and central scotoma (because atrophy occurs in the center of the retina).

How should you treat this patient?

Unfortunately, effective therapy is not available for dry ARMD. Consider antioxidants such as vitamin C, vitamin E, β-carotene, zinc, and copper. Also, monitor for disease progression with frequent dilated eye exams and the Amsler grid test.

The patient does not return for his follow-up appointment. He presents 2 years later with a 10-day history of line distortion (straight lines seem wavy). What is the most likely cause of his symptoms?

Line distortion that develops over days to weeks is most likely caused by wet ARMD (best assessed with the Amsler grid test). In addition to antioxidants, treatment options for wet ARMD are intravitreous VEGF inhibitors, thermal laser photocoagulation, and photodynamic therapy. Macular translocation surgery is an option for patients with refractory wet ARMD.

Alternative 16.1.1

Routine dilated eye examination of a 70-year-old man with hypertension and type 2 diabetes mellitus detects visual acuity of 20/100 that is not corrected with a pinhole mask. Dilated eye exam is performed (Fig. 16-2). Intraocular pressure (IOP) measured by tonometry is 25 mm Hg. Automated perimetry demonstrates marked decline in peripheral visual fields.

TABLE 16–1 Classification of Visual Acuity (best corrected visual acuity)

Mild impairment	20/20 to 20/60
Moderate impairment	20/60 to 20/200
Severe impairment	20/200 to 20/400
Profound impairment	<20/400

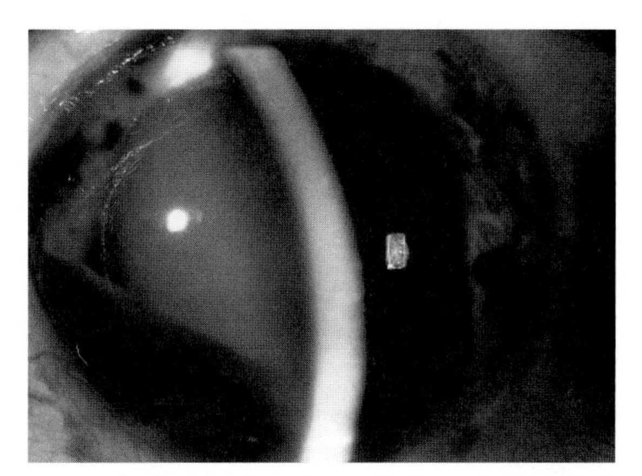

FIGURE 16–2 Eye image: Primary open angle glaucoma. From Tasman W, Jaeger E. *The Wills Eye Hospital Atlas of Clinical Ophthalmology*, 2nd ed. Lippincott Williams & Wilkins, 2001.

What diagnosis should you suspect?

The three characteristic features of primary open angle glaucoma (POAG) are:

1. **Optic nerve atrophy**: Suggested by increased hollow appearance of the central cup in the optic disk.
2. **Increased IOP**: Normal IOP is 11 to 21 mm Hg.
3. **Visual field**: Loss of peripheral vision gradually progresses to the center.

> **Visual field testing**: Automated perimetry is much more sensitive at detecting early peripheral vision loss due to glaucoma than confrontation testing with fingers.

What is the pathophysiology of POAG?

POAG accounts for 90% of glaucoma in adults. Impaired clearance of aqueous humor from the anterior chamber leads to gradual increase in IOP, which predisposes to optic nerve atrophy. Because visual loss begins in the periphery and progresses to the center, patients are often asymptomatic until late in the course. As a result, POAG is often termed the "sneak thief of sight."

> Some patients with glaucoma have normal IOP (normotensive glaucoma). Some patients with increased IOP and visual loss do not have signs of optic nerve atrophy.

How does open angle glaucoma differ from angle closure glaucoma?

Acute angle closure glaucoma results from rapid buildup of aqueous humor in the anterior chamber. Unlike POAG, presentation is acute onset of pain and visual loss.

> **Secondary glaucoma**: Causes include drugs (steroids), inflammation (uveitis), primary ocular disorders (e.g., pseudo-exfoliation), and ocular trauma/surgery.

What are risk factors for developing glaucoma?

The four major risk factors for glaucoma are older age, elevated IOP, black race, and first-degree family history of glaucoma. Consider screening eye examinations every 1 to 2 years after the age of 40 years in patients with any of these risk factors.

> **Screening patients without risk factors**: The American Academy of Ophthalmology and the American Optometric Association recommend comprehensive eye exam in all persons ≥40 years old. The U.S. Preventive Services Task Force (USPSTF) does not recommend for or against comprehensive eye exam in persons without risk factors.

How is POAG treated?

1. Medical therapy: First-line therapy for POAG is β-blocker eye drops (decrease aqueous humor production) or prostaglandin eye drops (improve aqueous humor clearance). Other medical options include cholinergic eye drops, adrenergic eye drops, or carbonic anhydrase inhibitor eye drops.
2. Laser therapy: Indicated if medical therapy is not effective.
3. Surgery: Indicated for glaucoma refractory to medications and laser therapy.

Alternative 16.1.2

A 70-year-old woman presents with a 6-month history of gradually worsening vision loss. She reports blurry vision and difficulty reading books as well as signs at night. She has had reading glasses since the age of 50 but mentions that she did not need to use them for a couple months before the visual loss began. Visual acuity is 20/100 in both eyes and is not improved with a pinhole mask. Ophthalmoscopy demonstrates an opacified lens and loss of red reflex.

What is the most likely cause of her symptoms?

Cataracts can cause gradually progressive painless visual loss. Patients often notice that near vision improves transiently before visual loss begins ("second sight"). Typical eye findings are corneal opacity and loss of red reflex. Surgery is very effective and is indicated for visual loss that significantly interferes with daily activities.

> **Risk factors**: age (most important), smoking, alcohol, diabetes, and steroids.

CASE 16–2 PAINLESS RED EYE

A 24-year-old man presents with a 3-day history of red eye with watery discharge and a gritty sensation in his eyes. Symptoms initially began in his left eye, but spread to his right eye a day later. He denies any photophobia. There is diffuse erythema of the bulbar and palpebral conjunctiva. Eye examination is otherwise unremarkable. There is a tender, enlarged pre-auricular node.

When is urgent referral to an ophthalmologist necessary in patients with red eye?

History and seven-step evaluation (Table 16-2) help identify alarm findings that warrant urgent ophthalmology referral (mnemonic: "***Please Find A Clever Ophthalmologist, HoNey!***"):

1. **P**hotophobia.
2. **F**oreign body sensation (objective): Inability to open the eye or keep it open.
3. **A**cuity of vision decreases (compared to baseline).
4. **C**iliary flush: Maximal erythema is in area surrounding cornea.
5. **O**pacification of the cornea.
6. **H**yphema (blood in anterior chamber), **H**ypopyon (pus in anterior chamber), and severe **H**eadache.
7. **N**onreactive pupil (dilated or constricted).

> **Subjective foreign body sensation**: "Grittiness" or "sandiness" in the eye does not necessarily warrant ophthalmology referral.

What is the most likely diagnosis?

Diffuse injection of both the bulbar and palpebral conjunctiva suggests that the patient has conjunctivitis. Both viral and allergic conjunctivitis can cause watery discharge, but a viral infection is more likely in this person with a tender pre-auricular node. Viral conjunctivitis

TABLE 16–2 Seven-step Primary Care Evaluation of the Red Eye

1. Visual acuity	Normal	Conjunctivitis Subconjunctival hemorrhage Pterygium
	Decreased	*"Angling KIT"*[a]
2. Conjunctiva injection	Diffuse	Conjunctivitis
	Localized	Subconjunctival hemorrhage, pterygium
	Ciliary flush	*"Angling KIT"*[a]
3. Discharge	Clear	Viral (conjunctivitis, keratitis, or iritis) Allergic conjunctivitis Acute angle glaucoma
	Reddish yellow	Trauma
	Purulent	Bacterial infection
4. Corneal opacity	Diffuse	Ultraviolet keratitis Acute angle closure glaucoma
	Localized	Herpes keratitis Corneal ulcer
5. Anterior chamber	Shallow	Acute angle closure glaucoma
	Hyphema	Trauma
	Hypopyon	Bacterial infection
6. Pupils	Constricted	Corneal abrasion, keratitis, iritis
	Dilated	Acute angle closure glaucoma
7. Other findings	Preauricular node	Viral conjunctivitis
	Colored halos	Acute angle closure glaucoma
	Itching	Allergic conjunctivitis
	Pain, photophobia	*"Angling KIT"*[a]

[a] Mnemonic: *"Angling **KIT**"*: **A**cute angle closure glaucoma, **K**eratitis, **I**ritis, and **T**rauma.
Adapted from Canadian Ophthalmological Society. http://www.eyesite.ca.

typically causes red eye, gritty sensation, and watery discharge in one eye 1 to 2 days before symptoms begin in the other eye. Treatment is symptomatic (warm or cool compresses and antihistamine decongestant eye drops).

> Red eye is the most common eye complaint in primary care settings. Conjunctivitis is the most common cause of red eye in the primary care setting.

Alternative 16.2.1

A 29-year-old woman presents with bilateral eye itching and watery discharge. Inspection demonstrates injection of both palpebral and bulbar conjunctiva. There are no alarm findings. There is no pre-auricular node.

What diagnosis is most likely?

The most likely diagnosis is allergic conjunctivitis. Unlike viral conjunctivitis, patients complain of itching rather than a gritty sensation. First-line agents to relieve symptoms are antihistamine/vasoconstrictor or antihistamine/mast cell stabilizer eye drops. The most important step to prevent future episodes is to identify and avoid precipitating allergens.

> Do not use antihistamine-vasoconstrictor eye drops for more than a few days at a time. Prolonged use leads to rebound conjunctivitis.

Alternative 16.2.2

A 37-year-old man presents with a 2-day history of red eye and a small amount of thick, yellow discharge in his right eye. When he wakes up, his right eye seems "glued shut." The right palpebral and bulbar conjunctiva is diffusely injected. A yellow discharge is evident at the tarsal margin. The left eye is unaffected.

What diagnosis is most likely?

Thick, yellow discharge and diffusely injected bulbar and palpebral conjunctiva typically result from bacterial conjunctivitis. Bacterial conjunctivitis is typically unilateral, although sometimes infection occurs bilaterally. In adults, *Staphylococcus aureus* is the most common pathogen implicated in bacterial conjunctivitis.

> **"Eyes glued shut in the morning":** Does not distinguish between viral, allergic, and bacterial conjunctivitis (common in all three types).

What is the next step in management?

Treat empirically with antibiotic eye drops (e.g., erythromycin or sulfa eye drops).

How would management differ if the patient with unilateral diffuse conjunctival injection had profuse purulent discharge and swollen pre-auricular lymph nodes?

Acute onset of copious purulent discharge should raise suspicion for *Neisseria gonorrhea* infection. Gonococcal conjunctivitis (hyperacute conjunctivitis) often causes marked pre-auricular lymphadenopathy. If you suspect gonococcal conjunctivitis, test the discharge with Gram stain and culture, hospitalize the patient, and administer intramuscular or intravenous ceftriaxone.

Alternative 16.2.3

A 52-year-old man presents with an asymptomatic red lesion in his right eye (Fig. 16-3). He has had the lesion for 6 months. He recently migrated from Barbados, where he worked as a fisherman.

What is the diagnosis?

The patient has a pterygium (Greek for "wing"). This lesion, which is often painless, classically appears as localized, wing-shaped erythema on the nasal side of the bulbar conjunctiva. People in tropical areas who spend a lot of time outdoors are at increased risk. Pterygia are usually a benign finding and do not require any therapy. Occasionally, pterygia can affect the cornea and cause astigmatism or visual loss. In this case, surgery is warranted.

> **Pinguecula**: Benign, wing-shaped, whitish-yellow lesion on nasal or temporal conjunctiva.

Alternative 16.2.4

A 60-year-old man presents with an asymptomatic red lesion in his left eye. He noticed the lesion this morning while shaving. On examination, there is bright red discoloration underneath a transparent conjunctiva.

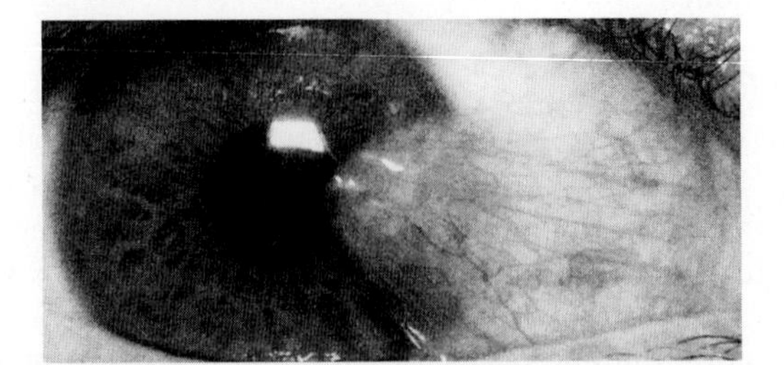

FIGURE 16–3 Eye image: Pterygium. From Willis MC. *Medical Terminology: A Programmed Learning Approach to the Language of Health Care*. Lippincott Williams & Wilkins, 2002.

What is the diagnosis?

The patient has a subconjunctival hemorrhage, which appears as a localized area of blood just beneath the surface of the cornea. Subconjunctival hemorrhage is typically a benign finding that resolves on its own. If the lesion persists for 2 to 3 weeks or reoccurs, consider referral to an ophthalmologist. Also, ask if the patient is taking any blood-thinning agents such as warfarin.

CASE 16–3 PAINFUL RED EYE

A 70-year-old man presents with 12 hours of severe right eye pain and redness. On entering the room, the lights are turned off. He is unable to keep the eye open. There is ciliary flush and pinpoint pupil. He is urgently referred to an ophthalmologist.

What is the differential diagnosis?

Common causes of painful red eye with foreign body sensation and constricted pupil are keratitis (inflammation of the cornea), uveitis, trauma, and corneal abrasion.

What diagnosis is most likely if the patient's symptoms began after a cold, sunny day of hiking in the snow and slit lamp demonstrates diffuse punctate fluorescein staining?

Diffuse punctate fluorescein staining on slit lamp examination is suggestive of keratitis. The history suggests that keratitis is caused by ultraviolet light exposure (sunlight reflects off snow and damages cornea). Treatment is pain relief with topical nonsteroidal anti-inflammatory drugs (NSAIDs), oral analgesics, and maybe a bandage contact lens. Most patients recover fully in 1 to 3 days.

> **Welder's eye**: Welding arc can cause ultraviolet keratitis if eye protection is not used.

What diagnosis is likely if slit lamp examination demonstrates the lesion in Figure 16-4?

Figure 16-4 demonstrates a dendritic corneal ulcer, which is the classic finding in herpes simplex keratitis. First-line therapy is acyclovir ointment or 1% trifluridine.

> **Cotton wisp test**: A hypoesthetic cornea is typically caused by herpes keratitis.

What diagnosis should you suspect if the patient has a history of ulcerative colitis and ankylosing spondylitis?

Painful red eye with alarm findings in a patient with ulcerative colitis or ankylosing spondylitis should raise suspicion for anterior uveitis (see Chapter 4: Gastroenterology). The diagnosis is usually confirmed with slit lamp examination (demonstrates white blood cells in the uvea).

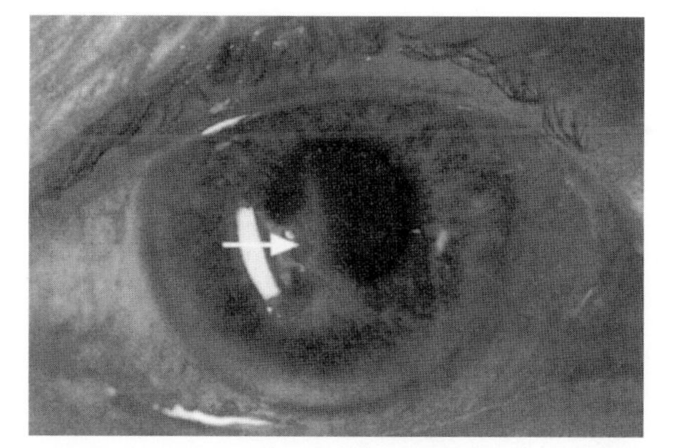

FIGURE 16–4 Eye image: Herpes simplex virus keratitis (dendritic corneal ulcer). From Ayala C, Spellberg B. *Boards and Wards*, 3rd ed. Lippincott Williams & Wilkins, 2006.

Anterior uveitis: inflammation of iris (iritis) or ciliary body (iridocyclitis).
Posterior uveitis: inflammation of the choroid or retina, or both (chorioretinitis).

How is uveitis treated?

1. **Infectious uveitis**: Treat the underlying infection.
2. **Noninfectious anterior uveitis**: First-line therapy is steroid eye drops.
3. **Noninfectious posterior uveitis**: First-line is steroid eye injections or oral steroids.

What diagnosis should you suspect if slit lamp showed the lesion in Figure 16-5 and the only pertinent finding on history is that he often wears daily soft contact lenses for weeks at a time before removing them?

Slit lamp demonstrates an area of increased fluorescein uptake by the corneal epithelium. This finding is suggestive of a corneal abrasion, which can result from trauma, foreign bodies, or contact lenses (the most likely cause in this patient). Treat with oral analgesics, antibiotic eye drops that cover Pseudomonas (e.g., ciprofloxacin, ofloxacin, or tobramycin), and monitor for corneal ulcers or infiltrates (white spots).

Eye patch: Use of an eye patch may benefit traumatic abrasions that involve less than half of the cornea. An eye patch is not indicated in other types of abrasions, and it is contraindicated in contact lens abrasions.

Alternative 16.3.1

A 75-year-old man presents with the "worse headache" of his life. He describes the pain as dull, right-sided pain. He also complains of right eye pain, blurry vision, and floaters. On examination, there is ciliary flush in the right eye. The right pupil is fixed and dilated. The cornea is opacified. There are no other focal neurological deficits.

What is the most likely diagnosis?

A fixed dilated pupil in a patient with acute onset of painful red eye should raise suspicion for acute angle closure glaucoma. Patients often complain of severe headache, photophobia, blurry vision, and floaters. IOP is usually elevated. Initial therapy for this ocular emergency is topical acetazolamide, β-blockers, and α-agonists to reduce IOP. If IOP decreases promptly, consider topical pilocarpine to relieve pupillary dilation and surgery (laser iridotomy) 1 to 2 days later. If IOP does not decrease with medical therapy, consider prompt referral for surgery.

The terms acute angle closure glaucoma, primary angle closure glaucoma, angle closure, and primary angle closure are often used interchangeably.

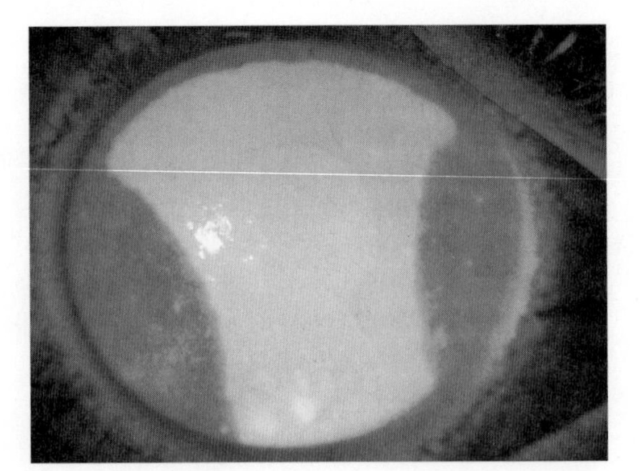

FIGURE 16–5 Eye image: Corneal abrasion. From Tasman W, Jaeger E. *The Wills Eye Hospital Atlas of Clinical Ophthalmology*, 2nd ed. Lippincott Williams & Wilkins, 2001.

Retinal tear or detachment: This condition presents with floaters, flashing lights with or without visual field deficits and does not usually cause red eye, ciliary flush, or pupil dilation.

Alternative 16.3.2

A 37-year-old woman presents with a 3-day history of deep bilateral eye pain and erythema. Pupils are equally round and reactive to light. Eye examination demonstrates the lesion in Figure 16-6.

What is the most likely diagnosis?

Scleritis presents with deep ocular pain and reddish purple sclera. Patients may also experience photophobia and excessive production of tears. The three subtypes of scleritis are nodular (localized erythema), diffuse (diffuse erythema), and necrotizing (severe diffuse scleritis). Almost two thirds of scleritis cases result from systemic disorders (especially rheumatological conditions). All patients should undergo detailed history and routine laboratory testing to search for an underlying cause (complete blood count, chemistry, urinalysis, erythrocyte sedimentation rate, C-reactive protein, anti-nuclear antibodies, radiofrequency, etc.). First-line therapy for nodular or diffuse scleritis is indomethacin (an NSAID). First-line therapy for necrotizing scleritis is oral steroids.

Episcleritis: Painless red eye and episcleral injection. Unlike scleritis, erythema usually resolves with phenylephrine drops (which can help differentiate the two when the diagnosis is not obvious). Treatment not usually necessary.

Alternative 16.3.3

A 45-year-old man calls 5 minutes after being splashed in both eyes with brake fluid. He reports that both eyes are red and painful.

What initial step should you recommend?

Chemical trauma to the eyes can cause pain and redness. The initial step is always copious irrigation with water or normal saline. After 20 to 30 minutes of irrigation, measure pH of the eye with litmus paper. Continue irrigation until pH is normal and refer the patient to an ophthalmologist.

Alkaline chemical trauma causes greater damage than acidic chemical trauma from solutions like brake fluid.

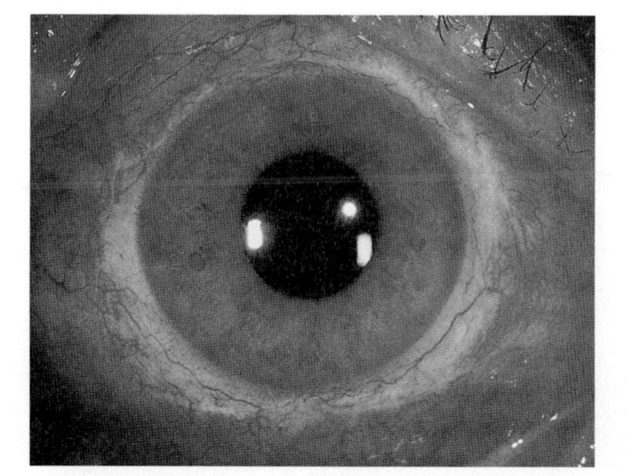

FIGURE 16–6 Eye image: Scleritis. From Tasman W, Jaeger E. *The Wills Eye Hospital Atlas of Clinical Ophthalmology*, 2nd ed. Lippincott Williams & Wilkins, 2001.

CASE 16–4 EYELID LESIONS

A 48-year-old man presents with the painful eyelid lesion in Figure 16-7.

What is the most likely diagnosis?

The patient has an external hordeolum (stye). Styes result from infection of a meibomian gland. *S. aureus* is the most common causative organism. First-line therapy is warm compresses. If the stye persists for a few weeks despite conservative measures, consider referral to an ophthalmologist for incision and curettage or steroid injections.

> **Chalazion:** This nodular eyelid lesion is caused by obstruction of a meibomian gland. Unlike stye, chalazions are typically painless. Most chalazions resolve within a few weeks, and treatment is usually not necessary. Warm compresses are an option for large chalazions.

Alternative 16.4.1

A 45-year-old man presents with a 7-day history of eye discomfort that he describes as a "gritty sensation" (Fig. 16-8).

What is the diagnosis?

The patient has blepharitis. Blepharitis is inflammation of the lid margin. The inflammation can subsequently spread to and obstruct the meibomian glands. Blepharitis typically presents with inflammation around the eyelashes. Gritty sensation and red eye are common because of decreased tear production. Blepharitis is a treatable but incurable condition. The most important step in management is eyelid hygiene. Many physicians also prescribe topical antibiotics.

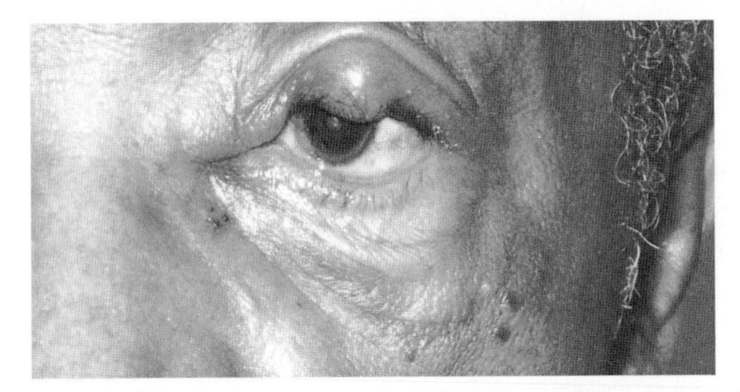

FIGURE 16–7 Eye image: Hordeolum (stye). From Ayala C, Spellberg B. *Boards and Wards,* 3rd ed. Lippincott Williams & Wilkins, 2006.

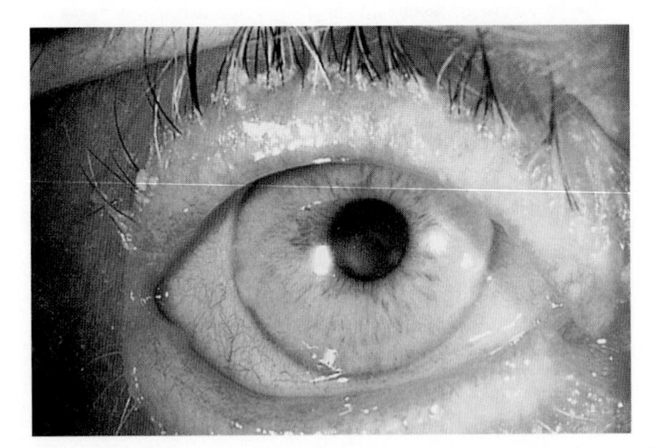

FIGURE 16–8 Eye image: Blepharitis. From Weber J, Kelley J. *Health Assessment in Nursing,* 2nd ed. Lippincott Williams & Wilkins, 2003.

Meibomian glands produce lipids required for tear production.

Eyelid hygiene: Soften the lid margin with a warm cloth, then remove lid margin debris.

Alternative 16.4.2

An 18-year-old man with a history of chronic sinusitis presents with erythema, pain, and swelling of the right eyelid and periorbital region. He also complains of blurry vision. On inspection, there is proptosis and cranial nerve 6 palsy. Temperature is 38.6°C.

What is the most likely diagnosis?

The most likely diagnosis is orbital cellulitis (postseptal cellulitis). Orbital cellulitis results from infection of fat and muscle within the orbit (posterior to the orbital septum). In addition to pain and erythematous swelling of the eyelids and periorbital region, patients may present with cranial nerve palsy and proptosis, which results in blurry vision. Fever may or may not be present.

What pathogens are most frequently implicated in orbital cellulitis?

The most common pathogens are *Streptococcus pneumoniae* and *S. aureus*.

Sinusitis: most important risk factor (due to contiguous spread).

How is orbital sinusitis managed?

Initial therapy is empiric broad spectrum intravenous antibiotics (e.g., vancomycin and piperacillin-tazobactam).

Orbital CT scan: Consider if the patient fails to respond to antibiotics within 24 hours to confirm the diagnosis and assess extent of infection.

What diagnosis would be more likely if the patient with eyelid and periorbital pain, swelling, and afebrile erythema, and he does not have blurry vision, proptosis, or cranial nerve palsy?

The presentation suggests preseptal rather than postseptal cellulitis. Preseptal cellulitis (periorbital cellulitis) results from infection anterior to the orbital septum. Although the microbiology is similar to orbital cellulitis, sinusitis is not as frequently implicated. Treatment is usually broad-spectrum oral antibiotics (e.g., amoxicillin-clavulanate).

It is often difficult to distinguish between periorbital and orbital cellulitis on the basis of clinical findings alone. If the diagnosis is in doubt, obtain orbital CT scan.

Orbital and periorbital cellulitis is much more common in children and young adults.

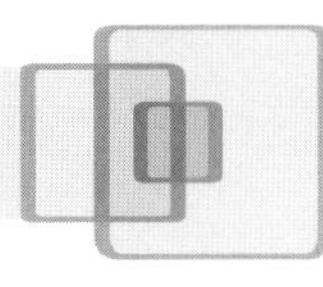

Index

C

D

E

I

J

K

L

M

N

O

S

T

U

V

W

X

Z